Medical
Anthropology

Medical Anthropology

Contemporary Theory and Method

Revised Edition

Edited by
CAROLYN F. SARGENT
and THOMAS M. JOHNSON

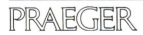
PRAEGER

Westport, Connecticut
London

The Library of Congress has catalogued the hardcover edition as follows:

Handbook of medical anthropology : contemporary theory and method /
  edited by Carolyn F. Sargent and Thomas M. Johnson.—Rev. ed.
      p.   cm.
  Includes bibliographical references and index.
  ISBN 0–313–29658–8 (hardcover : alk. paper)
  1. Medical anthropology.   I. Sargent, Carolyn Fishel.
  II. Johnson, Thomas M. (Thomas Malcolm).
  GN296.M423 1996
  306.4'61—dc20   95–40052

British Library Cataloguing in Publication Data is available.

A hardcover edition of *Medical Anthropology: Contemporary Theory and Method, Revised
Edition* is available from Greenwood Press, an imprint of Greenwood Publishing Group, Inc.,
under the title *Handbook of Medical Anthropology: Contemporary Theory and Method, Revised
Edition* (ISBN: 0–313–29658–8).

Library of Congress Catalog Card Number: 95–40052
ISBN: 0–275–95265–7 (pbk.)

First published in 1996

Praeger Publishers, 88 Post Road West, Westport, CT 06881
An imprint of Greenwood Publishing Group, Inc.

Printed in the United States of America

The paper used in this book complies with the
Permanent Paper Standard issued by the National
Information Standards Organization (Z39.48–1984).

10 9 8 7 6 5 4 3 2 1

Copyright Acknowledgment

The editors and publisher gratefully acknowledge permission for use of the following
material:

Chapter 4, ''Culture, Emotion, and Psychiatric Disorder'' is an adapted version from
Janis H. Jenkins, ''The Psychocultural Study of Emotion and Mental Disorder,'' ed.
Philip K. Bock. In *Handbook of Psychological Anthropology*. Reprinted with
permission of Greenwood Publishing Group, Inc., Westport, CT. Copyright © 1994 by
Philip K. Bock.

Contents

Contents

Illustrations

Introduction

Carolyn F. Sargent and Thomas M. Johnson

In the introduction to the first edition of this book, we commented on the increasing diversification of research interests in medical anthropology. This second edition reflects increasing division in theoretical approaches among the various authors, paralleling a major cleavage in the social sciences involving whether "facts" can be uncovered, empirically discerned, and analyzed, or whether they are produced through interaction between researcher and research subject. Much research in medical anthropology employs an empiricist orientation, but a powerful alternative position also prevails, focusing on the negotiation of meanings as key to understanding social life. This edition presents perspectives on this important theoretical debate, underscoring its relevance to the multiplicity of research concerns across the field.

As a whole, this book documents the significant contribution of medical anthropologists during the past decade to the development of a comprehensive theory of therapeutic process that connects therapeutic, political, and spiritual power and to an exploration of mind-body interactions, tracing the mediation of moral and physiological domains of experience. Several authors analyze the social, cultural, and historical construction of biomedicine and argue that anthropological and dominant biomedical ways of knowing are ultimately irreconcilable; others propose valuable linkages between cultural analysis and biomedical inquiry. Numerous authors challenge reductionist models, offering alternatives to bridge the biological and social, such as the biopsychosocial model that grounds the study of disease in historical and political-economic context and that links human behavior and biology or one that challenges the psychobiological universality of emotional life.

Together with the generation of theoretical debate, medical anthropologists have expanded the disciplinary repertoire of field methods. Many medical anthropologists continue to rely on standard ethnographic methodologies for field-work, but there is a growing reliance on specialized techniques generated by the increasingly interdisciplinary nature of much medical anthropological research.

This collection documents both the unique theoretical insights of medical anthropology and its relevance to public policy. From the research reported in these chapters, medical anthropology emerges in an increasingly important role, drawing on biological and social sciences, as well as clinical medical practice, to improve health status and health services worldwide. Anthropological research, sometimes controversial to policymakers, is shown to represent the possibility of a truly revolutionary form of inquiry, serving to combat the health consequences of social inequality.

This edition, like the first one, presents the state of the art in medical anthropology, capturing the range of theoretical orientations, research findings, and methods characterizing the discipline today. Although each chapter references key historical antecedents to the subject being discussed, the chapters are not intended to be exhaustive reviews. Rather, each chapter is designed to trace the developments in a major subarea of medical anthropology and to speculate about directions for future research and theoretical exploration. We include new chapters on emotion and psychopathology, nutrition, and bioethics. All the chapters from the first edition have been updated to reflect current trends and to include more recent references. Together these chapters represent the essence of medical anthropology providing, in one book, an introduction for those not trained in medical anthropology and defining the current parameters and future directions of the field.

The book is organized into five parts. The first five chapters address core theoretical issues in the discipline in order to present the breadth of theoretical concerns in medical anthropology. First, Thomas J. Csordas and Arthur Kleinman discuss the therapeutic process, clearly a fundamental theme for any cultural investigation of health and healing. They define the domain of active response to the universal realities of disease and distress and identify common elements of healing in diverse medical systems, from shamanism to surgery. In discussing the popular subject of symbolic healing, they question the assumption that some therapeutic interventions, particularly biomedical ones, are not symbolic. They suggest that we examine both the symbolic and nonsymbolic dimensions of different healing systems. A comprehensive theory of therapeutic process must explicate the connections between moral and physiological domains of experience in healing and may ultimately challenge the distinctions between body and self or physiology and mind. A theory of therapeutic process, they suggest, must distinguish healing as a form of oppression, healing as a response to powerlessness, and healing as a mode of empowerment.

Adopting an orientation that addresses both local and global power relations, Soheir A. Morsy discusses the political economy orientation in medical anthropology, which she describes as an expression of a more general, politically informed, historical development in the parent discipline. In sharing this approach with anthropology as a whole, medical anthropologists have brought into focus how global power relations pertain to local health systems. She argues that the systemic orientation of political economy, with its attendant blurring of disciplinary boundaries, does not deny cultural specificity. Rather, it promises to reinterpret the concept of culture. She reviews works addressing highly abstracted macroscopic and programmatic issues, as well as those focusing on the cultural expression of sickness in relation to political economic development. In concluding, Morsy considers both the status of political economy–oriented studies within medical anthropology and prospects for future research.

The past decade has witnessed a growing polemicism between the culturological and political-economic perspectives within medical anthropology. In Chapter 3, Margaret Lock and Nancy Scheper-Hughes offer a unified paradigm that challenges the discipline to reconcile these polarities. They propose a critical-interpretive approach, which recognizes the necessity of addressing experiences of illness and broader socioeconomic dynamics. From their perspective, medical anthropology should focus on the way in which all knowledge relating to the body, health, and illness is a cultural product undergoing constant renegotiation. Thus, medical anthropology is no longer only the study of alternative medical systems; biomedicine is itself subject to anthropological analysis as a product of particular historical and cultural processes. They reject the idea of a positivist social science, which seeks to discover "objective laws" of human behavior, asserting that the "culture of science" structures the kinds of questions being asked. In the critical-interpretive paradigm, the body assumes central theoretical significance as the "primary action zone of the late twentieth century," a theme explored throughout this chapter.

Research on the interrelations among psychiatric disorder, culture, and emotion also addresses the universal validity of biomedical constructs of psychopathology and the presumption of a "psychobiological universality of emotional life." In Chapter 4 on culture, emotion, and psychiatric disorder, Janis H. Jenkins urges anthropologists to explore how emotion and mental disorder are to be conceptualized. As biologically natural events or sociopolitically produced responses? Intrapsychic mental events or interrelational social processes? Discussing the relevance of the study of emotion to medical anthropology, she explores conceptual issues common to both medical and psychological anthropology, among these the current critique of Cartesian mind-body dualism (see also Chapters 3 and 9). In advocating increased attention to studies of culture and emotion, she observes that the domain of emotion historically has been subordinated to a focus on cognition in scholarly thinking influenced by Cartesian dualism. Cross-cultural research on emotion provides invaluable data for distinguishing "normal" and "pathological" emotion, for interpreting the expression of distress in varying cultural contexts, and for developing cross-culturally valid diagnoses of major mental disorders. Important research remains to be done to expand the analysis of emotional processes beyond the biological, psychological, and cultural to include an emphasis on power relations and the construction of affect.

Whereas these theoretical perspectives provide directions for analyzing medical systems, Noel J. Chrisman and Thomas M. Johnson describe the work of a growing number of applied medical anthropologists working in clinical settings. In contrast to anthropologists who condemn biomedicine reflexively, clinically applied medical anthropologists more often are accused of being apologists for the excesses of biomedicine. Chrisman and Johnson, however, describe how difficult it is to translate traditional anthropological knowledge into clinically useful data. The perils of the position of conceptual translator are also discussed; the authors highlight the necessity of studying biomedicine as another ethnomedicine in order to intervene effectively in clinical work. Similarly they respond to the criticism that clinically applied medical anthropologists neglect analysis of macrolevel concerns, essentially collaborating with those interested in maintaining the political and economic status quo, by discussing recent attempts to define a critical clinical anthropology.

Part II contains four chapters covering aspects of medical systems. The first three chapters consider various dimensions of ethnomedicine, a term that has connoted non-Western medical systems in a discipline that has traditionally dichotomized medical systems (traditional-modern, local-cosmopolitan, non-Western-Western, and so on). These first chapters, which cover ethnomedicine, ethnopsychiatry, and ethnopharmacology, hold great interest for medical anthropologists and focus on the most recent trends in the cross-cultural study of health and healing. The final chapter in this part deals with biomedicine; its inclusion in the same part with chapters on ethnomedicine is a conscious decision, reflecting the recent emphasis within medical anthropology not to consider biomedicine as separate but rather to subject it to the same scrutiny as other medical systems: that is, to study biomedicine as yet another ethnomedicine.

Arthur J. Rubel and Michael R. Hass provide a historical overview of ethnomedical studies in anthropology, looking at such issues as sickness etiology, healing and social control, and the recruitment and training of healers. Ultimately their goal is to show how ethnomedical studies can contribute to the development of theory and methodology in sociocultural anthropology. They also offer a provocative prescription for future anthropological research in health care: anchoring exploration in the interface between biology and culture. They suggest that the human body and its functioning, as a species-wide phenomenon, be used as the basis for comparative research on cultural practices.

Consistent with a biocultural approach, Charles C. Hughes's chapter on ethnopsychiatry briefly summarizes previous anthropological work that encompasses biological, social, and cultural levels of analysis. He then asks us to reexamine the semantics of the term *ethnopsychiatry*, warning that the cultural structuring of all knowledge and experience that the term implies is at risk of being "dulled through overuse and cursory familiarity." He deals with the cultural construction of normality and abnormality, discussing the culture-bound syndromes and extending his analysis to include the *Diagnostic and Statistical Manual of Mental Disorders*, third edition, revised (and by extension, the fourth edition, the updated official diagnostic classification system of the American Psychiatric Association) as an ethnopsychiatric artifact. Underlying his chapter is the theme that any distinction between ethnomedicine and ethnopsychiatry is artificial and that by using such terms medical anthropology is unwisely recapitulating the pervasive, institutionalized Western distinction between medicine and psychiatry.

Nina L. Etkin's chapter on ethnopharmacology also is rooted in a biocultural perspective, covering topics from plant taxonomy and phytochemistry to the sociocultural dimensions of plant use. Like Rubel and Hass, she raises the controversial issue of using a biomedical paradigm for analyzing ethnomedical data when she discusses the merits of studying medicinal plant use based on biomedical parameters. She also points out related areas in the literature not readily accessible to anthropologists, such as botany, pharmacology, nutrition, dietetics, and agriculture. For Etkin, ethnopharmacology promises to help us better understand the biological and behavioral dimensions of health and therefore to facilitate more cogent comparative health research.

Perhaps even more than they were a decade ago, medical anthropologists are working in biomedical settings, or studying problems such as AIDS or post-traumatic stress disorder that have been defined in biomedical terms. These medical anthropologists attempt what is exceedingly difficult: to study biomedicine itself, recognizing that it is the product of social-historical forces, while being members of societies in which biomedicine dominates the process of defining health problems. In "Studying Biomedicine as a Cultural System," Lorna Amarasingham Rhodes offers perspectives for medical anthropologists who are both participants in and observers of the culture of biomedicine. First, utilizing the theoretical writings of Foucault and Geertz, among others, she describes the historical embeddedness of biomedical knowledge and the cultural assumptions about science underlying biomedicine's "aura of factuality." Subsequently, she discusses how anthropological understandings of medical education and practice may reveal contradictions within biomedicine. She argues for greater attention to larger issues of class and gender inequality that are often obscured in biomedical theory and practice. She also addresses the theoretical pluralism within medical anthropology, suggesting that the epistemological differences within the discipline create discomfort yet must be embraced and discussed to ensure growth within the discipline.

All human populations exist in states of dynamic interaction with their natural and cultural environments. Part III contains five chapters, each addressing some aspect of this interaction that has been extensively studied by medical anthropologists. This part also takes a biocultural perspective, including the relationship between diseases and human behavior, cultural responses to human physiological processes throughout the life cycle, and the ways that people put themselves at risk for health problems through cultural practices and patterns such as drug use and urbanization.

Peter J. Brown, Marcia C. Inhorn, and Daniel J. Smith propose that the study of disease and human behavior from an ecological perspective is a fundamental but heretofore underdeveloped area of research in medical anthropology. They suggest an approach that illuminates the interaction of biology and culture in human evolution, aids in understanding the causes and distribution of diseases worldwide, and assists in anticipating the health consequences of technological change. They discuss basic concepts in the study of disease ecology, illustrating how human behavior plays a role in every major type of disease, particularly the infectious diseases. They delineate three complementary levels of disease causation: microbiological, cultural ecological (microsociological), and political ecological (macrosociological). They suggest that anthropological studies of disease ecology must be contextualized within larger historical and political-economic frameworks.

Carole H. Browner and Carolyn F. Sargent next argue that the domain of reproduction also bridges biology and culture, articulating with gender role issues and larger sociopolitical dynamics. They suggest that all human physiological processes are experienced through cultural filters and that anthropological studies of human reproduction should investigate linkages between a society's structural relationships and symbolic meanings and its paradigms of maternity, the products of sociocultural forces shaping maternal roles and reproductive activities such as menstruation, childbirth, abortion, and menopause. They employ case studies describing the ways societies manage obstetric events to show how such analyses of reproduction can enhance anthropological understandings of broader cultural and social principles.

Certain cultural practices put people at risk for health problems and yet are ubiquitous cross-culturally. One such practice is the use of psychoactive substances, which has been studied with purposeful relativism as a by-product of ethnographic studies in Latin America, Africa, and Oceania and among North American Indian and Eskimo societies. With the exception of these ethnic enclaves, drug use has either been a neglected research topic or studied as drug-specific examples of deviant, albeit culturally conditioned, behavior. Linda A. Bennett and Paul W. Cook, Jr., use this as a point of departure, discussing how many more anthropologists are studying substance abuse in interdisciplinary teams, with attention being given to problems associated with drug use (and development of solutions to drug abuse) rather than to only the ''normal'' use of substances in particular cultural settings. There is now an embryonic, distinctly anthropological tradition in the area of alcohol and drug studies. This tradition includes biocultural orientations, an emphasis on emic perspectives (such as that of street drug subcultures) relating substance abuse to larger political and economic processes, and an emerging applied-policy focus. Bennett and Cook describe how the AIDS epidemic has provided an impetus for medical anthropologists to apply alcohol and drug studies to the development of effective prevention programs. They also note that growing problems with cocaine provide opportunities to reassess old theoretical and research paradigms applied to the analysis of cocaine use. Paralleling the general awareness of gender issues in the discipline, the authors also address recent attention to gender as a factor in substance use and abuse.

William W. Dressler continues the theme that certain cultural practices put people at risk, focusing on the more general topics of stress, social support, and disease. These issues, which have been controversial in social medicine, are particularly important for medical anthropologists who are interested in studying the health effects of social changes such as migration, industrialization, and acculturation. The chapter discusses the concept of stress, reminding medical anthropologists that it is a process rather than a thing, and that stressors increasing the probability of pathology are counterbalanced by resources that lower the risk of diseases. Disease processes influenced by stressors include depression, hypertension, and coronary heart disease. The process by which stress influences health status is sociobiological, but unlike more reductionist models of stress and disease, Dressler argues that medical anthropology offers a perspective that stressors and adaptation are embedded in social relationships and historical circumstances. Special focus is given to the acute and long-term effects of migration, both voluntary and coercive. He notes that although the precise definitions of particular stressors vary by cultural context, there is a consistent and replicable effect of stressors on disease cross-culturally. Finally, Dressler describes how much research in this area focuses on disease as an outcome variable. Medical anthropology may make future contributions to the epidemiological study of stress and disease by focusing instead on illness and its relationship to macrosocial processes.

In Chapter 14 on nutrition in medical anthropology, Sara A. Quandt traces the roots of the field of nutritional anthropology and documents attempts to integrate studies of human behavior, social organization, nutritional status, and nutrient requirements and growth. Accordingly, she demonstrates the collaboration of both cultural and physical anthropology perspectives in the study of nutrition. Nutritional anthropology, she shows, has its theoretical foundation in nutritional science, as well as in cultural analyses of food. The field today draws heavily on both ecological theory and symbolic analyses to analyze human dietary behavior. Quandt explores two substantive issues in nutritional anthropology: the linkages between nutrition and reproduction and contributions by nutritional anthropologists to the understanding of malnutrition. In addition, she surveys the range of methods employed by anthropologists to study dietary intake, nutritional status, and other facets of human dietary patterns. She suggests important roles for anthropologists in both domestic and international health care arenas, as part of efforts to devise more appropriate models for food behavior, leading to innovative and effective food and health policy.

The fourth part of the book contains two chapters on methodology. The topics of preceding chapters clearly suggest that medical anthropologists increasingly need to have firm grounding in traditional anthropological techniques and understanding of specialized methodological approaches. This is particularly true as the politics of research funding have influenced anthropologists to participate in interdisciplinary research teams. Clearly the perspectives of funding agencies have had considerable influence in shaping the directions of research methods in medical anthropology. Although not all medical anthropologists will or should become experts in methodological specialties like epidemiology, successful involvement on research teams demands an ability to frame research questions, to conduct research, and to present conclusions in ways that are congruent with the expectations of other disciplines. At the very least, medical anthropologists can contribute to interdisciplinary research through their willingness to recognize the validity of multiple perspectives and to mediate interaction between the various specialists on such teams.

Pertti J. Pelto and Gretel H. Pelto contribute a chapter that is noteworthy for its rigorous delineation of current research questions, concepts, and methods of medical anthropology. While other chapters have emphasized the contributions that medical anthropology can make to theory in anthropology, Pelto and Pelto assert that medical anthropology is primarily an applied subdiscipline in that health problems throughout the world constitute a domain of research that leads directly to intervention. This research is, by definition, interdisciplinary, employing data from biological and social sciences, as well as clinical medicine. It demands refinement of conventional anthropological methods, including rapid ethnographic assessment procedures, specialized sampling techniques, use of microcomputers, and interdisciplinary team development strategies. They address an issue that is frequently left unstated in discussions of methodology: choice of method is strongly affected by national and international agencies sponsoring research, where proposals are often judged by interdisciplinary review dominated by biomedical scientists.

William R. True is a medical anthropologist who has utilized postdoctoral training in epidemiology in his work. His chapter on epidemiology is designed to contrast the logic of epidemiologic thinking with that of more traditional anthropological perspectives. In demonstrating how medical anthropologists can learn to think epidemiologically, True contends that we have not recognized that epidemiology shares with anthropology an interest in understanding how human health is directly affected by physical, social, and cultural environments. He asks medical anthropologists to specify research questions more precisely in terms of independent and dependent variables, to consider the advantages of methodologies designed to test directly associations between variables, and to improve the replicability (and hence the acceptability to other scientists) of anthropological research. The benefits of such methodologies include a greater ability to work with professionals from other disciplines characterized by quantitative rigor, which can be complemented by rich ethnographic description.

Many medical anthropologists join several of the contributors to this book in recognizing that the discipline has a strong applied tradition; one direction that this applied focus has taken is the area of policy and advocacy, the subject of Part V. There is a growing assertion that responsible researchers in medical anthropology must consider the implications of their research for the people and institutions they study and, further, that medical anthropologists can serve a useful role in translating research findings into policy statements. Many may even go further, adopting advocacy roles reflecting certain political orientations or policy objectives. Medical anthropologists who take such positions assert that their work is not only significant academically but ethically and has important implications for the delivery of health services and the health status of populations worldwide.

Patricia A. Marshall and Barbara A. Koenig argue that anthropological perspectives on bioethics have much to offer the education of health professionals and should inform the work of clinical bioethics practice. They observe that while the dramatic impact of medical (technological) innovations reinforces an ethos of scientific progress, there is at the same time a growing recognition of the moral dilemmas that accompany such achievements. Individual consumers of health care in industrialized societies expect access to complex therapies and technology but are troubled by the possibility of being maintained indefinitely on life support machines. The field of bioethics has evolved in this climate of technological promise and moral ambiguity. Medical anthropology challenges the universalizing discourse of basic science and biomedicine and holds the potential to transform bioethics by demonstrating the relevance of cultural analyses of locally situated moral conflicts, in their political and economic context, for clinical bioethics.

The impact of biomedical ideology and technology has long interested anthropologists engaged in research on health care delivery in Third World countries, as well as in the industrialized world addressed in Marshall and Koenig's chapter. Murray Last, in Chapter 18 on indigenous healers and their recruitment and training, discusses the struggles over professional recognition and dominance among practitioners of traditional medicine facing competition from other systems of medicine, most significantly, biomedicine. He argues that professionalization is one solution to the dilemmas healers face in confronting competition from alternative medical systems. His argument links the profession of medicine to the structure of the state and to cultural ideologies. Thus, national medical cultures are the products of dominant political philosophies, as well as cultural responses to health care needs. Competition from biomedicine represents a serious threat to the existence of flourishing systems of indigenous medicine, and there is a danger that intellectual insights into how societies function and their inner meanings and rituals may be forever lost with the disappearance of individual healers. Last argues that no country can afford to lose the insight and creative abilities of its indigenous practitioners; organizing healers professionally is one way to maintain their viability in health care delivery systems increasingly dominated by biomedicine.

While Last focuses on the policy of professionalization and the fate of indigenous healers, Sandra D. Lane and Robert A. Rubinstein expand the discussion to include other aspects of international health policy. They review the major health problems in the Third World, prior to describing specific international health projects and the roles of medical anthropologists in them. In discussing the potential for international health work by anthropologists, they state that such work is personally challenging and intellectually engaging but also potentially frustrating because local health problems and programs are inexorably linked to broader political and economic contexts, as well as to the culture of the international public health community. They discuss a broad range of public health issues, from clean water and sanitation to the health consequences of political repression, violence, and war. Significantly, they discuss the social, cultural, and health consequences of nuclear war. They also take the position that many of the health problems of the developing world result from inequality and that the greatest improvement in health will come through public health measures rather than technological advances. Historically, medical anthropologists have been both participants in and critics of public health programs. In defining future roles, Lane and Rubinstein urge medical anthropologists to work to eliminate the ethnocentrism involved in exporting health systems and to emphasize the critical role that political processes play in determining the health status of the world's population.

The chapters in this book demonstrate the creative expansion and diversity in medical anthropology over the past decade. Medical anthropology increasingly is characterized by interdisciplinary interaction, moving the field closer to achieving the type of biocultural synthesis that has long been among the major goals of anthropology as a discipline. The chapters also reaffirm a strong applied focus in the subdiscipline, illustrating how medical anthropologists continue to work at multiple levels, from individual involvement in clinical settings to team participation in international public health efforts. Cross-cutting applied and theoretical research in medical anthropology are recent efforts to link microdomains and macrodomains of analysis: to be able to examine the individual experience of sickness in the contexts of both local communities and global political and economic dynamics. Theoretical debate and epistemological conflicts notwithstanding, we believe the field of medical anthropology shows no signs of fragmenting but, rather, an impressive capacity to generate conceptual advances benefiting the discipline as a whole.

These issues and perspectives imply an array of challenges for future work in medical anthropology. This book is intended to provide the perspectives and methods needed if we are to continue to expand our abilities in cross-disciplinary collaboration. Significantly the growing diversity of interests demands even more attention to intradisciplinary cross-fertilization. Applied medical anthropologists face the added burden of competing with credentialed professionals from other recognized clinical fields, who claim greater legitimacy in clinically applied work. This dilemma requires our continued resolve to identify and assuage credibility issues in applied medical anthropology. One fact is clear: global efforts to eradicate disease and promote health present abundant opportunities, both applied and theoretical, for the continued development of medical anthropology and for medical anthropologists to confront problems of fundamental human import.

Part I

Theoretical Perspectives

1

The Therapeutic Process

Thomas J. Csordas and Arthur Kleinman

Therapy, treatment, and *healing* are terms that define the domain of active response to illness, disease, pain, suffering, and distress. At the broadest, they are a response to general conditions of life, as for the person who identifies the substance of her religious healing as a letting go of concerns and turning them over to God. At the narrowest, they are the application of a specific remedy to a specific and limited problem, as for the person who takes two aspirin for the relief of a headache. In this chapter we examine the domain of active response, with a view to how we can develop a comparative understanding that encompasses the global repertoire of folk and religious therapies alongside those of psychiatry and biomedicine.

The discussion will be pitched at a level more general than usual in anthropological discussions of symbolic healing. This concept has been useful in the past, but it has the unfortunate connotation that there are other forms of healing that are not symbolic. In fact, even conventional medical treatment has its symbolic component (Kleinman 1973). For this reason, rather than delineating symbolic healing as an abstract category, it would be better to examine symbolic and nonsymbolic aspects of concrete categories such as shamanism, faith healing, herbalism, New Age healing, Ayurvedic medicine, Chinese medicine, Western biomedicine, or psychotherapy.

Our strategy is to define the conceptual terrain on which we can develop a comprehensive understanding of therapeutic process, sketching out the most common distinctions and presuppositions that characterize this area of research. Next we distinguish the concepts of therapeutic process, procedure, and outcome and summarize the variety of ways in which therapeutic process has been defined and conceptualized in the scholarly literature. From there, we provide an account of four approaches to understanding therapeutic efficacy put forward by anthropologists. We then discuss analytic dimensions that define the form and effect of therapy, both of which must be included in any comprehensive account of process. Finally, we offer suggestions for future research on therapeutic process in medical anthropology.

CONCEPTUAL DISTINCTIONS AND CONVENTIONS

In introducing the topic of therapeutic process, we immediately encounter a set of conventional distinctions that we as anthropologists cannot take for granted because they encode some of our own cultural presuppositions about the nature of healing. First is the distinction between diagnosis and treatment, which separates identification of a problem from attempts to resolve it. This distinction, borrowed from clinical medical practice, breaks down almost as soon as it is applied in comparative studies of therapeutic systems. Not only is the search for diagnosis itself a form of active response, but it is widely recognized that naming a problem offers the sufferer and his or her family a degree of control through certainty that must itself be considered therapeutic. In some medical systems, diagnosis is so highly elaborated that it can be considered not just a gateway to therapy but part of the therapeutic process itself. In traditional Chinese medicine and homeopathic medicine, for example, diagnostic study of subtle variations in the patient's pulse and the description of symptoms are central to the therapeutic process. Clinical encounters in Chinese medicine are rarely private; the interaction with the doctor and other patients in the consulting room during the diagnostic session is also likely to play a therapeutic role. In other systems, diagnosis is either unimportant or dispensed with entirely, and the healer is neither required to ask patients to describe their problems (Finkler 1985) nor to identify the problem through examination.

In addition, some forms of healing appear to have the diagnostic function as their central concern. Contemporary North American astrologers serve a healing function by describing a person's life in terms of a celestial rationale. The treatment is the diagnosis, formulated as the elaborated statement, "This is what you are like and what your life is like." The Navajo who consults a hand trembler, crystal gazer, or other traditional diagnostician feels that he or she has done something about the illness through identification of its cause and the proper healing ceremonies needed to correct it. This is the case even if lack of money for the ceremony precludes holding the ceremony for extended periods of time. Meanwhile, the extensive diagnostic tests he or she receives at the Indian Health Service hospital remain unsatisfying because, while they may tell what is wrong with his or her body (such as cancer), they do not reveal the cause (such as killing a sacred animal or exposure to lightning).

To go beyond the issue of diagnosis in the strict sense to the cultural definition of illness, disease, and distress, it must be recognized that what counts as therapy depends first upon what is defined as a problem. A fundamental transformation of experience takes place when suffering is recast as disease in medical practice

(Kleinman and Kleinman 1991). Moral practice is made over into technical practice, and the latter then defines how the outcome will be defined, managed, and assessed. Historically, new problems can emerge, recede, be discovered, or even be created. In North American society, premenstrual syndrome, chronic Epstein-Barr virus infection, and hypoglycemia are medical reformulations of complaints that in other historical epochs may have been otherwise defined or may not have been defined as requiring active response. The chronic fatigue syndrome characteristic of the Epstein-Barr infection is strikingly similar to that associated with neurasthenia in the nineteenth century but carries a different cultural meaning insofar as it is conceived as a viral infection instead of a nervous disorder. That cultural meaning authorizes a particular way of framing and evaluating the course of this chronic condition (Ware 1992; Ware and Kleinman 1992). Bulimia, or binge-purge syndrome, is now identified as a pathological behavior, whereas it was a refined aristocratic practice in the Roman Empire. The definition of specific psychiatric diseases in the American Psychiatric Association's *Diagnostic and Statistical Manual* (DSM IV) (1994) is a constant subject of debate and revision, with unavoidable implications for the therapeutic process.

Cross-culturally, the same objective condition may be perceived as one of distress or as one to be taken for granted. Some contemporary Christians define the experience of having an abortion as a trauma that requires healing, and some regard the habit of masturbation as a problem equally in need of healing. Chronic parasitic infections in some parts of the world are so common that they are not regarded as in need of treatment. Latah, long regarded by scholars as a culture-bound psychotic syndrome unique to Malaysia (Kenny 1978), is on closer inspection a condition not always thought to require treatment by people in the region of its prevalence, and in fact it has been proposed to be essentially a variant of the common startle response (Simons 1985a).

A second conventional distinction is that between medical and nonmedical healing. Encoded in this distinction are several presuppositions, not least of which is that medical healing is scientific while nonmedical healing is nonscientific. We will not take issue here with medicine's claim that it is scientific, although medical research might be said in the strict sense to be more scientific than medical treatment (see Kleinman 1993:15–23). A more salient point is that by extension, nonmedical, nonscientific healing is considered to be nonempirical. That is, it is thought to be based on pure imagination or superstition and to be efficacious only as a placebo. One need only read Sudhir Kakar's (1982) account of how an Indian Muslim *pir* described the empirical evidence for demonic possession or Erik Erikson's (1950) description of the intrapsychic forces dealt with by a shaman of his acquaintance to realize that nonmedical healing is empirical in the sense that it is often based on systematic observation and interpretation of symptoms, suffering, cause, effects, and response to treatment. It is this empirical basis that establishes the ground for comparative study of healing systems.

Another embedded distinction related to that between scientific and nonscientific is that between technological and nontechnological. Although it is only recently that medicine has become high tech, it is important to include cultural attitudes toward technology and the tendency of technology to dictate or encourage particular practices as an influence on the therapeutic process (Eisenberg 1988). For example, the introduction of elaborate technology for fetal monitoring has not only contributed to the medicalization of pregnancy and childbirth by subjecting women to an intensified clinical gaze; it has also created a more vivid cultural image of the fetus as a being independent of its mother, thereby contributing to the ethical debate over abortion (Kenneth Bassett, personal communication). At the opposite end of the life course, the therapeutic process encounters new illness problems as technology prolongs the life span. The role of technology in the therapeutic process must therefore be considered independent of its popular association with science, from which it obtains much of its prestige.

Yet another distinction taken for granted is that medical treatment is Western, while nonmedical treatment is non-Western. Are there such things as non-Western medical systems? Yes—for example, the Ayurvedic medicine of India and the traditional medicine of China. Part of why they are considered ''medical,'' however, is based on yet another implicit distinction: that between professional and nonprofessional treatment. The Indian and Chinese systems have institutionalized formal training, their practitioners are full-time specialists, and they are organized in a way that sociologically qualifies them as true professions (Freidson 1970). The surprise that one feels at first learning that non-Western treatment can count as professional medicine has its counterpart in the realization that Western treatment includes far more than professional medicine. Physicians themselves are likely to be unaware of the wide range of alternative treatment sought by their patients; one study documented over 130 forms of alternative and religious healing in a single suburban New Jersey county (McGuire 1987). Lack of physician interest, often combined with active prejudice against such treatments, is perceived by patients. The patients then refrain from discussing the alternatives with their physicians, who comfortably conclude that nonmedical treatment is not so common after all.

On the other hand, ''professional'' in the sense we have just used it is not the same as full-time or even fee-for-service practice. Nonmedical healers often practice full time, and some make a living as healers. In the United States, medical doctors are typically paid; religious healers are not. The situation is reversed among Navajo Indians, where one pays quite dearly for the services of a traditional medicine man but receives professional medical services free at the Indian Health Service clinic. Among participants in the contemporary charismatic renewal movement, Christian counselors and clinicians who combine psychotherapy and faith healing are sometimes caught in a conflict between the roles of healer operating for free and therapist charging a fee.

When we turn to the domain of nonmedical treatment, we find that it too is defined in ways that implicitly distinguish it from medical treatment. Foremost among assumptions about nonmedical treatment is that it is essentially religious, whereas medical treatment is nonreligious. If religion is defined in terms of encounter with the sacred, this assumption is problematic since nonmedical practitioners such as herbalists or bonesetters may operate in a very instrumental, purely technical idiom (Kleinman 1980:4, 63–64). It is equally in error to read religious meaning into forms of healing that are not religious or to reduce the religious meaning of sacred healing to its medical or clinical significance. The latter error is by far more common. In fact, a paradoxical situation has come about in medical anthropology in which nonmedical forms of healing are explicitly acknowledged as religious but analysis then abandons the explicitly religious to focus on therapeutic aspects of healing. Moreover, this is more true of Anglo-American than of French anthropology (Csordas 1987), indicating that the empirical question of religion in healing is clouded by methodological predispositions of varying schools. A valuable corrective would be development of a theory of religion in relation to health.

Another categorical presupposition is that nonmedical forms of healing are more characteristic of stable, traditional societies than of complex industrial societies. Recent advances in the study of complex health care systems that stress the relations among professional, folk, and popular forms of healing (Kleinman 1980) and analyses of medical pluralism (Janzen 1978; Mullings 1984) appear to transcend this simplistic view. Yet the shaman operating in a ''pristine'' tribal ambience remains the prototype for scholars writing on these forms of healing. An important consequence for the study of therapeutic process is failure to distinguish clearly between traditional forms of healing such as shamanism and healing movements such as faith healing. The latter are not exclusive to industrialized, developed societies but are distinct from traditional healing in that they recruit adult participants. Unlike the prototypic case of a small-scale society where people take for granted and are familiar from birth with the shaman as healer (although they may be ignorant of the shaman's specialized knowledge), adult recruits to healing movements may never before have considered the possibility of divine healing, requiring secondary socialization to establish a predisposition toward such healing. In addition, unlike healing in traditional societies, such movements typically attract two quite distinct groups—one consisting of committed disciples and the other of marginal participants seeking relief for particular complaints.

PROCEDURE, PROCESS, OUTCOME

Having introduced the topic in terms of a broad network of concepts, we will begin to narrow the focus of our discussion by distinguishing therapeutic process from therapeutic procedure on the one hand and from therapeutic outcome on the other. As a first pass at elaborating these distinctions let us consider the relatively common situation of a bacterial infection. In the category of *proce-*

dure, we would include the diagnostic blood test and urine culture and the subsequent administration of an antibiotic medication. Successful *outcome* in this instance would be elimination of the bacterial infection; unsuccessful outcome would be continuation or worsening of the infection. Therapeutic *process* can then be understood as all the meaningful activity that mediates procedure and outcome.

Procedure (actions taken) and outcome (results obtained) are relatively easy to define, and we will deal with them first. We then turn to the concept of process, inherently more complex and used in a variety of ways. Typically for medical and psychiatric anthropology, these ways are cultural and psychological, though there is no necessary a priori reason to exclude biological process from consideration. Indeed, Browner, Ortiz de Montellano, and Rubel (1988) have called for ethnomedical studies to pay more attention to biologically definable diseases and physiologically identifiable processes that occur in both healing and pathology. In our example of the bacterial infection, fever is part of the physiological effort to overcome infection, as stomach upset is often part of the reaction to antibiotic treatment. Given the relative lack of emphasis on the physiological dimension of therapeutic process, however, we will review four common conceptions of therapeutic process as (1) the course of a treatment event, (2) a sequence of experiential or intrapsychic phenomena, (3) the course of an illness episode, and (4) social and ideological control exercised through healing practice.

Therapeutic procedure can be defined in terms of who does what to whom with respect to medicines administered, physical techniques or operations carried out, prayers recited, symbolic objects manipulated, altered states of consciousness induced or invoked. It is the organized application of techniques with some goal in mind. The shaman may go into trance and take a mystic journey to retrieve the soul of the afflicted or suck on an afflicted part of the patient's body in order to remove an intrusive spiritual object. The Native American patient may be treated with a combination of sweat emetic, herbal teas, and ritual chants in order to achieve purification. The psychoanalytic patient is instructed to say whatever comes to mind, and this free association is expected to bring important repressed contents of the unconscious into the scrutiny of the clinical gaze. The surgeon grafts a portion of a vein from the leg into a patient's aorta and coronary arteries, and this coronary bypass is expected to renew the restricted blood flow to the patient's heart. The patient at the temple of Asclepius in ancient Greece offered sacrifices and fell into a sleep during which the god appeared, and this "incubation" was expected to heal the person spontaneously or reveal instructions to follow for a healing. The anthropological literature is replete with descriptions of therapeutic procedures, and in fact such descriptions are much more common than are descriptions of what we shall define as therapeutic process in a strict sense. Familiarity with the ethnographic inventory of therapeutic procedures is essential, but a comprehensive survey of such procedures is beyond the scope of this chapter.

Therapeutic outcome refers to the disposition of participants at a designated end point of the therapeutic process, with respect to both their expressed (high or low) satisfaction and to change (positive or negative) in symptoms, pathology, or functioning. In biomedical terms, a successful outcome is elimination of a disease or disorder; in sociological terms it is termination of what Talcott Parsons called the "sick role" (Alexander 1982; Parsons 1958). Outcome is a remarkably complex phenomenon to study due to the immense number of factors to be taken into account and the difficulty of controlling observer effects. Models for such studies from clinical research include double-blind clinical trials of drugs and comparative studies of psychotherapy, but these are only marginally appropriate for studies by anthropologists in which outcome is invariably linked to cultural context and the meaning attributed to therapeutic change. To the standard concern with transformation in individual experience, anthropologists add concern for how cultural representation and collective experience alter individual states. The methodological problems are evident in a study that attempted to determine the therapeutic outcome of healing by prayer by means of a double-blind clinical trial (Joyce and Welldon 1965). For the sake of controlling the effect of suggestion, the researchers eliminated direct contact between the prayer group and their patient, thereby fundamentally altering the natural context of therapy in a way unacceptable to anthropological research. The results were inconclusive.

Psychotherapy researchers have executed systematic comparative outcome studies on different forms of psychotherapy (Luborsky et al. 1985, 1986). Anthropologists' analyses of efficacy in ritual healing paint a much broader picture, ranging from the conclusion that healing is invariably and necessarily effective due to the manner in which its problems are defined (Kleinman and Sung 1979) to the conclusion that it fails to fulfill its claims insofar as it is more a treatment of lifestyle than of symptoms (Pattison, Lapins, and Doerr 1973). Anthropologists have only recently and very tentatively attempted systematic studies of outcome, and these are based on patient reports of symptom improvement (Finkler 1985) or expression of their degree of satisfaction with treatment (Kleinman and Sung 1979; Kleinman and Gale 1982). The finding that those treated sometimes maintain their symptoms while at the same time claiming satisfaction bespeaks fundamental conceptual difficulties in the very definition of outcome. Thus it is necessary to take a step backward from assessment of outcome to more systematic descriptive analysis of therapeutic process. In this way, anthropologists may come to a more systematic understanding of what might count as efficacy across diverse forms of healing.

Having defined therapeutic procedure and outcome, we can identify at least four distinct senses in which the concept of therapeutic process has been used. The first is process as the unfolding of a specific treatment event. For anthropologists, this has typically been a ritual event, and much anthropological literature on healing can be seen as a subset of the literature on ritual. In the genre, the idea of therapeutic process is analogous to the idea of ritual process, the prototype of which is the rite of passage (Turner 1969). Process is understood as the sequence of actions, phases, or stages undergone by the participants. For most contemporary researchers on psychotherapy, on the other hand, process within therapeutic events is constituted by elements of verbal interaction (Labov and Fanshel 1977) and interpersonal relationship between therapist and client (Rogers et al. 1967). Psychotherapy researchers have argued that the relationship between therapist and client is critical for success (Gelso and Canter 1985; Rogers et al. 1967), while some anthropologists point out that the relationship between ritual healers and their clients is frequently superficial (Finkler 1985).

A second conceptualization is in terms of experiential process, with a focus on the sequence of mental states, the emergence of insight, interpretation of religious experience, and endogenous symbolic or somatic processes. To date, most work from this perspective by anthropologists has focused on the experience of the healer (Noll 1983; Peters and Price-Williams 1980; Peters 1981), although the experience of the patient is beginning to be addressed (Csordas 1988a, 1994; Hollan 1994). While some work in this perspective remains event based, it is more disposed to recognize that therapeutic process often extends beyond the event itself. This is certainly the case in insight-oriented therapies, where the significance of some part of the event may become clear only later and in any therapy where change is dependent on the response of others in the social milieu of the afflicted. Also, writing from this standpoint is increasingly inclined to conceive experience not as intrapsychic but as intersubjective. This is evident in the subtleties of shared perception and attention observable between healers and patients in a variety of traditions (Csordas 1993). In Chinese medicine, which emphasizes that all experience is intersubjective, practitioners have resisted the introduction of herbal remedies in pill form since it is recognized that ritual preparation of teas and infusions is part of the therapeutic process, with the smell of brewing medicine alerting neighbors to the presence of illness and thus attracting community support for the afflicted person.

In the work of Janzen (1978b, 1987) and others, therapeutic process is taken in a third sense: that of progression or course of an illness episode, defined by a sequence of decisions leading to diagnosis and treatment. This work broadens the notion of process to include not only the patient and therapist but the network of people who may be engaged with varying degrees of responsibility in the decision-making process, termed the *therapy management group*. This work also places therapeutic process squarely in the context of medical pluralism, emphasizing the way therapy management groups negotiate about the use of multiple health resources and, by extension, the interaction or complementarity among those resources. Along with other work on "hierarchies of resort" (Romanucci-Ross 1969) and the "social course of the illness experience" (Kleinman et al. 1995), it represents the actors' perspective on navigating through a sea of therapeutic choices. The complementary perspective of social organization is represented by analyses of health care systems as complexes of health care resources in a society that may interact in ways that are complementary or contradictory (Fabrega 1976; Field 1976; Kleinman 1980; Leslie 1976; Leslie and Young 1992; Feierman and Janzen 1992). Arthur Kleinman has described the typical structure of health care systems in complex societies in terms of the relation among sectors composed of professionalized healing forms, folk or traditional specialities, and popular health care, including the knowledge and practices of communities, families, and individuals.

A final sense of process that we shall consider is political, that is, the sense in which therapy and healing articulate with broader social issues and concerns. The role of therapy management groups is not only one of support and assistance for the afflicted but one of social control of the patient and ideological control of the values implicit in therapy and illness behavior. This is worked out in the process of deciding which treatments to use and in which order, as well as which are inappropriate and to be ruled out. Victor Turner's (1964) early work on Ndembu healing also emphasized that the process was one of intervention in community relationships as much as attention of the problems of a specific afflicted individual. Devisch (1993) offers an even deeper account of such sociosomatic processes.

A more macrosocial understanding of therapeutic process as political begins when one recognizes the existence of broader economic and social regulatory constraints on the structure of a therapeutic system. These constraints become most evident in situations of radical restructuring of a health care system, such as in the changes in Nicaragua following the 1979 overthrow of the dictator Somoza (Donahue 1986a). In other situations, sociopolitical constraints may not be explicit and may even be invisible on the level of specific therapeutic action. Hence they constitute an important challenge to cultural analysis and critique, which often focus on interpersonal interaction in discrete events.

The opposite possibility is that a reaction to and commentary on the human world in which affliction arises can be built into the structure of therapy itself. Such a perspective is offered in Michael Taussig's (1987) analysis of shamanistic healing in Colombia and Jean Comaroff's (1985) of evangelistic healing in South Africa. Both vividly set against the background of colonial oppression, these works show the inevitable reflection of ambient social conflict and power relations in practices ostensibly directed at individual suffering. Again, in the domain of gender relations, healing may be an enactment of a status quo of male dominance but may also be a mode of redistributing power into the hands of female healers, as well as a mode of empowerment when the rhetoric of affliction articulates the resistance of the afflicted (Lewis 1971; Boddy 1989; McLain 1989). Just as the therapeutic process extends beyond specific events into the broader social world of the participants, so also the world is embedded in the therapeutic process.

MODELS OF THERAPEUTIC EFFICACY

Anthropological studies of therapeutic outcome are in a very early stage of development. Lack of progress in determining the degree of success of traditional therapies, however, has not precluded analyses of how those therapies might work. Indeed, despite the inability of researchers to determine definitive outcomes, the very fact that people continue to have recourse to such forms of treatment suggests that they produce some kind of effect, and it remains relevant to search for definitions of that efficacy. In this section we outline the principal anthropological approaches to this problem. One or more of these approaches underlies virtually any anthropological analysis of healing. They should be seen not as mutually exclusive alternatives but as emphases that have appeared in various combinations in the literature.

The *structural* emphasis posits the existence of interrelated analytic levels, such as body-emotion-cognition or person-society-culture. The classic example of this approach is Claude Levi-Strauss's (1963c) discussion of how a Cuna pregnancy chant recapitulates on a symbolic level the physiological process of childbirth. The chant includes a narration in which the characters represent reproductive organs, and their actions represent the progression of the fetus through the birth canal. The principle of efficacy in this interpretation is the inherent power of a correspondence of homology between symbolic acts and objects, metaphors, or cosmological structure, and the thought, emotions, or behavior of those treated. Lyon (1990) suggests the possibility of interconnected orders, such that an ordering of an organism in one domain may be seen to be parallel to or a transformation of the ordering process in another domain, be it cognitive or physiological (see also Roseman 1991; Devisch 1993; Laderman 1991). Researchers in this tradition are often successful in demonstrating the existence of a homology but not in establishing why or whether the homology has an effect.

In a variant of this model, efficacy is said to derive from a transaction of symbol, meaning, or emotion between structural levels. In James Dow's (1986) influential formulation, therapeutic process begins with the particularization of mythic symbols to the level of the person—in effect, that healing makes sense of individual distress in terms of broader cultural meanings. The critical therapeutic transaction that ensues is an abstract transaction of emotions between self and somatic levels of the structural hierarchy (cf. Kleinman 1988a). Note that while usually the term *transaction* pertains to exchange between actors, in this context transaction is a form of internal communication. This internal communication is predicated on a tendency in the structural approach to reify the social, self, and somatic conceptually, such that one must then specify mechanisms of bridging and transacting between them. An alternative to separating self and body in this manner is to conceptualize a nondualistic body-self (Scheper-Hughes and Lock 1987; Kleinman 1988a; Csordas 1990, 1994b). In such an approach, the theoretical need for bridging and transacting mechanisms would be reduced to the extent that research could identify unitary body-self processes like the ''somatic modes of attention'' described by Csordas (1993b).

This abstract character creates a difficulty with the structural emphasis when it is not combined with any of the others we shall be discussing. It appears better suited to explain the efficacy of types of ritual such as rites of passage, where what the rite brings about is either a social fait accompli (such as marriage) or a biological inevitability (such as puberty). Using the structural approach, data can be collected primarily from observation of rituals and interviews with ritual specialists, ignoring the concrete experience of the person in distress and his or her therapy management group. To claim that establishing a homology or carrying out a symbolic transaction is inherently efficacious does not go far beyond the indigenous explanation of healing based solely on the inherent spiritual or supernatural forces mobilized by the healing process. One must actually show mediation across different levels or domains.

The *clinical* emphasis is based on the analogy between the traditional healer and a doctor who is treating an individual patient for a specific illness with a specific treatment in expectation of a definitive outcome. A paradigmatic example is Raymond Princes's (1964) analysis of indigenous Yoruba psychiatry as practiced by ritual specialists in which the analogy to psychiatry is tightly drawn in terms of specific techniques and elements of efficacy. In a broader cross-cultural survey or ritual therapeutic procedures and their variations, Prince (1980) includes sleep, rest, isolation, dreams, meditation and mystical states, dissociation, and shamanic ecstasy. Despite the existence of such a broad repertoire of techniques, however, arguments about efficacy typically fall back on properties of nonspecific mechanisms, such as suggestion (Calestro 1972), catharsis (Scheff 1979), or placebo effect. This inability to identify specific effect in clinical terms begs the question of whether traditional healing has its own forms of specificity.

Except when ethnopharmacological treatment is used, definitive outcomes are rarely observed. Yet rather than being nonspecific, it may better be said that the results of ritual healing are often incremental and inconclusive. That is, quite specific but small and step-by-step effects may be documented, with the result remaining open-ended and characterized by some change but no definitive "cure" (Csordas 1988a). This kind of change at the margin of disability is easily overlooked if the focus is on "therapeutic aspects" of ritual healing (Murphy 1964; Messing 1958; Kennedy 1967), following a clinical model in which distress is systematically medicalized as sickness, while the essential character of ritual healing as religious experience is deemphasized (Csordas 1987). If indeed there is a specificity to ritual healing, it may be discovered precisely in its religious rather than its clinical therapeutic dimension.

Another interpretation, or group of interpretations, are those that attribute therapeutic efficacy to *social support*. The classic example is V. Turner's (1964) analysis of Ndembu healing in which he shows that therapeutic efforts are directed at conflictual social relationships that have engendered symptomatic manifestations. In this analysis it can be said that the social group, not the individual, is the "patient." The mirror image of this argument is Vincent Crapanzano's (1973) demonstration that a distressed individual is cured by the Moroccan Hamadsha cult by being absorbed into a new social group. Here, healing is a form of social support so encompassing as to constitute a symbiotic relationship among participants and between the afflicted person and a possessing spirit or demon.

Beyond these paradigmatic statements, a substantial body of work examines the proposition that religious commitment (Larson and Larson 1994; Mathews et al. 1993) or participation in the religious milieu (Levin and Vanderpool 1987) has a beneficial effect on health. Since many of these studies ask nonspecific questions, they often come up with broadly general conclusions, such as that ritual healing is a treatment of lifestyle rather than of organic pathology (Pattison et al. 1973) or that religious practices in general have a therapeutic effect on a globally defined existential demoralization (Ness 1980). Studies of religious healing among immigrant groups in the United States, particularly Hispanic Americans, examine the circumstances of resort to and the range of illnesses treated by religious healing (Koss 1975; Harwood 1977a, 1977b; Garrison 1977a; Halifax and Weidman 1973; Sandoval 1979). While the religious dimension of these healing forms is explicitly recognized, there is typically an implicit functionalist orientation so that religion is seen almost exclusively in terms of its promotion of community solidarity and social support of suffering individuals.

The *persuasive* emphasis owes much to Jerome Frank's (1973) formulations concerning the cultivation of expectant faith through the personal influence of a healer or the ideology of the healing form and the rhetorical devices that bring about a shift in the person's "assumptive world," or set of assumptions about the nature of the world that allow a person to predict both the behavior of others and the outcome of his or her own actions. In this approach, the primary effect of therapeutic process is to transform the meaning of an illness for the sufferer (Bourguignon 1976). Healing ritual is understood not as liturgical repetition but as intentional social action directed toward the quality and content of experience.

Continuous with Frank's insight is the work in interpretive anthropology that analyzes rituals not as text but as performance (Csordas 1983; Kapferer 1979a, 1979b, 1983; Schieffelin 1985; Tambiah 1981). These works raise issues of subjective experience among ritual participants, impacts of utterance and action carried out within specific ritual genres, and performative transformation of context as well as of meaning. The form of healing ritual is understood in terms of rhetoric and language, and its content is understood in terms of image and symbol. In the past, much of the work in the performative tradition has been restricted to demonstrating transformations on the level of the text or ritual action, basing conclusions about therapeutic efficacy on the aesthetic postulate that aesthetic transformation has the inherent capacity to persuade and move people. Recent studies in this tradition, however, have given increasing attention to issues of bodily experience, self-transformation, and the engagement of emotion (Csordas 1990b, 1994a, 1994b; Desjarlais 1992; Devisch 1993; Laderman 1991; Roseman 1991; Turner 1992; Laderman and Roseman 1995).

These methodological approaches are by no means mutually exclusive. For example, in the article by Levi-Strauss (1963c) cited as paradigmatic of the

structural approach, we also find the clinical interpretation invoked in his identification of the psychological defense mechanism of abreaction. Levi-Strauss
argues that the patient relives fundamental intrapsychic conflicts evoked in ritual
performance, thereby resolving them. Stanley Tambiah's (1977) interpretation
of a Thai Buddhist healing cult invoked the homology between personal aspects
of illness and an "enduring cosmic paradigm of theodicy and tranquility" (p.
123) yet at the same time acknowledged the persuasive experience of mystical
power among participants. Prince (1982) searches for the biomedical, or more
precisely psychophysiological, sources of shamanistic healing in the release of
endogenous opiates, but in his discussion of endogenous processes he also suggests links among physiological, intrapsychic, and cultural domains (Prince
1976). New permutations continue to appear based not only on the methodological predispositions of ethnographers but on the actual diversity among healing forms that invites a diversity of analytic emphases.

DIMENSIONS OF THERAPEUTIC PROCESS

In this section we examine two dimensions of process relevant across all four
of the above approaches to therapeutic efficacy: (1) discursive-presentational
form, referring to the manner in which participants become engaged in therapeutic process, and (2) specificity-generality in *effect,* referring to the manner
in which therapy formulates and addresses problems or illnesses.

The distinction between discursive and presentational form stems from the
work of Suzanne Langer (1957). Discursive form is that of language, understood
as a succession of interrelated concepts with consistent internal logic and rationality. Presentational form is characteristic of symbol and metaphor, wherein
the meanings are simultaneous and integral and of that kind of intuitive knowledge "which the mind reads in a flash, and preserves in a disposition or an
attitude" (1957:98). Therapeutic process can be conceived along a continuum
between these forms, with, for example, the "talking cure" of psychoanalysis
occupying the discursive pole and healing based on a symbolic gesture such as
"laying on of hands" occupying the presentational pole.

Any particular type of healing may make use of both forms in succession or
combination, as in Sinhalese exorcism rites that alternate discursive narrations
and conversational sequences with presentation of demonic characters and symbolic objects (Kapferer 1979a, 1979b, 1983). In Catholic Pentecostal religious
healing, methods range from purely discursive sequences of counseling, to narrative unfolding of affectively rich sensory imagery, to the nondiscursive motor
dissociation and submergence in the healing sense of divine presence known as
"Resting in the Spirit" (Csordas 1983, 1988a). In traditional Navajo medicine,
healing ceremonies or "sings" require the patient's participation in as many as
nine consecutive nights of chants, prayers, and the rich symbolism of sacred
sand paintings, while in the relatively nondiscursive "sucking cure," the medicine man removes a piece of bone or flint allegedly inserted to do harm by a

witch who typically remains anonymous (Sandner 1979; Kunitz and Levy 1981). It is also the case both that the distinction between discursive and presentational form does not map precisely onto the distinction between verbal and nonverbal communication and that the same feature of the healing process may simultaneously have discursive and presentational aspects. For example, among American Indians, the altar fire of the Native American church is a nonverbal ritual element in the prayer meeting that exhibits both aspects: in its presentational form it is a symbol condensing meanings of power, social relations, and cosmology, and in its discursive form it can be said to speak in an inspirational way through its flickering flames and coals.

Related to the analysis of discursive and presentational form is the issue raised by Jerome Neu (1977) of the degree and nature in which different forms of therapy engage the thought processes of the participants. Neu contrasts psychoanalysis with electroconvulsive shock therapy in this respect, but it is not enough to understand the thought-nonthought continuum as simply one between verbal or cognitive modes and nonverbal or somatic modes. Psychoanalysis and behaviorist therapies also contrast in these terms insofar as the former attributes therapeutic efficacy to insight and the latter to conditioning. In addition, it is not enough to focus on the engagement of thought processes alone to the exclusion of emotional and self processes. Indeed the critical question about engagement in therapeutic process may be the way in which thought, emotion, self, and other are integrated.

The dimension of specificity and generality in effect has been cogently presented by Daniel Moerman (1979b). The prototype of specific treatment is, of course, the pharmacologic agent that reverses an organic condition or destroys a pathogen. Moerman defines general treatment empirically in terms of a patient's perceiving a field of symbols created by a healer, whether shaman or psychiatrist, and theoretically in terms of the relationship between mind and body, symbol and substance. He cites research on psychosomatic illness, biofeedback, and immunology, as well as links among the body's neural, endocrine, and autonomic systems, to suggest not only the existence of pathways linking body and mind but that these pathways are the locus for broad-based influence of metaphor and symbol on biological processes.

The prototypes for identification of nonspecific dimensions of therapeutic process are voodoo death and the placebo effect. W.B. Cannon (1942) explained death by witchcraft as a generalized reaction of the central nervous system ("fight-or-flight response") to the severe trauma provoked in someone who believed that he or she was bewitched. This analysis was strengthened by Hans Selye's (1956) definition of the body's response to stress (general adaptation syndrome) and refined in subsequent analyses of the destructive interaction in such cases between sympathetic and parasympathetic nervous systems (Lex 1974). The inverse of voodoo death as a nonspecific response is the placebo effect. A placebo is typically defined as an inert substance or practice that has a general effect, although in fact it is general not for lack of a detectable or measurable therapeutic impact but in that there is no definite causal link between the treatment and its effect. The placebo effect can be understood as an effect of interpersonal communication, activating endogenous healing processes inherent in all human beings (Prince 1980; Hahn and Kleinman 1983a; Moerman 1983b). Among these endogenous processes, one that has been singled out in both medical studies of placebo analgesia (Levine, Gordon, and Fields 1978) and anthropological studies of religious healing (Prince 1982) is the release of endorphins or endogenous opiate substances by the body itself. Nevertheless, as Howard Brody (1980) has argued, the placebo effect remains an anomaly of a magnitude that has in the history of science led to serious challenges to basic presuppositions and assumptions.

Daniel Moerman (1979b) has shown that even surgery, commonly regarded as a highly specific medical treatment, has a great deal of metaphoric meaning and that in some instances its effectiveness appears due in part to a generalized placebo effect. His observation that the surgical "laying on of steel" is in some ways parallel to the ritual laying on of hands requires us to acknowledge that contemporary biomedicine has a symbolic dimension (cf. Kleinman 1973). However, it is less frequently acknowledged that religious healing and even psychotherapy may have their own forms of specificity. When the issue is broached, the terms remain ambiguous. With regard to psychotherapy, for instance, C. H. Patterson (1985) has argued that while the therapist variables of perceived expertness, attractiveness, and trustworthiness are essentially placebos, empathic understanding, warmth or respect, and genuineness have quite specific effects. With regard to religious healing, discussion of therapeutic specificity remains limited to certain kinds of transformations in meaning (Bourguignon 1976; Csordas 1988a; Kapferer 1983) and resolutions of social conflict (Turner 1964, 1968).

Catharsis, or the discharge of negative emotional energy, is another widely reported psychological process that can be understood as specific or nonspecific. While it is most often described as nonspecific, this may be due more to lack of detailed data about therapeutic process in the kinds of healing typically described by anthropologists. Thomas Scheff (1979) has attempted to formulate catharsis more concretely as contingent on the creation in the therapeutic process of an aesthetic distance between the person and the problematic emotion, such that he or she is neither overinvolved nor detached from that emotion. Such a precondition for successful catharsis implies specificity about the relation between emotion and life situation, but this relation is in turn dependent on the relation of thought and emotion in therapeutic process.

Do some forms of general treatment only appear to be so because our research methods are not sophisticated enough to capture their specificity? Are we hopelessly muddled about our own definitions of what counts as a specific effect? Perhaps some treatments are irreducibly general because they treat a problem that is itself generalized and diffuse. This answer is given for both psychotherapy and religious healing in J. Frank's (1978) formulation of the demoralization hypothesis. Demoralization is understood to characterize all persons who come to the therapeutic process and is characterized by the inability to cope with a life situation, leading to constriction of the life space and preoccupation with threat, depression, self-blame, guilt, and shame. Frank argues that all forms of healing contain elements that counteract this condition, as well as elements that address specific symptoms. However, culturally specific values and ethnopsychologies of emotion might account for both modulations in the nature of demoralization across cultures (Jenkins 1994) and how different therapies counter particular aspects of the demoralization syndrome.

AN AGENDA FOR RESEARCH

To date there has been little progress toward a comprehensive theory of therapeutic process that could embrace the cross-cultural repertoire of healing modalities ranging from South American shamanism (Langdon and Baer 1992) to biomedical surgery (P. Katz 1990). Ideally, such a theory would be built up through complementary empirical studies of different types of healing. Finkler (1985, 1991, 1994) has begun such a program in successive studies of spiritualist healing and biomedical treatment in Mexico. Csordas has also taken such a step in examining therapeutic process in different forms of religious healing among Catholic charismatics and Navajo Indians (1994, n.d.). More such studies by individuals or teams of researchers would begin to fill this important lacuna in medical anthropological knowledge.

Perhaps the most frequently encountered comparative assertion in the literature on therapeutic process is that there exists an analogy between psychotherapy and religious or folk healing. In contemporary medical anthropology, this analogy can be traced back at least as far as Leighton and Leighton's (1941) discussion of psychotherapeutic elements in Navajo religion. Messing (1958) described the Ethiopian *zar* cult as an equivalent of the group therapy then achieving popularity in the United States. The touchstone work for authors invoking the psychotherapy analogy in the 1960s and 1970s was Frank's (1973; Frank and Frank, 1991) analysis of the role of assumptive worlds, expectant faith, placebo effect, and demoralization. The seminal work for the 1980s became Scheff's (1979) analysis of catharsis in ritual and therapy. While these works offer valuable theoretical formulations, most studies make use of them only to invoke the psychotherapy analogy. In addition to studies that empirically examine the analogy between psychotherapy and religious healing, cross-cultural studies of psychotherapy per se are much needed. This is an area that has been virtually neglected, with the exception of a few accounts of therapies in Japan (Lebra 1982; Murase 1982; Reynolds 1989; Fujita 1986), India (Singh 1977; Kapur 1979; Kakar 1982), Africa (Sow 1980), China, and Hong Kong (Cheng et al. 1993; Tseng and Hsu n.d.; Zhong 1988). Such research must include comparison of institutional settings, characteristics of interpersonal interaction among participants, characteristics of practitioners and patients, idioms of therapeutic communication, definitions of clinical reality, and therapeutic stages or mechanisms (see Kleinman 1988a for an elaboration of this comparative analytical framework).

A comprehensive theory of therapeutic process must also elaborate modes of mediation between moral and physiological domains of experience in healing. While language has frequently been recognized as such a mediator, increasingly sophisticated anthropological studies of sensory experience (Feld 1982; Howes 1991; Stoller 1989; Classen 1993) suggest that this is also a direction in which to look. Indeed, going well beyond the early work by Needham (1967), works by Rouget (1980), Roseman (1991), and Laderman (1991) have begun to demonstrate the importance of sound and music as mediators in this sense. Likewise, the importance of imagination as a mediating process has begun increasingly to come to the fore in works on healing (Price-Williams 1987; Stephen 1989; Csordas 1994a). Some of this work challenges the idea of mediation itself by rendering problematic the distinctions between domains to be mediated, such as body and self or mental or biological (Csordas 1993b, 1994a, 1994b). These developments in turn offer the opportunity for broadening the avenue of mutual interest that has recently begun to open between anthropologists and neuroscientists and that may lead toward a nonreductionistic account of mediating processes.

The search for specificity of effect should also be intensified with respect to patient experience, patient-healer interaction, and the performative elements of treatment. In the past, anthropologists have paid far more attention to the words, actions, and experience of healers than to those of patients. Extrapolation from these kinds of data to the effect on patients leads to the invocation of global mechanisms such as those discussed above and to conclusions that healing is either grossly effective or ineffective. Much welcome and likely more realistic would be increasingly fine-grained accounts of incremental efficacy (Csordas 1994a)—that uncertain domain in which the degree of disability may vary depending on the perceptions by the patient and those around him or her of a wide range of cultural and motivational factors.

Such studies of incremental change at the margin of disability must go hand in hand with an analytic of power. This analytic would recognize the intimate connection among therapeutic, political, and spiritual power in both the practice of healers and the experience of the afflicted. It would also work toward recognition of distinctions among healing as a form or reinforcement of oppression, healing as a meager stop-gap attempt to address the misery of poverty and powerlessness, and healing as a mode of empowerment wherein small changes can mean the difference between effective coping and defeat, between endurance as the remoralization of lived experience and the passive acceptance of despair.

Perhaps more important than any other principle for guiding research is the observation that the therapeutic process does not begin and end with the discrete therapeutic event. This is so in at least two ways. First, therapeutic systems and the events of therapy they generate exist in historical and social context, as both products of that context and performances that construct it. The trajectory of therapy, whether religious, psychiatric, or biomedical, may be to facilitate a person's adaptation to society or, on the other hand, to criticize societal demands and motivate the person toward creative personal change and social reform. Second, the therapeutic process cannot be understood as bounded by the therapeutic event precisely because it is ultimately directed at life beyond the event. If there is to be therapeutic transformation, it must occur not only in the event but in a person's life between events, as a social and experiential process. It is at this point that the study of therapeutic process rejoins the study of everyday life and takes its place in perspective alongside the range of social processes that constitute the human world.

ACKNOWLEDGMENTS

Thanks to Carolyn Sargent, John Garrity, and the students in the first author's seminar on psychological anthropology at Case Western Reserve University for helpful suggestions on revising this chapter for the second edition.

2
Political Economy in Medical Anthropology

Soheir A. Morsy

> The statement that anthropological subjects should be situated at the inter-
> sections of local and global histories is a statement of a problem rather than
> a conclusion. The problem imposes upon scholars who attempt to under-
> stand particular conjunctions a constant theoretical and methodological
> tension to which oppositions like global/local, determination/freedom, struc-
> ture/agency give inadequate expression. They must avoid making capitalism
> too determinative, and they must avoid romanticizing the cultural freedom
> of anthropological subjects. The tension defines anthropological political
> economy, its preoccupations, projects, and promise. (Roseberry 1988:174)

The past decade has witnessed a significant increase of studies in political economic medical anthropology (PEMA). Some publications specify political
economy in their very titles; others are not similarly explicit. Still other works
carry the label critical medical anthropology (CMA) (compare, for example,
P. J. Brown 1987; Chavez, Flores, and Lopez-Garza 1992; Frankenberg 1988c;
Morgan 1989a; Schoepf 1991b; Stebbins 1991, 1993; Whiteford 1993). Banners
aside, these studies represent recent expressions of a long-lived intellectual tradition, dating back to the scholarship of Abdul Rahman Muhammad Ibn Khaldun. Among other distinctions, this fourteenth-century North African is
considered the Father of Political Economy (Battah 1988).

Consistent with Ibn Khaldun's recognition of knowledge as "dependent on
the social, economic, and political conditions of society" (Battah:215), political
economy has been subjected to selective emphasis of one or another of its
constituent conceptual elements. Over the centuries this analytical orientation
has been adapted to a multitude of intellectual concerns. In addition to the major
paradigms of classical political economy and related Euro-centered intellectual

traditions, variants of this perspective have informed the works of contemporary scholars of the Third World.

With the development of academic disciplinary compartmentalization, the integrity of political economy as a systemic analytical orientation was compromised (Wolf 1982). For anthropology, the integrative disciplinary ideal of holism represents a potential deterrent in this regard. While anthropological political economy bears a conceptual kinship to other contemporary variants of this intellectual tradition, it is privileged by a grounding in comparative cultural analysis. As William Roseberry has remarked in relation to Eric Wolf's work,

Although the anthropological project Wolf envisions might be called a global and historical political economy, it has little in common with some forms of global social science . . . , especially the "world-system" theory. . . . [These forms] tend to obliterate cultural difference and interpret social processes in various parts of the world in terms of processes occurring in the developed centers of the world economy. As an anthropologist, Wolf starts with the multiform and various societies studied by other anthropologists and attempts to explore their histories in a way that connects them with processes occurring elsewhere. . . . History as cultural difference and history as material social process . . . have important critical things to say to a more traditional, "ahistorical" anthropology. (Roseberry 1989:12)

Far from rendering ethnographic detail and the study of individual human experience obsolete, anthropological political economy regards culturally informed interactions between social actors and political economic relationships as dialectically related (Comaroff and Comaroff 1992; Worsley 1984:179–80; Fields 1988). As such, this integrative, systemic approach is not a simple expansion of eclectic holism or a particular micro-macro mix. As an approach to history and culture, including the culture of health and sickness, anthropological political economy "sees the Other as different but *connected,* a product of a particular history that is itself intertwined with a larger set of economic, political, social and cultural processes to such an extent that analytical separation of 'our' history and 'their' history is impossible" (Roseberry 1989:13, original emphasis; compare Asad 1987; Ortner 1984). Neither is there a distancing of culture as a system of symbols from society as an institutional order. Interpretation of symbols simultaneously involves consideration of their political context.

For PEMA, its partaking of intellectual elements of the political economy of health (PEH) tradition proceeds from a foundation of cross-cultural knowledge of health and sickness. The very identification of political economy as the "missing link in medical anthropology" (Morsy 1978, 1981; see also Frankenberg 1980) occurred in conjunction with the study of cultural specificity and social dynamics. Medical anthropologists have gone beyond the general proposition that the "mix of traditional and modern medicine" is a function of "political economy [and] cultural hegemony" (Elling 1981). In addition to the base of cultural construction and historically specific social contextualization,

PEMA studies address the experiential particularities surrounding sickness and healing, medical pluralism, and the process described by Frankenberg (1980: 199) as the "making social of disease" (for example, Crandon-Malamud 1991; Frankel and Lewis 1989; Morsy 1993a).

Although macroanalysis is associated with political economy, it does not define this analytical tradition. As a focus of proposals of analytical rigor, the persistent concern with micro-macro linkages threatens PEMA with confused formulations of the problematic. PEMA is distinguished from conventional medical anthropology not simply by its scope of analysis but more fundamentally by its priority of embedding culture in historically delineated political-economic contexts. Accordingly, the relevance of culture is not restricted to ethnomedical conceptions but extends to issues of power, control, resistance, and defiance surrounding health, sickness, and healing (Comaroff 1985; Morsy 1978, 1993a; Schiller 1992).

Far from denying the importance of microanalytic studies of the existential particularities of sickness and healing—in essence, discarding the anthropological baby with the bath water—PEMA promotes an analytic strategy whereby "the medical anthropologist has to situate his/her work in the context of three processes—development, the making social of disease, *and in the more general concepts of anthropological analysis*" (Frankenberg 1980:197, emphasis added).

In following Frankenberg's advice, medical anthropologists have illuminated both ethnomedical and biomedical constructs as historically situated social products. Far from neglecting culture, or "writing against culture" (Abu-Lughod 1991), culturally meaningful constructs are examined in sociohistorical context. Thus, spirit possession, for example, is freed from its conventional status of reified engendered "culture-bound syndrome" (see, for example, Morsy 1978; Ong 1988; Sharp 1993). Other forms of "folk" medicine, which have long served as gatekeeping concepts in conventional anthropological discourse, have been "reconsidered in terms of problems of subalternity, the dynamics of social classes, the intrinsic relationship between the history of the subaltern and the culture of the subaltern" (Pandolfi 1992:163), including the culture of resistance to medical modernization within the framework of alien political and economic domination (Janes 1995; Morsy 1991; Stoller 1994). Similar liberation from another form of reductionism, that of medicalization, now extends to biomedically constructed states of compromised health, such as alcoholism (Singer 1986b), AIDS (El-Bayoumi and Morsy 1993; Farmer 1992; Schoepf 1991b), infertility (Inhorn 1994), leprosy (Gussow 1989), and hypertension (Janes 1990).

PEMA AS ANTIDOTE TO MEDICAL ANTHROPOLOGY'S SOCIOCULTURALISM

As illustrated by a collection of papers published in the mid-1950s, "The Peoples of Puerto Rico" (Steward et al. 1956), the political economy perspective in the parent discipline long predates its incorporation in anthropological studies of health and sickness. This is understandable in relation to the early development of medical anthropology when its very mission was rendering comprehensible the Other's distinct cultural construction of health and sickness.

Rooted in applied research, medical anthropology was expected to facilitate the introduction of Western biomedical health care into impoverished communities of the allegedly developing world. Following the post–World War II modernist tendency of studying the condition of underdevelopment apart from its processual attributes, medical anthropology tended to emphasize the cognitive dissonance between indigenous and biomedical constructs. Accordingly, the anthropological approach "defined the problem of resistance [to modern health care] . . . as lying largely with the recipient people" (Foster and Anderson 1978: 8). Although the "problem" of "acceptability" was later redefined as "resistances in scientific medical bureaucracies" (Foster and Anderson 1978:233), the historically derived global structural determinants of sickness in "developing" societies remained unscrutinized (see Cameron 1960; Darity 1965; Gould 1965; Polgar 1962; Shiloh 1968).

Critical review of the medical anthropological literature revealed that the discipline's "doctrine of the maintenance function of ideology" (Asad 1979:621) had been incorporated in its health-focused subdiscipline (for example, see Fabrega 1979; Foster 1958; Foster and Anderson 1978; compare, for example, Frankenberg 1974; Kunstadter 1975). Accordingly, materially based authoritative discourse generally remained beyond the concerns of meaning-focused medical anthropology.

The African anthropologist Omafume Onoge rejected the socioculturalism manifested in the field's emphasis on cultural determinism, and its localized microanalytic focus, which left unelaborated global political-economic relations (Onoge 1975). Other anthropologists also criticized medical anthropology for shunning what Janzen (1978a) has termed the "macrolevel of analysis," which extends beyond the family or the local community. Adoption of socioculturalism meant that "phenomena other than those covered by the model are ruled out of the court of specialized discourse" (E. Wolf 1982:10). In the field as a whole, this resulted in the neglect of the historical political-economic context of the development of health systems.

In short, synchronic emphasis on the cognitive, affective, and behavioral dimensions of local health systems in medical anthropology has been deemed analytically restrictive, ignoring the relationships between local and global power relations pertaining to the production and shaping of sickness and the initiation and management of healing (Hopper 1975; Singer and Baer n.d.; Susser 1985:562; Taussig 1980a:12–13; Young 1982:269). Traditional analytical emphasis in the field undermines the idea that power—a central concept in the ethnography of health and sickness (Glick 1967; see Morsy 1978)—originates and resides in arrangements between social groups that are not defined simply by local boundaries.

MEDICAL ANTHROPOLOGY AND THE SOCIAL
PRODUCTION OF KNOWLEDGE

Epistemologically, PEMA controverts claims of scientific objectivity and ethical neutrality by explicitly acknowledging that both anthropological and medical knowledge are socially informed products of particular historical and cultural contexts (Morsy 1993a; see also, for example, Martin 1987; Taussig 1980b; A. Young 1980, 1988). Indeed, from the perspective of the "political economy of knowledge" (Keesing 1981), the development of PEMA in the 1970s was not simply the result of anthropologists' intellectual creativity or skill as "disciplinary brokers" (Baer 1986b). Medical anthropologists' interest in health-related variants of the political economy tradition represented a specific expression of a more general, politically informed development in the parent discipline. Appreciation of global orientations in social science research was an outcome of the protracted struggles of the legendary Other, which forced the "reinvention" of the discipline (Leacock 1982; Mafeje 1976; Nader 1969; Schoepf 1979; Scholte 1983).

Among Third World scholars, there was a call for "decolonializing Anthropology" (Stavenhagen 1971; see also, for example, Asad 1973; Banaji 1970; Harrison, ed., 1991; Magubane 1971). Critical reviews of health research in Latin America (Bonfil-Batalla 1966), India (Banerji 1984), and the Middle East (Morsy 1981) sensitized anthropologists working around the world to the material determinants of health status and brought into focus local and global power relations (see also, for example, Laurell 1989; Asad 1987:596).[1]

While developments in the anthropological periphery continue to provide raw material for theory (see, for example, Nzimiro 1977; Peiris 1969; Shukri 1985), the declaration of the "coming of age of critical medical anthropology" (Singer 1989) also rests on studies of the "dominative medical system" (Baer 1989; see, for example, Frankenberg 1988b; Lazarus 1988a, 1988b; Singer et al. 1984). Some medical anthropologists now extend explicit attention to the connectedness of "Western" and "non-Western" health issues within the framework of global political economy (Baer 1982; Martin 1988:19–20; Young 1982; Morsy 1993b). With biomedicine conceptualized as a social system, medical anthropologists have demonstrated that anthropology's traditional idea of fit ("dialectics" in PEMA) between medicine and society in non-Western settings is equally valid for the heartland of scientific medicine (compare, for example, Foster 1958:7; Singer 1987).

In sum, PEMA's intellectual genealogy ties this health-focused analytical perspective to the Other not as the passive object of anthropological scrutiny but as a source of intellectual enrichment of the field. It was the determined resistance and protracted struggle of "our" people and the related 1960s antiwar movement in the United States (Sider 1974) that precipitated the ferment in which political-economic analysis took root as a legitimate, but not uncontested, anthropological orientation. In relation to the latter status, the designation "critical medical anthropologist," erroneously distinguished from medical anthropologists who "focus on developing practical solutions" (Backstrand 1994), serves to rationalize exclusion from the academy, Western democracies' bastion of "free speech." Less belligerent expressions of gatekeeping sometimes take the form of sarcastic commentaries on the "whining" and "ideological roars" of political economy theorists (Estroff 1988:421–23, 426).

As a serious scholarly pursuit, it is worth giving consideration to the idea that the medical anthropological research process, like other forms of sociomedical investigations, is more than merely a set of methods for gathering and treating data. When viewed as a socially constituted system of inquiry, it becomes clear that this process in fact consists of a series of interconnected and interactive decision points, each of which requires a subjective, value-laden choice by the researcher as he or she confronts several possible alternatives. This means that issues of analytical rigor are not simply technical but political-ideological value commitments underlying the choices made by researcher (Ratcliffe and Gonzalez-del-Valle 1988).

PEMA'S INTELLECTUAL ANCESTRY

While PEMA's current popularity is traceable to changes within "the world order of Anthropology" (Stocking 1982), consideration of its specific intellectual constitution and origins takes us back to the wisdom of ancient medical traditions and historically antecedent scholarship. We are indebted to a variety of ancestral intellectual traditions that emphasize the social production of health and sickness. For example, from ancient Egyptians we learn that the "conditions of life" are the major determinants of health status. Similarly, a reading of Al-Suuyti's medieval medical treatise leads us to recognize deprivation as a cause of poor health (Elgood 1962).

As a serious scholarly pursuit, interest in political economy links us to Ibn Khaldun. As illustrated in the Prolegomena, his analytical orientation, also known as the "science of culture," addressed the "interaction and interdependence of political and economic factors, and their effects on cultural and social phenomena" (Battah 1988:12). Although power and hegemony were central to Ibn Khaldun's analysis of society and history (Salame 1989), they were not isolated from culture. Within the analytical map of the Khaldunian systemic perspective, custom, the parent of humanity, was linked to historically situated political-economic developments.

In relation to more recent intellectual developments, PEMA relates to Rudolf Virchow's nineteenth-century work, which, in addition to demonstrating the social etiology of compromised health, including powerlessness, insists on the understanding of contradictory social forces that obstruct reform (Taylor and Rieger 1985).

As a corrective to cultural reductionism in medical anthropology, PEMA is indebted not only to Virchow's vision but also to contemporary derivative variants of PEH that emphasize the social relations of sickness and healing (see, for example, Elling 1981; Navarro 1986; Turshen 1989).

PEMA has also been informed by the Marxist variant of PEH, which directs attention to historical context and the centrality of class relations within the framework of global capitalism. This analytical orientation also sensitized medical anthropologists to the role of the state, the commodification of health care, illness-generating social conditions (including labor), the ideological nature of medical knowledge, and the micropolitics of medicine (Navarro 1986; Turshen 1989; Waitzkin 1989).

Medical anthropology has also benefited from Marxist cultural theorizing, notably that of Luckas (Taussig 1980a), Gramsci (Frankenberg 1988c), and E. P. Thompson (V. Adams 1988). Humanist Marxism, which focuses on experience as mediating between social structure and the individual, has also been incorporated into medical anthropology (Scheper-Hughes and Lock 1986). In addition, under the label CMA, researchers have made explicit their indebtedness to Marx's critical theory and the work of the Frankfurt school. Lazarus and Pappas (1986:136) define the goal of critical theory in medical anthropology as "understand[ing] the way in which medical science and medical practice take shape, and the way that possibilities for change and improvement are limited and circumscribed" (see also Baer 1986b).

Many medical anthropologists who advocate political-economic analysis have been influenced by the "dependency" or "world system" variant of the PEH (L. Morgan 1987). This global perspective inspired a significant modification in medical anthropology's conventional ahistoric outlook and cultural reification. It brought into focus the relatively neglected, although locally influential, effects of national and international asymmetric power relations (Elling 1981; Janzen 1978a, C. Smith 1983).

Aside from the all-too-familiar limitations of the dependency perspective in relation to cultural specificity and social dynamics, this perspective remains significant for having made explicit the sociopolitical nature of the connectedness between us and other. This dialectical relationship had been effectively obscured in medical anthropological discourse by models that juxtapose "Western" and "non-Western" medical systems and straightforwardly connect poor health to the inaccessibility of "Western" medicine.

Undoubtedly, the analytical limitations of the dependency perspective are worthy of serious consideration by medical anthropologists (L. Morgan 1987), as they have been by other scholars, anthropologists included. However, it must be emphasized that these limitations are not automatically applicable to culturally informed medical anthropological studies, which have benefited from the expanded analytical scope of the dependency perspective.[2] The fact that medical anthropologists are taking into account global structural relations, after years of neglect, does not preclude concern with the cultural, social, and experiential particularities of sickness and healing, the mainstay of the field (Inborn 1994; Janes 1995; Morsy 1993a).

MEDICAL ANTHROPOLOGY AS EXPANDED ANALYTICAL TERRAIN

Informed by variants of the PEH orientation, PEMA transcends traditional disciplinary boundaries, integrating, for example, "sociological [and anthropological, or political science] contributions to the political economy of health" (Baer 1986b) rather than confining medical anthropologists to "cultural contexts" or sociologists to "social contexts" (Foster 1974:4–5). Thus PEMA research is not limited by medical anthropology's conventional methodology—informant-focused knowledge production—freeing us to address such nontraditional concerns as the effects of national revolutionary transformation on health services (Donahue 1986a), the impact of regional political and economic developments on the incidence of spirit possession (Morsy 1991), transnational cigarette companies' "making a killing" in Mexico and Guatemala (Stebbins 1994), the "medicalization of homelessness" in New York City (Mathieu 1993), "biomedicine in relation to the political economy of science" (Singer 1992a), and biomedicine's cultural authority (Martin 1987).

Attention has also extended to the discourses of medical sciences and international health programs (Morsy 1993b, 1993c; Morsy and El-Bayoumi 1993; Nash and Kirsch 1988; Rapp 1988a). Analytical scrutiny now also includes the historically specific authoritative discourses that had been effectively obscured by desocialized "emic" accounts. As for historically and socially situated "emic analysis," this certainly has a place in PEMA. For example, in relation to Sandanistan Nicaragua, it has been identified as the means by which researchers would be able to observe how specific health strategies are negotiated among several interest groups within the same political economy and how the outcome conforms to the stated goals of the political system (Donahue 1984:70).

Methodologically, the expansion of anthropology's conventional analytical field (Koptiuch 1985) required revision of the notion of holism. The ideal that each investigator study every facet of a designated phenomenon is unattainable in practice. To safeguard holism as an integrative disciplinary approach, it has become necessary for individual researchers to specify the scope, and linkages of their studies, and to consider the commensurability of related paradigms and research emphases (DeWalt and Pelto 1985:11; Young 1982:279; Lett 1987; Comaroff 1985).

While selective emphasis of level of analysis is expected to vary from one study to another, even when undertaken by the same researcher, this does not necessarily compromise the overall integrity of the political-economic framework of analysis (compare, for example, Ferguson 1981 and 1986; Morsy 1988b and 1991). For example, Van der Geest (1987a), in a methodological note that has relevance well beyond his specific concern with unequal access to pharmaceuticals in southern Cameroon, illustrates the explicit delineation of the multidimensional scope of medical anthropology's expanded analytical purview. He reasons that "because it is virtually impossible to deal with the whole gamut of relevant contexts, [it is necessary to restrict oneself] to considering contextual forces which seem of particular political and economic importance in the rapidly modernizing state of Cameroon" (p. 142). This selective emphasis on the part of the researcher necessarily leaves out "further linkages with the social, domestic, and individual cognitive domain of drug consumers [which although] not discussed are [recognized as] equally important" (p. 155). In another publication devoted to the local perspective in studies of pharmaceuticals in the Third World, Van der Geest urges researchers to consider these "cognitive and domestic factors" (Van der Geest 1987b; see also Alubo 1987; Ferguson 1981; Stock 1987).

Although varying from highly abstracted programmatic statements to concrete case studies, studies in anthropological political economy share a characteristic historical specificity and a dialectical orientation. Thus, they contrast with conventional anthropology, which renders all societies temporally equal by placing them in an imaginary, timeless space (Saa 1986; Worsley 1966:5), which is based on integrative models of society, to the neglect of conflict (Firth 1975: 30), and pursues the illusory search for cultural authenticity, thereby compromising social and historical variation.

Political-economic anthropological studies also contrast with the traditional anthropological preoccupation with systems of "authentic meaning" presumed to be shared by ideologically defined communities, without regard to historical variations in political activity and economic conditions (Asad 1979:614). Political-economic anthropology, far from ignoring ideology, considers it to be a type of socially constituted knowledge: the product of evolving social forces. This perspective seeks to analyze the historically specific social conditions or structures of society that are associated with certain types of ideologies. For recent human history, the structures of society extend inevitably to global economy and power relations.

Regarding material correlates of health and sickness, PEMA is distinguished not by singular variables but by the analytic scheme within which variables are integrated. For example, the concept of social class has been addressed in both conventional and political-economic studies in medical anthropology. Whereas a conventional meaning-centered study might focus on how interclass differences relate to understanding a medical concept (Foster and Anderson 1978: 231), PEMA accords social class (in the form of class-linked power differentials) a central role in the study of social relations of sickness and healing (see, for example, Beardsley 1987; Ferguson 1986; Navarro 1986).

Nancy Scheper-Hughes's (1984b) study of infant care in northeast Brazil also sheds light on PEMA as an explanatory scheme. Among the multiple factors that are detrimental to child survival in this part of the world, Scheper-Hughes includes ecological and psychocultural variables. While this study shows that PEMA is capable of accommodating a variety of health-relevant factors, it demonstrates that the distinctiveness of this orientation pertains to its explanatory priority. Scheper-Hughes identifies the "macroparasitism of class exploitation" as the social mechanism whereby morbidity and mortality are generated.

In sum, PEMA's purposeful divergence from established modes of anthropological investigation enables researchers to expose fundamental social processes that are hidden from easy view in locally grounded, empiricist social analysis (Leacock 1972:60–61). In addition to benefiting from developments in other disciplines, this endeavor involves drawing on the knowledge base of anthropology's sister fields. Relevant issues include political anthropology's investigations of the role of the state, economic anthropology's elaborations of the labor process, including child labor, in the context of development, and linguistic anthropology's significance as a probe of the nature of social relations. For example, in a study focused on health, nutrition, and development in the Cauca Valley of Colombia Michael Taussig's analysis (1978) is clearly informed by concerns that are ordinarily associated with economic anthropologists' investigations of agrarian transformation in the context of regional and global development (see also Dewey 1989; Laurell et al. 1977; Morsy 1986c:367, 370–71, 1993a). Similar linkage to other specializations in the discipline is reflected in Ellen Gruenbaum's (1981) study of health policy and the state in the Sudan, in Morsy's (1988b) account of health services within the framework of state policies of economic liberalization, in Lynn Morgan's (1989b) emphasis on the role of the state in primary health care, and in Nancy Scheper-Hughes's (1992) account of child hunger and death in the context of regional agrarian developments in Brazil. In the same vein, Merrill Singer (1992b) underscores the importance of linguists in his research team's efforts to develop culturally specific AIDS prevention programs.

RESEARCH, DIALOGUE, AND DEBATE

As in the case of the parent discipline, medical anthropology has been affected by the proposal that "anthropologists can creatively deal with the theoretical and methodological tensions imposed by the attempt to place anthropological subjects at the intersections of local and global histories" (Roseberry 1988:179; see also Frankenberg 1980; Morsy 1993a; Mullings 1984; Scheper-Hughes 1984b; Young 1982). In operationalizing the basic tenets of the political economy perspective, medical anthropologists have addressed a number of topics of current concern in the parent discipline, including issues of development, gender, and praxis. Critical medical anthropologists have also engaged in dialogue and debate with ecologically oriented colleagues who partake of the biocultural orientation, and clinically oriented medical anthropologists (compare, for example Baer 1990, 1993a; Heurtin-Roberts 1995; Leatherman, Goodman, and Thomas 1993; McElroy 1990; Morgan 1993a; Press 1990; Scheper-Hughes 1990; Singer 1995; Wright and Johnson 1990), as well as proponents of the "interpretative-constructivist" persuasion in medical anthropology (Baer 1993b).

Third World Development, Health, and Medicine

In relation to health and development in the global perspective, PEMA spans such topics as health care within the framework of colonial and neocolonial relations, as well as socialist transformation (Taussig 1987; Gruenbaum 1981; and New 1975, respectively). By situating analysis of the role of colonial health services "within a larger societal analysis" and "link[ing] medical care to the structures of power," PEMA researchers bring into focus "inequities in health care delivery" and show how "health systems . . . serve nonmedical goals of a society's dominant groups" (Lasker 1977; see also Gruenbaum 1981; Pearce 1980.

Research on the social production of sickness also has been undertaken in conventional anthropological research settings: contemporary impoverished and underdeveloped parts of world. Studies range from investigation of the colonial medical legacy in Nigeria (Alubo 1987), to consideration of the health consequences of the marginalization of Andean populations in national development schemes (Leatherman et al. 1986). In these studies of the social production of morbidity and relations of healing, underdevelopment and its resultant health problems are defined as structural rather than conjunctural (Navarro 1985:537). With this reformulation, attention is given to the articulation of local developments and global political economy, a relation heretofore not perceived as problematic in conventional medical anthropology (DeWalt and Van Willigen 1984; Foster 1984b; compare Banerji 1984; Lane 1988; Low 1985b; Stebbins 1986).

The concern with contextuality is also manifest in a number of studies emphasizing the interpretation of ethographically derived data in the light of global, national, or regional political-economic developments. These studies address a variety of issues, including the distribution and use of pharmaceuticals (Van der Geest 1987a), rural health services (Morsy 1993a), the role of the state in primary health care programming (Morgan 1989b), and the cultural specificity of biomedical hegemony (Adams 1988; Morsy 1988b; Hammady 1989). As Myntti's (1988) Yemen study demonstrates, this hegemony of modern Western medicine may well be upheld within the framework of traditional repositories of power.

While shedding light on the social control functions of modern medicine, PEMA research on medical modernization represents an alternative to postmodernist vilification of biomedicine as "discourse." In opposition to this posture, and postmodernist indeterminacy (Tesh 1988), it is arguable that

capitalist medicine is controlling medicine because it is effective, not vice versa. To think otherwise—as the antimedicine positions do— . . . is tantamount to believing that medicine is a complete falsification that people have swallowed in their ignorance. (Navarro 1986:242)

Also in contrast to postmodernists, whose admonishment of medical modernity as "discourse" proceeds from the privileged terrain of modern comforts, for activists of the South, scientific knowledge, including its medical variants, has been an important tool of political resistance in relation to such modernizing projects as the introduction of nuclear power, human experimentation, and the dumping of hazardous pesticides (Morsy 1993c). For the United States, Scheder has encouraged access "to the tools or . . . knowledge [of biological disease etiology] to influence the system whose effects we often bemoan" (Scheder 1988:277). In relation to international health, partaking of such knowledge enables medical anthropologists to transcend the conventional status of handmaidens-translators to biomedicine. We are enabled to assess critically the implications of global health strategies such as the child survival mandate (Morsy and El-Bayoumi 1993; Nichter and Cartwright 1991), the call to action on maternal mortality by the World Health Organization (WHO) (Morsy 1995), and its cross-cultural studies of psychiatric epidemiology (Hopper 1991).

PEMA, Advanced Capitalism, and Socialist Transformation

No longer limited to the part of humanity targeted for the civilizing mission of development expertise (Escobar 1987), medical anthropological studies now include investigations of health and medicine in the context of industrial capitalism and within the framework of socialist transformation (for example, Baer 1989; Hopper 1988; Lock 1986a; Martin 1987; Scheper-Hughes and Lovell 1986).

Studies of health and medicine in North America have directed medical anthropology's comparative gaze to the very medical system about which researchers hold "emic" views. The intellectual consequence of this new direction has been positive, undermining the assumption of a "monolithic and inflexible organization . . . , [bringing] into view 'peripheral specialties,' the subcultures of biomedicine, . . . and the tensions within American medicine over issues such as power and control, different types of knowledge, and dependency and autonomy" (Lock 1986a:931; see also Lock 1988a:210; Lock and Gordon 1988).

As medical anthropologists stepped on the once-sacrosanct terrain of biomedicine, they addressed the field's initial, and yet-to-be-abandoned, concern with patient compliance. Following Brooke Schoepf's seminal study of doctor-patient communication in the United States (Schoepf 1975), anthropologist-physician Michael Taussig, partaking of Marxist cultural theorizing, presented a critical analysis of biomedicine that clearly diverged from medical anthropology's "clinical mandate." He illuminated the ideological nature of medicine and addressed the mechanisms whereby it contributes to the reproduction of social power relations in capitalist society (Taussig 1980a; see also Leslie and Taylor 1973; Waitzkin 1983; Young 1980).

Following the disciplinary trend of studying one's own society and apart from concern with the issue of "clinical relevance," Hans Baer and Merrill Singer have been active contributors to the study of medicine in the United States (and also, in the case of Baer, in the United Kingdom) in both its "dominative" and "heterodox" forms (Baer 1984, 1989; Singer et al. 1984; Singer 1986b). Political economy informed–critical medical anthropologists have also addressed class, racial-ethnic, and gender relations as reflected in the "dominative" medical system of the United States (Baer 1989; Campell 1988; Chavez 1986; Morgen 1986). As in PEMA research focused on the Third World, attention has been extended to issues of medical pluralism within the framework of historically specific political-economic developments in the United States (Baer 1989).

In PEMA studies influenced by the Marxist variant of PEH and the "rediscovery of the relationship between work and health," analysis transcends the important but limiting concern with the exposure of individual workers to harmful physical, chemical, and psychological agents. Instead of the individual-environmental dichotomy implied in this focus, researchers address the "social relations that determine both the individual worker and the environment" (Navarro 1985:535). From this perspective, the workplace is but a microcosm of social contradictions expressed in the labor process. Thus informed, analysis of "occupational health" involves consideration of a variety of social relations, including those that govern the deployment of labor and the allocation of its product (Wolf 1982:4). Analytical scrutiny also involves class-based power relations and associated ideological orientations, extending from the level of management to that of the state (MacLennan 1988; Michaels 1988; Siskind 1988).

Researchers' attempts to demystify the nature of social etiology and medicalization extend to the social production of disease within the framework of agrarian capitalist relations. This is illustrated by Jo Scheder's (1988) study of type II diabetes mellitus among Mexican-American farmworkers. Her analysis of the social issues fundamental to the etiology of the disease demonstrates the relationship between stressful life events and life change, social inequality and psychological stress (inherent in the migrant lifestyle), and physiological responses culminating in hyperglycemia.

In short, as a result of PEMA research over the past two decades, Onoge's observation that capitalism is a neglected theme in medical anthropology is less valid today. In fact, it is socialism, the often-proposed alternative for better health, that remains understudied by medical anthropologists. The establishment of a national unified health system in Nicaragua following the Sandinista revolution in 1979 offered "medical anthropologists a unique opportunity to study the dynamics of political economy, decision-making structures, class conflict, and health care delivery" (Ripp 1984:68).

On a socialist political agenda, health care development is not a matter of projects, selective health strategies, medical technology transfer, or international medical aid. Instead, health care becomes part of a comprehensive strategy of social transformation (Navarro 1985) that increases people's access to the means of production (land for food production, for example), increases health consciousness through educational campaigns, encourages popular participation in the delivery of health care, and, more basic, assigns the state a central responsibility for providing health for all.

As anthropologists have demonstrated for socialist-oriented Cuba (Guttmacher and Garcia 1975) and the Indian state of Kerala (Rosenfield n.d), John Donahue shows that socialist development in Nicaragua is correlated with more equitable allocation of health resources (Donahue 1986a, 1986b). Beyond this general observation, Donahue advises against the ''ideal-type'' approach that classifies health systems as capitalistic or socialistic apart from historical analysis, which considers the concrete conditions of the political economy. Indeed, the susceptibility of Sandanistan Nicaragua to U.S. political and military influences in Central America demonstrates that ''taking account of world historical political economy'' is equally important in the study of socialist-oriented societies as in any other.

Women and Health

Among other sociopolitical manifestations, PEMA is a scholarly expression of the current concern with issues of power, control, and alienation brought to the fore within the framework of social movements. Notable among these is the international struggle waged by women in pursuit of self-empowerment (Fee and Krieger 1994; Koblinsky 1993). As PEMA, studies of women and health have been influenced by the theoretics of social power relations, by the cultural critique variant of political economy, and by international health development concerns (Browner 1989b; Inhorn 1994; Lazarus 1994; Morsy 1978; Morsy and El-Bayoumi 1993).

In addition to reflecting medical anthropology's general emphasis on issues of reproductive health (see Browner and Sargent, this volume) and the increasing concern with the spread of AIDS among women (El-Bayoumi and Morsy 1993: 3–4; Schoepf 1991b, 1993), PEMA studies of engendered bodies, health, and sickness cover other areas that connect medical anthropology to the general disciplinary interest in the cultural construction of gender. Informed by historical specificity and characterized by explicit social contextualization, these studies have addressed health issues in relation to culturally variable forms of gender differentiation (Inhorn 1994; Kim 1993; Morsy 1993a; Singer, Davison, and Gerdes 1988), to class as a correlate of risk to health (Ferguson 1986; Lazarus 1994; Handwerker 1994; Morsy and El-Bayoumi 1993), to the role of the state (Gruenbaum 1989; Morgen 1986; Morsy 1993a), and to development programming (Kamal 1994; Morsy 1995; Whiteford 1993).

In short, PEMA expands the horizon of analytical scrutiny, bringing into focus women's role in production and social reproduction as these relate to health. This is the case whether a study focuses on the cultural construction of gendered bodies in scientific discourses of biological reproduction (Martin 1987), health care management (Browner 1989b), maternal mortality (Morsy 1995), or AIDS (Schoepf 1991b).

Medical Anthropology and Praxis

Advocating a theory of practice as alternative, the author of one of the earlier criticisms of anthropological political economy contends that this analytical orientation is deficient as an account of "real people doing real things" (Ortner 1984). Contradicting this assertion, Ida Susser's extension of the "political economy of health into the ethnologic domain of community research," highlights the role of "real people" doing the "real thing" of community action in a Puerto Rican industrial community (Susser 1985). On the mainland, concern with "real people" covers a number of health issues, ranging from industrial health (Nash and Kirsch 1986) to genetic counseling, which illuminate "not only medical information but also structural power arrangements, social knowledge, and popular meanings about medically defined disability" (Rapp 1988a: 143).

In spite of the invalidation of Ortner's assertion through a simple review of the literature, (see, for example Hopper 1988; Morsy 1993c; Taussig 1979, 1980a:xiii) her criticism is useful. Critical appraisals such as Ortner's, or an analogue articulated by a medical anthropologist in relation to CMA (Gaines 1991, cited by Baer 1993b), are significant for leading to debate surrounding the issue of praxis.[3]

With studying still the predominant modus operandus of the field, it is indeed important to lay bare the theoretical-philosophical-political implications of "applied" and "critical–political economic" medical anthropology. This exercise is now part of an embryonic debate involving critical–political economic medical anthropologists on the one hand and cultural constructivists on the other. As this debate develops and becomes informed by the ample social science literature on the social production of knowledge, we need to go beyond evaluation of the effectiveness of individual doers and thinkers in alleviating the suffering of members of social collectivities or working toward a synthesis of critical and constructivist perspectives. Particularly deserving of serious consideration is the social context in which one or another analytical approach is operationalized. Given the social nature of transformative activism, it cannot be assumed that acquisition of relevant knowledge, including that assembled within the framework of applied medical anthropology research, will necessarily result in action conducive to human well-being.

As the praxis debate proceeds, it would be useful to consider basic questions, ranging from some that address the very construction of health research agendas internationally to others related to the beneficiaries of health development research. Whether in relation to critical–political economic theoretical studies or their constructed applied opposite, it is important to specify the nature of the application of anthropological knowledge.

To those who shun theoretical talk in favor of the action of applied health research[4] and the promotion of development, it is worth considering the social reservoir into which actions are channeled. In other words, the excitement of doing should not blind us to the general framework of infliction of harm on the targeted Other within which some applied research and development programming is undertaken. In relation to the latter, Kenyon Stebbins (1991) reminds us of the use of tobacco in the U.S. government international development program known as Food for Peace. Another case in point is applied research surrounding selective health strategies, which are executed within the framework of structural adjustment programs, and international medical aid (Barker and Turshen 1986).

Our ''intra- and cross-cultural examinations of problems associated with medical ethics and bioethics'' (Marshall 1992) should certainly consider cultural constructions, but not as essentialism and reductionism, which obscure sociopolitical context. Whether in relation to family planning under the supervision of the Indonesian military (Hartmann 1987:80), or the testing of the efficacy of a topical niclosamide on Egyptian peasants in a project supervised by a U.S. Army general (El-Mofty n.d), it is important to investigate the relation between applied research and what anthropologist-physician Paul Farmer (1995) has described as the ''political economy of brutality,'' which structures the majority of human rights violations in the world. Selected as sample and control, people of the South have been described as ''exploitable populations'' who are at risk of being targeted as means for the ends of others within the framework of marked asymmetrical global power relations (Mariner 1993).

Also worthy of anthropological investigation is the short- and long-term outcomes of applied research projects, other than those popularized as success stories and rewarded as such (Wulff and Fisk 1987). Instructive in this regard is a comment that appeared in the November 8, 1982, edition of the Egyptian weekly *Al-Ahram al-Iqtisadi*. Its author is a researcher who participated in a 1978 Aid for International Development (AID) national health survey with the understanding that the research would improve the health situation in Egypt. He explains that ''the stage of data collection has been over for four years. . . . But unfortunately we know nothing about the fate of the [data]. . . . Where did this information go? Whom has it benefitted?. . . Why was [the research] showered with [such a large amount of] financial support?'' (author's translation from the Arabic text).

A response to such inquiries as those documented for Egypt might be discerned in the work of Michael Taussig. Based on his investigation of an AID-funded applied nutrition research project in Colombia, Taussig (1981:145) concludes,

Appearances are what count. . . . The projects are little more than a triple play in desperation—the desperation of the poor, the desperation of the governments to act in a way that does not threaten their power, the desperation of the local and foreign professionals for the grants and international connections by which their careers can be furthered—leaving rational social change an empty promise.

Attention to the sociopolitical context of applied research is equally important for nongovernmental organizations (NGOs). Increasingly, anthropologists are serving as resource persons or members of such grass-roots organizations. To some of us, such affiliations may be viewed as solidarity with Others, on *their* own terms. As such, this form of praxis may be regarded as an alternative to the international development lobby's efforts to "empower" the peoples of "developing" societies. While this may well be the case for some NGOs, it is important to caution against the blanket romanticization of these organizations. As Gyatri Spivak (1995) has observed in relation to the 1994 UN-sponsored International Conference on Population and Development (ICPD) held in Cairo, some NGOs serve nothing more than a token function, providing the stamp of legitimacy on what might otherwise appear to be "scary" development projects, such as experimental trials on human subjects or population control measures.

Anthropologists have the opportunity to investigate the social character and viability of NGOs, particularly in terms of the variable effectiveness of civil society and in relation to the role of the state, including the erosion of its welfare variants. Noteworthy with regard to the role of the state in relation to health are research projects undertaken in Egypt by two anthropologist-physicians, Kamran Ali (1994) and Montasser Kamal (1994).

CONCLUSION

We are told that talk of large-scale forces, of poverty, structural violence or (heaven forbid) imperialism. turns people off. But the people turned off by discussion of the political economy of brutality are quite often ourselves: people of good will who want to make a difference but who are indebted to powerful institutions. We need to think locally and globally and to act in response to both levels of analysis. This realization implies a commitment to study, to do analysis, to link our scholarly work to efforts among and on behalf of those most at risk of having their rights violated. We must take on the task of studying the political economy of brutality and then challenge the powers and structures that ensure its maintenance. (Farmer 1995)

In addition to mirroring the general anthropological interest in political economy, PEMA has benefited from transdisciplinary developments in sociomedical research. Transcending the limitations of conventional meaning-focused anthropological approaches, PEMA takes into account local and global historically specific social forces, relations, and processes surrounding collective health and sickness (see, for example, Laurell 1989).

A review of PEMA research indicates that this genre of medical anthropology spans a range of substantive and analytical concerns. Examples range from the social production of illness in relation to class-based power asymmetry in industrial settings (Nash and Kirsh 1988; Siskind 1988; Susser 1985) to issues of power relations surrounding women's reproductive health defined biomedically (Inhorn 1994; Lazarus 1988b; Morgen 1986; Morsy 1993b) and ethnomedically

(Singer, Davison, and Gerdes 1988). Far from exhibiting a fixed micro-macro ratio, PEMA studies reflect different levels of analysis, from the consciousness of the patient (Taussig 1980b), to community organization (Susser 1985), to the cultural and political context of patient dissatisfaction in clinical encounters (O'Neil 1989), to regional political economy (Morsy 1988b), and international corporate power (Stebbins 1994). Irrespective of the level of analysis and substantive focus, historical contextualization is central to PEMA. This characteristic contextual specificity is equally applicable to the study of "school refusal syndrome" in Japan (Lock 1986b:110) as to possession illness in Madagascar (Sharp 1993).

PEMA represents a significant epistemological development that has already shown promise in addressing medical anthropology's acknowledged theoretical sterility (see, for example, Browner, Ortiz de Montellano, and Rubel 1988). Indeed, this orientation may well be judged as constituting the most important paradigm shift in medical anthropology to date. Political-economic considerations are no longer automatically excluded from phenomenological studies of health systems. Even medical anthropologists whose work has generally been identified with the explanatory model approach have begun to utilize the conceptual tool kit of PEMA (for example, Good and Good 1988; Kleinman 1986). Also noteworthy is Horacio Fabrega's recent "plea for a broader ethnomedicine" in which he advises consideration of the "organization and political economy of the society" (Fabrega 1990a). Similarly, an "autocritique" by Alexander Alland (1987), a prominent proponent of the ecological perspective in medical anthropology, recognizes "traditional societies" as "part of a world system." Extended to medical ecology's central concept of adaptation, Alland's "hindsight" ties this phenomenon to "social and economic forces."

Without doubt, PEMA research is relevant to central analytical concerns within social science, the parent discipline, and its specialized fields. However, there remains a need for serious attempts at rendering this connection more explicit. While some studies manifest a concerted effort in this direction (for example, Morsy 1993c; Singer 1990a; Schoeph 1991b), there is still ample room for generalization of the endeavor toward preserving (and contributing to) the "anthropology" in "medical anthropology." As is the case for medical anthropology in general, PEMA research stands to benefit from intellectual developments related to such health-relevant issues as development and globalization, agrarian transformation, the labor process (including often neglected child labor), the role of the welfare state and the impact of its erosion, gender differentiation in historical context, human rights, and technological developments.

As for the debate surrounding academic and applied medical anthropology (Johnson 1994), this too would be enriched by existing disciplinary and transdisciplinary intellectual productions related to the political economy of knowledge, paradigm commensurability, the history of anthropology, and, not least, the philosophical-theoretical grounding of praxis (Lett 1987; Borofsky 1994; Tesh 1988). As the late Roger Keesing reminds us, the genuine transformation of social systems—not simply the cosmetic treatments that often pass for "development"—places the ultimate demands on the adequacy of our theories. Commitment to improving the world is no substitute for understanding it. . . . If we do not have the power to see beneath the surfaces of things, to see processes rather than symptoms, to see whole systems rather than separate parts, then our individual efforts and energies will be dissipated; our voices will add to the confusion that surrounds us. (Keesing 1981:497)

The understanding Keesing called for takes us well beyond the rhetoric of civilizing missions, whether that of the "white man's burden," "sustainable development," "participatory development," or "women in development," to consider the sociopolitical context of the practice of social engineering. As we attend to the miseries and sufferings of what Tom Johnson (1994) describes as the "global village,"[5] we should not lose sight of the reality of "global pillage" during this age of "downward leveling" of environmental, labor, and social [including health] conditions" (Brecher and Costello 1994).

While one would readily agree with Tom Johnson's observation of the numerical increase of "applied" medical anthropologists, his characterization of this development as an "applied revolution in anthropology," comparable to a Kuhnian "scientific revolution," is, to say the least, an exaggeration. What would be truly revolutionary is a shift of applied research "towards a new structure of inquiry in which the practices and culture of the wealthy and powerful, and not those of the starving, were the subject of investigation" (Taussig 1979:1; see also Pottier, ed., 1993). It is such a redirection of the anthropological gaze that would constitute a radical departure from a long-standing tradition established by Malinowski. As far back as 1929, he called for "bridging over" the gap between the "theoretical concerns of the anthropology of the schools" and "various Colonial interests in their practical activities" (Malinowski 1929 as cited by James 1973; compare, for example, Escobar 1987; Frank 1975).

Decades of experience of anthropologically assisted colonial "practical activities," and their many neocolonial variants, have demonstrated the ineffectiveness of "their" agendas, whether labeled "progress," "development or "empowerment" (Escobar 1987; Frank 1975; Navarro 1986). Human welfare is best served when people engage in direct collective action rather than expect "them" to do things for "us" (IFDA 1980). With or without the benefit of anthropological knowledge, praxis, unlike Machiavellian pragmatism, is a dialectical process. It is not a standardized prescription of tactics and strategies that can be acquired by way of an academic curriculum or professional affiliation; its framework is collective, protracted social engagement, also known as political struggle. Noteworthy in this regard is the orientation adopted by the president of the Italian Society of Medical Anthropology:

In his view, the anthropologist is called upon to mediate the widest range of social demands. Between the Gramcian roles of intellectual and cultural worker in the field, he has fostered medical anthropology as ideological choice and political militancy, an experience unique in Italy and hard to match elsewhere in the world. (Pandolfi 1992:165)

Closer to home, inspiration is provided by the activism of an African-American intellectual ancestor, W. Montague Cobb. Rankin-Hill and Blakey (1994:92) remind us that in "applying anthropology, Cobb was not limited by the traditional parameters of professional concerns. He chose activism, an applied anthropology directed against the effects of social inequality and discrimination." No matter the label we choose to attach to such activism, it remains a challenging part of the contradictory nature of our anthropological heritage.

NOTES

1. Global power relations are equally deserving of attention in relation to the politics of citation (Harrison 1991:7). For example, the authors of a medical anthropology textbook acknowledge only the work of First World scholars in a discussion of the significance of taking account of social power relations, and worldwide political economic forces (McElroy and Townsend 1989:68).

2. It is important to stress once again that PEMA is *not* reducible to the dependency variant of PEH, or any other variant for that matter. It is also worth noting that the analytical limitations of the dependency orientation, which have been elaborated in the development literature for years, have been long recognized by some of its earliest promoters, including André Gunder Frank himself (Frank 1977).

3. I consider praxis to be dialectically articulated to theoretical productions, which are themselves inseparable from political dynamics.

4. Applied social research, whether medical anthropological or otherwise, is also theoretically informed. This is so even if the privileged theoretical basis of a given research project remains unstated.

5. In Johnson's "global village" "formerly isolated, indigenous people [have been incorporated], forcing us to examine and even intervene in the process of change."

3

A Critical-Interpretive Approach in Medical Anthropology: Rituals and Routines of Discipline and Dissent

Margaret Lock and Nancy Scheper-Hughes

It is well to establish the position of the body from the outset.
—Samuel Beckett, *The Unnamable*

PROLOGUE: THINKING WITH THE BODY

We wish to suggest at the outset that it is medical anthropology's engagement with the body in context that represents this subdiscipline's unique vision as distinct from classical social anthropology (where the body was largely absent) and from physical anthropology and the biomedical sciences (where the body is made into a universal object). In the history of social anthropology—as in sociology—with a few notable exceptions such as Benthall and Polhemus (1975), Blacking (1977), and Needham (1973), the body made only occasional and cryptic appearances, and most debates about human relations and social life swirled around an analytic gap at the core of the discipline: the absence of the body (Lock 1993a).

Insofar as it was treated at all, the body figured in the writings of social anthropologists and sociologists as a medium on which to inscribe symbols and homologies of the social order. The body "naturalized" the social order, making society and its social categories and hierarchies appear unquestionably real, certain, and existentially given. In many of these early social anthropological monographs in which the body in health and illness appears, the authors were ostensibly studying religion, ritual, witchcraft, comparative modes of thinking, and so on, and they discovered that the body was "good to think with." The best-known examples are undoubtedly E. E. Evans-Pritchard's *Witchcraft, Oracles and Magic among the Azande* (1937), Victor Turner's *Forest of Symbols* (1967) and *Drums of Affliction* (1968), and *Purity and Danger* by Mary Douglas

(1966). Though the body was invoked in these studies, it was conceptualized as little more than a passive participant, part of the domain of the natural sciences but attached to a lively, responsive, nomadic mind, the true agent of culture.

Had social anthropologists taken the study of Durkheim on anomie theory, Marx on alienation theory, or even Freud on conversion hysterias more seriously, or had they anticipated the insights of Foucault or the rise of feminist and literary criticism, they might have participated in the emergence of the body as the primary action zone of the late twentieth century. As it was, however, social anthropology's belated awakening to the theoretical significance of the body came largely through the empirical studies of medical anthropologists laboring in the clinics, hospitals, fields, and factories among people whom sickness, madness, pain, disability, and distress had rendered critically reflexive as well as often negatively and oppositionally situated in relation to a given social and moral order. It was in these "clinics" that medical anthropologists, often criticized by other anthropologists for their lack of theoretical sophistication, developed concepts such as sickness as cultural performance (Frankenberg 1986), body praxis (Scheper-Hughes 1993), local biologies (Lock 1993b), illness as aesthetic object (Good 1994), and body mnemonics (Comaroff 1985; Boddy 1989) in understanding the social and political relations of illness.

TOWARD A CRITICAL-INTERPRETIVE PERSPECTIVE IN MEDICAL ANTHROPOLOGY

A major division in theoretical approach has crystalized over the past twenty years or more within the social sciences around the question of whether "facts" about the world are uncovered or whether, on the other hand, they are produced as a result of interaction between researcher with the subject of research. Much of the work in contemporary medical anthropology, along with the classical social anthropological monographs, falls into the first of these two camps. That is, it is assumed by conventional medical anthropologists that rigorous empirical research will lead to a truthful representation of the objects under study (D'Andrade 1995). While much of this research may be culturally sensitive and designed to show that nonliterate peoples, immigrants, and refugees are rational beings, there is a striking lack of awareness in these "objectivist" studies of the ways in which the culture of science structures the kind of questions asked. As Allan Young pointed out, "Epistemological scrutiny is suspended for Western social science and Western medicine" (1982:260). Whereas one can nurture a cultural analysis of traditional medical systems, biomedicine by virtue of its "scientific" nature is held privileged and exempt from such an analysis. How could an anthropology of religion have developed if Christianity were exempt from cultural analysis and its premises left unexamined and unquestioned? Yet this is precisely what happened to medical anthropology. Critical research on the body, illness, and healing was stymied for many generations by a prohibition against examining, and therefore "bracketing," some of the most essentializing and universalizing Western epistemological assumptions underlying the theory and practice of biomedicine.

When medicine is exempt from cultural analysis, several assumptions usually follow: that nature and culture are dichotomous categories, that it is possible to understand the natural world logically and rationally through the application of science, and that technological mastery will eventually be obtained over nature including the human body. With respect to health and illness, this objectivist perspective assumes that the entire range of human explanations and practices regarding health, illness, disease, and death, from evil eye beliefs to the chanting of sutras in a temple, can be rendered superfluous through universal education in public health and human biology and through the availability of affordable Western medical care. The objectivists would agree with Susan Sontag that "the most truthful way of regarding illness—and the healthiest way of being ill—is one purified of, most resistant to metaphoric thinking" (1978:3).

Here we wish to advance an alternative theoretical position, one that begins from a recognition of the fundamental epistemological irreconcilability of anthropological and dominant biomedical ways of knowing and seeing. Most anthropological knowledge is fundamentally esoteric (concerned with difference, basic strangeness, and Otherness), local (in the Geertzian sense), symbolic, and doggedly relativist. Much biomedical knowledge remains intrinsically universal, objectivist, and radically materialist/reductionist—the result of its lingering Cartesian heritage. Whereas biomedicine, in theory if not always in practice, presupposes a universal, a historical subject, critically interpretive medical anthropologists are confronted with rebellious and "anarchic" bodies—bodies that refuse to conform (or submit) to presumably universal categories and concepts of diseases, distress, and medical efficacy.

This other side of the theoretical divide is less concerned with orderly explanations and more with the understanding of social life as the "negotiation of meanings" (Marcus and Fisher 1986:26). It is part of a broader movement in which reductionist science as a whole, including biomedicine, has been reappraised as a product of its specific historical and cultural contexts (Lock and Gordon 1988; Mulkay 1979; Toulmin 1982). Here, rather than simply the study of "alternative" medical systems and practices, medical anthropology becomes a much more radical undertaking: the way in which all knowledge relating to the body, health, and illness is culturally constructed, negotiated, and renegotiated in a dynamic process through time and space.

Every attempt is made to avoid a conversion of the dialogue that takes place between informants and the anthropologist into categories that originate in Western medical thought, although ultimately it is usually recognized that it is important to go beyond a position of extreme cultural relativism. Moreover, the anthropologist is highly sensitive to the way in which representation of the other is, in effect, a fiction, a document created out of an ongoing dialogue. Rabinow sums up this approach in the following way: "The ethical is the guiding value. This is an oppositional position, one suspicious of sovereign powers, universal truths, overly relativized preciousness, local authenticity, moralisms, high and low. Understanding is its second value, but an understanding suspicious of its own imperial tendencies. It attempts to be highly attentive (and respectful of) difference, but is also wary of the tendency to essentialize difference'' (1986: 258). To this extent, medical anthropology is no different from the general field of critical-interpretive anthropology. But one ever-present constraining and irreducible fact is rather special to medical anthropology: that of the sentient human body.

Metaphorically, flights of fancy come crashing down in the face of the anguish and pain that often surround birth, illness, and death. The relationship between theory and practice takes on special meaning in such a context. The medical anthropologist is repeatedly studying situations where drama is commonplace and action deemed imperative. Hence, the work of the medical anthropologist rarely stops at an ethnographic description of medical theories and practice but extends willy-nilly into the world of decision making and action. Biomedical technology (some of it equal or superior to traditional therapies) is available to some extent in most parts of the world today. Clearly everyone should have an opportunity to benefit from this technology. One of the biggest challenges for medical anthropology is to come to terms with biomedicine, to acknowledge its efficacy when appropriate while retaining a constructively critical stance. At the same time it is necessary to be critical, at times, of the cultural values and tradition of the societies under study. The webs of culture that people spin and have spun about them are essential for the functioning of humankind in social groups. We cannot strip all metaphor away, as Sontag suggests. However, wherever inequalities and hierarchy are institutionalized, they will of necessity be imposed by means of a dominant cultural ideology, which is likely to inflict a negative self-image, distress, and often ill health on the underprivileged and disenfranchised. Today we have the intellectual freedom and impetus to sort out harmful discourse from that indispensable to the continuity of cooperative social groups. The medical anthropologist must tread lightly between the poles of cultural interpreter and cultural critic, defender of tradition and broker for change.

The task of a critical-interpretive medical anthropology is, first, to describe the culturally constructed variety of metaphorical conceptions (conscious and unconscious) about the body and associated narratives and then to show the social, political, and individual uses to which these conceptions are applied in practice. By this approach, medical knowledge is not conceived of as autonomous but is rooted in and continually modified by practice and social and political change. Medical knowledge is, of course, also constrained (but not determined) by the structure and functioning of the human body. A medical anthropologist therefore attempts to explore the notion of ''embodied personhood'' (Turner 1986:2): the relationship of cultural beliefs and practices in connection with health and illness to the sentient human body.

In this chapter we will set out a critical-interpretive perspective in which we draw for inspiration upon some facets of general anthropological discourse about the body. We believe that insofar as medical anthropology fails to consider the way in which the human body itself is culturally constructed, it is destined to fall prey to certain assumptions characteristic of biomedicine. Foremost among these assumptions is the much-noted Cartesian dualism that separates mind from body, spirit from matter, and real (that is, measurable) from unreal. Since this epistemological tradition is a cultural and historical construction and not one that is universally shared, it is essential that we begin by examining this assumption.[1]

THE THREE BODIES

> The body is the first and most natural tool of man.
>   —Marcel Mauss (1979 [1950]).

Essential to our task is a consideration of the relations among what we will refer to here as the "three bodies."[2] At the first and perhaps most self-evident level is the individual body, understood in the phenomenological sense of the lived experience of the body-self. We may reasonably assume that all people share at least some intuitive sense of the embodied self as existing apart from other individual bodies (Mauss 1985[1938]). However, the constituent parts of the body—mind, matter, psyche, soul, self—and their relations to each other and the ways in which the body is experienced in health and sickness are highly variable.

At the second level of analysis is the social body, referring to the representational uses of the body as a natural symbol with which to think about nature, society, and culture (Douglas 1970). Here our discussion follows the well-trodden path of social, symbolic, and structuralist anthropologists who have demonstrated a constant exchange of meanings between the natural and the social worlds. The body in health offers a model of organic wholeness; the body in sickness offers a model of social disharmony, conflict, and disintegration. Reciprocally, society in "sickness" and in "health" offers a model for understanding the body.

At the third level of analysis is the body politic, referring to the regulation, surveillance, and control of bodies (individual and collective) in reproduction and sexuality, work, leisure, and sickness. There are many types of polity, ranging from the acephalous groupings of "simple" foraging societies, in which deviants may be simply ignored or else punished by total social ostracism and consequently by death (see Briggs 1970; Turnbull 1962), through to chieftainships, monarchies, oligarchies, democracies, and modern totalitarian states. In each of these polities the stability of the body politic rests on its ability to regulate populations (the social body) and to discipline individual bodies. A great deal has been written about the regulation and control of individual and social bodies in complex, industrialized societies. Michel Foucault's work is exemplary in this regard (1973, 1975, 1979, 1980c). Less has been written about the ways in which preindustrial societies control their populations and institutionalize means for producing docile bodies and pliant minds in the service of some definition of collective stability, health, and social well-being.

The following analysis will move back and forth between a discussion of "the bodies" as a useful heuristic concept for understanding cultures and societies, on the one hand, and for increasing knowledge of the cultural sources and meanings of health and illness, on the other.

THE INDIVIDUAL BODY

How Real Is Real? The Cartesian Legacy

A singular premise guiding Western science and clinical medicine (and one, we hasten to add, that is responsible for its efficacy) is its commitment to a fundamental opposition between spirit and matter, mind and body, and (underlying this) real and unreal. We are reminded of a presentation that concerned the case of a middle-aged woman suffering from chronic and debilitating headaches. In halting sentences the patient explained before the large class of first-year medical students that her husband was an alcoholic who occasionally beat her, that she had been virtually housebound for the past five years looking after her senile and incontinent mother-in-law, and that she worried constantly about her teenage son, who was flunking out of high school. Although the woman's story elicited considerable sympathy from the students, one young woman finally interrupted the professor to demand, "But what is the real cause of the headaches?"

The medical student, like many of her classmates, interpreted the stream of social information as extraneous and irrelevant to the real biomedical diagnosis. She wanted information on the neurochemical changes, which she understood as constituting the true causal explanation. This kind of radically materialist thinking is the product of a Western epistemology extending as far back as Aristotle's starkly biological view of the human soul in *De Anima*. As a basis for clinical practice, it can be found in the Hippocratic corpus (ca. 400 B.C.)[3] Hippocrates and his students were determined to eradicate the vestiges of magicoreligious thinking about the human body and to introduce a rational basis for clinical practice that would challenge the power of the ancient folk healers or "charlatans" and "magi," as Hippocrates labeled his medical competitors. In a passage from his treatise on epilepsy, ironically entitled "On the Sacred Disease," Hippocrates (Adams 1939:355–56) cautioned physicians to treat only what was observable and palpable to the senses: "I do not believe that the so-called Sacred Disease is any more divine or sacred than any other disease, but that on the contrary, just as other diseases have a nature and a definite cause, so does this one, too, have a nature and a cause. . . . It is my opinion that those who first called this disease sacred were the sort of people that we now call 'magi.' ''

The natural-supernatural, real-unreal dichotomy has taken many forms over the course of Western history and civilization, but it was the philosopher-mathematician René Descartes (1596–1650) who most clearly formulated the ideas that are the immediate precursors of contemporary biomedical conceptions about the human organism. Descartes was determined to hold nothing as true until he had established the grounds of evidence for accepting it as such. The single category to be taken on faith was the existence of the thinking being, expressed in Descartes' dictum: "Cogito, ergo sum" ("I think, therefore I am"). He then used the concept of the thinking being to establish "proof" for the existence of God whom, Descartes believed, had created the physical world. Descartes, a devout Catholic, stated that one should not question that which God had created; however, by creating a concept of mind, Descartes was able to reconcile his religious beliefs with his scientific curiosity. The higher "essence" of man, the rational mind, was thus extracted from nature, allowing a rigorous objective examination of nature, including the human body, for the first time in Western history. This separation of mind and body, the so-called Cartesian dualism, freed biology to pursue the kind of radically materialist thinking expressed by the medical student, an approach that has permitted the development of the natural and clinical sciences as we know them today.

The Cartesian legacy to clinical medicine and to the natural and social sciences is a rather mechanistic conception of the body and its functions and a failure to conceptualize a "mindful" causation of somatic states. It would take a struggling psychoanalytic psychiatry and the gradual development of psychosomatic medicine in the early twentieth century to begin the task of reuniting mind and body in clinical theory and practice. Yet even in psychoanalytically informed psychiatry and in psychosomatic medicine, there is a tendency to categorize and treat human afflictions as if they were either wholly organic or wholly psychological in origin: "it" is in the body or "it" is in the mind (Kirmayer 1988). In her analysis of multidisciplinary case conferences on chronic pain patients, for example, Kitty Corbett (1986) discovered the intractability of Cartesian thinking among sophisticated clinicians. These physicians, psychiatrists, and clinical social workers "knew" that pain was "real," whether or not the source of it could be verified by diagnostic tests. Nonetheless, they could not help but express evident relief when a "true" (single, generally organic) cause could be discovered. Moreover, when diagnostic tests indicated some organic explanation, the psychological and social aspects of the pain tended to be all but forgotten, and when severe psychopathology could be diagnosed, the organic complications and indexes tended to be ignored. Pain, it seems, was either physical or mental, biological or psychosocial—never both or something not quite either.

As both medical anthropologists and clinicians struggle to view humans and the experience of illness and suffering from an integrated perspective, they often find themselves trapped by the Cartesian legacy. We lack a precise vocabulary with which to deal with mind-body-society interactions and so are left suspended in hyphens, testifying to the disconnectedness of our thoughts. We are forced to resort to such fragmented concepts as the "biosocial" or the "psychosomatic" as altogether feeble ways of expressing the many forms in which the mind speaks through the body and the ways in which society is inscribed on the expectant canvas of human flesh. As Milan Kundera (1984:15) observed: "The rise of science propelled man into tunnels of specialized knowledge. With very step forward in scientific knowledge, the less clearly he could see the world as a whole or his own self." Ironically, conscious attempts to temper the materialism and reductionism of biomedical science often end up inadvertently recreating the mind-body opposition in a new form. For example, a distinction between disease and illness was elaborated in an effort to distinguish the biomedical conception of "abnormalities in the structure and/or function of organs and organ systems" (disease) from the patients' subjective experience of malaise (illness) (Eisenberg 1977). While this paradigm has certainly helped to sensitize both clinicians and social scientists to the social origins of sickness, one unanticipated effect has been that physicians now often claim both aspects of the sickness experience for the medical domain. As a result, the illness dimension of human distress is being medicalized and individualized rather than politicized and collectivized (see Scheper-Hughes and Lock 1986; Lock 1978b). Medicalization inevitably entails a missed identification between the individual and the social bodies and a tendency to transform the social into the biological.

Mind-body dualism is related to other conceptual oppositions in Western epistemology, such as those between nature and culture, passion and reason, individual and society—dichotomies that social thinkers as different as Emile Durkheim, Marcel Mauss, Karl Marx, and Sigmund Freud understood as inevitable and often unresolvable contradictions and as natural and universal categories. Although Durkheim was primarily concerned with the relationship of the individual to society, he devoted some attention to the mind-body, nature-society dichotomies. In *The Elementary Forms of the Religious Life* Durkheim wrote that "man is double" (1961[1915]:29), referring to the biological and the social. The physical body provided for the reproduction of society through sexuality and socialization. For Durkheim society represented the "highest reality in the intellectual and moral order." The body was the storehouse of emotions that were the raw materials, the stuff, out of which mechanical solidarity was forged in the interests of the collectivity. Building on Durkheim, Mauss wrote of the "dominion of the conscious [will] over emotion and unconsciousness" (1979[1950]:122). The degree to which the random and chaotic impulses of the body were disciplined by social institutions revealed the stamp of higher civilizations.

Freud introduced yet another interpretation of the mind-body, nature-culture, individual-society set of oppositions with his theory of dynamic psychology: the individual at war within himself. Freud proposed a human drama in which natural, biological drives locked horns with the domesticating requirements of the social and moral order. The resulting repressions of the libido through a largely painful process of socialization produced the many neuroses of modern life. Psychiatry was called on to diagnose and treat the disease of wounded psyches whose egos were not in control of the rest of their minds. *Civilization and Its Discontents* may be read as a psychoanalytic parable concerning the mind-body, nature-culture, and individual-society oppositions in Western epistemology.

For Marx and his associates the natural world existed as an external, objective reality that was transformed by human labor. Humans distinguish themselves from animals, Marx and Engels wrote, "as soon as they begin to produce their means of subsistence" (1970:42). In *Capital* Marx wrote that labor humanizes and domesticates nature. It gives life to inanimate objects, and it pushes back the natural frontier, leaving a human stamp on all that it touches.

Although the nature-culture opposition has been interpreted as the "very matrix of Western metaphysics" (Benoist 1978:59) and has "penetrated so deeply . . . that we have come to regard it as natural and inevitable" (Goody 1977:64), there have always been alternative ontologies. One of these is surely the view that culture is rooted in (rather than against) nature, imitating it and emanating directly from it. Cultural materialists, for example, have tended to view social institutions as adaptive responses to certain fixed, biological foundations. M. Harris (1974, 1979) refers to culture as a "banal" or "vulgar" solution to the human condition insofar as it "rests on the ground and is built up out of guts, sex, energy" (1974:3). Mind collapses into body in these formulations.

Similarly, some human biologists and psychologists have suggested that the mind-body, nature-culture, and individual-society oppositions are natural (and presumed universal) categories of thinking insofar as they are a cognitive and symbolic manifestation of human biology. R. E. Ornstein (1973), for example, understands mind-body dualism as an overly determined expression of human brain lateralization. According to this view, the uniquely human specialization of the brain's left hemisphere for cognitive, rational, and analytic functions and of the right hemisphere for intuitive, expressive, and artistic functions within the context of left hemisphere dominance sets the stage for the symbolic and cultural dominance of reason over passion, mind over body, culture over nature, and male over female. This kind of biological reductionism is, however, rejected by most contemporary social anthropologists, who stress instead the cultural sources of these oppositions in Western thought.

We should bear in mind that our epistemology is but one among many systems of knowledge regarding the relations held to obtain among mind, body, culture, nature, and society. For example, some non-Western civilizations have developed alternative epistemologies that tend to conceive of relations among similar entities in monistic rather than in dualistic terms. Representations of holism in non-Western epistemologies in defining relationships between any set of concepts or principles of exclusion and inclusion come into play. Representations of holism and monism tend toward inclusiveness. Two representations of holistic thought are particularly common. The first is a conception of harmonious wholes in which everything from the cosmos down to the individual organs of the human body is understood as a single unit. This is often expressed as the relationship of microcosm to macrocosm in which the relationship of parts to the whole is emphasized. A second representation of holistic thinking is that of complementary (not opposing) dualities in which contrasts are made between paired entities within the whole. One of the better-known representations of balanced complementarity is the ancient Chinese yin-yang cosmology, which first appears in the *I Ching* somewhat before the third century B.C. In this view, the entire cosmos, including the human body, is understood as poised in a state of dynamic equilibrium, oscillating between the poles of yin and yang, masculine and feminine, light and dark, hot and cold. The tradition of ancient Chinese medicine acquired the yin-yang cosmology from the Taoists and from Confucianism a concern with social ethics, moral conduct, and the importance of maintaining harmonious relations among individuals, family, community, and state. Conceptions of the healthy body were patterned after the healthy state. In both there is an emphasis on order, harmony, balance, and hierarchy within the context of mutual inter-dependencies. The health of individuals depends on a balance in the natural world, and the health of each organ depends on its relationship to all other organs. Nothing can change without changing the whole (Unschuld 1985).

Islamic cosmology, a synthesis of early Greek philosophy, Judeo-Christian concepts, and prophetic revelations set down in the Qur'an, depicts humans as having dominance over nature, but this potential opposition is tempered by a sacred worldview that stresses the complementarity of all phenomena (Jachimowicz 1975; Shariati 1979). At the core of Islamic belief lies the unifying concept of Towhid, which Shariati argues should be understood as going beyond the strictly religious meaning of "God is one, no more than one" to encompass a worldview that represents all existence as essentially monistic. Guided by the principle of Towhid, humans are responsible to one power, answerable to a single judge, and guided by one principle: the achievement of unity through the complementarities of spirit and body, this world and the hereafter, substance and meaning, natural and supernatural, and so on.

The concept in Western philosophical traditions of an observing and reflexive "I," a mindful self that stands outside the body and apart from nature, is another heritage of Cartesian dualism that contrasts sharply with a Buddhist form of subjectivity and relation to the natural world. In writing about the Buddhist Sherpas of Nepal, Robert Paul suggests that they do not perceive their interiority or their subjectivity as "hopelessly cut off and excluded from the rest of nature, but [rather as] . . . connected to, indeed identical with, the entire essential being of the cosmos" (1976:131). In Buddhist traditions the natural world (the world of appearances) is a product of mind, in the sense that the entire cosmos is essentially "mind." Through meditation, individual minds can merge with the universal mind. Understanding is reached not through analytic methods but rather through an intuitive synthesis, achieved in moments of transcendence that are beyond speech, language, and the written word.

The Buddhist philosopher Suzuki (1960) contrasted Eastern and Western aesthetics and attitudes toward nature by comparing two poems, a seventeenth-century Japanese haiku and a nineteenth-century poem by Alfred Tennyson. The Japanese poet wrote:

> When I look carefully
> I see the nazuna blooming
> By the hedge!

In contrast, Tennyson wrote:

> Flower in the crannied wall,
> I pluck you out of the crannies,
> I hold you here, root and all, in my hand,
> Little flower—but if I could understand
> What you are, root and all, and all in all,
> I should know what God and man is.

Suzuki observes that the Japanese poet, Basho, does not pluck the nazuna but is content to admire it from a respectful distance; his feelings are "too full, too deep, and he has no desire to conceptualize it" (1960:3). Tennyson, in contrast, is active and analytical. He rips the plant by its roots, destroying it in the very act of admiring it. "He does not apparently care for its destiny. His curiosity must be satisfied. As some medical scientists do, he would vivisect the flower" (Suzuki 1960:3). Tennyson's violent imagery is reminiscent of Francis Bacon's description of the natural scientist as one who must "torture nature's secrets from her" and make her a "slave" to mankind (Merchant 1980:169). Principles of monism, holism, and balanced complementarity in nature, which can temper perceptions of opposition and conflict, have largely given way to the analytic urge in the recent history of Western culture.

Person, Self, and Individual

The relation of individual to society, which has occupied so much of contemporary social theory, is based on a perceived "natural" opposition between the demands of the social and moral order and egocentric drives, impulses, wishes, and needs. The individual-society opposition, while fundamental to Western epistemology, is also rather unique to it. Clifford Geertz has argued that the Western conception of the person "as a bounded, unique . . . integrated motivational and cognitive universe, a dynamic center of awareness, emotion, judgment, and action . . . is a rather peculiar idea within the context of the world's cultures" (1984:126). In fact, the modern conception of the individual self is of recent historical origin, even in the West. It was only with the publication in 1690 of John Locke's *Essay Concerning Human Understanding* that we have a detailed theory of the person that identifies the I or the self with a state of permanent consciousness that is unique to the individual and stable through the life span until death (Webel 1983:399).

Though not as detailed perhaps, it would nonetheless be difficult to imagine a people completely devoid of some intuitive perception of the independent self. We think it reasonable to assume that all humans are endowed with a self-consciousness of mind and body, with an internal body image, and with what neurologists have identified as the proprioceptive or sixth sense, our sense of body self-awareness, of mind-body integration, and of being-in-the-world as separate and apart from other human beings. David Winnicot regards the intuitive perception of the body-self as "naturally" placed in the body, a precultural given (1971:48). While this seems a reasonable assumption, it is important to distinguish this universal awareness of the individual body-self from the social conception of the individual as "person," a construct of jural rights and moral accountability (LaFontaine 1985:124). *La personne morale,* as Mauss (1985[1938]) phrased it, is the uniquely Western notion of the individual as a quasi-sacred, legal, moral, and psychological entity whose rights are limited only by the rights of other equally autonomous individuals.

Modern psychologists and psychoanalysts (Winnicot among them) have tended to interpret the process of individuation, defined as a gradual estrangement from parents and other family members, as a necessary stage in the human maturation process (see also Johnson 1985; DeVos, Marsella, and Hsu 1985:3–5). This is, however, a culture-bound notion of human development and one that conforms to fairly recent conceptions of the relation of the individual to society.

In Japan, although the concept of individualism has been debated vigorously since the end of the last century, the Confucian heritage is still evident today in that it is the family that is considered the most natural, fundamental unit of society, not the individual. Consequently, the greatest tension in Japan for at least the past four hundred years has been between one's obligations to the state and one's obligations to the family.

The philosophical traditions of Shintoism and Buddhism have also militated against Japanese conceptions of individualism. The animism of Shinto fosters feelings of identification with nature, and many of the techniques of Buddhist contemplation encourage detachment from earthly desires. Neither tradition encourages the development of a highly individuated self.

Japan has been repeatedly described as a culture of social relativism, in which the person is understood as acting within the context of a social relationship, never simply autonomously (Lebra 1976; Smith 1983). One's self-identity changes with the social context, particularly within the hierarchy of social relations at any time. The child's identity is established through the responses of others; conformity and dependency, even in adulthood, are not understood as signs of weakness but rather as the result of inner strength (Reischauer 1977: 152). But one fear haunts may contemporary Japanese: that of losing oneself completely, of becoming totally immersed in social obligations. One protective device is a distinction made between the external self *(tatemae)*—the persona, the mask, the social self that one presents to others—and a more private *(honne)*, that "natural" hidden self. Clifford Geertz has described a similar phenomenon among the Javanese and Balinese (1984:127–28).

Kenneth Read argues that the Gahuku-Gama of New Guinea lack a concept of the person altogether: "Individual identity and social identity are two sides of the same coin" (1955:276). He maintains that there is no awareness of the individual apart from structured social roles and no concept of friendship, that is, a relationship between two unique individuals that is not defined by kinship, neighborhood, or other social claims. Gahuku-Gama seem to define the self, insofar as they do so at all, in terms of the body's constituent parts: limbs, facial features, hair, bodily secretions, and excretions. Of particular significance is the Gahuku-Gama conception of the social skin, which includes both the covering of the body and the person's social and character traits. References to one's "good" or "bad" skin indicate a person's moral character or even a person's temperament or mood. Gahuku-Gama seem to experience themselves most intensely when in contact with others and through their skins (see also LaFontaine 1985:129–30).

Such sociocentric conceptions of the self have been widely documented for many parts of the world (see Shweder and Bourne 1982; Devisch 1985; Fortes 1959; Harris 1978) and have relevance to ethnomedical understanding. In cultures and societies lacking a highly individualized or articulated conception of the body-self, it should not be surprising that sickness is often explained or attributed to malevolent social relations (that is, sorcery), to the breaking of social and moral codes, or to disharmony within the family or the village community. In such societies therapy, too, tends to be collectivized. The !Kung of Botswana engage in weekly healing trance-dance rituals that are viewed as both curative and preventive (Katz 1982). Lorna Marshall has described the dance as "one concerted religious act of the !Kung [that] brings people into such union that they become like one organic being" (1965:270).

In contrast to societies in which the individual body-self tends to be fused with or absorbed by the social body, there are societies that view the individual as comprising a multiplicity of selves. The Bororo (like the Gahuku-Gama) understand the individual only as reflected in relationship to other people. Hence, the person consists of many selves: the self as perceived by parents, by other kinsmen, by enemies, and so forth. The Cuna Indians of Panama say they have eight selves, each associated with a different part of the body. A Cuna individual's temperament is the result of domination by one of these aspects or parts of the body. An intellectual is one who is governed by the head, a thief governed by the hand, a romantic by the heart, and so forth.

Finally, the Zinacanteco soul has thirteen divisible parts. Each time a person "loses" one or more parts, he or she becomes ill, and a curing ceremony is held to retrieve the missing pieces. At death the soul leaves the body and returns to whence it came—a soul "depository" kept by the ancestral gods. This soul pool is used for the creation of new human beings, each of whose own soul is made up of thirteen parts from the life force of other previous humans. A person's soul force and his or her self is therefore a composite, a synthesis "borrowed" from many other humans. There is no sense that each Zinacanteco is a "brand-new" or totally unique individual; rather, each person is a fraction of the whole Zinacanteco social world. Moreover, the healthy Zinacanteco is one who is in touch with the divisible parts of himself or herself (Vogt 1969:396–374).

While in the industrialized West there are only pathologized explanations of dissociative states in which one experiences more than one self, in many non-Western cultures, individuals can experience multiple selves through the practice of spirit possession and other altered states of consciousness. Such ritualized and controlled experiences of possession are sought after throughout the world as valued forms of religious experience and therapeutic behavior. To date, however, psychological anthropologists have tended to "pathologize" these altered states as manifestations of unstable or psychotic personalities. The Western conception of one individual, one self effectively disallows ethnopsychologies that recognize as normative a multiplicity of selves.

Body Imagery

Closely related to conceptions of self (perhaps central to them) is what psychiatrists have labeled body image (Schilder 1970 [1950]; Horowitz 1966). Body image refers to the collective and idiosyncratic representations an individual entertains about the body in its relationship to the environment, including internal and external perceptions, memories, affects, cognitions, and actions. The existing literature on body imagery (although largely psychiatric) has been virtually untapped by medical anthropologists, who could benefit from attention to body boundary conceptions, distortions in body perception, and so on.

Some of the earliest and best work on body image was contained in clinical studies of individuals suffering from extremely distorted body perceptions that arose from neurological, organic, or psychiatric disorders (Head 1920; Schilder 1970 [1950]; Luria 1972). The inability of some so-called schizophrenics to distinguish self from other or self from inanimate objects has been analyzed from psychoanalytic and phenomenological perspectives (Minkowski 1958; Binswanger 1958; Laing 1965; Basaglia 1964). Oliver Sacks (1973[1970], 1985) also has written about rare neurological disorders that wreak havoc with the individual's body image, producing deficits and excesses, as well as metaphysical transports in mind-body experiences. Sacks's message throughout his poignant medical case histories is that humanness is not dependent on rationality or intelligence—that is, an intact mind. There is, he suggests, something intangible, a soul force or mind-self that produces humans even under the most devastating assaults on the brain, nervous system, and sense of bodily or mindful integrity.

While profound distortions in body imagery are rare, neurotic anxieties about the body, its orifices, boundaries, and fluids are quite common. S. Fisher and S. Cleveland (1958) demonstrated the relationship between patients' ''choice'' of symptoms and body image conceptions. The skin, for example, can be experienced as a protective hide and a defensive armor protecting the softer and more vulnerable internal organs. In the task of protecting the inside, however, the outside can take quite a beating, manifested in skin rashes and hives. Conversely, the skin can be imagined as a permeable screen, leaving the internal organs defenseless and prone to attacks of ulcers and colitis.

Particular organs, body fluids, and functions may also have special significance to a group of people. The liver, for example, absorbs a great deal of blame for many different ailments among the French, Spanish, Portuguese, and Brazilians, but to our knowledge only the Pueblo Indians of the Southwest suffer from ''flipped liver'' (Leeman 1986). The English and the Germans are, by comparison, far more obsessed with the condition and health of their bowels. Allan Dundes takes the Germanic fixation with the bowels, cleanliness, and anality as a fundamental constellation underlying German national character (1984), while Jonathon Miller writes that ''when an Englishman complains about constipation, you never know whether he is talking about his regularity, his lassitude, or his depression'' (1978:45).

Blood is a nearly universal symbol of human life, and some people, both ancient and contemporary, have taken the quality of the blood, pulse, and circulation as the primary diagnostic sign of health or illness. The traditional Chinese doctor, for example, often made his diagnosis by feeling the pulse in both of the patient's wrists and comparing them with his own, an elaborate ritual that could take several hours. Loudell Snow (1974) has described the rich constellation of ethnomedical properties attached to the quality of the blood by poor black Americans, who suffer from ''high'' or ''low,'' fast and slow, thick and thin, bitter and sweet blood. Uli Linke (1986) has analyzed the concept of blood as a predominant metaphor in European culture, especially its uses in political ideologies, such as during the Nazi era. Similarly, the multiple stigmas suffered by North American AIDS patients include a preoccupation with the ''bad blood'' of diseased homosexuals (Lancaster 1983).

Mother's milk assumes new cultural and symbolic meanings wherever subsistence economies have been replaced by wage labor. Scheper-Hughes (1992: 316–326) found that culture of breast feeding unraveled over a brief historical period in northern Brazilian sugar plantation society, including poor women's beliefs in the essential ''goodness'' of what comes out of their own ''dirty,'' ''disorganized,'' and ''diseased'' bodies compared to what comes from ''clean,'' ''healthy,'' ''modern'' objects, like cans of Nestlé's infant formula and clinic hypodermic needles and rehydration tubes. In terms of the ''bricolage'' that governs family formation in the shantytowns of Brazil, the ritual that creates social fatherhood relocates baby's milk from mother's breasts, disdained by responsible, loving women, to the pretty cans of powdered milk formula (bearing corporate and state warnings about the dangers of the product that these illiterate women cannot read) carried into the homes by responsible, loving men. Paternity is transacted today through the gift of ''male milk,'' that is, powdered milk. Father's milk, not his semen, is his means of conferring paternity and symbolically establishing the legitimacy of the child. Similarly Farmer (1988) has discussed the relationship between moral order and concepts of spoiled milk and bad blood in Haiti.

In short, ethnoanatomical perceptions, including body image, offer a rich source of data on both the social and cultural meanings of being human and on the various threats to health, well-being, and social integration that humans are believed to experience.

THE SOCIAL BODY

The Body as Symbol

Symbolic and structuralist anthropologists have demonstrated the extent to which humans find the body ''good to think with.'' The human organism and its natural products of blood, milk, tears, semen, and excreta may be used as a cognitive map to represent other natural, supernatural, social, and even spatial relations. The body, as Mary Douglas observed, is a natural symbol supplying some of our richest sources of metaphor (1970:65). Cultural constructions of and about the body are useful in sustaining particular views of society and social relations.

Rodney Needham, for example, pointed out some of the frequently occurring associations between the left and that which is inferior, dark, dirty, and female, and the right and that which is superior, holy, light, dominant, and male. He called attention to such uses of the body as the convenient means of justifying particular social values and social arrangements, such as the ''natural'' dominance of males over females (1973:109). His point is that these common symbolic equations are not so much natural as they are useful, at least to those on the top and to the right.

Ethnobiological theories of reproduction usually reflect the character of their associated kinship system, as anthropologists have long observed. In societies with unilineal descent, it is common to encounter folk theories that emphasize the reproductive contributions of females in matrilineal and of males in patrilineal societies. The matrilineal Ashanti make the distinction between flesh and blood that is inherited through women and spirit that is inherited through males. The Brazilian Shavante, among whom patrilineages form the core of political factions, believe that the father fashions the infant through many acts of coitus, during which the mother is only passive and receptive. The fetus is ''fully made,'' and conception is completed only in the fifth month of pregnancy. As one Shavante explained the process to David Maybury-Lewis, while ticking the months off with his fingers: "Copulate. Copulate, copulate, copulate, copulate a lot. Pregnant. Copulate, copulate, copulate. Born" (1967:63).

Similarly, the Western theory of equal male and female contributions to conception that spans the reproductive biologies from Galen to Theodore Dobzhansky (1970) probably owes more to the theory's compatibility with the European extended and stem bilateral kinship system than to scientific evidence, which was lacking until relatively recently. The principle of one father, one mother, one act of copulation leading to each pregnancy was part of the Western tradition for more than a thousand years before the discovery of spermatozoa (in 1677) and the female ova (in 1828) and before the actual process of human fertilization was fully understood and described (in 1875) (Barnes 1973:66). For centuries the theory of equal male and female contributions to conception was supported by the erroneous belief that females had the same reproductive organs and functions as males, except that, as one sixth-century bishop put it, "theirs are inside the body and not outside it" (Laqueur, 1986:3). To a great extent, talk about the body and about sexuality tends to be talk about the nature of society.

Of particular relevance to medical anthropologists are the frequently encountered symbolic equations between conceptions of the healthy body and the healthy society, as well as the diseased body and the malfunctioning society. John Janzen (1981) has noted that every society possesses a utopian conception of health that can be applied metaphorically from society to body and vice versa. One of the most enduring ideologies of individual and social health is that of a vital balance and harmony such as are found in the ancient medical systems of China, Greece, India, and Persia, in contemporary Native American cultures of the Southwest (Shutler 1979), and also the holistic health movement of the twentieth century (Grossinger 1980). Conversely, illness and death can be attributed to social tensions, contradictions, and hostilities, as manifested in Mexican peasants' image of the limited good (Foster 1965), in the hot-cold syndrome and symbolic imbalance in Mexican folk medicine (Currier 1969), and in such folk idioms as witchcraft, evil eye, or "stress" (Scheper-Hughes and Lock 1986; Young 1980). Each of these beliefs exemplifies links between the health or illness of the individual body and the social body.

The Embodied World

One of the most common and richly detailed symbolic uses of the human body in the non-Western world is the personification of the spaces in which humans reside. The Qollahuayas live at the foot of Mt. Kaata in Bolivia and are known as powerful healers, the "lords of the medicine bag." They "understand their own bodies in terms of the mountain, and they consider the mountain in terms of their own anatomy" (Bastien 1985:598). The human body and the mountain consist of interrelated parts: head, chest and heart, stomach and viscera, breast and nipple. The mountain, like the body, must be fed blood and fat to keep it strong and healthy. Individual sickness is understood as a disintegration of the body, likened to a mountain landslide or an earthquake. Sickness is caused by disruptions between people and the land, specifically between residents of different sections of the mountain: the head (mountain top), heart (center village), or feet (the base of the mountain). Healers cure by gathering the various residents together to feed the mountain and to restore the wholeness and wellness that was compromised. Bastien concludes that Qollahuaya body concepts are fundamentally holistic rather than dualistic. He suggests that ''the whole is greater than the sum of the parts. . . . Wholeness (health) of the body is a process in which centripetal and centrifugal forces pull together and disperse fluids that provide emotions, thoughts, nutrients, and lubricants for members of the body'' (p. 598).

Possibly the most elaborate use of the body in native cosmology comes from the Dogon of the western Sudan, as explained by Ogotemmeli to Marcel Griaule (1965) in his description of the ground plan of the Dogon community. The village must extend from north to south like the body of a man lying on his back. The head is the council house, built in the center square. To the east and west are the menstrual huts, which are ''round like wombs and represent the hands of the village'' (1965:97). The body metaphor also informs the interior of the Dogon house:

The vestibule, which belongs to the master of the house, represents the male part of the couple, the outside door being his sexual organ. The big central room is the domain and the symbol of the woman; the store-rooms each side are her arms, and the communicating door her sexual parts. The central room and the store rooms together represent the woman lying on her back with outstretched arms, the door open, and the woman ready for intercourse. (1965:94–95)

Other well-known examples of the symbolic use of the human body in cosmological classification include the western Apache (Basso 1969), the Indonesian Atoni (Cunningham 1973), the Desana Indians of the Colombian-Brazilian border (Reichel-Dolmatoff 1971), the Pira-Pirana of the Amazon (Hugh-Jones 1979), the Zinacantecos of Chiapas (Vogt 1970), and the Fali of northern Cameroon (Zahan 1979).

Peter Manning and Horatio Fabrega (1973) have summarized some of the major differences between non-Western ethnomedical systems and modern biomedicine. In the latter, body and self are understood as distinct and separable entities; illness resides in either the body or the mind. Social relations are seen as partitioned, segmented, and situational—generally as discontinuous with health or sickness. By contrast, many ethnomedical systems do not logically distinguish body, mind, and self, and therefore illness cannot be situated in mind or body alone. Social relations are also understood as a key contributor to individual health and illness. In short, the body is seen as a unitary, integrated aspect of self and social relations. It is dependent on, and vulnerable to, the feelings, wishes, and actions of others, including spirits and dead ancestors. The body is not understood as a complex machine but rather as a microcosm of the universe.

As Manning and Fabrega note, what is perhaps most significant about the symbolic and metaphorical extension of the body into the natural, social, and supernatural realms is that it demonstrates a unique kind of human autonomy that seems to have all but disappeared in the modern, industrialized world. The confident uses of the body in speaking about the external world convey a sense that humans are in control. It is doubtful that the Colombian Qollahuayas or the Desana or the Dogon experience anything to the degree of body alienation, so common to Western civilization, as expressed in the schizophrenias, anorexias, and bulimias or the addictions, obsessions, and fetishisms of life in the postindustrialized world.

The mind-body dichotomy and body alienation characteristic of contemporary society may be linked not simply to reductionistic post-Cartesian thinking but also to capitalist modes of production in which manual and mental labors are divided and ordered into a hierarchy. Human labor, thus divided and fragmented, is by Marxist definition "alienated." E. P. Thompson discusses the subversion of natural, body time to the clockwork regimentation and work discipline required by industrialization. He juxtaposes the factory worker, whose labor is extracted in minute, recorded segments, with the Nuer pastoralist, for whom the "daily timepiece is the cattle clock" (Evans-Pritchard 1940:100), or the Aran Islander, whose work is managed by the amount of time left before twilight (Thompson 1967:59).

Similarly, Pierre Bourdieu describes the "regulated improvisations" of Algerian peasants, whose movements roughly correspond to diurnal and seasonal rhythms. "At the return of the Azal (dry season)," he writes, "everything without exception, in the activities of men, women and children is abruptly altered by the adoption of a new rhythm" (1977:159). Everything from men's work to the domestic activities of women, to rest periods, and ceremonies, prayers, and public meetings is set in terms of the natural transition from the wet to the dry season. Doing one's duty in the village context means "respecting rhythms, keeping pace, not falling out of line" (1977:161) with one's fellow villagers. Although, as Bourdieu suggests, these peasants may suffer from a species of false consciousness (or "bad faith") that allows them to misrepresent to themselves their social world as the only possible way to think and to behave and to perceive as "natural" what are, in fact, self-imposed cultural rules, there is little doubt that these Algerian villagers live in a social and a natural world that has a decidedly human shape and feel to it. We might refer to their world as embodied.

In contrast, the world in which most of us live is lacking a comfortable and familiar human shape. At least one source of body alienation in advanced industrial societies is the symbolic equation of humans and machines, originating in our industrial modes and relations of production and in the commodity fetishism of modern life, in which even the human body has been transformed into a commodity. Again, Manning and Fabrega capture this well: "In primitive society the body of man is the paradigm for the derivation of the parts and meanings of other significant objects; in modern society man has adopted the language of the machine to describe his body. This reversal, wherein man sees himself in terms of the external world, as a reflection of himself, is the representative formula for expressing the present situation of modern man" (1973: 283).

We rely on the body-as-machine metaphor each time we describe our somatic or psychological states in mechanistic terms, saying that we are "worn out" or "wound up" or when we say that we are "rundown" and that our "batteries need recharging." In recent years the metaphors have moved from a mechanical to an electrical mode (we are "turned off," "tuned in," we "get a charge" out of something), while the computer age has lent us a host of new expressions, including the all-too-familiar complaint: "my energy is down." Our point is that the structure of individual and collective sentiments down to the "feel" of one's body and the naturalness of one's position and role in the technical order is a social construct. Thomas Belmonte described the body rhythms of the factory worker: "The work of factory workers is a stiff military drill, a regiment of arms welded to metal bars and wheels. Marx, Veblen and Charlie Chaplin have powerfully made the point that, on the assembly line, man neither makes nor uses tools, but is continuous with tool as a minute, final attachment to the massive industrial machine" (1979:130). The machines have changed since those early days of the assembly line. One thinks today not of the brutality of huge grinding gears and wheels but rather of the sterile silence and sanitized pollution of the microelectronics industries to which the nimble fingers, strained eyes, and docile bodies of a new, largely female and Asian labor force are now melded. What has not changed to any appreciable degree is the relationship of human bodies to the machines under twentieth-century forms of industrial capitalism.

Non-Western and nonindustrialized people are "called upon to think the world with their bodies" (O'Neill 1985:151). Like Adam and Eve in the Garden, they exercise their autonomy, their power, by naming the phenomena and creatures of the world in their own image and likeness. By contrast, we live in a world in which the human shape of things (and even the human shape of humans with their mechanical hearts and plastic hips) is in retreat. While the cosmologies of nonindustrialized people speak to a constant exchange of metaphors from body to nature and back to body again, our metaphors speak of machine-to-body symbolic equations. O'Neill suggests that we have been "put on the machine" of biotechnology, some of us transformed by radical surgery and genetic engineering into "spare parts" or prosthetic humans (1985:153–54). Lives are saved, or at least deaths are postponed, but it is possible that our humanity is being compromised in the process.

THE BODY POLITIC

The relationship between individual and social bodies concerns more than metaphors and collective representations of the natural and the cultural. They are also about power and control. Mary Douglas (1966) contends, for example, that when a community experiences itself as threatened, it will respond by expanding the number of social controls regulating the group's boundaries. Points where outside threats may infiltrate and pollute the inside become the focus of regulation and surveillance. The three bodies—individual, social, and body politic—may be closed off, protected by a nervous vigilance about exits and entrances. Douglas had in mind witchcraft crazes, including the Salem trials, contemporary African societies, and even recent witch-hunts in the United States, to which we must now add the current concern about ritual abuse of children. In each of these instances, the body politic is likened to the human body in which what is "inside" is good and all that is "outside" is evil. The body politic under threat of attack is cast as vulnerable, leading to purges of traitors and social deviants, while individual hygiene may focus on the maintenance of ritual purity or on fears of losing blood, semen, tears, milk, or even one's life.

Threats to the continued existence of the social group may be real or imaginary. Even when the threats are real, however, the true aggressors may not be known, and witchcraft or sorcery can become the metaphor or the cultural idiom for distress. Shirley Lindenbaum (1979) has shown, for example, how an epidemic of kuru among the South Fore of New Guinea led to sorcery accusations and counteraccusations and attempts to purify both the individual and collective bodies of their impurities and contaminants. Leith Mullings suggests that witchcraft and sorcery were widely used in contemporary West Africa as "metaphors for social relations" (1984:164). In the context of a rapidly industrializing market town in Ghana, witchcraft accusations can express anxieties over social contradictions introduced by capitalism. Hence, accusations were directed at individuals and families, who, in the pursuit of economic success, appeared most competitive, greedy, and individualistic in their social relations. Mullings argues that witchcraft accusations are an inchoate expression of resistance to the erosion of traditional social values based on reciprocity, sharing, and family and community loyalty. She suggests that in the context of increasing commoditization of human life, witchcraft accusations point to social distortions and disease in the body politic generated by capitalism.

When the sense of social order is threatened, boundaries between the individual and political bodies become blurred, and there is a strong concern with matters of ritual and sexual purity, often expressed in vigilance over social and bodily boundaries. For example, in Ballybran, in rural Ireland, villagers were equally guarded about what they took into the body (as in sex and food) as they were about being "taken in" (as in "codding," flattery, and blarney) by outsiders, especially those with a social advantage over them. Concern with the penetration and violation of bodily exits, entrances, and boundaries extended to material symbols of the body: the home, with its doors, gates, fences, and stone boundaries, around which many protective rituals, prayers, and social customs served to create social distance and a sense of personal control and security (Scheper-Hughes 1979).

In addition to controlling bodies in a time of crisis, societies regularly reproduce and socialize the kind of bodies that they need. Body decoration is a means through which social self-identities are constructed and expressed (Strathern and Strathern 1971). T. Turner developed the concept of the "social skin" to express the imprinting of social categories on the body-self (1980). For Turner, the surface of the body represents a "kind of common frontier of society which becomes the symbolic stage upon which the drama of socialization is enacted" (1980:112). Clothing and other forms of bodily adornment become the language through which cultural identity is expressed.

In our own increasingly "healthist" and body-conscious culture, the politically correct body for both sexes is the lean, strong, androgenous, and physically fit form through which the core cultural values of autonomy, toughness, competitiveness, youth, and self-control are readily manifest (Pollitt 1982). Health is increasingly viewed in the United States as an achieved rather than an ascribed status, and each individual is expected to "work hard" at being strong, fit, and healthy. Conversely, ill health is no longer viewed as accidental, a mere quirk of nature, but rather is attributed to the individual's failure to live right, to eat well, to exercise, and so forth. We might ask what it is our society wants from this kind of body. Lloyd DeMause (1984) has speculated that the fitness-toughness craze is a reflection of an international preparation for war. A hardening and toughening of the national fiber corresponds to a toughening of individual bodies. In attitude and ideology, the self-help and fitness movements articulate both a militarist and a social Darwinist ethos: the fast and fit win; the fat and flabby lose and drop out of the human race (Scheper-Hughes and Stein 1987). Robert Crawford (1980, 1984), however, has suggested that the fitness movement may reflect instead a pathetic and individualized (also wholly inadequate) defense against the threat of nuclear holocaust.

Rather than strong and fit, the politically (and economically) correct body can entail grotesque distortions of human anatomy, including in various times and places the bound feet of Chinese women (Daly 1978), the sixteen-inch waists of antebellum southern societies (Kunzle 1981), and the tuberculin wanness of nineteenth-century romantics (Sontag 1978). Crawford (1984) has interpreted the eating disorders and distortions in body image expressed in obsessional jogging, anorexia, and bulimia as a symbolic mediation of the contradictory demands of postindustrial American society. The double-binding injunction to be self-controlled, fit, and productive workers and to be at the same time self-indulgent, pleasure-seeking consumers is especially destructive to the self-image of the American woman. Expected to be fun-loving and sensual, she must also remain thin, lovely, and self-disciplined. Since one cannot be hedonistic and controlled simultaneously, one can alternate phases of binge eating, drinking, and drugging with phases of jogging, purging, and vomitting. Out of this cyclical resolution of the injunction to consume and to conserve is born, according to Crawford, the current epidemic of eating disorders (especially bulimia) among young women, some of whom literally eat and diet to death.

Cultures are disciplines that provide codes and social scripts for the domestication of the individual body in conformity to the needs of the social and political order. Certainly the use of physical torture by the modern state provides the most graphic illustration of the subordination of the individual body to the body politic (Foucault 1979). The history of colonialism contains some of the most brutal instances of the political uses of torture and the "culture of terror" in the interests of economic hegemony (Taussig 1984, 1987; Peters 1985). Elaine Scarry suggests that torture is increasingly resorted to today by unstable regimes in an attempt to assert the "incontestable reality" of their control over the populace (1985:27).

The body politic can, of course, exert its control over individual bodies in less dramatic ways. Foucault's (1973, 1975, 1979, 1980c) analyses of the roles of medicine, criminal justice, psychiatry, and the various social sciences in producing new forms of power-knowledge over bodies are illustrative in this regard. The proliferation of disease categories and labels in medicine and psychiatry, resulting in ever more restricted definitions of the normal, has created a sick and deviant majority, a problem that medical and psychiatric anthropologists have been slow to explore. Radical changes in the organization of social and public life in advanced industrial societies, including the disappearance of traditional cultural idioms for the expression of individual and collective discontent (such as witchcraft, sorcery, rituals of reversal, and travesty), have allowed medicine and psychiatry to assume a hegemonic role in shaping and responding to human distress.

In all, Foucault has explored the "negativity" of the body, particularly the *destructive* effects of power relations on the socially and politically constituted body. In "Body/Power" Foucault (1980c:55) dismisses the conventional social anthropological notion of the body as socially constituted through a convergence of wills: "The phenomenon of the social body is the effect, not of social consensus, but of the materiality of power operating on the bodies of individuals." He demonstrates this most forcefully in his histories of medicine and psychiatry with their overproduction of medicalized bodies and psychologized and defeated sexualities (Foucault 1980a, 1980b).

The "Foucauldian body," as the nexus of power struggles originating in the "state" of things, is readily transferred to critically interpretive medical anthropology, where the body in question is more often afflicted, alienated, and suffering than it is ecstatic, decorated, and affirming. The Foucauldian question— "What kind of body does society want and need?"—has stimulated a great deal of critical thinking in contemporary medical anthropology.

But the body of Foucault's imagining is still, to a great extent, a body devoid of subjectivity and lacking the experience of power and powerlessness. What is missing is the existential, lived experience of the practical and practicing human subject. Foucault's negative notion of the body leaves us with a project that is essentially "self-defeating" in that it ignores the lived experience of the body-self. It is this dimension, the self-conscious, often-alienated individual and collective experiences of the body-self that critically interpretive medical anthropology returns to anthropology in the form of the "mindful body." It does so through the pressure exerted by its very subject matter: suffering bodies that refuse to be merely aestheticized or metaphorized. In returning the missing, subjective body to the center of their inquiries, critical medical anthropologists invert the Foucauldian question to ask: "What kind of society does the body need, wish, and dream of?"

BODY PRAXIS

When illness and distress are conceptualized as conditions that occur to real people as they live out their lives in the context of specific social and cultural milieus, it becomes easier to envision distress as just one of the numerous everyday forms of resistance to what for many is the oppressive and monotonous daily round of labor and service. James Scott has pointed out that most subordinate classes throughout history have rarely been afforded the "luxury of open, organized political activity" (1985:xv). This argument can, of course, readily be extended to the situation of the majority of women. Political activity is in fact positively dangerous for most people; nevertheless, those who are relatively powerless put up a remarkable assortment of resistance, including "foot dragging, dissimulation, desertion, false compliance, pilfering, feigned ignorance, slander, arson, sabotage, and so on" (Scott 1985:xvi), to which we would add those types of institutionalized behavior that appear with great frequency in medical anthropological writings: accusations of witchcraft, sorcery, or the evil eye, gossip, the use of trance or organized rituals of reversal, and fantasy play. Physical distress and illness can also be thought of as acts of refusal or of mockery, a form of protest (albeit often unconscious) against oppressive social roles and ideologies. Of all the cultural options for the expression of dissent, the use of trance or illness is perhaps the safest way to portray opposition—an institutionalized space from which to communicate fear, anxiety, and anger because in neither case are individuals under normal circumstances held fully accountable for their condition (Boddy 1988, 1989; Lewis 1971; Comaroff 1985).

Of course, not all illness episodes are recognized as having political significance; mere ailments thought to be of no significance are recognized everywhere. Gilbert Lewis tells us, for example, that the Gnau of New Guinea say of some illnesses: "They just come," "he is sick nothingly," "he died by no purpose or intent" (Lewis 1975:179). The reductionistic, mechanistic explanations characteristic of mainstream biomedicine routinely ignore the social origins of illness problems (Taussig 1980a), and so too do the explanations often made use of in the traditional medical systems of East Asia where a hypothesized imbalance of the body is said to originate in a lack of personal vigilance (Lock 1980).

If, however, one starts with a notion of "bodily praxis," of someone living out and reacting to his or her assigned place in the social order, then the social origins of many illnesses and much distress and the "sickening" social order itself come into sharp focus. It is then possible to interpret incidents of spirit possession in multinational factories in Malaysia, for example, as part of a complex negotiation of reality in which women factory workers are reacting by bringing production to a halt through the use of possession (Ong 1988). Or again, a traditional interpretive approach would perhaps lead one to believe that Japanese adolescents who refuse to go to school, who lie mute and immobile in their bed all day, often medicated, are reacting against pressures of the Japanese school system or the aspirations of their parents. A critical-interpretive analysis, in contrast, indicates that this situation is part of a much larger national concern about modernization and cultural identity of which the school system, parental values, and the culturally constructed form of resistance of the children is only one small part (Lock 1988b). The experiences of women in connection with menstruation, childbirth, and menopause and the variety of ways in which they either embrace, equivocate about, or downright reject dominant ideologies in connection with these life-cycle events provide other telling examples of the dynamic, contested relationship between the three bodies, in connection with the politics of reproduction and aging (Lock 1993b, 1993c; Martin 1987). Similarly, the large body of research on nerves in medical anthropology can be interpreted not merely as a culturally constituted idiom for the expression of individual distress but also as a dominant, widely distributed, and flexible metaphor for expressing malaise of social and political origin and for negotiating relations of power (Lock 1990; Van Schaik 1989; Scheper-Hughes 1988).

Apart from anarchic forms of street violence and other forms of direct assault and confrontation, illness somatization becomes a dominant metaphor expressing individual and social complaint. A limitation, however, of the conventional somatization model is that while it pretends to advocate an indissoluble unity of mind and body, individual and social bodies, and of nature and culture, it has, in practice, failed to overcome the dualisms of biomedicine (Kirmayer 1988). Illnesses are understood as the subjective, transparently psychological manifestation of real, identified physical diseases, or else they are nothing at all, except perhaps the illusory traces, figments of imagination, and "bits of undigested beef" Charles Dickens attributed to the apparition of the ghost of Scrooge's dead partner, Marley. But if mind and body are truly one, as even the most conventional medical anthropologists assert, then *all* diseases and bodily distress, without exception, are and must be psychosomatic because all are "somatized" as well as "mentalized." But here medical anthropology has rarely lived up to the full strength of its convictions and has not been prepared to support so radical and consequential a thesis.

In referring to the "somatic culture" of the displaced and marginalized sugarcane workers of northeast Brazil, Scheper-Hughes (1992) has suggested that theirs is a social class and a culture that privileges the body and instructs them in a close attention to the physical senses and to the language of the body as expressed in symptoms. Here she follows the lead of Luc Boltanski (1984), who has argued that somatic thinking and practice is frequently found among the working and popular classes who extract their subsistence from physical labor. Boltanski noted the tendency of the French working classes to communicate with and through the body so that, by contrast, the body praxis of the bourgeois and technical classes appears impoverished.

Among the agricultural wage laborers living on the hillside shantytown of Alto do Cruzeiro, in the plantation zone of Pernambuco, Brazil, who sell their labor for as little as a dollar a day, socioeconomic and political contradictions often take shape in the "natural" contradictions of angry, sick, and afflicted bodies. In addition to the wholly expectable epidemics of parasitic infections and communicable fevers, there are the more unexpected outbreaks and explosions of unruly and subversive symptoms that will not readily materialize under the microscope. Among these are the fluid symptoms of *nervos* (angry, frenzied nervousness): trembling, fainting, seizures, hysterical weeping, angry recriminations, blackouts, and paralysis of face and limbs. These nervous attacks are in part coded metaphors through which the workers express their dangerous and unacceptable condition of chronic hunger and need and in part acts of defiance and dissent that graphically register the refusal to endure what is, in fact, unendurable, and their protest against their availability for physical exploitation and abuse at the foot of the sugarcane. And so rural workers who have cut sugarcane since the age of seven or eight years will sometimes collapse, their legs giving way under an *ataque de nervos* (a nervous attack). They cannot walk, they cannot stand upright; they are left, like Oliver Sacks (1984), without a leg to stand on.

The nervous-hungry, nervous-angry body of the cane cutter offers itself as metaphor and metonym of the nervous sociopolitical system and for the paralyzed position of the rural worker in the current economic and political disorder. In "lying down" on the job, in refusing to return to the work that has overdetermined their entire lives, the cane cutters' body language signifies both surrender and defeat. But one also notes a drama of mockery and refusal. For if the folk ailment *nervos* attacks the legs and the face, it leaves the arms and hands intact and free for less physically ruinous work. Those who suffer from nervous attacks press their claims as sick men on their various political bosses and patrons to find them alternative work—explicitly "sitting-down" work: arm work, not clerical work, for these men are illiterate.

The analysis of *nervos* does not end here, for nervous attack is an expansive and polysemic form of disease. Shantytown women, too, suffer from *nervos*— both the *nervos de trabalhar muito,* the "overwork" nerves from which male cane cutters suffer, and also the more gender-specific *nervos de sofrir muito,* the nerves of those who have endured and suffered much. Suffers' nerves attack those who have endured a recent, especially a violent, tragedy. Widows of husbands and mothers of sons who have been abducted and violently disappeared are prone to the mute, enraged, white-knuckled shaking of suffers' nerves. Here Taussig's (1991) linking of the "nervous system," anatomical and sociopolitical, is useful. One could read the current "nervousness" of shantytown residents as a response to the nervous and unstable democracy emerging in Brazil after more than twenty years of repressive, military rule. Many vestiges of the military state remain intact, and on the Alto do Cruzeiro, the military presence is most often felt in the late-night knock on the door, the scuffle, and the abduction of one's husband or teenaged son.

The epidemic of *nervos, sustos* (fright sickness), and *pasmos* (paralytic shock) signifies a state of alarm, of panic. The people of the shantytown, thrown into a state of nervous shock, set off the alarm, warning others in the community that their bodies and their lives are in danger. The epidemics of *nervos* among the wives and mothers of the politically disappeared is a form of resistance that publicizes the danger, the fright, the "abnormality of the normal," while not exposing the sufferers to further political reprisals. The political nature of illness and the communicative subversive body remains an only partly conscious, and thereby protected, form of protest. One can hardly reduce this complex, creative, somatic, and political idiom to the vapid biomedical discourse on patient "somatization." Whatever else illness is, and it is many different things—an unfortunate brush with nature, a fall from grace, a social rupture, an economic contradiction—it is also, at times, an act of refusal. The refusal can express itself in various ways: a refusal to work, a refusal to struggle under self-defeating conditions, a refusal to endure, a refusal to cope. This is the case with the nervous collapse of those paralyzed sugarcane cutters who have had enough and reached the end of their rope.

Refusal is available, however, for shaping and transformation by doctors and psychiatrists into symptoms of "diseases" such as PMS (premenstrual syndrome), depression, or attention deficit disorder (Martin 1987; Lock 1986a; Lock and Dunk 1987; Rubenstein and Brown 1984). In this way, exhaustion, misery, rage, and school phobias can be recast as individual pathologies rather than as socially significant signs (Lock 1988b, 1988c). This funneling of diffuse but genuine complaints into the idiom of sickness has led to the problem of medicalization and the overproduction of illness in contemporary advanced industrial societies. In this process, the role of doctors, social workers, psychiatrists, and criminologists as agents of social consensus is pivotal. As Kim Hopper (1982) has suggested, health professions are predisposed to "fail to see the secret indignation of the sick." The medical gaze is, then, a controlling gaze, through which active (although furtive) forms of protest are transformed into passive acts of breakdown.

The debate as to how cultural categories can best be subsumed under biomedical categories of disease becomes a red herring in a critical-interpretive approach. The transformation of a culturally rich form of communication into the individualizing language of physiology, psychology, or psychiatry is inappropriate. What is crucially important for the medical anthropologist is to demonstrate the way in which polysemic constructs such as *nevra, solidao, hara,* stress, and menopause and the language of trance, ritual, dreams, carnival, and so on can be made use of in order to facilitate the bringing to consciousness of links between the political and social orders and physical distress. If this form of communication that keeps body metaphorically linked to both mind and society is reduced to the "truthful" language of science, then one of the most impressive "weapons of the weak" (Scott 1985) is rendered useless in the struggle for relief from oppression. Similarly, a culturally relativistic approach that relies exclusively on local explanations or narratives is inadequate because involved actors are often unable to distance themselves and take a reflexive stance about their own condition. Not only oppressors but the oppressed are likely to accept their lot as natural and inevitable, even when human social relations are grossly distorted and unjust. A critical-interpretive approach seeks to go beyond a culturally sensitive presentation to reveal the contingency of power and knowledge in both their creation of and relationship to the culturally constructed individual body.

While the medicalization of life (and its political and social control functions) is understood by critical medical social scientists as a fairly permanent feature of industrialized societies (Freidson 1972; Zola 1972; Roth 1972; Illich 1976; deVries et al. 1982) few medical anthropologists have yet explored the immediate effects of medicalization in areas of the world where the process is occurring for the first time (but see Nichter 1989), although an old Kabyle woman explained to Bourdieu (1977:166) what it meant to be sick before and after medicalization became a feature of Algerian peasant life:

In the old days, folk didn't know what illness was. They went to bed and they died. It's only nowadays that we're learning words like liver, lung . . . intestine, stomach . . . , and I don't know what! People only used to know [pain in] the belly; that's what everyone who died died of, unless it was the fever. . . . Now everyone's sick, everyone's complaining of something. . . . Who's ill nowadays? Who's well? Everyone complains, but no one stays in bed; they all run to the doctor. Everyone knows what's wrong with him now.

An anthropology of relations between the body and the body politic inevitably leads to a consideration of the regulation and control not only of individuals but of populations and therefore of sexuality, gender, and reproduction—what Foucault (1980b) refers to as biopower.

The medicalized body is not simply the result of changing medical knowledge and practice; neither is it simply the product of medical self-interest. A medicalized body represents more than an individual body, for it is also a manifestation of potent, never settled, partially disguised political contests about how aging and rebellious bodies should be managed. The female body, as is well known, is frequently targeted for control, and one recent manifestation of this phenomenon is the aggressive medicalization of female aging, particularly in North America, evidence of which is the creation of a new population characterized as "postmenopausal" women. As the baby boomers age, increasingly the postmenopausal woman is targeted as a potential burden on the health care system, and it is now recommended by the gynecological associations of the United States and Canada that virtually all women should, as they enter middle age, imbibe powerful hormone replacement therapy daily, for the rest of their lives, in order to feed their "estrogen-depleted" bodies. Thus, it is assumed, they will avoid contracting major diseases twenty or thirty years down the road. No extended controlled trials have been conducted with this medication, the effects of long-time usage are not known, and furthermore, the existence of simple cause-and-effect associations between estrogen levels, heart disease, and osteoporosis is hotly debated (Lock 1993c). Moreover, increased risk for cancer is implicated from extended medication use, which also produces unpleasant side effects in many women. The perpetration of this debate depends on the vulnerable "postmenopausal" woman whose body is classed as "unnatural." Older women have been described in both the biological and gynecological literature as "cultural artifacts," where it is argued that menopause is evolutionarily nonadaptive (Lock 1993b). The bodies of young women are set up as the gold standard, to which postmenopausal women must be returned with medical help. Cooperation with this regime, offered in terms of "risks" and "benefits," is regarded as socially responsible. Clearly the addiction to youth, characteristic of much North American culture, ensures that many people are willing to cooperate; indeed, they seek out medical help to counter the process of aging. For a small proportion of women, the physical distress associated with menopause is such that use of medication is entirely appropriate; however, the experiences of these women are increasingly taken as representative of the population at large. Menopause is constructed as a universal fact, a dismal time that augurs badly for the future; the postmenopausal body becomes a synedoche for middle-aged women in all their variety, who are reduced to potential burdens on society (Lock 1993b). In comparing female middle age in Japan and North America, Lock found that "local biologies" have contributed historically and in contemporary times to both subjective experience and discourse production (Lock 1993b), indicating that the biopolitics of normalization and control and the construction of vulnerable populations is an exceedingly complex process, which must be interpreted in context.

We would like to think of medical anthropology as providing the key to the development of a new epistemology and metaphysics of the body and of the emotional, social, and political sources of illness and healing. If and when we tend to think reductionistically about the mind-body, it is because it is "good for us to think" in this way. To do otherwise, that is, employing a radically different metaphysics, would imply the "unmaking" of our own assumptive world and its culture-bound definitions of reality. To admit the "as-ifness" of our ethnoepistemology is to court a Cartesian anxiety: the fear that in the absence of a sure, objective foundation for knowledge, we would fall into the void, into the chaos of absolute relativism and subjectivity (see Geertz 1973a: 28–30).

We have tried to show the interaction among the mind-body and the individual, social, and body politic in the production and expression of health and illness. Sickness is not just an isolated event or an unfortunate brush with nature. It is a form of communication—the language of the organs—through which nature, society, and culture speak simultaneously. The individual body should be seen as the most immediate, the proximate terrain where social truths and social contradictions are played out, as well as a locus of personal and social resistance, creativity, and struggle.

NOTES

1. This chapter is not intended to be a review of the field of medical anthropology. We refer interested readers to a few excellent reviews of this type: Landy (1983a); Worsley (1982); Young (1982). With particular regard to the ideas expressed in this chapter, however, see also Comaroff (1985), Csordas (1994), Devisch (1985), Estroff (1981), Good (1994), Good and Good (1981), Hahn (1985), Helman (1985), Kleinman (1986, 1988b); Laderman (1983, 1984), Lindenbaum and Lock (1993), Low (1985a), Morgan (1993b), Nichter (1981), Obeyesekere (1981), and Taussig (1980a, 1984).

2. Mary Douglas refers to "The Two Bodies," the physical and social bodies, in *Natural Symbols* (1970). More recently John O'Neil has written *Five Bodies: The Human Shape of Modern Society* (1985), in which he discusses the physical body, the communicative body, the world's body, the social body, the body politic, consumer bodies, and medical bodies. We are indebted to both Douglas and O'Neil and also to Bryan Turner's *The Body and Society: Explorations in Social Theory* (1984) for helping us to define and delimit the tripartite domain we have mapped out here.

3. We do not wish to suggest that Hippocrates' understanding of the body was analogous to that of Descartes or of modern biomedical practitioners. Hippocrates' approach to medicine and healing can be described only as organic and holistic. Nonetheless, Hippocrates was, as the quotation from his work demonstrates, especially concerned to introduce elements of rational science (observation, palpation, diagnosis, and prognosis) into clinical practice and to discredit all the "irrational" and magical practices of traditional folk healers.

4

Culture, Emotion, and Psychiatric Disorder

Janis H. Jenkins

The study of the interrelations among culture, emotion, and psychiatric disorder is central to the fields of medical and psychological anthropology.[1] This has become evident with the convergence between the recent wave of psychocultural studies of emotion (Abu-Lughod 1986, 1993; Gaines and Farmer 1986; Good and Good 1988; Jenkins 1991b; Hollan 1988; Hollan and Wellenkamp 1994; Kleinman and Good 1985; Lutz 1985b, 1988, 1990; Lutz and White 1986; Kitayama and Markus 1994; Matthews 1992; Myers 1986; Ochs and Schieffelin 1989; Rosaldo 1980b; Roseman 1991; Scheper-Hughes and Lock 1987; Schieffelin 1976; Shweder and LeVine 1974; Wellenkamp 1988; Wikan 1990) and a long-standing interest in psychological and medical anthropology in studies of ethnopsychiatry (Caudill 1958b; Devereux 1969; Edgerton 1966, 1969, 1971a, 1971b; Hughes this volume; Hallowell 1938, 1955; Kennedy 1974; Sapir 1961; Scheper-Hughes 1979; Sullivan 1953; Wallace 1961). Taken together, these studies argue that since virtually every aspect of illness experience is mediated by personal and cultural sentiment, the study of emotion is necessarily of relevance to medical anthropology.

The domain of emotion has recently been elaborated as a cultural problem in the light of anthropological challenges to the presumption of a psychobiological universality of emotional life (Gaines 1992; Kitayama and Markus 1994; Rosaldo 1984; Kleinman and Good 1985; Lutz 1988; Schwartz, White, and Lutz 1992; Shweder and LeVine 1984; Stigler, Shweder, and Herdt 1990). Revitalization of the study of psychopathology in culturally interpreted terms has occurred in the wake of the "new cross-cultural psychiatry" (Hopper 1991; Kleinman 1977, 1980, 1988a; Littlewood 1990) and "meaning-centered medical anthropology" (Good and Good 1982; Good 1994; Good 1995). This chapter explores these developments in the anthropological study of emotion and mental disorder by drawing out conceptual issues common to each.

While implicit claims about emotion abound in classic ethnographies (Bateson 1958; Benedict 1934; Mead 1935; Hallowell 1955), explicit and sustained theorizing on emotion has emerged only recently. Where studies of culture and personality once held sway, studies of culture and emotion are now numerous. In psychological anthropology, previously suitable topics would likely include, for example, motivation, cognition, perception, dreams, and values but not emotion (Bock 1980; Barnouw 1973; LeVine 1974; Spindler 1978).[2] Where subdisciplines of "cognitive anthropology" or "cognitive psychology" appeared, similar attention was not granted to "affective anthropology" or "affective psychology."

The relative valuation of cognition at the expense of emotion is embedded in the mind-body dualisms that structure scholarly thinking on the issue. Feminist theories of gender, emotion, and social relations (Lutz 1988, 1990; Lutz and Abu-Lughod 1990; Rosaldo 1984; Miller 1993) shed light on this dualism by revealing symbolic associations of emotion with the irrational, uncontrollable, dangerous, natural, and female (Lutz 1988).[3] Catherine Lutz's (1988) analysis of these complex cultural logics reveals contradictions among the cherished presuppositions that constitute the domain of emotion in scientific and popular discourse. For example, while emotional expression is generally devalued in favor of a rational, controlled demeanor, failure to demonstrate "basic" human emotions renders one "estranged" from an innate human capacity for feeling (Lutz 1986). The particular associations of emotion, the body, and women has also been examined by Emily Martin (1987).

The historic anthropological ambivalence and neglect of the cultural category of "emotion" can therefore be understood in relation to how some scholarly topics are deemed worthy or otherwise (Ortner 1974; Lutz 1990). Emotion has emerged as an explicit problem in cultural anthropology only recently because the passions have been considered secondary cultural artifacts relative to more "cognitively" conceived objects such as beliefs, propositions, and values. With the expansion of the conceptual horizons of medical and psychological anthropology, however, emotion is now regarded as properly situated within a cultural repertoire. This problem will be addressed further below in relation to the question of how the construct of culture suggests (or constrains) questions about emotion.

Current studies by psychological anthropologists cover a range of emotion topics that include child-rearing practices and the socialization of emotion (Clancy 1986; Ochs and Schieffelin 1986; Weisner 1983; LeVine 1990); the cultural constitution of the self (Csordas 1994; Hallowell 1955; Marsella, DeVos, and Hsu 1985; Shweder and Bourne 1990; White and Kirkpatrick 1985); cross-cultural variations in the experience and expression of emotion (Briggs 1970; Edgerton 1971b; Shweder and LeVine 1984; Levy 1973; Myers 1979; Schieffelin 1983; Wikan 1990; Roseman 1991); cognitive approaches to emotion

(D'Andrade 1987; Holland 1992; Lakoff and Kovecses 1987; Lutz 1982; White 1992); linguistic studies of emotion (Beeman 1985; Ochs and Schieffelin 1986; Lutz 1988; Matthews 1992; Solomon 1984; White and Kirkpatrick 1985); violence, sexual abuse, and child development (Korbin 1987; Scheper-Hughes 1992); and theoretical examination of Western scientific discourse on emotion (Lutz 1988; Lutz and Abu-Lughod 1990; Rosaldo 1984).

In contrast to the case of emotion, mental disorder has long been the subject of study in both medical and psychological anthropology. This interest stems in large measure from the collaboration of Edward Sapir (1961) and Harry Stack Sullivan (1962) for whom the study of mental disorder was considered essential to an understanding of fundamental (and divergent) human processes. Sullivan and Sapir insisted that a person with a psychiatric disorder must be studied in interpersonal contexts, with particular attention paid to the emotional atmosphere (Jenkins 1991a). Although their collaborative program for the study of culture and mental disorder never fully reached its potential in psychological anthropology (Darnell 1990; Perry 1982; Kennedy 1974), their works still stand as an important foundation for current studies in this area. To draw a parallel between emotion and psychopathology, the early conceptualization of mental disorder as socially transacted has as its counterpart the contemporary formulation of affect as interactive construction (Jenkins 1991).

Reconsideration of relations among culture, emotion, and psychopathology therefore requires examination of enduring and previously unexplored questions: What is particularly cultural about emotion and psychopathology? How are emotion and mental disorder to be conceived: as intrapsychic mental events or intersubjective social processes? As biologically natural events or sociopolitically produced reactions? Can cognitively comprised "emotion" be differentiated from bodily "feeling"? How is "illness" to be distinguished from "pathology"? In what sense might an emotion be termed "abnormal"? How are emotions to be probed in relation to "mental" disorders such as schizophrenia or depression?

CULTURE, ETHNOPSYCHOLOGY, AND ETHNOBIOLOGY

Before proceeding further, it will be helpful to provide a working definition of culture as used in this chapter. This is so not merely because I wish to introduce my particular use of the term *culture* as a basis for my discussion of emotion and psychopathology but also because the concept of culture has become so controversial that some may prefer to abandon it altogether. Identification of problems with the notion of culture has resulted in a significant movement to substitute the term *discourse*. Some find that the concept of culture presumes an uneasy coherence, a static and ahistorical notion that excludes agency (Abu-Lughod and Lutz 1990; White and Lutz 1992). The term *discourse*, however, has a variety of quite specific meanings in fields ranging from literary criticism to conversational analysis, and the new role for discourse sacrifices this specificity for the sake of a linguistic and textual slant on the domain sub-sumed under the term *culture*. It will do just as well to be clear about what counts as culture, taking advantage of the sustained revision of culture theory over the past several decades.

I take culture to be a context of more or less known symbols and meanings that persons dynamically create and recreate for themselves in the process of social interaction. Culture is thus the orientation of a people's way of feeling, thinking, and being in the world—their unself-conscious medium of experience, interpretation, and action. As a context, culture is that through which all human experience and action—including emotions—must be interpreted. This view of culture attempts to take into consideration the quality of culture as something emergent, contested, and temporal (White and Lutz 1992), thereby allowing theoretical breathing space for individual and gender variability and avoiding notions of culture as static, homogeneous, and necessarily shared or even co-herent. I would argue that such a conceptualization of culture is crucial for comparative studies of psychopathology (Jenkins and Karno 1992:10). It encom-passes the indeterminacy of experience and subjectivity that are submerged both by restricting the debate to discourse and by reducing it to a generalized baseline from which individuals and groups may, and often do, deviate.[4]

An essential step toward culturally informed models of emotion is the inves-tigation of indigenous ethnopsychologies. Ethnopsychological issues include the constitution of the self; indigenous categories and vocabularies of emotion; the predominance of particular emotions within societies; the interrelation of various emotions; identification of those situations in which emotions are said to occur; and ethnophysiological accounts of bodily experience of emotions. These ele-ments of ethnopsychology will mediate both the experience and expression of emotion, presuming the existence of an actively functioning (or dysfunctioning) psyche in transaction with the social world.

Whether labeled as ethnopsychology or as cultural psychology, compared to psychologists' definitions of emotion within a framework of stimulus properties, physiological manifestations, and behavioral responses (Fridjda 1987), anthro-pological frameworks appear considerably more broad ranging (Shweder 1990). Consider Michelle Rosaldo's anthropological definition of emotion: "self-concerning, partly physical responses that are at the same time aspects of moral or ideological attitudes; emotions are both feelings and cognitive constructions, linking person, action, and sociological milieu" (see Rosaldo in Levy 1983: 128). In general, the anthropological conception of emotion as inherently and explicitly cultural (Lutz 1982, 1988; Rosaldo 1980b, 1984) is designed to en-compass a broader social field than psychological definitions of emotion as in-dividual response to stimulus events. What is cultural about emotion is that emotion necessarily involves an interpretation, a judgment, or an evaluation (Soloman 1984; Rosaldo 1984). However, as Lila Abu-Lughod (1990:26) has recently cautioned, there may be a problem with privileging cultural-cognitivist accounts of emotion "such as understanding, making sense of, judging, and interpreting, [since] these theorists may be inadvertently replicating that bias toward the mental, idealist, or cognitive that Lutz (1986) points out is such a central cultural value for us.''

On the other hand, anthropologists have also disputed essentialist claims of basic, universally shared emotions based on innate, uniform processes where "brute, precultural fact" is bedrock (Geertz 1973a).[5] The presumption of biological regularity and similarity of human emotional life has been challenged by several ethnographic accounts (Lutz 1988; Kleinman 1986; Rosaldo 1980b). Robert Plutchik (1980:78) exemplifies the natural science approach to the psychological study of emotion in his search for a set of basic emotions that are the equivalent to Mendeleyev's periodic table in physics or Linnaeus's system of classifications in biology. In contrast, anthropological studies are likely to highlight the cultural specificity and situatedness of emotion. The conceptualization of emotion as situationally constituted in social settings has been firmly established in the theoretic formulations of Lutz (1988, 1990). Her analyses of the emotional repertoire of the Ifaluk serve as a powerful retort to the notion of basic, universally recognizable emotions. It is also within this Ifalukian ethnographic light that emotion is found not to reside within hearts or minds of individuals but in the mutually transacted terrain of social and political space.

James Russell (1991:445) has taken issue with Lutz's assertion that Ifaluk emotion terms (*song* [or justifiable anger], for example) do not refer to a person's internal state but rather to something external. He cites Lutz's finding that Ifaluk terms sometimes define emotions as "about our insides" and raises "the conceptual issue of how a word in any language that does not refer to an internal state could be said to be an emotion word. If *song* were a member of a class of words that, like *marriage* or *kinship,* referred to a relationship, then the reason for calling *song* an emotion word is unclear" (Russell 1991:445). Russell interprets the problem as a conflation of sense and reference and suggests that the proper interpretation is that *song* refers to an internal state created when certain external circumstances occur. There are two problems with this critique. First is a conceptual difficulty with the equation of marriage, kinship, and emotion in that the last is inherently evaluative and interpretive (as formulated by Lutz), whereas the former are things that emotions are about. The assertion that emotions are located in social space (rather than individual, internal space) does not "externalize" emotion in such a way to render it conceptually similar to marriage or kinship. Second, there may be a difficulty with just what kind of self is premised here. Should the self be ethnopsychologically conceived as private, bounded, and separate, the notion of "internal" states may make cultural sense. However, if the self is more social-relationally conceived, the "internal" and "external" dichotomy may prove an unsatisfactory point of comparison.

Yet Russell's concern with the theoretic representation of the ethnographic fact that Ifaluk emotion words are sometimes defined as "about our insides" may suggest a genuine dilemma: the need for the representation of subjective experience in anthropological constructs for emotion. This problem is significant since emotion necessarily involves subjectivity (and intersubjectivity) in presupposing some object about which the subject is feeling (Shweder 1985; Fridja 1987). The socially constructed object might be not only a human person (or group) but also a deity, demon, animal, or landscape. The role of subjectivity for emotion cannot be confined to one ethnopsychological version of emotion but can instead be productively employed in comprehensive studies of emotion cross-culturally. At present the problem of emotion as subjective experience is still mostly neglected by anthropologists, a difficult area not much advanced beyond the pioneering work by A. Irving Hallowell (1938, 1955). The difficulty, however, should not dissuade us from investigation of what must be regarded as a crucial dimension of emotion realms.

Psychological and cognitive researchers have tended to distinguish between emotion, on the one hand, and feeling, on the other (Levy 1984). By *emotion,* psychologists have tended to mean cognized, behavioral response, whereas by *feeling* they have tended to mean physiologically based sensation. In contrast to the mental nature of emotion, the contemporary distinction dualistically construes feelings as physical. The consequences of this scientific dichotomy are that (1) feelings are understood as biological while emotions are constructed as cultural and (2) feelings as biological are further construed as universal and immutable, whereas emotions alone may reasonably be thought of as cross-culturally variable. Because feelings are immutable, they are no longer problematized. However, the very notion that emotion is cultural, cognitive, and interpretive while feeling is homogeneous, biological, and universal is inherently problematic. An enduring contribution of William James (1884) and more recently of Michelle Rosaldo (1984) is the observation that a disembodied emotion is a nonentity. Emotion and feeling cannot be separated; emotion must involve feeling.

MEDICAL ANTHROPOLOGY, EMOTION, AND SOCIOPOLITICAL ANALYSES

In medical and psychiatric anthropology, researchers have examined cultural dimensions of dysphoria generally and affective and psychotic disorders in particular. An abbreviated sampling from domains of inquiry in this area would include cultural meanings and indigenous conceptions of distress and illness (Gaines and Farmer 1986; Good and Good 1982; Good 1994; Jenkins 1988; Kirmayer 1984; Low 1985a; Lutz 1985b; Tousignant 1984); "culture-bound syndromes" (Carr and Vitaliano 1985; Simons and Hughes 1985); comparative treatments of the cultural validity of psychiatric syndromes cataloged in the American Psychiatric Association's *Diagnostic and Statistical Manual* (DSM) (Gaines 1992; Good, Good, and Moradi 1985; Good 1992; Hopper 1991, 1992; Kleinman 1980, 1986, 1988a; Manson, Shore, and Bloom 1985); emotional climates and the course of mental disorder (Corin 1990; Karno 1987; Jenkins 1991a; Jenkins and Karno 1992); epidemiological studies of affective and anxiety disorders (Guarnaccia, Good, and Kleinman 1990; Beiser 1985; Manson,

Shore, and Bloom 1985); phenomenological accounts of embodiment and illness experience (Csordas 1990b, 1993b; Frank 1986; Good 1993; Kleinman 1988b; Ots 1990; Scarry 1985), and the medicalization of social problems and human suffering in Western scientific discourse (Fabrega 1989; Kleinman 1988a; Kleinman and Good 1985; Scheper-Hughes and Lock 1987).

Another area that has very recently emerged concerns sociopolitical analyses of emotion (Feldman 1991; Jenkins 1991a, Jenkins and Valiente 1994; Nordstrom and Martin 1992; Scheper-Hughes 1992). Mary-Jo DelVecchio Good and Byron Good (1988) have introduced the idea of the "state construction of affect," or the production of sentiments and actions by the nation-state. They argue for the importance of the "role of the state and other political, religious, and economic institutions in legitimizing, organizing, and promoting particular discourses on emotions" (Good and Good 1988:4). Lutz and Abu-Lughod's (1990) analysis of the interplay of emotion talk and the politics of everyday social life is also significant here. They redirect scholarly attention away from largely privatized and culturalized representations of emotion to examination of emotion discourse in the contexts of sociability and power relations. Another important formulation in this area comes from Kleinman's (1986) studies of affective disorder. His analysis of case studies from China in the period following the upheaval of the Cultural Revolution provides a convincing argument for the social and political production of affective disorders. In a case study of El Salvador, Jenkins (1991a:139) seeks to extend current theorizing on emotion "by examining the nexus among the role of the state in constructing a 'political ethos,' the personal emotions of those who dwell in that ethos, and the mental health consequences for refugees." Other recent literature on the mental health sequelae of sociopolitical upheaval includes treatment of Latin America (Farias 1991; Suarez-Orozco 1989), Southeast Asia (Mollica, Wyshak, and Lavelle 1987; Westermeyer 1988), and South Africa (Swartz 1991).

Emphasis on sociopolitical aspects of affectivity expands the parameters of emotion theory beyond the biological, psychological, and cultural. Closely related to much of this current thinking is feminist theory, which has long been analytically concerned with power relations and inequities (rather than differences) in global context (Rosaldo and Lamphere 1974; Miller 1993). Feminist analyses also question the limits of cultural relativism through grounded locational perspectives on human experience and the human condition (Haraway 1991). The argument here is that the emerging agenda for studies of emotional processes and experience must take political dimensions into account in any of an array of intentional worlds large and small.

"NORMAL" AND "PATHOLOGICAL" EMOTION: DISCONTINUOUS CATEGORIES OR POLES ON A CONTINUUM?

In what sense can we draw a distinction between "normal" and "pathological" emotion? If normal emotions are those commonly shared within cultural settings, are abnormal emotions those outside the range of normal human experience within a particular community? Or within the range of normal experience but inappropriate to a particular setting or event? What criteria would render an emotion or emotional state "abnormal"? Here we encounter the enduring question of whether the normal and pathological are discontinuous categories or poles of a continuum. In the study of emotion and psychopathology we have yet to resolve the problem of what Georges Canguilhem (1989) defined as the ontological versus positivist conceptions of disease. Is there, as the ontological view would have it, a distinct qualitative difference between depression as a normal emotion and depression as a pathological state? If so, is this based on some pathogenic alteration or on some "inborn error" of biochemistry with a genetic origin? Or, as the positivist view would hold, is there only one depression, the intensity of which can vary quantitatively from total absence to a degree that becomes so great as to be pathological? In this view, abnormality is defined as "more" of what otherwise might be considered within the bounds of normal human experience. Canguilhem (1989:45) quotes Nietzsche as follows: "It is the value of all morbid states that they show us under a magnifying glass certain states that are normal—but not easily visible when normal."

In a more contemporary vein, Sullivan argued that there is no definitive threshold distinguishing healthy from ill individuals. The inability to recall a name that is "right on the tip of one's tongue" is a mental disorder in the same sense as is schizophrenia, albeit much less severe. Sullivan maintained that schizophrenic illness could productively be considered as a paradigmatic case for the analysis of fundamental human processes (Sullivan 1962).

In theory, contemporary psychiatry and medicine have for some time been dominated by the quantitative perspective, with its corollary that since they are essentially the same, studies of the pathological can help us understand the normal, and vice versa. However, in actual diagnostic practice, a curious mixture of quantitative and qualitative criteria is characteristic in psychiatry today. The qualitative criteria revolve around the specific symptoms that comprise the symptom cluster or syndrome for a given diagnostic category. Yet the DSM-IV (American Psychiatric Association 1987) is unhesitatingly organized in quantitative terms according to three kinds of criteria: (1) intensity or severity of specific experiences/symptoms (generally exceeds normal range); (2) duration of the experiences (generally longer than usual); and (3) occurrence of the symptom along with one or more other affective, cognitive, and behavioral phenomena that form a particular configuration or symptom profile. It should be obvious that the particular psychiatric symptoms selected for attention as well as the cutoff points for cooccurring symptoms, their duration and severity, are somewhat arbitrary. Failure to meet criteria of enough symptoms of sufficient duration is a failure to meet the parameters of particularly defined syndromes. Therefore, patients who meet some but not all of the designated classificatory category are considered "subclinical." Most persons have at least some experience of the myriad of diverse symptoms cataloged in the DSM. Whether this observation provokes anxiety or amusement, it is evidence of the continuous nature of such definitions of psychopathology. Much normal range experience is cataloged in those 567 pages.

According to psychiatric diagnostic procedure, emotions are unusual or abnormal not because they are unrecognizable features of human experience but because they appear more severe and prolonged, and they often cooccur with an array of other behavioral or cognitive disturbances that (as a syndrome) are outside the range of culturally prescribed orientations to the world. On the other hand, when we move from diagnosis to the etiology and ontology of psychiatric disorder, the dominant paradigm argues that there is a qualitative gulf between normal and pathological. Pathology is a result of a genetically based "inborn error of metabolism," a qualitative anomaly, or even a kind of lesion.

There are other more specific ways in which the continuity or discontinuity between normal and pathological is incorporated in our thinking. Take, for example, the delusional fear that a university president wants a given male faculty member dismissed from his position. Quantitatively, such a person might find this fear becoming increasingly intense or being just a passing notion that is extinguished when it is shrugged off as silly. On the other hand, qualitatively there would be a definite discontinuity between a mistaken idea and a fixed delusion about a university president, for given the proper evidence, the former can be changed or corrected and the latter cannot. Again, although delusions can become quantitatively more or less intense and rigid, true delusions have the qualitative feature of exfoliating into a system, adding more and different and even absurd elements. The delusion that the president of the university wants one dismissed from his position can become the idea that the president, provost, dean, and department chair are in a conspiracy and can come to include the fact that they especially want his parking space taken away. Again, depending on the way an emotion is formulated, it may presuppose a quantitative or qualitative notion of normal versus pathological. For example, one might conceive a qualitative continuum between happiness and sadness, with clinical mania and depression at the pathological extremes of the continuum. On the other hand, when it comes to the symptomatic "flat affect" of schizophrenia, one thinks of a quantitative continuum between flatness and expressiveness. Could one formulate a qualitative distinction between normal flat affect and pathological flat affect? The differences between quantitative and qualitative, continuous and discontinuous, easily become quite tangled. As Canguilhem observed, "the continuity between one state and another can certainly be compatible with the heterogeneity of these states. The continuity of the middle stages does not rule out the diversity of the extremes" (1989:56).

EMOTION AND PSYCHIATRIC DISORDER

Systematic study of emotion and psychopathology requires examination of the following questions: How are the phenomenological worlds of persons with major mental disorder culturally elaborated? What consequences ensue for cross-culturally valid diagnoses if emotions are considered as cultural objects? Are there cross-cultural variations in emotions expressed by kin about a relative with a major mental disorder? Does emotional response on the part of kin mediate the course and outcome of a psychiatric disorder? This section explores these issues in the context of the major disorders of schizophrenia and depression. A cogent rationale for the productive use of specific DSM diagnostic categories (as opposed to generalized distress) in anthropological studies of culture and psychopathology has been already provided by Byron Good (1992). Good agrees that although they are plainly grounded in Western cultural assumptions, they are systematic enough to be used as the basis for cross-cultural research and to be subject to critique as the result of that research.

With respect to the cross-cultural study of the phenomenology of psychosis, little is known about the processes whereby selves and emotional atmospheres constitute worlds of experience for persons living with schizophrenia. At issue is the fundamental question of how psychiatric illness is emotionally experienced. Is schizophrenic psychosis, for example, nearly always and everywhere devalued as a terrifying experience? While many feel this is likely to be the case, we cannot know with certainty since the cross-cultural ethnographic and clinical record is notably thin with respect to phenomenological accounts of mental disorder (Kennedy 1974; Kleinman 1988a, 1988b). Jenkins (1991a) has summarized cross-cultural studies of ''emotional atmospheres'' to document not only the variation in everyday experience but also the importance of that emotional experience in mediating the course and outcome of major mental disorder.

For theoretical orientation to future phenomenological studies of psychosis, it may be useful to reconsider ideas long ago introduced by Sullivan (1953). Recall that for Sullivan, mental disorder is properly conceived not as a discrete disease entity but as an interactive process. This has major implications if used as a cross-cultural starting point for investigation since it would appear to require that mental disorder be examined within the arena of everyday social life rather than in the brain scan or clinic. For Sullivan, psychiatry ''is not an impossible study of an individual suffering mental disorder; it is a study of disordered interpersonal relations nucleating more or less clearly in a particular person'' (p. 258). Not sick individuals but ''complex, peculiarly characterized situations'' are then the target of cross-cultural research and therapy. Sullivan's theory is premised on a notion of the ''self-system'' as a constellation of interpersonal mechanisms in the service of emotional protection against a noxious emotional milieu (Sullivan 1953). Here the self is not a discrete and fixed entity but instead a constellation of interpersonal processes developed during childhood and adolescence. This view of self as intersubjective creation leaves behind the more usual intrapsychic and individuated configuration in psychiatric science. Thus these early theoretical formulations by Sullivan provide a bridge between the subjective experience of the afflicted self and the world of everyday social interaction.

Emotion and Schizophrenic Disorders

In this section, emotion issues are examined in relation to the content and form of diagnostic symptom criteria for schizophrenia and illness processes relevant to the experience, manifestation, and the course and outcome of schizophrenia. Exploration of the emotional dimensions of schizophrenia serves to underscore the point that emotion should be considered no less central to so-considered thought disorders (i.e., the schizophrenias) than to mood disorders (i.e., affective disorders).

The cross-cultural evidence appears to support the notion of important variation in both the content (e.g., delusions about witches rather than about popular performing artists) and form (e.g., visual, auditory, or tactile hallucinations) of schizophrenic symptomatology. An early report from HBM. Murphy et al. (1963) lists four schizophrenic symptoms as common cross-culturally: (1) social and emotional withdrawal, (2) auditory hallucinations, (3) delusions, and (4) flatness of affect. In addition, the early transcultural psychiatric reports provide documentation of significant differences in the manifestation of symptomatology. For example, "falling toward the quiet, nonaggressive end of the continuum appear to be patients from India, the Hutterites, and the Irish. Toward the noisy, aggressive side would probably come the Africans, Americans, and Japanese" (Kennedy 1974:1148–49). Cross-cultural variation in the subtypes of schizophrenia, such as paranoia, hebrephenia, and catatonia, has also been widely noted (WHO 1979b). The pathoplasticity of symptom formation and expression has been interpreted by Kennedy (1974:1149) as providing evidence not only of the cultural shaping of the disorder but also of the likelihood that "schizophrenia" does not denote a single disease process. It is probable that as a research and clinical construct, schizophrenia is better conceived as a plurality of disorders rather than a unitary diagnostic category.

Anthropological analysis of the specific symptoms from the American Psychiatric Association's most recent edition of the DSM (DSM IV) for the category of schizophrenia makes it evident that all prodromal, actively psychotic, and residual symptoms must be evaluated with reference to the patient's cultural context. Failure to do so can result in misdiagnosis. Broadly conceived, symptom criteria include the patient's sense of self, behavioral repertoire, beliefs, cognitive style, and affects. Narrowly conceived, and for the purposes of differential diagnosis, the DSM IV symptom criteria are (1) delusions, (2) hallucinations, (3) disorganized speech, (4) grossly disorganized or catatonic behavior, and (5) negative symptoms (i.e., affective flattening, alogia, or avolition). While delusions, hallucinations, disorganized speech, or behavior might all arguably be affective in nature (i.e., how can these have no culturally specific affective coloration?), culture in relation to the so-called negative[6] symptoms is of particular interest to this analysis. This is particularly so in the case of flat affect, long thought to be pathognomonic for schizophrenia.

"Flat" or "blunted" affect is defined as a "disturbance of affect manifest by dullness of feeling tone'' (Freedman, Kaplan, and Sadock 1976:1280). To examine this symptom cross-culturally, I turn to cross-cultural data on schizophrenic symptomatology as collected by the World Health Organization's (WHO) International Pilot Study of Schizophrenia (IPSS). The IPSS conducted a longitudinal study of schizophrenic symptomatology and course of illness. Psychiatric assessments were completed for 1,202 patients in nine countries (United Kingdom, Soviet Union, United States, Czechoslovakia, Denmark, China, Colombia, Nigeria, and India). Two-year follow-up data (WHO 1979b) across all sites provide a striking range in the presence of flat affect: from 8 (Ibadan, Nigeria) to 50 percent (Moscow, Russia) of patients were so rated.[7] A slight tendency for flat affect to be more common among patients from the more industrialized countries was noted. In addition, flat affect was recorded as the second most common symptom.[8] While these longitudinal data suggest important cross-cultural differences in the presence of flat affect, methodological questions remain as to precisely how flat affect was assessed. The lack of systematic discussion by IPSS investigators on this point is troubling. The cross-cultural variation in emotional experience and expression generally and in schizophrenic symptomatology specifically render the culturally valid assessment of flat affect a complicated undertaking.

The other two DSM IV negative symptoms of schizophrenia—alogia[9] and avolition—have been subjected to even less systematic cross-cultural examination. Alogia (speechlessness that may be resultant from psychotic confusion) is of particular cultural and sociolinguistic concern insofar as the language and ethnicity of the individual conducting the psychiatric assessment may differ from those of the patient. Certainly the symptom of avolition can be expected to vary substantially in relation to culturally constituted capacities such as self, agency, motivation, and the meaning of purposeful action (Karno and Jenkins 1995).

A second area of research concerns emotion and schizophrenic illness processes. This processual approach to affective components of schizophrenic illness can be considered in relation to the experience of emotion, on the one hand, and the expression of emotion, on the other. With respect to experience, questions arise in regard to everyday phenomenological constitution of affect in relation to schizophrenic illness. While a full range of affects may be experienced by the patient, fear and terror have often been a large part of schizophrenic experience (Glass 1989). The question of the illness experience of families has been more systematically investigated in relation to emotional expression about the patient and his or her illness. The suggestion that kin and community emotional response to schizophrenic illness may vary cross-culturally is certainly present in early reports from transcultural psychiatry. Nancy Waxler (1974, 1977), for instance, has maintained a greater tolerance for schizophrenic illness in non-Western settings. Following a systematic analysis of the WHO (1979a) data on recovery from schizophrenia, Edgerton (1980) points out that the findings of better prognosis in non-Western settings may not reflect especially salutary conditions in those settings but instead noxious features within more industrialized nations. Cohen (1992) also disputes Waxler's claim and raises questions about her findings. (See Hopper 1992 and Warner 1992 for critical commentaries on Cohen's article.) (For additional reviews and critiques of the WHO studies, Hopper (1991) and Edgerton and Cohen (1994) identify specific methodological shortcomings.)

Three decades of research on "expressed emotion" serve as confirmation that emotional response to schizophrenic illness not only varies substantially cross-culturally but also mediates course and outcome (Brown, Birley, and Wing 1972; Vaughn and Leff 1976a; Vaughn et al. 1984; Karno et al. 1987; Jenkins and Karno 1992). In particular, the "expressed emotion" factors of criticism, hostility, and emotional overinvolvement[10] show considerable variability (Brown, Birley, and Wing 1972; Vaughn and Leff 1976a; Karno et al. 1987; Vaughn et al. 1984). Lower levels of criticism and emotional overinvolvment have been found observed among Indian, British, and Mexican-descent families than among Euro-American families (Jenkins and Karno 1992). Moreover, persons suffering from a schizophrenic illness who reside with critical, hostile, or emotionally overinvolved relatives are far more likely to suffer a relapse or exacerbation of symptoms compared to their counterparts who reside in households noteworthy by virtue of the relative absence of such factors.

To account for the link between "expressed emotion" and schizophrenic outcome, the hypothesis of a heightened vulnerability to negatively constituted family atmospheres has been put forward (Vaughn 1989). This formulation is merely general, however, and much remains to be examined with respect to the specific mechanisms of how such processes unfold. In addition, the specifically cultural basis of the "expressed emotion" construct has yet to be fully appreciated by psychiatric researchers (Jenkins 1991a; Jenkins and Karno 1992). Certainly the emotional response to schizophrenic illness must be understood as mediated by cultural conceptions of the nature of the problem (for example, "witchcraft," "*nervios,*" "laziness," or "schizophrenia"). Such analyses draw our attention to the inherently affective nature of conceptions of mental disorder (Jenkins 1988; Fabrega 1982). To the extent that cultural conceptions of illness may partially determine which affects surround the illness and, conversely, which emotional stances may suggest the saliency of particular conceptions of the problem, we must be concerned with how such reciprocally constructed responses mediate the course of disorder.

The IPSS also provides evidence of a cross-culturally variable course of schizophrenia. The IPSS concluded that "on virtually all course and outcome measures, a greater proportion of schizophrenic patients in Agra (India), Cali (Colombia), and Ibadan (Nigeria) had favorable, non-disabling courses and outcomes than was the case in Aarhus, London, Moscow, Prague, and Washington" (Sartorius, Jablensky, and Shapiro 1978:106). While the IPSS investigators believed that this variation was probably accounted for by social and cultural factors, they could not submit their hypothesis to examination since sociocultural data were not systematically collected. Insights into the possible cultural sources of variation are offered in two especially careful and critical reanalyses of these data of the IPSS and "expressed emotion" data recently published by Hopper (1991, 1992). Additional evidence for the important role of the emotional environment on the course of schizophrenia comes from Ellen Corin's (1990) research in Montreal on "positive social withdrawal." Patients who regularly inhabit behavioral environments with few social demands evidence less psychotic symptomatology and a greater personal functioning.

Emotion and Major Depressive Disorders

When viewed cross-culturally, depression is more commonly manifest in somatic than in psychological forms (Kleinman 1986, 1988a; Kleinman and Good 1985). This finding necessarily calls into question the validity of DSM symptoms such as "depressed mood" or "loss of pleasure" as pathognomonic symptoms of the disorder. Cultural propensities toward "psychologization" versus "somatization" are more fully reviewed elsewhere (Kirmayer 1984, 1992; Ots 1990; Kleinman 1986). Jenkins, Kleinman, and Good (1991:67) have argued that "insofar as this dichotomous approach distinguishes psyche and soma, it reproduces assumptions of Western thought and culture, [but] must from the outset be suspended in formulating a valid comparative stance." A key cross-cultural question is whether the clinical-research construct of depression can validly include both somatic and psychologized forms of depressive symptomatology or whether these are better considered as essentially different disorders.

Somatized versus psychologized expressions of depressive affect suggest a cultural specificity to "sadness" and "suffering" (Kleinman and Kleinman 1991). Cultural styles of dysphoria are perhaps best understood as elements of indigenous or ethnopsychological models of emotion (Lutz 1988; White and Kirkpatrick 1985). An understanding of local ethnopsychological models of depression is crucial to specification of everyday depressive affects, on the one hand, and more severely distressing depressive states, on the other.

As pointed out by Kleinman and Good (1985), there are methodological problems in differentiating depression as emotion, mood, and disorder. The parallel observation by Sullivan has already been made for normal-range behavior and that characteristic of schizophrenia. An extension of Sullivan's approach to schizophrenia as "complex, peculiarly characterized situations" was adopted by George Brown and Tirril Harris (1978) in their studies of depression. They find that cases of depressive illness, apparently very common among working-class women in the London area, can be predicted not by individual factors but instead by a specific set of situational factors: unemployment, dilapidated housing conditions, caring for three or more small children, the lack of a confiding relationship, and the death of mother before age eleven. Taken together, these factors can be observed to produce depressive reactions in these English women. This careful empirical study provides powerful evidence for the conclusion that depression is more diagnostic of women's social and economic situations than women's psychobiological vulnerability.

The sociocultural context that may be most important to cross-cultural studies of depression is gender. The relationship between depression and gender is well known: epidemiological evidence documents that women disproportionately suffer from depression relative to men (Nolen-Hoeksema 1990). This epidemiological fact with reference to North American women has also been confirmed cross-culturally in virtually every case that has been investigated. Strickland (1992) has recently summarized these data. Jenkins, Kleinman, and Good (1991) critically review the available literature on cross-cultural susceptibility to depression to conclude that the disproportionate degree of depression among women is likely to be universal. This disturbing conclusion must be accounted for in the light of gender inequality conferring less power and status to women relative to men in both Western and non-Western countries (Miller 1993; Rosaldo and Lamphere 1974). Lower socioeconomic status also must be examined since several studies have linked adverse life events and conditions to a vulnerability to depression, with again a disproportionate effect on poor women and children (Brown and Harris 1978). Migration (of immigrants and refugees) and social change are also implicated in the onset of a major depressive episode (Farias 1991; Jenkins 1991b; Kinzie et al. 1984; Mollica, Wyshak, and Lavelle 1987; Westermeyer 1988, 1989).

Cultural variations in socialization practices, marital discord, as well as "expressed emotion" may also contribute to differential rates of depression (Vaughn and Leff 1976a; Hooley, Orley, and Teasedale 1986). In summary, there is evidence that culture plays a strong role in the formation of the experience of depressive affects and disorder, the meaning of and social response to depression within families and communities, and the course and outcome of the disorder (Jenkins, Kleinman, and Good 1991:68).

CONCLUDING REMARKS

In this chapter I have drawn together two critical but often separate areas within medical and psychological anthropology, the study of the relation between culture and emotion and the study of psychopathology, in order to suggest that there is a great deal of commonality in the conceptual issues raised by each. My argument has encompassed the methodological orientations of ethnopsychology and cultural psychology, interpersonal and intrapsychic accounts of the theory of emotion, the conceptual distinction between emotion and feeling, and the problem of continuity and discontinuity between normal and pathological. I have summarized studies of dysphoric affects and emphasized the importance of experiential accounts of the emotional distress and disorder in the context of power relations and considerations of the state construction of affect, formulated in intersubjective interpersonal terms, and premised on a relational notion of self. Finally, I have considered cultural variability in the phenomenology, course, and outcome of two major mental disorders, schizophrenia and depression, and examined contemporary psychiatric diagnostic conventions in the light of anthropological theories of emotion.

Anthropological approaches to the study of emotion have come a great distance in a relatively short period of time. Nevertheless, we have yet to see the full development of the intersection of culture, emotion, and illness processes. Along with Western traditional views of the superiority of mind over body, there is currently a strong bias toward cognitive science. While "cognitive anthropology" has made a powerful scientific contribution to the anthropological endeavor, relatively less anthropological attention has been directed toward the full range of emotion phenomena.

I conclude with suggestions for future anthropological directions in the study of emotion. First, as feminist theory has taught us, situated knowledge of emotion will continue to be critical to avoid decontextualized accounts of the passions (Haraway 1991). Psychological and medical anthropologists have long been naturally inclined toward this end. However, as Lila Abu-Lughod (1993) and others (Brown 1991; Edgerton 1992) have recently cautioned, anthropological enthusiasm for the particular should not be allowed to obscure the likelihood of shared features of human emotional experience. Second, in contrast to studies of emotion based on lexicon, discourse, ethnopsychological category, communication, and expression, we are in rather short supply of studies based on intersubjective and experiential dimensions of culture and emotion (Hallowell 1938, 1955 was a notable exception). Signs are beginning to be observable, however, that this is about to change (Csordas 1994; Shweder 1990a; Wikan 1990). Kleinman and Kleinman (1991:277) have recently offered a definition of experience as "an intersubjective medium of social transactions in local moral worlds. It is . . . the felt flow of that intersubjective medium." Theodore Schwartz, Geoffrey White, and Catherine Lutz (1992), who had previously endorsed a "distributive" theory of culture, now call for an "experience-processing" model of culture. Byron Good (1994) provides a compelling argument of the specific need in medical anthropology for the study of culture and experience in relation to affective and illness realities. Third, studies of emotion need to expand in scope beyond local and intrapsychic analyses and toward a concomitant consideration of state and global forces in mediating the experience and expression of emotion. Initial steps in this direction are evident in the work of Mary-Jo DelVecchio Good and Byron Good (1988) on the state construction of affect and Jenkins (1991) on political ethos. Fourth, the recent cultural interest in emotion would benefit from a renewed interest in naturalistic observation in tandem with interpretive analyses of emotion. A methodologically greater ethnographic emphasis on the interactive, nonverbal behavioral and symbolic dimensions of emotion would go far in complementing the current focus on linguistic and verbal dimensions of emotion.

NOTES

1. This chapter is a slightly adapted version of a chapter by Jenkins (1994) entitled "The Psychocultural Study of Emotion and Mental Disorder," published in *Handbook of Psychological Anthropology,* ed. P. Bock (Westport, Conn.: Greenwood Press).

2. Much of the discourse on emotion was subsumed under the rubric of "personality" studies (Rosaldo 1984; White 1992). A notable exception is Hildred Geertz's excellent 1959 article on the "vocabulary of emotion" published in the journal *Psychiatry.* Another important exception is Gregory Bateson's (1958:118) notion of ethos defined as "the expression of a culturally standardized system of organization of the instincts and emotions of the individuals."

3. The counterpart of cognition (and thought) as rational, controlled, safe, cultural, and male is obvious. The scientific suitability of these adjectival descriptors has long been assumed in anthropological and psychological discourse.

4. For theoretical discussion of culture, deviance (including psychopathology), and ambiguity, see Edgerton (1985). For review of a controversial thesis concerning the notion of societally widespread or institutionalized forms of deviance as constitutive of a "sick society," see Edgerton (1992). For a discussion of "explanatory models" of discrete illness episodes as necessarily complex, dynamic, contradictory, and ambiguous, see Kleinman (1980). Both of these theorists have been preoccupied with how culture theory can account for change, heterogeneity, and disagreement in the context of individual and subgroup variability.

5. Lutz and Abu-Lughod (1990) and Kirmayer (1992) provide thorough accounts of issues surrounding essentialist presumptions in social scientific discourse.

6. So-termed negative symptoms in schizophrenia are noteworthy by virtue of their absence: e.g., lack of appropriate affect, speech and volition.

7. The differences between the nonindustrialized and more industrialized countries are not uniform, however: only 9 percent of London patients and 11 percent of Washington patients displayed flat affect at the time of follow-up.

8. The observation of "lack of insight" as the most common symptom might be indicative of a clash between professional psychiatric and popular lay formulations of the problem (e.g., as a psychiatric, nervous, mental, or personality problem). If the psychiatric interviewer had accorded a legitimacy to popular illness categories, this "symptom" might not have been recorded so frequently. Failure to anthropologically appreciate these cross-cultural differences in what Kleinman (1980) has termed "explanatory models" can result in an array of methodological difficulties in the assessment of symptoms.

9. Alogia can also be present in relation to intellectual deficit.

10. Methodological definitions of these affects have been provided elsewhere (Vaughn and Leff 1976b). Briefly, criticism is any verbal statement indicating dislike, resentment, or disapproval. Emotional "overinvolvement" is indexed by a set of particular attitudes, emotions, and behaviors that are culturally determined to include overprotective or intrusive behaviors. Although affects of warmth and praise are also undoubtedly important to many qualitative dimensions of family life, these have yet to be significantly predictive of recovery from major mental disorder. The relationship between criticism, hostility, and emotional overinvolvement has also been found for depressive illness at even lower thresholds than for schizophrenia (Hooley, Orley, and Teasedale 1986; Vaughn and Leff 1976a).

5

Clinically Applied Anthropology

Noel J. Chrisman and Thomas M. Johnson

More than forty years ago, William Caudill noted in the first review paper encompassing medical anthropology that "social anthropologists and other social scientists have recently been doing some unusual things" (1953:771). He went on to examine a number of these behaviors: working closely with physicians, teaching in medical schools, collaborating with the public health service, studying hospitals and patients, and conducting psychotherapy with American Indians. Since that time the unusual things have continued, but until 1979 little explicit was said about them. Anthropology was expanding dramatically during the 1960s and 1970s, and although anthropologists were working in clinical settings, more attention was focused on theoretical concerns within the discipline and on the expansion of such academic subfields as urban, psychological, and medical anthropology. Little was being written about collaboration between anthropologists and health practitioners.

In the preface to *Clinically Applied Anthropology,* Noel Chrisman and Thomas Maretzki (1982) noted that it was time for a systematic examination of these unusual behaviors—to move beyond the informal dinner conversations among colleagues at professional meetings and to write about what these anthropologists had been doing for more than a decade. That volume became one of a number of published discussions about what some heralded as a new subfield of anthropology. This chapter provides an overview of how anthropologists have approached working with health practitioners. After examining the debate about what the subfield is called, we discuss how anthropologists currently fit into health science settings, their reliance on holism and system advocacy, the need for theoretical approaches, and the anthropological knowledge frequently used in clinical settings.

THE SCOPE AND NATURE OF CLINICAL INVOLVEMENT

There have been difficulties deciding how to define what anthropologists do in clinical settings. Certainly when Caudill wrote, anthropological attention to matters of health and health care systems was sporadic. There was no need to distinguish the cross-cultural study of health-related phenomena from the activities of anthropologists in health science centers because so few engaged in the latter. In the late 1960s and early 1970s, however, education in the health professions witnessed revolutionary changes, in which social science became a far more important part of the curriculum than previously. Some anthropologists became involved in health science centers at this time. In addition, the twin pressures of increasing numbers of anthropologists and a shrinking academic job market, coupled with post-1960s conviction that anthropology should be applied to solving practical problems, have made the differentiation between academic and applied medical anthropology all the more meaningful. Anthropologists' current desires to become visible and marketable for professional positions outside academia in clinical settings continue to be a major impetus for defining a new and different kind of anthropological endeavor and discussing how to do it.

In Caudill's time and up until the mid-1970s, it made sense to include anthropological activities in clinical settings simply as part of medical anthropology. In fact, in Norman Scotch's 1963 review, much of medical anthropology was involved with Western medicine and its introduction in cross-cultural settings. Many anthropologists who were beginning to work in health science centers at the time were traditionally trained members of academic anthropology faculties experiencing serendipitous changes in professional focus. Now, however, there are more specially trained applied medical anthropologists, and those who work in clinical settings are able to document unique contributions to both Western medicine and anthropology. With this emerging anthropological role differentiation, a kind of academic-versus-applied distinction within medical anthropology has emerged.

We see medical anthropology as the study of health-related phenomena. These phenomena range from individual-level biological studies, such as those examining cultural influences on hypertension and malnutrition, to microlevel studies of health care choices and illness beliefs, to macrolevel research on health care systems and their political and economic contexts. In short, medical anthropology is anthropological theory and methods devoted to the topics of health, illness, and health care. These interests have a long history within academic medical anthropology.

The type of anthropology found in health science centers is part of a growing applied arm of the discipline: anthropology devoted to helping health practitioners do their work better. One medical educator has noted that applied medical anthropology is "properly distinguished and distinguishable from medical anthropology and other social sciences by virtue of this focus on using the concepts of anthropology to explain and suggest changes for the health care system and patients within the systems'' (Swartz 1983:21). Our experience and that of others is that anthropologists in clinical settings apply all of anthropology to the problems presented—educational, research, and therapeutic (Chrisman and Maretzki 1982).

At the individual level, the scope and nature of involvement by applied anthropologists in clinical settings always is an ongoing negotiation, as much determined by health practitioner expectations as by anthropologists' desires or disciplinary traditions (Ablon 1980). Although often not labeled or identified as such, the methods and theories applied anthropologists bring to clinical settings often are very much those of anthropology. In fact, the utility of our presence among health practitioners is based on this covert, unlabeled difference in perspective. Some anthropologists in clinical settings eschew defining their identity as anthropologists in those settings, while maintaining their anthropological identity through continuing involvement in scholarly publication and reliance on peers in the discipline for intellectual response. This may be advantageous, for as nursing found in its history, at the disciplinary level it is problematic for one field to define itself primarily in terms of its relation to another. Medical anthropology has been able to develop new areas of research stimulated by actual clinical problems and work with clinicians (Weidman 1983), creating unique opportunities to make contributions to both anthropology and patient care without defining medical anthropology in some rigid way vis-à-vis medicine or nursing.

Recognition of the importance of anthropology and the work of medical anthropologists within health science centers gradually has ameliorated problems with identity and role definition among health practitioners. The discipline also is beginning to grapple with the anthropological uncertainties about role definition alluded to by Scotch (1963:33): "On the other hand, there are those anthropologists who, in working in a medical setting, like to get overinvolved; like to play the role of the doctor or psychiatrist; prefer to play an active role rather than the role of the detached scientist. . . . Their publications suffer accordingly." We unapologetically argue against anthropologists in clinical settings confining themselves to the role of detached scientist, for this may both inhibit understanding of health science professionals and waste opportunities for making anthropological knowledge relevant to clinical concerns.

Although anthropologists working in medical settings will be expected to be involved in the clinical activities, they also must be aware of both the costs and benefits of allowing system demands for therapeutic activism to determine their roles. For example, Thomas Johnson (1987b) pointed out how important for rapport building and acceptance it is to pass the "tests" demanding clinical involvement that physicians typically pose for anthropologists (not unlike being expected to partake of indigenous cuisine in traditional anthropological fieldwork), but cautions against becoming seen primarily as a clinician. While reducing role ambiguity may be personally less stressful, "going native" in clinical settings may reduce objectivity and preclude some potentially unique and powerful contributions. Mark Nichter, Gordon Trockman and Jean Grippen (1985), Linda Alexander (1979), Atwood Gaines (1982), Chrisman (1988), and Johnson (1987b, 1991b) are anthropologists who constantly struggle to maintain both their clinical involvements and their identities as anthropologists.

A MATTER OF TERMINOLOGY

Up to this point, we have been relatively careful to avoid naming the anthropology carried out in health care settings because there is still debate about what to call it. Some simply refer to this practice as *applied medical anthropology* (Hill 1984; Shiloh 1980). The two most popular alternatives are *clinical anthropology* (Golde and Shimkin 1980; Shimkin and Golde 1983) and *clinically applied anthropology* (Chrisman and Maretzki 1982). The former has the advantage of being shorter and snappier and has the same connotations as clinical psychology, which claims its own independent clinical mandate. The difficulty with the "clinical anthropology" appellation is that it may not accurately describe the activities of the anthropologist and may imply a more extensive therapeutic role than is desirable or can be accomplished following traditional anthropological training (Ablon 1980).

It is largely unrecognized, however, that anthropology has strongly clinical—and sometimes even therapeutic—roots. Alfred Kroeber completed psychoanalytic training and practiced analysis, first at the Stanford Clinic in 1918 and later in private practice. Although recently anthropological methodology has become increasingly quantitative and ascribed to the myth of "objective" science, Margaret Mead actually viewed anthropological research as a clinical skill, emphasizing good listening, sensitivity to nuances, and extracting patterns from data. Mead has been remembered as operating from the clinician's notion of disciplined subjectivity, a notion very similar to a psychotherapist's attention to countertransference responses (emotional reactions to patients), when she advocated that ethnographers bring their subjective responses to the field setting into consciousness so they become part of the available data to be considered (Bateson 1980).

Both because of the analogy with clinical psychology and the tenor of some of the early writing associated with the term, *clinical anthropology* implies that medical anthropologists are using anthropology to solve clinical problems—for example, to cure or care for somebody (Todd and Clark 1985). Peggy Golde (1983a, 1983b), a major early writer on the subject who was trained in both anthropology and counseling, described herself as a clinical anthropologist. Hazel Weidman (1980, 1982b) would describe such colleagues with dual training as anthropologist-clinicians. Some anthropologists do take care of patients, but this activity occurs primarily because they also have clinical training as a physician, nurse, or counselor (Tripp-Reimer 1983b; Dougherty 1985). All contend that although anthropologist-clinicians bring to their work more than traditional clinicians without training in anthropology, their clinical practices are based primarily on their other profession, not on anthropology.

A number of writers, usually health practitioners themselves (Swartz 1983), have been strongly supportive of the move of anthropology into clinical settings but have warned against attempting to become clinicians based solely on anthropological training. One argument is that anthropology is a research, not a clinical, discipline. We study culture, and although our research insights into the nature of a culture might help understand a patient, conducting research does not prepare us to take care of individuals. A second problem is that anthropology is a discipline without a therapeutic mandate (Chrisman and Maretzki 1982b): not possessing interventions, ethical standards, or societal sanction to treat people.

Chrisman and Maretzki (1982b) argued that anthropologists in health care settings teach, do research, and consult with clinical colleagues. Anthropologists in clinical settings, like anthropologists in any other applied setting, help analyze and resolve problems facing specialists (Weidman 1983). Clinically applied anthropologists direct their attention toward health care much as other applied anthropologists might direct their efforts toward economic development or agrarian change. *Clinically applied anthropology* is a more cumbersome appellation than *clinical anthropology* but does not carry the connotation of clinical practice and its implicit threat to the many more traditional clinicians who constitute the medical care system. When we are not directly involved with the care of patients, clinicians need not worry about our presumed lack of clinical skills—or our potential effectiveness—in working with patients (Johnson 1987b). In addition, we are removed in large measure from competition for increasingly difficult-to-obtain health care dollars (Barnett 1980).

A second concern in defining clinically applied anthropology is whether to include the topic of applied anthropology in public health. There is much to recommend its inclusion, especially given the long history and central position that anthropology in public health has had in medical anthropology. The earliest text easily identifiable as medical anthropology was Benjamin Paul's *Health, Culture, and Community* (1955), a series of case studies of the application of anthropology in public health projects. Nonetheless, most of the writers about clinically applied anthropology have discussed their roles in health care institutions and/or working with clinicians (Kaufman 1980; Johnson 1991a, 1991b). Most of the writing in the area of applied anthropology in public health is not explicit about collaboration with practitioners. One exception is discussion in *Clinical Anthropology* about a public health project, parts of which refer to relationships with clinicians (Shimkin et al. 1983).

Currently, this situation is changing; clinicians who previously toiled only in hospitals and clinics are beginning to focus their attention on community settings. Primary care practitioners are discovering the necessity of learning to work with as well as in communities. The specialties of community-oriented primary care in medicine and community health nursing are examples. In addition, community-based research and intervention projects are gaining in stature in both areas.

Clinically applied anthropology is seen here as the application of anthropological data, research methods, and theory to clinical matters. Weidman and others who have discussed the word *clinical* refer to care of patients in some fashion. This does not mean that the clinically applied anthropologist must be seeing patients, though a number of these specialists do. It refers to the involvement of anthropologists with the everyday tasks of formal health practitioners: seeing patients, teaching students, carrying out research with and on health practitioners, and the like.

ALTERNATIVE CONCEPTIONS AND CRITIQUES

There have been two notable alternative views of clinically applied anthropology. The first was termed *therapeutic anthropology* by its major proponent, Ailon Shiloh (1977, 1980). Shiloh, commenting primarily about mental health care, asserted that most clients seeking help from community mental health centers do not have problems with either their neurochemistry or their intrapsychic functioning but rather simply have "problems of living." In other words, because many patients cannot cope with the demands of life in modern society, mental health professionals need to be experts on culture rather than on psychology. Shiloh went on to advocate for special training in interpersonal skills for anthropologists, followed by prescribed steps to licensure and certification similar to psychologists and social workers, although it is not clear exactly what such therapeutic anthropologists might do differently from the more traditionally recognized mental health practitioners.

A second alternative vision of clinically applied anthropology has come from a more recent emphasis in medical anthropology, critical medical anthropology. This perspective has never been thought of as explicitly clinical but rather as theoretical: understanding health issues in the "light of the larger political and economic forces that pattern human relationships, shape social behavior, and condition collective experience, including forces of institutional, national, and global scale" (Singer 1986a:128). The principal assertions of advocates of this position are that critical medical anthropology promotes a concern for the relationship between microlevels and macrolevels of analysis and that the qualities of class, race, ethnicity, and gender are fundamental to understanding health, illness, and health care (Baer 1993). This important analytic approach has been successful in promoting a much stronger consideration of the ways in which macrolevel political and economic forces affect health in all societies. That is, critical anthropology is influencing theory and research in medical anthropology.

Devotees of the critical approach have soundly criticized clinically applied anthropology on the grounds that it does not consider the inherent power and class differentials between patients and practitioners. Perhaps the initial and most direct challenge came from Michael Taussig (1980a:12), a physician-anthropologist who charged that, by helping physicians to understand patients better, anthropologists who work directly in patient care activities are unwittingly perpetuating the existing class structure and exploitation by helping to "make the science of human management all the more powerful and coercive." Although both Taussig's and Shiloh's approaches are theoretically compelling, their practical nonspecificity makes questionable their individual-level efficacy for resolving patient problems, medical as well as social.

A CRITICAL CLINICALLY APPLIED ALTERNATIVE?

Recently, critical anthropologists have begun to describe actual critical praxis (Singer 1995), indicating that proponents of a critical approach have a more encompassing vision that recognizes the need for clinical strategies: "Ultimately critical medical anthropology will need to combine theory and practice if it is to liberate human beings from political economic structures that exploit and oppress them" (Baer 1993a:300). The first approach to praxis has been a suggestion that among clinical anthropologists, a

shift from the individualistic approach to a collective one that forms an alliance with other progressive medical social scientists, physicians, patients, and even administrators is required. Critical clinical anthropologists will need to inform patients that their health problems are not unique but are shared by others of their class, race, ethnicity, and gender and that social action can serve as a form of therapy. In short, clinical anthropologists who wish to adopt a critical perspective will need to accept patient advocacy. (Baer 1993:310)

Baer and others recognize that clinically applied anthropologists see themselves as translators of cultural knowledge for clinicians so that the medical care system can become more responsive to patient and societal needs. However, they see this as being trapped in a restricted role and that "clinical anthropologists may be forced to downplay the social origins and reification of illness, the increasingly medical interpretation of social problems, and inequities in the availability and quality of health care" (Baer 1993a:303). For the clinically applied anthropologist, two issues are central to this debate: the theoretical stance of the anthropologist and the professional role of the clinically applied anthropologist.

The central theoretical propositions of critical anthropology have been important, but not always salient, in social science analysis for more than a century. How critical theory is constructed, and its utility for analyzing culture and society, including the health care system, continue to be debated in the literature (Morgan 1987; Morsy, this volume). Critical anthropological analyses of health care systems are illuminating the importance of political and economic processes in health status and health care. In this way, these analyses will affect the body of knowledge on which the clinically applied anthropologist must draw for working with clinicians. Although many clinically applied anthropologists do not sound like critical anthropologists, they are grappling with the issues (Kleinman 1985:69; Wright and Johnson 1990; Johnson 1995; Stein 1995).

The key concern for critically informed clinically applied anthropology is not so much the validity of a macrolevel political and economic approach. That will be decided on the basis of its utility for understanding society. Rather, it is the particular sort of advocacy position that critical anthropologists expect clinically applied anthropologists to take (to advocate for social action as a form of therapy). Regarding the latter, we already have argued that anthropologists are not typically trained as therapists and need to leave those decisions to people who are, such as the physicians Waitzkin (1986) or Taussig (1980a) or the nurse Thompson (1981). For the former, patient advocacy, this chapter stresses the notion of clinical anthropologists as system advocates: helping to resolve the problems of patient and practitioner alike.

Critical medical anthropologists point out that patients are caught in an inferior position, that practitioners' treatment decisions promote an undesirable status quo, and that the health care system is one element in an oppressive capitalist economic system. When the clinically applied anthropologist can introduce this knowledge into the conduct of a clinical case or set of cases so that all participants have an opportunity for a better outcome, then the critical approach will have served its useful function. This kind of approach is not absent now. For example, Lazarus's (1988a) analysis of a prenatal clinic provides strong evidence of the need for restructuring simply on humanitarian grounds. Pointing out to residents that they can do little in the clinic for their poor and minority patients not only may restrain the physician from trying to do too much (the massive injection of penicillin rather than a course of pills, sometimes out of compassion, but sometimes punitively as a result of displaced anger) but also may open up opportunities for social welfare interventions. We recognize that these fall short of the agenda of the critical medical anthropologists, but they may move clinician viewpoints beyond the narrow confines of the clinic to consider health care system effects on all participants.

RATIONALE AND METHODS FOR CLINICALLY APPLIED MEDICAL ANTHROPOLOGY

Perhaps the key question for clinically applied anthropology is: What can anthropologists do with and for health practitioners? There has been some agreement about what is needed from anthropologists who have a long association with health science schools (Leighton 1983) related to the set of topics discussed here. In addition, anthropologists and clinicians have been jointly committed to improving the quality and efficacy of care. Patients have been dissatisfied with high cost, low personal attention, and the related problems of class, race, and cultural differences. For example, Harold Swartz (1983:17) feels that practitioners "need to develop better understanding of the factors that affect an individual's perception and response to health, illness, and therapy.... [Anthropologists] can increase the understanding and use of anthropological concepts in the activities of traditional providers of health care." Practitioners have been dissatisfied with difficulties in providing care that meets patient needs (and, just as important, their own needs) and have noticed that many of their difficulties are related to patients' cultural backgrounds. This recognition has been conditioned strongly by the civil rights and consumer movements of the 1960s, which called attention to group demands for more culturally sensitive care. In addition, some cities have experienced an influx of Southeast Asian refugees whose special needs are visible enough to heighten sensitivity to cultural issues in patient care.

Thus, a key issue in medical care has become the cultures of particular groups and the relationship of culture to the care of patients (Weidman 1983). Anthropologists have been the logical professionals to turn to for help on such problems, and they have been available because of their presence on or near the faculties of medical and nursing schools for decades. A number of topics has drawn anthropologists and health practitioners together over the years: defining which behaviors are normal and which are abnormal among humans using cross-cultural research; delineating specialized cultural diagnoses such as the culture-bound syndromes; contributing ethnographic research on health care settings to expand clinician understanding of their own environments; exploring the cultural dimension in human relationships; participating in public health projects overseas; and collaborating in community psychiatry (Chrisman and Maretzki 1982a). Through these years, anthropological contributions have been seen as important, but anthropologists have not always been involved in the daily functioning of health science schools. (This is certainly the case when the anthropologist is present only because of a research grant.)

Medical faculties are accustomed to using "basic scientists" to provide the specialized information for medicine to carry out its mission (Hughes and Kennedy 1983; Hasan 1975). For example, physiologists, microbiologists, anatomists, and physical anthropologists are on these faculties to teach about the body, and psychologists (usually called behavioral scientists) are present to teach human behavior. Cultural anthropologists have been present (as another kind of behavioral scientist) to accomplish these same ends (Polgar 1962). For example, Robert Ness (1982) teaches short courses encompassing single topics, such as child abuse or alcoholism, as electives for medical students.

Many anthropologists, however, find it difficult to assume the limited and specialized role of providing information narrowly: to package their information to fit the time demands of clinical settings and to be congruent with the dominant information-processing style of their clinician colleagues (Johnson 1981, 1991a, 1991b). Howard Stein (1985a), for example, has complained about the "ethnic cookbook" approach that clinicians frequently seem to demand from anthropologists, in which they want to learn only a series of clinically relevant cultural characteristics of a particular ethnic group. Discussions among clinically applied anthropologists suggest that they prefer a broader mandate, teaching about cultural processes. Conflict can be illustrated by the reciprocal dissatisfaction of a hypothetical anthropologist and physician: the physician asks the anthropologist during hospital rounds to explain about the manifestations of grief among Ethiopians, and the anthropologist provides a fifty-minute lecture on Ethiopian culture. The clinician is frustrated by such "information overload" (vowing never to ask a question like that again), and the anthropologist complains in frustration that all physicians want is a "cookbook."

An important dynamic in the relationship between clinicians and anthropologists has to do with the paradigm into which information concerning the care of patients will be put (Friedman 1983; Phillips 1985). Physicians, and to a lesser extent nurses, possess a biological and reductionist way of thinking about health and illness that is satisfying to them. The scheme they use to interpret information usually is successful in the care of patients and, like other belief systems, not easily susceptible to challenge. Although most anthropologists are able to provide ethnic lore for clinical use, they are uncomfortable with its use as immutable fact. We know that these "facts" are subject to wide variation among members of ethnic groups because of diversity of context.

Nevertheless, anthropologists are invited to many health care institutions to provide the information necessary to help physicians and others deal with cultural issues as clinicians see them emerging (Poland 1985). Thus, a key issue in clinically applied anthropology is how to formulate anthropological theory and data in ways that will be responsive to the imperatives of clinical settings: time consciousness and direct relevance to patient care (Johnson 1991a, 1991b). This is difficult, for while social scientists are trained to tolerate ambiguity and uncertainty in data (von Mering 1985), effective clinicians must strive to achieve a state of "optimal ignorance" (knowing enough to make effective decisions but not so much that they become paralyzed by ambiguities and uncertainties). Put another way, anthropologists are trained to elaborate and understand reality in all its nuances; physicians strive to simplify and explain reality parsimoniously.

Like clinicians who must always make decisions based on inadequate data, clinically applied anthropologists often are expected to deliver anthropological information when they have too few data for their own comfort (von Mering 1985). Their primary challenges, then, are to translate anthropology into something usable for clinical practice (Chrisman and Maretzki 1982b) and to be comfortable with that style. Arthur Kleinman (1985:70) says, "We need to make ourselves useful in order to make ourselves heard." What this requires of the anthropologist is that he or she know anthropology well enough to transform it into something it was not necessarily designed for and, simultaneously, to know one or another of the health sciences well enough as a cultural system to phrase this information so it will be accepted and incorporated into clinical practice. It is a process very much like culture brokering, especially since mutual goodwill and respect become significant in the process (Weidman 1982b).

There are broader or narrower ways for the anthropologist to conceive of this task, depending on the degree of commitment to the clinical setting. A narrow construction of the translation need might be offered by anthropologists who only occasionally consult about one ethnic group and its behavior and are likely to learn over time which information is most useful and the ways in which it can best be presented. A broader translation is more likely to arise among anthropologists who spend a significant segment of time with clinicians and feel the necessity for more integrated approaches that might encourage actual change in the practice of that group of clinicians.

THE ROLE OF HOLISM AND A SYSTEMS PERSPECTIVE

There is debate about the kind of role that a clinically applied anthropologist should have in a health science setting. Actual roles range from that of clinician or researcher, with somewhat singular responsibilities; through roles as teacher or consultant, with broader responsibilities; to roles that may encompass the former and even include patient advocacy. Linda Alexander (1979) and Howard Stein (1980a) point out that clinical anthropologists must be extremely wary of the tendency to be advocates for patients, families, or specific ethnic groups in a fashion analogous to traditional anthropologists' predisposition to be ''on the side of the natives.'' Such a tendency leads to a focus on the power differential between doctors and patients, and a reflexive bashing of physicians while cheering for patients as underdogs. In addition, they tend to introduce cultural information to the clinician from the patient's perspective, as is the practice in ethnographies. As logical as this inclination seems to many anthropologists, it contradicts another strongly held position within anthropology: holism. Alexander argues that anthropologists should not lose track of this central theoretical perspective simply because they are working in nontraditional settings.

For Alexander, the advantage of holism is that it forces clinically applied anthropologists to take a systems perspective. When they are able to stand back and analyze the entire system, both clients and clinicians stand to gain. To a large degree, anthropologists are better prepared to use a systems perspective than are their psychology colleagues, and thus they have an additional skill to offer in clinical settings. Psychology shares with biomedicine a relatively narrow focus on the individual. Frequently the anthropologist's assessment and intervention at a systems level can create many new options for treatment.

A holistic perspective has the practical advantage of reducing the chance of alienating clinical colleagues by appearing to favor one side or the other (a reputation for working effectively with all participants is essential in clinical settings [Johnson 1987a]). As much as clinicians may want or need patient information, they do not need to have their authority or expertise undermined by a patient advocate who is seemingly working against them. Nichter, Trockman, and Grippen (1985), Johnson (1987b, 1991a) and Alexander (1979), who have described their "clinical" practices in some detail, mention the need to maintain positive relationships with clinicians while working closely, and frequently confidentially, with their patients. Practitioners are tremendously protective of their control over patients and are reluctant to let outsiders in. Once in, clinically applied anthropologists have a better chance of staying in if they can be seen as systems therapists rather than as patient advocates.

Howard Stein has provided a number of good examples of how the systems perspective works. In an article written for family physicians, Stein (1985e) directs them to distinguish between patient wants and needs: needs are seen as the patient's medical requirements as judged by practitioners, yet wants may be just as important for care. Stein's stance is clearly sympathetic with physicians. He mentions the logical ways in which family doctors can become drawn into meeting patient demands even when they are not the most helpful for the patient. In another paper (1982c), he explains how he was able to discern patient meaning regarding an X-ray and thus facilitate communication between doctor and patient. In this example, Stein is behaving much more like a patient advocate, but he sees his actions as facilitating systemic goals. In a third article (1985c), Stein suggests that the clinicians' focus on the culture of patients may be a red herring. First, not all problems of ethnic patients are the result of cultural background. Second, the clinician may call upon the anthropologist to give lengthy explanations of why the person's culture leads him or her to act a particular way when, in fact, difficulties in the doctor-patient relationship or other personally threatening matters are the real issues.

THE IMPORTANCE OF ETHNOGRAPHY

Contributing to anthropologists' holistic view of the world is their central interest in ethnography, which must be an important aspect of their work in clinical settings. For example, their naturalistic descriptions can be the delight of clinicians as long as these are not perceived as overly negative. The early work of William Caudill (1958b) and the more recent work of Robert Edgerton (1967) can be of great value to clinicians. However, as in teaching other aspects of anthropology, clinically applied anthropologists need to do more than simply carry out ethnographies and hand them to clinicians.

An important advantage of anthropology's ethnographic approach for work with clinicians is attention to context (Johnson 1987a; Press 1985). Anthropologists are unlikely to view the patient, or even the patient's immediate family, in isolation. Hospital social organization profoundly influences patient behavior, as well as the behavior of practitioners. Moving beyond the walls of the hospital, community economic and political issues are extremely important to the provision of health care, and anthropology can expand clinicians' understanding of these factors. Sim Galazka and J. Kevin Eckert (1986) show how such contextual features can be taught and can make a difference in primary medical care.

Ethnography is also a valuable tool for understanding clinicians and the clinical setting. Some have reasoned (Johnson 1987b; Stein 1982c) that anthropologists are accustomed to moving in with the natives to learn their culture. Given the importance of knowing clinician culture well enough to avoid mistakes and to become accepted, it makes sense to use ethnographic skills for this task (Weidman 1983). The benefits of thinking in an ethnographic way about one's job are manifold. (We are not suggesting carrying out a formal ethnography, though our physician and nurse colleagues frequently ask us whether we are doing so.) As all of us learned in field situations, the process of asking purposefully naive or empathic questions about any setting aids in creating rapport with those who work therein. This is especially true of hospitals or other health care facilities, where clinicians can be overly sensitive to criticism by adversarial social scientists. Moreover, explicit examination of the environment can produce understandings that may not emerge with a less methodologically explicit approach. For example, subtle status differences between types of colleagues may be discovered.

Finally, ethnography might be used as the basis for a process of reconciling different cultural systems, as between practitioners and patients. Michael Agar (1986) sees ethnography as an encounter among different traditions. Perhaps a clinically applied anthropologist can accomplish this reconciliation through carrying out good ethnography (which includes establishing rapport and maintaining status and role ambiguity), communicating its results to patients and practitioners, and acting as an advocate for the entire system. Clifford Barnett (1985) has suggested that anthropological research is the best avenue for influencing clinicians. Yet such research cannot be reported as it would be to anthropology colleagues. It is necessary to use a culturally sensitive approach in communicating the results of research to practitioners. In short, ethnography is a legacy of traditional anthropology that must not be abandoned simply because we assume we are working in our own culture.

DEVELOPMENT OF PRESCRIPTIVE THEORY

One of the most significant issues facing clinically applied anthropologists is the matter of theory. Theory may be considered in two ways: as anthropological concepts and their relationships that constitute the core of our discipline (Galazka and Eckert 1986) and as perspectives on how to use these concepts in clinical settings (Friedman 1983). We are able to take the first for granted since anthropological concepts and theories, along with methodology, define much of what anthropologists do. The second, how to apply the discipline, is undeveloped and requires much more thought and practice among clinically applied anthropologists.

Anthropologists must be able to contribute a theoretical perspective to health practitioners since we argue, implicitly or explicitly, that new approaches are needed in medicine. This means that we need to have an explicit rationale for how to provide culturally sensitive care. Sue Donaldson and Dorothy Crowley (1978) refer to this as "prescriptive theory." One aspect of prescriptive theory relates to the clinician question: "Under what circumstances should this anthropological approach be used?" Implicit here is the assumption that anthropological approaches are somehow akin to carrying out a medical procedure, such as a patient history or an ophthalmoscopic examination. In medicine, there are some indications for carrying out one procedure and others that suggest a different one.

What are some of the indicators that might lead clinicians to respond with an anthropological approach? One is the presence of patients identified as ethnically different. Health practitioners, who tend to view anthropology as a basic science to provide background data for their practices, are stimulated to think about the need for cultural knowledge when they work among ethnically distinct patients. We receive calls two to three times a year asking for information about specific ethnic groups. Frequently, the inquirer says that he or she is treating more people from that group and wants to know about their culture so as not to offend them or treat them improperly. This is a positive step for a practitioner to take. From an anthropological viewpoint, however, it is too exclusive. Rather than seeing ethnic diversity among patients as the sole stimulus to culturally sensitive care, we hope that this type of care would be used with every patient.

A second situation that motivates practitioners to seek specific cultural information is when a particular patient complaint seemingly can be tied to ethnicity. When there is a problem with an "ethnic" patient, anthropological knowledge makes sense, particularly to clinicians who have had prior positive experiences with anthropology in patient care. It is interesting, and quite unfortunate, that for the same complaint in a "nonethnic" patient, practitioners usually turn to a psychologist for behavioral information or a biological scientist for biological data. One of the major battles for clinically applied anthropologists is to assert continually that cultural data and a culturally sensitive approach are relevant to all patients, not just to those whose ethnic background happens to be different from the practitioner's.

Although clinically applied anthropologists argue that a culturally sensitive approach is always necessary in health care (Tripp-Reimer 1983b), we have not always been clear or in agreement with each other about what that approach should be. If clinically applied anthropology is to have some validity as a field, development of an anthropological approach to patient care and its dissemination to health practitioners is essential. In other words, we need to develop a prescriptive theory. There are certainly consistencies in what clinically applied anthropologists do in clinical settings. Here we outline what medical anthropologists see as core information for use by clinicians.

Topics that frequently are considered by clinically applied anthropologists include a focus on ethnocentrism, eliciting patient perspectives, the disease-illness distinction, holism, the importance of context when understanding behavior, and the concepts of culture, values, beliefs, customs, ethnic group, and the like. Perhaps what they add up to is a statement of a theoretical view in clinically applied anthropology. How these concepts are used may be the basis for prescriptive theory.

RELEVANT KNOWLEDGE

There are two general bundles of information that clinically applied anthropologists use in their dealings with clinicians. First, in response to clinicians' felt needs for culture-specific information, anthropologists provide data on a variety of subjects about specific ethnic groups—"the ethnic cookbook" (and there are some excellent ones: Barker and Clark 1992; Clark 1983; Harwood 1981; Spector 1991). Second is a set of topics that would be presented in any introductory course in cultural anthropology (Weidman 1983:3). This latter information is not necessarily well received in undigested form by practitioners, but it is an important part of developing a culturally sensitive approach to health care. For example, the concept of culture presented in an academic and abstract debate is of little interest to clinicians. Interestingly, some nonanthropologists who write about ethnic health care for clinician audiences include these same topics (Louie 1985).

Culture is an essential concept for anthropologists to introduce because it is so central to the discipline and because a concern with problems evidently caused or exacerbated by culture is a major reason that anthropologists are consulted by health practitioners. However, our lack of clarity about the difference between "Culture" (generalized patterned behavior or rules) and "culture" (a specific culture or subculture) frequently leads to confusion among practitioners, just as it does among managers in organizations (Morey and Morey 1994).

Definitions of culture utilized clinically are those traditionally used in anthropology. For example, Toni Tripp-Reimer, a nurse-anthropologist, defined culture in a chapter for undergraduate nursing students as the "total lifeways of a human group. It consists of learned patterns of values, beliefs, customs, and behaviors that are shared by a group of interacting individuals. More than material objects, culture is a set of rules or standards for behavior" (1984a:226). Chrisman uses a shortened version in which culture is defined as a "learned, shared, symbolically transmitted design for living" (Chrisman 1986:62). Rather than transmitting strict definitions, however, clinically applied anthropologists must convey a number of key qualities about culture. The most important of these is that culture supplies a way of perceiving the world, creating different realities across cultures, and thereby provides guidelines for action.

Explicit discussions of culture as an approach to life and its variability across members of the same culture are critical for health practitioners (Isaacs 1983). Practitioners clearly carry around their own versions of reality—tacit understandings of the world built on a foundation of biomedical knowledge that are concrete in many ways. Certainly physiological processes and anatomy are "real" and observable for them, and even abstractions like diseases are similarly real (Taussig 1980a). Culture can also be seen as concrete—like a virus or bacterium—implying to practitioners that knowledge about the cultural pattern of a group will be valid for each individual in the group and will "explain" a particular malady or patient behavior. This may lead to stereotyping, a problem that clinically applied anthropologists aim to reduce. In fact, clinicians sometimes criticize anthropologists for stereotyping when we talk about patterns of group behavior because their tendency is to hear us talking about individual behaviors.

The features of culture as learned and shared are significant aspects of the concept for practitioners. The first, that culture is learned, is clinically important in at least two ways. First, the anthropologist can make the point that not all members of an ethnic group, for example, will share the same culture because of variations in enculturation or acculturation processes. This may reduce problems such as the difficulty created by one clinician who knew about Hispanic health beliefs. He complained that his patient did not know her own culture when she failed to explain her illness in hot and cold terms. Second, if culture can be learned, new perspectives can also be learned from the health practitioner. In fact, we discuss patient teaching with our students as a process of presenting new cultural patterns as options for patients rather than a matter of truth divulged by the clinician.

The notion that culture is shared is also clinically relevant. One of the most difficult problems for both clinicians and anthropologists is deciding whether culture is playing a role in a health problem or in its presentation to a practitioner (Stein 1985c). This is most striking in psychiatry and is one reason that anthropologists have been associated with that medical specialty for so long. Most clinicians now accept the possibility that cultural differences may help explain seemingly bizarre behavior when it occurs, and this may stimulate a telephone call requesting a consultation. One call concerned an Asian man who had attempted suicide, stating that his action was part of his religion. That is, he had hoped to speed up the process of achieving higher spiritual status by living his lives quickly. One response would be to say that although we may not have personal knowledge about that as part of Buddhism, the psychiatrist should call a Buddhist priest and ask. Clinicians should use a different approach when a behavior can be located toward the culturally prescribed and shared end of a theoretical continuum than when a behavior can be placed on the idiosyncratic and pathological end of it.

A second important anthropological concept is custom: those observable behaviors exhibited by members of a culture. Discussions of such culturally patterned behaviors are easy for clinicians to appreciate, especially if our own customs are contrasted with similar ones from other groups. Clinicians want information about customs since they include such behaviors as dietary practices, communication patterns, religious behaviors, and health and illness practices. Specific guidelines for altering these behaviors may be given to practitioners. Learning pragmatic techniques constitutes an important portion of health practitioner training so this activity on the part of anthropologists fits with the educational expectations of most health science students and clinicians; in fact, such guidance may be demanded of anthropologists. For example, practitioners find it useful to learn how to adapt ethnic dietary practices to biomedical requirements for diabetes. Alternative healing practices have been promoted in hospital situations, as when folk healers are invited to practice in a Western hospital. At the very least, it can be helpful to remind clinicians of the relative imperviousness of customs to change so that they will not view noncompliant patients as purposefully defying them and resort to punitive or neglectful treatment strategies.

Another important concept is value, referring to societal evaluative standards. The idea of value constitutes an important concept for health practitioner use since value differences affect patient and family relations with practitioners. Specifically, varying value orientations (like varying health beliefs) influence care seeking, the style of practitioner interaction preferred by patients, the degree to which practitioner suggestions will be followed, and the kinds of self-care that the patient and family will carry out. It is useful to introduce values to practitioners in terms of how they influence the practitioners' own lives. In fact, the clinician's ability to know his or her own values and beliefs is a critical portion of culturally sensitive care. One approach used by a number of writers (Tripp-Reimer 1984a; Hartog and Hartog 1983; Fong 1985) is to discuss the value orientations that Clyde Kluckhohn and Fred Strodtbeck delineated. These broad orientations present ways that societies organize a variety of values that relate to situations of daily life. One orientation popular during the culture of poverty discussions of the 1960s referred to time orientation: past, present, and future. Although there are problems with ethnocentric bias in applying the orientations to specific cases (see Liebow 1967 for a critical evaluation of the misuse of a "present time orientation"), these global perspectives are useful in helping clinicians to comprehend how values pervade everyday life. For example, groups with a future orientation can be seen as more likely to engage in disease prevention efforts.

Beliefs constitute another core concept useful to practitioners. Goodenough's definition—beliefs are propositions accepted as true (1963)—is succinct. However, like culture, beliefs are invisible and thus difficult for clinicians to deal with. The anthropologist must emphasize that patient beliefs need constant attention by clinicians. Most practitioners recognize the possibility that patients may have beliefs that differ from theirs, whether health related or not. It is useful to discuss a variety of beliefs—not only health beliefs—with clinicians so they can begin to recognize the general utility of the term. Case examples about how beliefs can strongly affect behavior are helpful in getting the point across. Experienced clinically applied anthropologists collect a repertoire of cases in which beliefs have affected patients' illness behavior and practitioner care (Kleinman, Eisenberg, and Good 1978) and transmit them in ways that are culturally accepted in medicine as "war stories" and "clinical pearls." The former are almost mythological accounts of particularly difficult patients or disastrous outcomes that reveal truths and are passed on as part of the informal socialization process in medicine. The latter are succinct and often pithy aphorisms delivered with such conviction that they also convey truth.

Discussions of health beliefs identified with particular populations (such as ethnic groups) seem to be enjoyable for health practitioners, just as they are for anthropology students. Beliefs form part of the esoteric lore that anthropologists are famous for repeating. The literature in anthropology is replete with detailed analyses of such interesting beliefs as spiritual sickness, witchcraft, hot and cold imbalances, vital energy, and the like (Snow 1974; Harwood 1971, 1981; Kleinman et al. 1975. Harwood 1981 is a particularly good source for a large number of ethnic groups). It is valuable for practitioners to be acquainted with folk beliefs characteristic of the ethnic groups with which they work so that patients are not referred for psychiatric help when they convey "odd" beliefs to practitioners. In addition, these data may help practitioners learn to work with beliefs and behaviors that seem deviant to them. This ability constitutes the kind of challenge that health practitioners sometimes need in order to maintain interest in their work. We have been surprised on occasions when the residents have already engaged the use of indigenous healers to help care for their patients.

The anthropological love affair with esoteric beliefs also needs to be tempered in clinical settings. A culturally appropriate approach to health care requires that all patient beliefs should be attended to, and in primary care settings the types of health beliefs that will arise are not typically exotic. Clinically applied anthropologists need to discuss everyday beliefs about colds, flu, or appendicitis with the same enthusiasm as spirit possession. Clinicians can learn from this approach that popular culture health beliefs are as important as the more esoteric beliefs for understanding patients. In fact laypeople's use of biomedical terminology may be more misleading to clinicians than folk beliefs.

It is not surprising that ethnocentrism and allied ideas such as cultural relativism should be a routine part of the clinically applied anthropologist's repertoire. Their centrality within anthropology is related to the need to understand peoples' diverse beliefs and behaviors without imposing judgments from one's own culture. Their relativist implications, however, contrast strongly with the universalist and action orientations in biomedicine and may threaten some clinicians. Nonetheless, they are the fundamental lessons that anthropologists have to contribute.

One of the difficulties that clinically applied anthropologists must face is that a relativist perspective is, in itself, relative: that is, a relativist posture may increase the anxiety level of clinicians, who are asked to make decisions based on inadequate data and therefore reflexively strive to reduce, rather than increase, ambiguity and relativity. Practitioners are often uncomfortable with a relativist position because inquiry in clinical settings must lead to action, but relativism easily can cause doubt and promote inaction bound up with reflection.

One way around this problem when working with practitioners is to point out circumstances under which ethnocentrism is and is not appropriate in practice. For example, ethnocentrism may impede taking an accurate history if significant information is dismissed because it is "wrong." Patients likely will refuse to divulge important information if their revelations about folk beliefs or practices have previously elicited negative reactions from practitioners. Practitioners do not like to think of themselves as less than thorough in gathering data, particularly when those data might be "cultural" and thus interesting. Anthropologists can take advantage of this aspect of clinical culture to introduce the necessity of a more relativist approach during the history taking or assessment portion of a clinical encounter (Tripp-Reimer 1983b).

Treatment, on the other hand, requires the confidence, risk taking, and rejection of uncertainty that are hallmarks of clinical practice. For this element of clinical care, ethnocentrism, with its accompanying confidence in the "rightness" of a particular cultural world, is essential. Thus, a kind of ethnocentrism can be promoted for this set of tasks. Anthropological recognition of differences in the diagnosis and treatment activities of clinicians can ease the insertion of a new perspective into a traditional behavior.

A useful way to operationalize the concept of cultural relativism (or the avoidance of ethnocentrism) is the notion of eliciting patient perspectives. Cultural relativity manifested at the individual level is more closely allied to the way clinicians think than is cultural relativism at a societal level. In addition, practitioners are accustomed to listening to their patients. Unfortunately, much of what the patient says is considered to be subjective, with the connotation of "not real" or not as important as "objective" data, such as findings from the physical examination or laboratory tests. Demonstrating that eliciting patients' perspectives on their symptoms can provide equally valuable data makes sense to most clinicians and is usually accepted.

An important related construct for many clinically applied anthropologists is the illness-disease distinction (Fabrega 1972). This seminal idea is related to a relativist point of view and is crucial for the anthropologist who is trying to demonstrate how elicitation of patient perspectives is critical to culturally sensitive care. The past decade has seen more agreement on how to describe the distinction. Illness is identified with the perspective of the popular or folk sectors of the health care system (Kleinman 1980), and thus to the patient; disease is tied to the perspective of the professional sector and its practitioners. In the Western world, disease is a perspective of sickness that refers to some biophysiological abnormality that can be objectively demonstrated by Western scientific means. We teach illness as a view of sickness that refers to distress as experienced, described, and explained by the patient and/or the family (Chrisman 1986:60).

The disease-illness distinction is taught to clinicians so they will be able to recognize multiple ways of experiencing and explaining symptoms and the implications of this for care, to recognize that their way of seeing sickness is not necessarily the only way. For clinicians, neither the words nor the idea of such a contrast is new. As is true for many laypeople as well, disease and illness are seen as different. In addition, the meaning of the contrast seems to be similar. For most Americans, disease refers to the biological process, and illness refers to the experience of the disease. The anthropological contribution is not to restate the contrast in different words but to be able to point to differences in beliefs about sickness as a fundamental property of culture. In addition, anthropologists point out that these beliefs influence the behavior of patients and providers alike.

The concept of an explanatory model (Kleinman, Eisenberg, and Good 1978) aids in concretizing the disease-illness distinction for clinicians. Although there is a great deal of debate within anthropology about what an explanatory model (EM) is and how it should be used (Young 1982), the set of questions used to elicit an EM and the idea that it constitutes important data to gather from a patient are easy to transmit to health practitioners. This should not be surprising; Kleinman and Eisenberg are physicians, and the questions strongly resemble questions used in normal primary care encounters. In brief, eliciting an EM involves asking open-ended questions about the patient's notions of symptom etiology, onset, pathophysiology, severity, course, and appropriate treatment.

We try to use the similarity of EM questions and primary care questions as the means to introduce the value of eliciting a patient's EM. We argue that good clinicians obtain most of this information anyway. The requirement for higher cultural sensitivity is to elicit and process the information—the patient's cultural perspective—as an essential step in patient care and not merely as an oddity. In addition, as Kleinman (1988b:chap. 15) points out, these questions and others about family, occupation, and the like promote a fuller view of the patient in ways that may not be obvious on the first encounter but may be crucial later in the practitioner-patient relationship. Medical and nursing students have difficulty recognizing that when they are in practice, their relationships with patients will often last longer than the examples experienced in their training.

Like other anthropological ideas, the notion of an EM has become modified in its usage among health practitioners (Like and Steiner 1986). For example, the family practice residents with whom we work seem to refer to an explanation of cause(s) for symptoms only when they use the term. By ignoring the richness of EM information—for example, the range of treatments already used, whether the health problem is chronic, and the fears associated with the sickness—much of the point that illness is embedded in social life can be lost. Graduate students in nursing are susceptible to attending to the model aspect of the concept and use the term to refer to a model of thinking about patients in which culture is taken into account.

The degree to which anthropological ideas and terminology can be tuned to serve the needs of clinicians is nicely illustrated in a paper by Robert Like and R. P. Steiner, "Medical Anthropology and the Family Physician" (1986; see also Galazka and Eckert 1986). These physicians, sophisticated in the clinical applications of anthropology and the other behavioral sciences, make a similar distinction to the one we made earlier in this chapter between medical and clinically applied anthropology:

The anthropology of family medicine can be considered to represent a subdiscipline within family medicine, and will be defined here as the academic field which specializes in the study of the cultural dimensions of family health and illness in the context of primary care medical practice. The anthropology of family practice, or clinically applied anthropology, focuses on the ways in which family practitioners employ anthropological knowledge and techniques in the everyday care of patients and their families. (Like and Steiner 1986:88)

They go on to state the basics of a culturally sensitive approach to patient care. Other authors have reported similar success with culturally sensitive care (Capers 1985; Fong 1985), and their work should encourage clinically applied anthropologists to formulate our roles with clinicians so that they reflect the broad strength of anthropology, including its unique perspectives on the world.

SUMMARY AND CONCLUSIONS

We use the same set of ideas in single lectures to clinicians, to structure whole classes, or to organize our thoughts when collaborating on clinical cases. Having this conceptual framework in mind helps us to be consistent over time and with a variety of practitioners. For example, we teach nurses at graduate and undergraduate levels; physicians during medical school, residencies, and as fellows; and other health practitioners, such as social workers and occupational therapists; and we work with epidemiologists and biostatisticians in public health settings. Chrisman refers to his contribution as "Culture-Sensitive Care" (Chrisman 1986, 1991a, 1991b) in order to identify it clearly for clinicians. It is based on the notion of culture as a way of imputing meaning to the world. Values and beliefs are analytically distinct aspects of culture that are useful in understanding health-related behavior. Legitimate variation in perception is the fundamental message. Closely linked to these ideas is a discussion of ethnocentrism and cultural relativism, phrased as cautions about losing data or misunderstanding the patient. We see a narrow construction of the health care system and a restriction in understanding of sickness simply to disease as strong contributors to medical ethnocentrism. To counteract this, we introduce Kleinman's more complex view of the health care system with folk, popular, and professional sectors (Kleinman 1980) and the disease-illness distinction.

We use the health-seeking process (Chrisman 1977; Chrisman and Kleinman 1983) as the means to introduce a broad perspective of an illness episode. The idea of an EM and how to elicit one is introduced as part of the patient's perception of the health care problem and is seen as part of the symptom definition element of health seeking. Moreover, for clinicians who work in heterogeneous urban settings, we talk about illness belief systems (Chrisman 1986).

There are four types of illness beliefs: equilibrium (hot-cold) beliefs or germ-theory beliefs are two of them. These identify major illness beliefs in a variety of cultures and serve to acquaint clinicians with beliefs in a way that is usable. We relate the various beliefs with treatments. A key approach is to provide enough information about a variety of healers, including Western practitioners, so that the clinician will recognize strengths as well as weaknesses. This is particularly important with clinicians who worry about quacks (see Chrisman 1991a).

We also attempt to include the patient's immediate social environment—seen in terms of family, social network, and community—in a discussion of lay consultation and referral. Finally, we examine the concept of sick role and make two major points. One is that clinicians tend to focus on only one aspect of the sick role—release from normal social obligations—without attending to other aspects, such as feelings of responsibility. This approach stresses the negotiation aspects such as feelings of responsibility that occur between patients and their social environment. The second aspect of sick role refers to the chronic sick role. American culture has not yet adopted a cultural definition of chronic illness, and this hampers both practitioners and patients as they work together (see Kleinman 1988b). In a short presentation, we may conclude with the negotiation process (Katon and Kleinman 1980); in other situations, this approach is discussed more or less continuously.

We see negotiation as the culmination of skills and attitudes that are strongly promoted with an anthropological approach: cultural relativism or valuing the patient perspective as a major attitude and open-ended questioning to achieve a native view as a major skill. In addition, we consider the overall approach of valuing alternative realities, expanding the clinical view to encompass much of the social environment, and being willing to negotiate as essential parts of culturally sensitive care.

Clinically applied anthropology emerged from the ongoing activities of anthropologists working in clinical settings. In the beginning, each may have felt somewhat isolated since there was little discussion. Over the past two decades, however, discussions of these activities have been published; clinically applied anthropologists have discovered that we do have some things in common and we can enunciate a set of skills and perspectives from successful clinical work. Now there is a need to go beyond the scope of this chapter and formulate more prescriptive theory. Categorizing such theories will greatly simplify training for clinically applied anthropology. More important, is the opportunity to design clinical trials of culturally appropriate care to test systematically what many of us assume to be true based on rewarding clinical experiences: that an anthropological approach changes health care delivery in positive ways.

Part II

Medical Systems

6

Ethnomedicine

Arthur J. Rubel and Michael R. Hass

In this chapter we discuss some of the more salient approaches taken by anthropologists in their analyses of illness, healing, and those who provide assistance when sickness strikes. We discuss an anthropological interest that has evolved from curiosity about exotic beliefs and customs related to health and illness into a robust, rapidly growing, anthropological specialization. We will emphasize the evolving approach to attributions of sickness, the social use of sickness and healing for purposes of social control, and the recruitment and training of healers. We hope to demonstrate how these studies have contributed to the development of general theory and methodology in sociocultural anthropology, in addition to the emergence of the subfield of ethnomedicine. The chapter concludes with recommendations for the kinds of research necessary for the continued healthy growth of ethnomedicine.

HISTORICAL OVERVIEW OF ETHNOMEDICAL APPROACHES

Healing, shamanism, and the relationship between illness and supernatural forces have captured the interest of ethnologists and the public from anthropology's earliest days (Tylor 1871; Seligmann 1910; Frazer 1911). These early classics reported from the far corners of the earth seemingly bizarre notions of the causes of illness and diagnostic procedures that invoked supernatural spirits or machinating spouses or neighbors. Accounts of the recruitment of diviners and counter-witchcraft specialists to discover the causes of illness had strong appeal for turn-of-the-century readers, whose own beliefs about health had just been radically altered by the industrial and scientific revolutions (Osherson and Amarasingham 1981; Starr 1982; Freidson 1970).

By the 1930s research in the origins and provenance of the cultural components of medical systems was a prominent dimension of American cultural anthropology (Clements 1932). Since ideas and behavior related to sickness and
healing were considered a significant part of culture, efforts to reconstruct the
processes of culture building included close study of the tools and other para-
phernalia of healers. In this effort, the distribution of culture traits related to
health and the control of sickness were mapped and analyzed by Clements,
resulting in the identification of five major causes of disease in the nonindustrial
world: sorcery, soul loss, breach of a taboo, intrusion by a disease object, and
intrusion by a spirit. It was concluded that a society can be characterized by the
disease cause most prominently reported for it (e.g., as a spirit-intrusion society
or a soul-loss society). In addition, Clements sought to infer from the spatial
distribution of these traits how long they had been a part of a particular culture
under study (cf. Kroeber 1947).

Clements's work was roundly criticized by researchers who saw more promise
in the configurationist approach being advanced by Ruth Benedict in her *Patterns of Culture*. A major argument, forcefully pursued (Ackernecht 1971:31),
contended that a configurationist approach placed medicine in its cultural context: "What counts are not the forms but the place medicine occupies in the
life of a tribe or people, the spirit which pervades its practice, the way in which
it merges with other traits from different fields of experience." His critique was
a harbinger of a radical shift from a historical approach to research on health
phenomena to an ahistorical, empirical orientation. The emerging functionalism
viewed society as comprising interrelated parts, concepts of disease and its
causes, and the characteristic of healers being interdependent (Ackernecht 1971:
31, 54, 55; Wellin 1977:50–51; Beals 1980:289–91).

One of the earliest (Rivers 1924) and, subsequently, most prominent ways in
which ethnomedicine contributed to the development of theory and method in
sociocultural anthropology was to show the functional integration of the components of health care institutions within society's cultural matrix, its social
organization, or political system. The functional integration approach, together
with what have become known as the cognitive and symbolic approaches, have
become the dominant theoretical approaches to institutions of health care for the
approximately half-century since Clements published his major work.

As anthropology became more systematic and research more sophisticated,
ethnomedicine became one of the essential dimensions of culture investigated.
As the community study method increased in popularity, especially in studies
of Mexico and Guatemala (Chambers and Young 1979), greater prominence
was given to a society's conceptualizations of illness (the causes and cures), the
role of healers, and the relationship between concepts of disease and cosmology.
Links were identified between what had appeared to be bizarre health beliefs
and practices and other aspects of the culture or social organization (Cassel
1955; Rubel 1960, 1966a; Marwick 1965; Lieban 1967; O'Nell and Selby 1968;
Garrison 1977b; Lindenbaum 1979). These findings contributed to a more

culturally relativistic attitude toward other peoples' health practices and understandings (Lewis 1975:201). Even the most exotic-appearing health beliefs and
behaviors are made understandable in the cultural context in which they are
found.

For example, the many productive studies of the attribution of sickness and
death to witchcraft or sorcery identify them as prime sources for students seeking
information on cultural interpretations of how and why sickness and death are
visited on some members of a group but not others. The assumption that people
become ill because they have been victimized by neighbors transformed into
animals was rendered more accessible by the reports of Villa Rojas (1947) and
others that in some societies, transgressions of social norms are believed to be
sanctioned by illness visited on the transgressor.

Villa Rojas utilized the structural-functionalist approach to good advantage in
analyzing the causes of sickness among Tzeltals of southern Mexico. That analysis appeared in the forefront of a number of important works in which associations were drawn between the social norms governing behavior and the
attribution of sickness to supernatural forces charged with maintenance of those
norms (Dillon-Malone 1988; Vogt 1969; Stratmeyer and Stratmeyer 1977:135–
36; Holland 1963a; Adams and Rubel 1967). Sometimes those who use illness
to punish a failure to follow the social norms are those holding official positions;
sometimes it is the deceased or supernatural figures who play this role (Nadel
1952; Rubel 1960; Marwick 1964:263–68; Turner 1967:282; Vogt 1969; Bahr
et al. 1974; Evans-Pritchard, cited by Lewis 1975:200; Howell 1984).

The connection is elegantly developed (Whiting 1950) in a study of a small
society of Native Americans, the Harney Valley Paiute. These Paiute have few
formal mechanisms of social control (police, army, courts, or judges) but a well-
developed fear of sorcery. Sickness attributed to sorcery is hypothesized as representing a societal sanction of socially unacceptable behavior rather than
interpersonal enmity. This explanation seems plausible and does elucidate the
fear of sorcery as a mechanism for maintenance of social order among the people
of Harney Valley. But its even more vital contribution is to test the hypothesis
that the attribution of illness to sorcery may contribute to the more successful
functioning of some kinds of society with social organizations, like the Harney
Valley Paiute, but not other kinds. As a result, we now know that in societies
in which formal institutions of social control are absent or weak, sorcery attributions are more frequent. In societies in which institutions like a police force,
courts, or an army are prominent, attributions of sickness to sorcery are less
frequent.

In a subsequent examination of that hypothesis in connection with a Filipino
Christian group under the hierarchical control of the modern Philippine Republic, sorcery allegations are found to be rampant (Lieban 1967). These allegations
prove, however, to be associated with social discord that is not clearly assigned
to a formal social control agency (e.g., police or army). Competition for a lover,
conflict between spouses, broken verbal agreements, and arguments over own-

ership of land in which title is not unequivocally vested fall between the cracks, not being clearly in the domain of a provincial or federal court or clearly under familial control. In these cases, sickness is a form of punishment presumed exacted by means of sorcery. In other words, sorcery fills the void when responsibility for the resolution of conflict has not been clearly assigned (cf. Gluckman 1965:viii; Marwick 1965; Lindenbaum 1979).

Although anthropological interest in the attribution of sickness and other health phenomena dates from at least 1915 (Rivers, republished 1979; Ackernecht 1958:4–5), it was not until 1968 that the term *ethnomedicine* was applied (Hughes 1968; cf. Ackernecht 1971:11). In that year Hughes applied the term to "those beliefs and practices relating to disease which are the products of indigenous cultural development and are not explicitly derived from the conceptual framework of modern medicine." Subsequently *ethnomedicine* was applied more broadly to refer to "culturally oriented studies of illness," and it was argued that the concern of the ethnomedical investigator was to explain "an illness—its genesis, mechanism, descriptive features, treatment, and resolution—as an event having cultural significance" (Fabrega 1974:39–43). One year later, ethnomedicine was defined as the "study of how members of different cultures think about disease and organize themselves toward medical treatment and the social organization of treatment itself" (Fabrega 1975:969). More recently, Nichter (1992:x) described ethnomedical inquiry as the "study of how well-being and suffering are experienced bodily as well as socially, the multivocality of somatic communication, and processes of healing as they are contextualized and directed toward the person, household, community and state, land and cosmos."

Consideration of ethnomedical matters in the holistic investigation of the cultural life of communities gave increasing prominence to the group's conceptualizations of illness, its causes and cures, the role of healers, and the relationship between concepts of disease and cosmology. Additional studies more narrowly analyzed specific ethnomedical issues (Cooper 1933, 1934; Hallowell 1934; Honigmann 1947; Teicher 1960; Aberle 1952; Gussow 1960; Wallace 1960). That large amount of attention paid ethnomedical observations in the first half of this century contrasts with a view (Landy 1977) that anthropologists had paid little attention to medical matters in the first half of this century.[1]

Ethnomedical Systems in Comparative Perspective

The effort to contrast and oppose "other" kinds of medicine with the increasingly dominant allopathy as practiced by medical physicians represents a serious problem, long impeding comparative medical studies. The difficulty contributes to a befuddlement as to the appropriate way to refer to allopathy, much less how to refer to those "other" systems so as to avoid invidious comparisons. It has been essential to find a nonpejorative term with which to describe biomedicine—the ethnomedicine in which medical physicians are trained—so as to be able to compare and contrast that ethnomedical system with others without making a priori value judgments. We will refer to the former henceforth as *cosmopolitan medicine* to distinguish it from other ethnomedicines (Dunn 1976: 135–37). To do otherwise is to fall prey to absurdities (Leslie 1976). For example, to describe the practices of curing among American, Mexican, or German laypersons as not modern when they are widely practiced in the year this is written is foolish. Similarly problematic is to label as non-Western those diagnoses or healing procedures extensively practiced today in suburban New Jersey or in the neighborhoods of Detroit or Los Angeles (Mcgoire 1988). To refer to allopathy as the uniquely university-based medicine is to fail to account for the tens of thousands of physicians in India or Sri Lanka trained in the many university medical schools in which Ayurvedic medicine is the subject of lectures, laboratory training, and clinical preparation, to say nothing of the thousands of licensed doctors of osteopathic medicine produced in the past decade by American medical schools. For the reasons just indicated we will henceforth refer to the medicine practiced by physicians trained in biomedicine as *cosmopolitan medicine,* and other ethnomedicines will be referred to by the name of the group of which it forms part of the culture (e.g., Bontoc medicine, Chinantec medicine, Zulu medicine).

Critiques of the Ethnomedical Approach

Critiques of the rapidly growing field of ethnomedical studies (Fabrega 1974; Rubel 1983a) draw attention to its peculiarly mentalistic orientation. Fabrega (1974:40) wrote:

The implicit assumption adopted by the researcher is that he is dealing with a disorder that is either typically psychiatric or at least psychiatric-like. Excessive preoccupation with this dimension on the part of culturally oriented anthropologists has tended to obscure the influences that biological components have on [culturally defined] illnesses. Consequently, the potential of examining the reciprocal influences that psychocultural and biological factors have on instances of illness occurrence [as defined and categorized by subjects] has been missed.

Indeed, ethnomedical studies are often conducted in societies in which such killer diseases as infant diarrhea, pulmonary tuberculosis, "river blindness," and schistosomiasis are rampant with little, if any, attention to the local population's cultural response to these diseases. Instead, research fastens on concepts, prevention, and curing of folk diseases or diseases with psychiatric implications (see reviews by Lieban 1973; Wellin 1977).

As a consequence of this emphasis, the impact of ethnomedical ethnographies on cosmopolitan medicine and, in particular, the culturally relativistic analyses of health institutions and practices in diverse societies have been primarily in broadening and making more flexible the psychiatric categories of the *Interna-*

tional Classification of Disease and the *Diagnostic and Statistical Manual* (Devereux 1956; Simons and Hughes 1985; Hufford 1988; Kapur 1987; Prince and Tcheng-LaRoche 1987). The growing number of cosmopolitan physicians engaged in studies of how illness in other ethnomedical systems is constructed and responded to by patients promises new efforts to examine the implications of comparative studies for the diagnosis and treatment of patients (Lewis 1975; Helman 1978; Like and Ellison 1981).

Current Controversies: The Case of Humoral Medicine

Humoral medicine, one of the most thoroughly studied topics in ethnomedicine, remains a subject of controversy. The concept of opposing humoral qualities' affecting health is a prominent premise of Latin American and other ethnomedicines. According to this theory, health is a matter of balance between the opposites "hot" and "cold," "wet" and "dry" (Browner 1985a; Escobar, Salazar, and Chung 1983; Graham 1976; Hart 1969; Kay 1977; Kendall, Foote, and Martorell 1983; Nations and Rebhun 1988; Rubel, 1960, 1966a; Schreiber and Homiak 1981; Scheper-Hughes 1988).

One orientation to the widespread humoral concepts among Amerindians is to attribute their origins to the pre-Christian eras of Greek and Arab history (Foster 1953, 1978a, 1978b). Proponents consider that this humoral theory of health and illness was introduced to indigenous America in the sixteenth century by the Spanish conquerors. Four humors—hot, cold, wet, and dry—constituted this important system. A person's state of health was to be attributed to a state of balance between such opposite qualities as hot and cold, and wet and dry. Reference to these humoral qualities appears again and again in ethnographic accounts of Spanish and Portuguese-speaking people's efforts to engage in preventive health and to cure themselves or others of disease.

Compelling data have, however, been marshalled to show that prior to the arrival in America of Europeans, the concept of opposite qualities played a prominent role in health care of indigenous American societies (Colson and de Armellado 1983; Lopez Austin 1975, 1980; Ortiz de Montellano 1986, 1987, 1992). Other, more radical criticisms question whether such understanding of opposite qualities was systematically distributed among these populations, much less systematically applied as measures of preventive and curative health (Weller 1983).

Although no one disputes that the concepts of hot and cold are remarkably widespread in Latin America or that they undergird much of the diagnostic and healing practices of these populations, whether of Indian or non-Indian cultural background, our concern is the extent to which this critical system is systematically distributed and used within these groups. For instance, we know (Kay 1977a:162) that in one Spanish-speaking barrio of Tucson, Arizona, "no woman under 30 could make such a distinction [between qualities of hot and cold] or seemed to be aware of this system of classification." In Guatemala, although women recognize hot and cold conceptual categories and their application to nutritional and medicinal decisions are widespread (Weller 1983), they are simply not systematically distributed, and perhaps never were. On the other hand, the free recall task Weller used by which to make salient the respondents' own domains of illness may not have provided an adequate key to tap the women's concepts of humoral qualities. When the humoral categories of disease provided by a sample of urban Guatemalans are compared with those elicited from women who live in the countryside, "the disease terms that were categorized beyond the chance level by the rural women were not necessarily the same ones significantly categorized by the urban women, nor were they necessarily categorized in the same manner." Inasmuch as a reader might conclude that these women simply fail to order things or concepts, such as humoral qualities, into categories, it is important to realize that these same women did systematically agree in their assessments of the levels of "severity" and "contagion" associated with familiar disease names (Weller 1983:255; Young 1980; Logan 1977).

Among highland Chinantecs of Mexico, although the conceptualization and utilization of humoral categories is widespread (Browner 1985a), a more encompassing system cross-cuts that of hot and cold. This one is based on mechanical understandings of human physiological processes. In the Chinantec-speaking municipality of San Francisco, the physiological processes of reproduction are managed by the use of medicinal plants, some of which are of a hot quality, others cold. However, rather than using these qualities according to some arcane logic, townswomen pragmatically select humorally hot or cold plants to set off bodily mechanisms (e.g., to cause the uterus to evacuate its contents—whether the intent is to facilitate labor, prevent a conception, or cause a miscarriage—or to retain them—to prevent miscarriage or to arrest excessive menstrual flow or spontaneous menstrual hemorrhaging). This analysis is important because it interprets the use of hot and cold concepts as facilitators of an underlying system by means of which essential physiological mechanisms are regulated. Those results also provide reason to investigate similar efforts to manage physiological processes in other indigenous groups. However, in another Mexican group (Fabrega and Silver 1973:85), there are "no indications anywhere in Zinacanteco curing that h'iloletik [shamans] or their patients think or act about illnesses on the basis of concepts that involve the body as a system composed of functionally interrelated parts and processes—with the possible exception of body temperature." These investigations raise the question why the results and conclusions of so many investigations of the same humoral categories of disease are in conflict.

Several students of the problem have asked the same question (Logan 1977; Weller 1983). Logan suggests that the problems attaching to research in humoral qualities plague ethnomedicine in general:

Most ethnographic accounts of humoral medicine are descriptive, in that no specific hypotheses or set of relationships are central to the given research. It is of limited use simply to report that a given people classify certain items or conditions as hot and others as cold. For without explanation, that is, without relating the data to some fact of the group's culture, ecology, or biological adaptations, the data tell us little more than certain items and conditions are judged, by some informants, to be hot or cold. (1977:95)

It is possible that the questions researchers ask about humors are phrased ambiguously (Weller 1983), leading to different answers to apparently similar questions. Unfortunately, this cannot be evaluated, inasmuch as readers are seldom provided information as to the questions asked. Neither are readers provided the criteria by which respondents are included in the sample, the sample size, or how the data were collected (Logan 1977). In view of the fact that organizing hypotheses are not utilized, and interviews or information as to the constitution or size of the sample are commonly unavailable, collection of a cumulative body of data has been problematic. Furthermore, earlier studies mistakenly assumed homogeneous understandings of humoral categories, failing to account for intracultural variability or variation within individuals' accounts in the context of such life events as sickness, pregnancy, and lactation (Logan 1977:102, 104; Weller 1983:256). Until such methodological problems are resolved, it is too soon to conclude that ethnomedical domains are not systematically distributed within a social group (Weller 1983:255).

Current Use of Ethnomedical Paradigms

Much of the research on ethnomedical systems has focused on the questions of how ethnomedical phenomena are classified, how illness experiences are given meaning by patients and healers, and how ethnomedical knowledge influences health-seeking behavior. A recent development has been an increasing interest in the efficacy of traditional healing methods.

Access as to how a group classifies ethnomedical phenomena has been achieved by studying the language it uses to describe illness symptoms. In one pioneering study of Subanun diagnosis of skin disease (Frake 1961), it was assumed that cognitive structures underlying illness behavior and decision making were implicit in symptoms, which were systematically elicited from informants with standardized questions. That approach was subsequently improved by making the questions asked even more specific (Metzger and Williams 1963). In a study of curers and curing in highland Chiapas, Mexico, Metzger and Williams formulated their questions in terms of the informants' own concepts and categories rather than their own. They discovered unforeseen subtle distinctions in Tzeltal illness categories, illuminating a classificatory system far more complex than previously considered.

Other researchers, however, argue that not all of a people's knowledge about health and disease can be accurately represented by unidimensional semantic representations (D'Andrade et al. 1972). Using multidimensional scaling instruments, they show how members of different cultural groups cluster diseases on the basis of a number of attributes or features. Comparing English-speaking Americans' and Spanish-speaking Mexicans' disease classifications, these researchers found that for both subject groups, diseases were not organized conceptually on the basis of the features that formally defined them but on the basis of pragmatic dimensions, such as type of victim, consequence or impact of the disease, and kind of remedy indicated. This conclusion marked a shift away from features that define disease to the way people perceive the impact of disease on their lives.

THE MEANING OF ILLNESS

The influential concept of explanatory models of illness also recognizes the importance of context. Explanatory models are sets of beliefs or understandings that specify for an illness episode its cause, time, and mode of onset of symptoms, pathophysiology, course of sickness, and treatment. Explanatory models are "formed and employed to cope with a specific health problem, and consequently they need to be analyzed in *that* concrete setting" (Kleinman 1980:106, emphasis added). Although others have invoked the concept of an explanatory model of illness as a cultural construct (Friedl 1982), Kleinman makes it clear that his explanatory models are attributes of individuals, drawing upon general cultural knowledge but remaining at least partially idiosyncratic and situational. Kleinman's work, and that of many others influenced by his approach, however, fail to specify in any detail the extent to which individual explanatory models are shaped by culture and the extent to which they are idiosyncratic formulations.

A major innovative effort to analyze this important issue is found in a study of the Canadian Ojibway (Garro 1988). Combining in a single study the explanatory model and the cognitive approach to health understandings, Garro found an average of 78 percent of the personal explanations—explanatory models—reflect the shared Ojibway cultural model. Using this approach to understand Ojibway explanation of high blood pressure, we now know that individual Ojibway have explanatory models that draw from the group's shared cultural knowledge about high blood pressure.

Another limitation of the explanatory model approach is that models focusing on designation and classification do not inform us about the links between illness and social context. In contrast, on the basis of fieldwork in the Iranian city of Maragheh, Good examined the complaint of heart distress in its social and cultural context. Using information on the distribution of heart distress in a stratified sample of 750 persons from Maragheh and the surrounding area in conjunction with an explanatory model drawn from local traditions of Galenic-Islamic and sacred-Islamic medicine, he described the social and affective context of the experience in terms of a semantic illness network: the "words, situations, symptoms and feelings which are associated with an illness and give it meaning for the sufferer" (1977:39). In his view, heart distress not only served as a vehicle for the expression of social stress but was also used instrumentally to bring about action to relieve it.

Elsewhere, in another study about the ways in which a group speaks and thinks about sickness, it was observed (Bibeau 1981) that over the course of an illness episode, villagers change the labels assigned the signs and symptoms of the condition. In these observations among the Ngbandi of Zaire, Bibeau concluded that to understand medical language, one must examine it in context. Bibeau's observation that the Ngbandi name for a disease changed from one context to another (e.g., when discussing the site at which the condition is located, or the extent to which it resembles an animal, or if it is assumed to represent a social sanction for inappropriate behavior) led him to develop the idea of a network of names associated with a particular disease. Each name in the network refers to a different feature or characteristic of the disease, changing from one context to another. Bibeau discusses six principles that underlie the origins of the different labels used contextually, or what he refers to as "speech situations." Like D'Andrade, Bibeau emphasizes the productive or generative capacity of language systems. Bibeau attempts to contextualize verbalized medical categories and forge links between them and the social settings in which they occur. Yet another effort (Early 1982:1491) to contextualize health knowledge focused on therapeutic narratives—"commentary on illness progression, curative actions, and surrounding events"—that occur naturally among members of the lay therapy management group (an idea that appears to have been borrowed from Janzen's 1978b work in Zaire). Others (Lindenbaum 1979; Morsy 1978; Rubel 1960; Turner 1967) have also written of how symbols of ill health serve multiple social purposes.

Whereas ethnomedicine's insistence on providing the cultural context in which an illness is analyzed has enriched our understanding of how cultures construct illness and has expanded the forms that illness can assume, that emphasis has inhibited cross-cultural comparison. A methodology has recently been proposed (Browner, Ortiz de Montellano, and Rubel 1988) that might render certain types of cross-cultural comparison ethnographically valid and systematic. When cultural processes are anchored to physiological mechanisms, which are the same species wide, responses to those referents by different cultural groups can be more readily compared. For example, comparative ethnographic descriptions of illness in infants in which diarrhea is a salient physiological process illustrate what might be done with this approach. Many ethnomedical studies describe chronic infantile diarrhea, accompanied by a depressed fontanel, eyes seemingly sunken in the face, apathy, and sometimes vomiting. Cosmopolitan medicine refers to this congeries of symptoms as dehydration associated with diarrhea. Other cultural groups, such as the sixteenth-century Aztec; contemporary Hondurans, Peruvians, and Brazilians; Mexican Americans of Texas; Shona and Ndebele of East Africa; and East Indians respond in diverse ways to the same signs and symptoms of biological dysfunction.

Some of these ethnomedical systems attribute the condition to the escape of the infant's vital force through the still-open fontanel (Lopez Austin 1967; Ortiz de Montellano 1987:392). In others it is attributed to pressure or trauma, which depresses the fontanel, in turn causing the upper palate to block the oral passageway (Rubel 1960). Elsewhere the condition is attributed to the child's mother's breast feeding him or her too soon after she has been exposed to a woman who has recently experienced a miscarriage (Lozoff, Kamath, and Feldman 1975). In another system, biomedicine, the same condition is explained by intrusion of an enteric pathogen, causing the infant an infection, of which loose stools is a consequence (Jelliffe 1966), whereas in parts of Brazil it is a consequence of the evil eye (Nations and Rebhun 1988). It is striking that some ethnomedical systems explain the condition as dehydration, of which a depressed fontanel is a manifestation, while others understand the characteristic runny stool, fluid loss, sunken eyes, and fitfulness to be *caused by* the depression of the fontanel.

ETHNOMEDICINE AND HEALTH-SEEKING BEHAVIOR

Ethnomedical research has made a significant contribution to the understanding of how knowledge about illness influences health-seeking behavior. But recent investigations have emphasized that verbalized illness categories, explanatory models, and other knowledge are not predictive of consequent behavior. Two studies, one in urban Nepal and the other in rural Mexico, provide strong evidence that illness beliefs are not good predictors of the health-seeking strategies of patients and their families.

Nepalese, who have access to alternative forms of treatment, behave according to two basic patterns: illness specific, in which they seek out different kinds of therapy for different disorders, and multiple use, in which assistance is sought from a variety of different medical resources during a single episode of illness. When asked (Durkin-Longley 1984), informants expressed a preference for an illness-specific strategy; when observed, their behavior reflected a multiple-use strategy. The discrepancy may occur because therapeutic choices reflect the beliefs and preferences not only of the patient but of family and friends as well.

In rural Mexico, Young and Garro (1982) seized on an opportunity presented by two rural, Tarascan-speaking villages similar in medical beliefs but differing in degree of access to cosmopolitan medical facilities. In this quasi-experiment the researchers tested two competing explanations of why Indians fail to utilize cosmopolitan health services: (1) because it is too costly in time and money to gain access to those services or (2) because their health understandings are incompatible with those which guide clinic services. Those in the village with bus service to cosmopolitan health services proved to use them at approximately twice the rate of the other. Other studies seeking to weigh the influence of, respectively, a group's ethnomedical knowledge and the ease with which it can utilize cosmopolitan medical clinics have produced different results (Stock 1980; Pearson 1982). Apparently, the differences from Young and Garro may be attributed to the fact that the more recent studies are of patients with the socially stigmatizing disease of leprosy. To avoid becoming known and stigmatized as lepers by their neighbors, these Nigerian and Nepalese villagers bypassed local clinics, spending additional money and time to obtain care far from their home (Stock 1980:385–86; Pearson 1982:229–36).

The linkage between medical knowledge and social context becomes considerably more complicated the more medically pluralistic a society is. For example, in Belize there are a variety of medical resources available to residents (Staiano 1981): cosmopolitan medicine in the form of a hospital, outpatient clinic, and pharmacy; "bush medicine" consisting of traditional practitioners outside the cosmopolitian framework; Catholic or pentecostal spiritualist healers; and household lay knowledge. Staiano argues that in a pluralistic setting, such as Belize, there are alternative systems of interpretation from which the patient and healer can select. Two case studies serve to illustrate the continuing process of negotiation that goes on as the patient seeks therapies and etiologies consistent with his or her understanding of an illness. In both cases, the patients and their families accept some aspects of the cosmopolitian health care system as presented to them by a government physician, but they supplement this with information gathered in consultation with traditional healers.

The dynamic process by which patients accept, reject, and adapt information provided by health care providers is exemplified in research from Detroit (Hunt et al. 1989). In this study of middle-class women of Detroit, all of whom are diagnosed as hypoglycemic, the women incorporate the physician-provided diagnosis, adapt it to their preconceived concepts of disease, and utilize it to meet the needs and exigencies of their already established lifestyles.

Healers

From the earliest periods of anthropology, there has been a marked interest in the recruitment, training, and personality of traditional healers. Indeed, interest in the varied ways in which cultures permit the evidencing of psychopathology extended to speculation that the behavior of healers who cured their patients with dramatic ritual procedures was to be explained by emotional aberrance (Anisimov 1963:86, 102, 103, 120; Kroeber 1948:298–99). One authority (Sigerist 1951:172) has even defined shamanic procedures in Siberia as evidence of mental illness: "the Siberian shaman . . . undoubtedly is psychopathic. Mental illness plays a great part in his life and behavior." That view is no longer accepted.

Although many popular books and much of the medical literature make reference to "*the* traditional healer," it is abundantly clear that there is no such universal entity. In the following passages, some more accurate generalizations will portray traditional healers.

Traditional healers are recruited in several ways. One common way is by divine selection, in which an individual has a dream in which it is indicated that the dreamer is to undertake healing responsibilities (Joralemon 1985:5). Another form of divine selection is the normative obligation of a person who must accept such a responsibility in return for his or her recovery from an acute or life-threatening illness (Rubel 1966a; Turner 1967:282; Steedly 1988:855). An elected person who fails to become a healer is thought to be subject to divine sanctions, inclusive of serious illness and death. In many other societies, in contrast, an individual who aspires to healing apprentices to an established practitioner. The apprentice learns through didactics as well as observation of the master's conduct. In such situations, the student usually compensates for the training by assisting the senior healer and the latter's family. Sometimes a neophyte seeks out a noted healer, paying a fee to be trained (Rubel, field notes among Chinantec). Finally, there are some societies in which individuals who wish to embark on a curing career and possess the necessary self-confidence to engage in such risky behavior (Schweder 1965; Metzger and Williams 1963) initially test their abilities on household members and close family and subsequently expand their practice to nonrelatives.

There are several important differences between divine selection and formal training by means of apprenticeship. For one, people who are divinely selected or elect to learn by the seat of their pants are less subject to social control than those who undergo an apprenticeship or other formal training program. Inasmuch as traditional healing often includes considerable management of supernatural forces, the fear that healers who gain such control through efforts not publicly bestowed and largely unsupervised may use such potent forces for "antisocial" as well as helpful purposes (e.g., sorcery or witchcraft) is realistic (Brown 1988:102–20).

Some research has looked specifically at the relationship between healers' empirical knowledge and that of nonhealers (Garro 1986; Browner 1988). Anthropological attention has also focused on the personal characteristics that differentiate healers from nonhealers. For instance, in one ethnomedical study (Fabrega and Silver 1973), shamans and nonshamans who reside in the Tzotzil-speaking town of Zinacantan were compared using both projective tests and data such as economic level, participation in the *cargo* system, levels of formal classroom education, and acculturation to Spanish-speaking Ladino culture. The shamans identified less than laypersons with the sociopolitically dominant Ladino culture and were more likely to perceive human figures and themes of interpersonal conflict in ink blots. The (Fabrega and Silver 1973:83, 84, 87) knowledge about sickness utilized by shamans in Zinancantan proved not substantially distinct from the comprehensions of laypersons, but the former are more willing to utilize that knowledge (Garro 1986; Browner and Perdue 1988). In another provocative study of Zinacantan healers (Shweder 1965), it was concluded that there was little to differentiate laypersons and specialized healers in their store of healing knowledge and little differentiation in knowledge between healers, but a considerable cognitive difference between healers and nonhealers. The healers were more likely than laypersons to impose their own sense of order on ambiguous stimuli, presented in the form of blurred photographs: less frequently saying "I don't know," giving greater variety of responses, and tending to respond with their own categories rather than choices presented by the interviewer.

Elsewhere, among Tarascan-speakers in Mexico, whereas the medical knowledge of women curers and noncurers was substantially the same, the curers demonstrated far more consistency and agreement among themselves (Garro 1986).

Although there is little in these reports to indicate how healers acquire their knowledge, a study from South Africa reports an unusual learning process (Ngubane 1977):

Informal networks or associations of healers do exist, and these provide for the exchange of techniques and information, and monitoring of each other's behavior. . . . Meetings take place regularly between diviners to share ideas, experiences, and techniques. Each diviner has the opportunity to meet the ex-students, teacher, and neophyte of each other neighboring diviners, as well as more distant ones.

The extent to which knowledge is common among healers has received little attention, but in one interesting study, a Peruvian shaman was asked (Joralemon 1985) to comment on the symbolism employed in the altar of another local shaman:

His reaction was quick and definite: "He's a spiritist. The *mesa* [altar] doesn't have power, it's pure stone, with no herbs whatsoever. There aren't any images! Mine is superior; his isn't the half of mine."

When the other was shown photographs of his rival's altar, he called it "fetishistic" and implied that it was founded on superstitions:

With a disdain no less intense than Paz's, he asserted that Jose Paz does not really understand the illnesses he treats or the significance of the objects on his mesa. (5; cf. Levi-Straus 1963: 175–79)

In Thailand, those who aspire to study with an established curer must often travel great distances to find a willing teacher. Golomb (1986) described the social and economic factors leading to a geographically widespread network of traditional healers in Thailand. Consistent with his observation that within a particular geographic area there were considerable inconsistencies in diagnosis and recommended therapy among traditional healers, he noted that local healers rarely consulted with one another. Indeed, junior healers or patients visiting the home of a master healer usually traveled at least an hour by car from their own villages. Golomb argued that this lack of diagnostic consensus among local practitioners and the pattern of long-distance consultation were the result of intense competition among traditional healers for a limited patient pool. Competition from government-run clinics and the threat of competition from other healers made master healers loath to train local novices. This led aspirants to seek training from master healers who were geographically distant from their home villages. These long-distance networks were used for sharing knowledge and seeking consultation on difficult cases. By seeking assistance from geographically distant experts, healers did not reveal their limitations to the local community, thus preserving their status in the regions they serve.

The studies of how healers are recruited to serve crucial societal functions, how they acquire their knowledge, and how they practice medicine retain a central position in ethnomedicine.

Assessing Healing Successes

Another of anthropology's long-time interests, assessing the success of traditional healing practices, has received new interest and reformulation. For example, Kleinman (1980:312) describes the assessment of therapeutic efficacy as the central problem in the cross-cultural study of healing. This issue is beleaguered by unsecured impressions, strong opinions, and outright dismissiveness of traditional practices by some and undue romanticization by others (Ott 1993). Thus, it becomes vitally important to fashion ways to assess objectively the efficacy of traditional healing practices (Anderson 1991; Etkin 1988a, 1990; Kleinman and Sung 1979). As Etkin so usefully comments, "Plant use and other medical behaviors are effective if they effect or assist in producing the requisite, culturally defined outcomes" (Etkin 1988a:301). In Etkin's significant contribution to the study of ethnomedicine, she urges the importance of viewing traditional healing as a process containing several levels of success. The anthropologist can then determine the extent to which that process succeeds in returning the patient to normal well-being as well as assessing proximate successes achieved along the way. Proximate successes are the appearance of hopeful culture-specific indications that the effort is having a desired effect (e.g., inducement of high body temperature, expulsion of phlegm, stoppage of bleeding). Proximate successes are distinct from those that are ultimate, that is, the full restoration of well-being (Etkin 1988a:300–305).

These studies of healers and their practices represent some of the most traditional interests in anthropology. Yet our inability to make generalizable statements or predictions as to the kinds of sociocultural environments that will produce one or more category of healer and our difficulties in evaluating the successes of traditional healing remain challenges still to be achieved.

RESEARCH FOR THE FUTURE

Future ethnomedical research might profitably focus on some of the following themes.

1. *The interface between biology and culture.* Ethnomedical researchers have

shown a troubling "reluctance to explore the interface between biology and culture [which] derives from their belief that previous efforts to do so using the biomedical paradigm were failures because they forced rich, complex ethnographic data into artificial categories" (Browner, Ortiz de Montellano, and Rubel 1988:682). However, by building on the anthropological tenet that human physiological processes are the same species wide, studies of cultural responses to such physiological processes as maturation, aging, gestation, pregnancy and delivery, and disease offer the opportunity to maximize the equivalence of the processes to which cultural responses are being made (Browner, Ortiz de Montellano, and Rubel 1988:682). The effort is, first, to design standardized comparable units into which characteristics of, say, an illness, gestation period, or maturational changes can be placed and then to compare the response to them across cultural groups. Efforts to accomplish these goals have been few but noteworthy (Jordan 1978; Fabrega 1970b; Rubel, O'Nell, and Collado Ardon 1984; Clark and Anderson 1967; Lock, 1993b).

2. *The incidence and distribution of particular illnesses within a population.* Skewed distributions may be clues to underlying social or emotional mechanisms (Rubel 1964; Carey 1988). Is a stipulated illness widespread or confined to one or several segments of the population? Do women and men suffer from it in equal measure? Does it affect persons without respect to their social and political status? Is it confined to a particular ethnic group or social class? For example, in ethnically pluralistic villages in Nicaragua, susceptibility to the illness *grisi siknes* distinguishes the Miskito-speaking residents from others (Dennis 1981). In Guatemala, discovery (Logan 1979) that two Cakchiquel villages with a common understanding of *susto* suffered significantly different attack rates contributed to insightful analysis of the socioeconomic stresses each was experiencing.

3. *The effects of healing procedures.* It is vitally important to discover the extent to which healing procedures directed at the improvement of social relationships have succeeded. Where the healing of an individual's health is a metaphor for the alleviation of social difficulties that threaten to rupture structural ties or social solidarity of his or her membership group (e.g., Lindenbaum 1979; Marwick 1964, Steedly 1988), do participants feel or acknowledge that social ties are less threatened following the procedure? In societies whose social structures are otherwise similar, do those that possess such metaphoric healing mechanisms experience less threat or disruption than those that lack them?

4. *The healing implications of patient support groups.* Although it is conventionally accepted (Frank 1973; Pilisuk and Parks 1986) that healing procedures that include patient support groups have better outcomes, the importance of this assumption urges empirical assessment. Does social support in a healing ceremony ensure better results and, if so, in what kinds of social organizations?

Similarly, it is reasonable to question the extent to which the gender of either patient or healer influences the performance and success of treatment procedures. Future research can provide a corrective to earlier tendencies to present a group's healing procedures as virtually uniform no matter what the gender, social status, or other important social characteristics of the participants.

5. *Distinctions among types of healers. The choice of nonprofessional care when cosmopolitan physicians are available* (Harwood 1977a:201; Landy 1983a:235; Helman 1984b:49). Speculation that people prefer nonphysician healers because they share with them a paradigm of health and healing, or because lay healers take more time in treatment of patients than biomedical physicians, is unproductive. In several interesting studies (Finkler 1985; Kleinman and Sung 1979; Kleinman and Gale 1982) of the patient-healer relationship, it has been discovered that healers of whatever persuasion who are in great demand treat their patients impersonally and quickly. Furthermore, in one investigation, it is reported that these popular healers "generally fail to explain the etiology of the illness for which the patient is being treated, fail to share similar etiological beliefs with their patients, and frequently fail to uphold the patient's claim to the sick role" (Finkler 1985:6; see also pp. 54, 84–89). Similarly Kleinman writes of "Chinese-style doctors" on Taiwan that "unless a patient asks they rarely explain about cause, pathophysiology, or course of illness. They may not even name the illness" (Kleinman 1980:261; see also pp. 89, 262).

6. *The differences between healers locally identified by distinctive labels (e.g., curandero and empirica [midwife], espiritista and espiritualista, "Chinese-style doctor," tang-ki and ch'ien interpreters) should be specified, whether they are recruited from the same segments of society, gain healing power in the same manner, and undergo similar training.* Studies may eventually permit cross-cultural generalizations about categories of healers that can help guide fieldwork on the subject (Montgomery 1976:272–84; Topley 1976).

7. *Symptoms of sicknesses.* It is only through tabulation and description of the symptoms reported by all patients suffering a particular sickness that we can hope to discover a consistent assemblage of indicators and identify the relationships among them (Fabrega 1977; Marwick 1964:263–68; Prince and Tcheng-Laroche 1987). This kind of study can inform us whether individuals who complain of, for example, *susto* share more symptoms than a person who complains of *susto* and another who complains of *mal de ojo* (Fabrega 1970b). We need to know as well to what people are responding when complaining of illness. For example, Lewis (1975) comments that although the Gnau of New Guinea complained of being ill, they based their reports not on the signs and symptoms but on other characteristics of the sufferer, "since in their view causes were not discernible from the clinical signs, exact description of these [signs] was not relevant" (p. 142).

8. *The range of applicability of ethnomedical hypotheses.* Such studies as Lieban's test among Filipinos of B. Whiting's linking of attribution of sickness to form of social organization and O'Nell and Selby's (1968) test of Rubel's hypothesis of a relationship between failure to meet role expectations and heightened susceptibility to *susto* contribute to the comparative study of ethnomedical

systems and eventually to a testable theory of illness and healing. To sustain so valuable a direction, it is essential that the results of studies of ethnomedicine in one society be tested in other cultural groups to determine their general applicability.

ACKNOWLEDGMENTS

We wish to acknowledge the constructive help of Dr. Carole Browner and Barbara Metzger. We are most grateful to them both.

NOTE

1. In contrast, Landy's (1977) impression was that prior to 1960, "despite the fact that every human society faces critically and daily the often life-and-death questions of health and disease, coverage of institutional means of coping with these vital problems in most ethnographic reports had been generally unsystematic, often handled in a casual, fragmentary, and even confusing manner, and in some cases almost completely neglected. Of course, some classic ethnographies did include substantial accounts of the medical aspects of the cultures observed, but these were distinguished by their rarity. (p. 4)

Fabrega (1975:969) also concluded that "ethnomedicine as an area of inquiry has been either bypassed and neglected or handled indirectly."

7
Ethnopsychiatry

Charles C. Hughes

THE CONTEXT

Anthropology is ambitious in its theoretical scope, and has been so since the time of Aristotle. In its first appearance in an English text (1595) the term referred to the "science of man, or of mankind, in the widest sense" (*Oxford English Dictionary*). That holistic conception was undoubtedly reinforced when anthropology began to be institutionalized as an academic discipline following the appearance of Darwin's *On the Origin of Species* in 1859; for, comparable in orientation to other "natural history" disciplines—entomology, ichthyology, ornithology are examples—anthropology is species centered, the species in this case, of course, being the human animal, *Homo sapiens sapiens*. Such a "natural history" orientation takes a wide-ranging framework that includes biological evolution, modes of reproduction, forms of social organization, mechanisms of communication, methods of adapting to multiple levels of stimuli, and other features characteristic of the animal population of concern. Anthropology is similarly comprehensive (La Barre 1968). Key structural elements in its frame of reference include an ingrained, multilevel evolutionary and diachronic perspective; preference for natural settings in investigations of human behavior; recognition of the pervasiveness of ecologic imperatives; attentiveness to the power and varieties of symbolism in human behavior; and an implicit cross-cultural and comparative viewpoint in which the laboratory is the great variety of human behavior patterns.

Biologic phenomena manifest themselves in continua that are subject to analytic differentiation between "normal" and "abnormal" states or conditions in anatomic, physiologic, and developmental characteristics as these are influenced by genetic and environmental factors (Mayr 1982; Williams 1956). While abnormal somatic states and conditions—"disease"—have been investigated by anthropologists (Livingstone; see also Brown, Inhorn, and Smith, in this volume) so, too, have "psychological" abnormalities or disorders. Influenced, for example, by developments in psychology and particularly psychoanalysis, culture and personality studies began in the 1920s, especially in the United States (Kluckhohn 1944). Such inquiry represented a forthright assertion of the discipline's appropriate but certainly not proprietary application to questions of how the human personality, from the first babblings of infancy through the vicissitudes of adult life and old age, is shaped by diverse sociocultural contexts. Inevitably culture and personality studies presented data that raised the question of the normality or abnormality of various behavior patterns as these might be viewed in a Western psychiatric or psychological framework. The human infant being highly malleable in potential and dependent upon caretaking by others for a relatively long period of developmental time, one question raised was the long-range structural effects of the manner in which the personality is shaped and structured in the early and formative years through reward, punishment, coercion, or other modalities of interpersonal influence. For example, it is suggested that because of neglectful and inconsistent patterns of treatment in infancy, Alorese emerge as hostile, distrustful, and emotionally starved adults (DuBois 1944; Kardiner 1945:101–258).

From another domain of inquiry is the shaman, when performing the seance and acting in a decidedly bizarre and "nonnormal" manner, merely playing a role in a culturally familiar healing drama? Or is he (or she) acting out the deep-rooted tensions of the neurotic personality? How are "abnormal" or "deviant" thought and behavior—as contrasted to "normal" behavior and thought—culturally constituted and assessed from an insider's as well as an outsider's point of view? Indeed, are there "mental disorders" in other societies, such as small-scale, non-Western societies, that are often characterized as free from the emotionally disruptive pressures of a complex, industrialized milieu? If so, what cultural resources, social procedures, and special roles exist to ameliorate distress and disorder? Recognizing the power of the concept of cultural relativity, can one validly assess "craziness" in other societies by using the theoretical constructs of Western psychiatry? And what are these things called "culture-bound syndromes"? In the spirit of the species-centered nature of the discipline, these and numerous other questions have become embedded in the broad institutional fabric of anthropology as an academic discipline.

ETHNOPSYCHIATRY

The prefix *ethno-* derives from the Greek term *ethno,* referring to "tribe," and is illustrated in such usages as *ethnology* and *ethnography*—the comparative analysis or descriptive study of ways of life of different societies. The prefix has proliferated in the social and behavioral science literature, serving as a signal reminder of the pervasiveness of the cultural structuring of all knowledge and experience. Thus we have *ethnomedicine, ethnopharmacology, ethnologic, ethnosemantics,* and so many other "*ethno-*s" that one expects an article or chapter soon on "ethnoethnology."

Indeed, that would be an apt usage, for, as with its other instances, the reader may properly infer that the given substantive subject matter is being considered as a subset of the total way of life of a given people. Ethnocentrism is, of course, a predictable feature of any human society, and it is accompanied by traditional or conventional characterizations of other groups. In the case of ethnoethnology, the term would refer to a society's set of assumptions about and descriptions of people foreign to themselves—out-groups. To suggest examples that come to mind, how did the Zulus of southern Africa perceive, evaluate, and define the Boers who in the nineteenth century were encroaching upon their lands? Or what image did the Celts of King Arthur's time have of the Belgaic Angles and Saxons who were invading Britain in the sixth century A.D.? Or that of the European-descended American settlers, of the indigenous Americans whose lands they were seizing under the mandate of manifest destiny (unfortunately, the record is full of the disparaging and dehumanizing images used).

Thus the prefix *ethno-* structures a conceptual approach in which experience (or a selected aspect) is seen through the cultural lenses of a particular group—their "assumptive world," as Frank calls it (1973:24ff.). But beyond facile reiteration of the prefix in connection with a substantive subject matter, it does not necessarily follow that it is a simple matter for the investigator to step into that world, that unknown terrain, and experience in a fundamental way a world-view structured by different concepts. For the known has great tenacity in one's personality; the process of socialization lays down a firm structure (which, indeed, is necessary for viability and adaptation). Thus, in confronting the new, the novel situation, it is easier—and far more comforting—to render the unfamiliar into one's own familiar terms rather than approach the task with one's familiar cognitive categories suspended. This is well known from studies of culture change: the exotic is adapted, modified, transformed in label and perhaps even appearance to conform with what has existed up to this point. The behavioral rule appears to be: Fit the phenomenology to the familiar cultural category, cutting and trimming if necessary.

The preceding comments have been raised in the spirit of the by-now-familiar distinction between an emic and an etic approach to understanding human behavior, concepts drawn from linguistics that have come into widespread use in the anthropological and cognate literature over the past several decades. They are useful shorthand tools to reinforce the crucial theoretical dictum that the experienced world of the persons being studied, *as well as that of the researcher,* is culturally structured, and each must be accepted on its own terms and not be thought as interchangeable. Over the past couple of decades, there has been considerable discussion of the investigator's being aware of the implications of such a distinction, not only for the initiation of inquiry but also for analysis and interpretation of results.

An example of the difference this distinction makes will illustrate its importance in the study of any aspect of cultural behavior. More than a century ago, in the formative years of the discipline, anthropologists were confronted with the question of understanding the degree of correspondence between biologically created relationships and culturally structured kinship designations in a society different from one's own, and a research technique was developed to elucidate the issue systematically. The technique is the *genealogical method* for deriving indigenous kin terms (cf. *Notes and Queries* 1951:54ff.); its use led to the translation of the highly variable emic kin terms in different societies into a common idiom of structural categories that allow for theoretically productive comparative study of kinship systems.

As the anthropological readership recalls, the genealogical method reaches through the cultural facade defining kin and enables exploration of the widely varying ways in which human groups selectively define culturally constructed (as contrasted to biologically created) relationships. Using the method, rather than proceeding from an ethnocentric base by asking an informant, for example, "What is the name of your uncle?" (which assumes that the biological relative culturally labeled "uncle" in the investigator's own group is the same as "uncle" to the informant), one asks for the emic terms designating other males born to the informant's father's mother, the term for the man who married mother's sister, and so on. That is, a set of more abstract categories based on biological or affinal relationships is developed as the semantic niches used by societies to define social relationships and shape behavior. Simply to ask, "What are the names of your uncles?" is to be an unwitting prisoner of one's own cultural constructs; one might appropriately ask such a question in American society, where "uncle" refers to father's brother, father's sister's husband, mother's brother, or mother's sister's husband. In this instance, a single term, *uncle,* refers to four discriminably different biological relationships. But patterns elsewhere vary greatly.

It must be emphasized, however, that to remain only at the emic level is to be locked into a theoretical stance that appears to offer no possibility of reaching across that presumed impermeable barrier between "the world as I see it"—a quintessential phenomenological position—and the world as others see it (sometimes called the "objective" perspective). Generalization is stultified, if not made impossible. Yet the matter need not be left with such a simple, deconstructionist solipsism. MacLeod (1969:194) reminds us:

The task of the phenomenologist is to penetrate the world of the other person, to describe it and analyze it in such a way that its structure, properties, relations, and dimensions can then be correlated meaningfully with independently defined physical, biological and social variables. Phenomenology in this sense is always propaedeutic to a science, never the science in itself. Its scientific function is to generate questions, not to answer them.

These comments on the utility of the insider's perspective as against that of the outsider are as applicable to the study of mental disorders as of kinship categories, and the principal lesson they underscore is that *one must return to primary observational data in order to ground one's analyses*. In regard to both domains (indeed, all cultural domains) it is not suggested that in every case emic concepts must be translated into etic terms—or vice versa. What is needed is research acumen capable of either or both approaches when the issue being addressed requires such conceptual flexibility. The method of choice will depend on the nature of the problem being investigated and the level of analysis to which the results are intended to refer. But it is clear that for optimal understanding in many of the problems studied by anthropology and the other behavioral sciences, and especially with reference to the topic of this chapter, *the emic must inform the etic* (for an instructive example, see Weiss et al. 1992).

The reason the constructs *emic* and *etic* have been examined here in what to an anthropological readership may appear so prolix a manner is that, paradoxically, the difference implied between ethnomedicine and ethnopsychiatry in self-same chapter titles in this very book suggest separable domains of events and illustrate the need for a constant self-monitoring vigilance in order to avoid the insidious entrapments of one's own emic world. As McLuhan noted (1964), the medium is the message. To separate ethnopsychiatry from ethnomedicine when adopting a cross-cultural perspective on the conceptualization of diseases of any kind, on the labeling of disorders, and on the manifest as well as latent techniques of healing in societies other than one's own is to become hoist on one's own theoretical petard. The petard in this instance, of course, is the institutionalized distinction in Western societies between medicine (''real'' medical problems, meaning physiologic or somatic processes and structures) and psychiatry, that medical subspecialty dealing with disorders of the mind and behavioral abnormalities and deviations, which are typically given secondary consideration in any assessment of patient history after thorough examination of ''primary,'' that is, medical, causes of the presenting complaint have been ruled out.

In the Western world, psychiatry is formally included as one branch of science-based medicine, yet its status remains anomalous. While it, more than any other subdiscipline of medicine, is potentially capable of treating human illness and distress in a comprehensive, integrated psychobiological conceptual framework, many clinicians seem so intimidated by peers wedded to a philosophy of biomedical reductionism that the easier course of searching for disease ''entities'' and tissue- or molecular-level etiologies is chosen over a broader, multilevel conceptual framework for understanding the totality of human problems of adaptation and maintenance of a healthy self-system. While there are those who speak out in an attempt to counter the trend toward biomedical reductionism in current Western psychiatric clinical practice (e.g., Engel 1977, with his call for a ''biopsychosocial model,'' or White 1988), when compared to the comprehensive character of indigenous or ''folk psychiatry,'' Western psychiatry is often selectively equivocal in conceptual scope and etiological considerations. For example, sometimes common problems of living and adaptation are not given the formal diagnostic status (e.g., type A behavior in modern society), while in other instances, behavior patterns that, to be sure, may be harmful from some points of view, such as "specific arithmetic disorder," are included as formal diagnoses.

Overwhelmingly non-Western, indigenous medical systems—those not based on Western science-derived concepts and techniques—are holistic in scope and basic premises. Not for them the seductive Cartesian division between body and mind. Rather, an affliction, a discomfiture of mind, or an accident of nature is seen in a context of not only ailment in body but also of possible soul loss, spirit intrusion, taboo violation, malevolent acts of other persons or supernatural agents, or any number of other constructs that define a world of unseen powers (Clements 1932). To be sure, non-Western disease constructs and treatment techniques also include "empirical" causes (Ackerknecht 1943, 1944, 1946; Foster and Anderson 1978:51 ff.), but critical weight is given to transempirical causative factors.

Thus, to speak of ethnomedicine and ethnopsychiatry separately when considering the majority of the world's medical systems is, in effect, to take two different points of entry (of our own contriving) into what for the vast span of human history has been and remains phenomenologically a unitary continuum: illness-disease-sickness, pain, anxiety, foreboding, gnawing, frustration, anger, grief, or the many unfulfilled wishes that characterize human life. But to the extent that either one of these conceptual points of entry becomes rigidly fixed and presumed to reflect natural as contrasted to social categorizations, it can quickly obfuscate rather than help, thus becoming another instance of the mischief created by uniformed emic projection.

An example is useful here. A native healer in Sokoto, Nigeria, advertises that he can provide "medicine" for over fifty listed human problems, afflictions, desires, and quandaries. Some of these are:

scorpion medicine, market medicine, learn medicine, medicine for prevention of evil powers, medicine to drive witchcraft, medicine for gonorrhea, medicine for ring worm, medicine for motor accident, medicine for record pen, medicine for promotion, medicine for progress, medicine for general love, medicine for examination, medicine for guinea worm, medicine for prevention of bad dreams, for measles, for information [sic] disease or "coughous" disease, chest pain and nerviousness [sic], commanding tongue, eye sight prevention, stomach trouble, medicine for office love, medicine for within, to prevent bad juju, medicine for fever, medicine for woman conciption [sic], medicine for life aboundant [sic], medicine to play ball, medicine to drive away poverty, medicine to catch thieves, medicine for tired penies [sic], medicine for cough, medicine for backache, medicine for headache disease. (Hughes, printed advertisement, Nigerian fieldwork)

The intent of this chapter is to comment on the evidence from "folk" societies about what can be termed topics of psychiatric interest as viewed in an ethnopsychiatric perspective. These include "abnormal" behaviors, thoughts, and emotions; ethnotheories regarding diagnosis, labeling, and causation; and modes of treatment for such deviant instances or patterns of behavior. It will sketch the most salient of the interests that have driven research into the question, What are the essential semantics of the term *ethnopsychiatry,* and how do they differ from *ethnomedicine?*

"NORMAL" AND "ABNORMAL" BEHAVIOR

All human societies have notions of what constitutes normal behavior patterns expected—indeed, demanded—of group members, as contrasted to abnormal behavior—behavior that is not only different but often also socially disvalued. The most comprehensive rubric for such behavior is deviance from norms in any institutionalized sector of society, whether that be the division of labor ("He's just a lazy slob"), exchange of goods and services, behavior toward kinsmen, marital obligations, reverence to the spirits conceived to constitute the very basis of empirical reality, or any of the multitudinous obligations that are the costs standing in dialectic relationship to the benefits of belonging to a social group. Shared norms of behavior are essential to the survival of any society (Aberle et al. 1960), although there are reports in the ethnographic literature of groups that would appear to be dangerously close to approximating the Hobbesian state of anarchy, the "war of all against all" (perhaps the Ik of East Africa or the Yanomamo of the Brazilian rain forest).

Like the more general sick role as a "legitimated" form of deviance (Parsons 1951:436ff.), "behavioral disorders," "mental disorders," or "psychopathology" represent a subset of the broad category of social deviance. But the clear specification of when a pattern of norm-violating behavior passes from being mere forgetfulness or outright criminality to that of pathology is one of the most vexing issues in psychiatry and social deviance (cf. "sociopaths" and in forensic psychiatry the McNaughton rule of not guilty by reason of insanity). However, any attempt to devise a universalistic specification or listing of patterns of abnormal behavior, whether representing pathology or not, quickly becomes blunted when held against a cultural relativistic framework. Drawing upon the extensive cross-cultural data on human behavior, a major figure in American anthropology commented that cultural "anthropology has the healthiest of all skepticisms about the validity of the concept of 'normal behavior.' ... [It] is constantly rediscovering the normal" (1949:514, 515). Yet, ironically, the terms *normal* or *normality* are rarely even indexed, much less discussed, in psychiatric textbooks. This suggests that either such a crucial concept is so well understood in that professional group and its meaning and reference so widely accepted that there is no reason even to discuss it or that a discussion is missing because of the difficulty of specifying its operational indicators. However, when the question requires taking a cross-cultural perspective on the concept, it is essential that there be an attempt to develop a core conceptual meaning to avoid emic projection and guide researchers through that murky domain of differentiating between "normal" and "abnormal" behavior.

Beyond Sapir, another influential figure in American anthropology who conducted pioneering research in culture and personality, A. Irving Hallowell underscored the need for an outsider studying "deviant" or "abnormal" behavior to know the normative baseline against which such acts or patterns are being assessed. He stipulated that such an investigator should have an

[intimate] knowledge of the culture as a whole, he must also be aware of the normal range of individual behavior within the cultural pattern and likewise understand what the people themselves consider to be extreme deviations from this norm. In short, he must develop a standard of normality with reference to the culture itself, as a means of controlling an uncritical application of the criteria that he brings with him from our civilization. (1934:2)

Deviant behavior is a major research field in sociology, a subfield that includes not only such topics as criminality but also illness and behavioral disorders that depart from the functional norm. Much literature has developed that points to varying patterns of nonadherence to norms, structural motivations for noncompliance, and the types of sanctions brought against offenders (Blake and Davis 1964). Curiously, although individual behavioral deviations from prescribed norms are discussed in the anthropological literature, there appears to be no established rubric in cultural anthropology comparable to that in sociology. One significant marker of this is the lack of indexing of "deviance" or "social deviance" in the last couple of decades of a major compendium of review articles, the *Annual Review of Anthropology*. But quite aside from rubric, the existence of norms and the failure to live up to those norms (and the consequences of such failure) is abundantly documented in the anthropological literature.

THE "PSYCHIATRY" OF "ETHNOPSYCHIATRY"

Psychiatry deals with abnormal behavior and mentation, and no society is free from mental disorders (cf. Murphy 1982b). Thus, when we speak of ethnopsychiatry, the need for some specification of "abnormality" that can carry meaning across cultural barriers becomes paramount. In a classic article Wegrocki (1953) drew a distinction critical for understanding the difference between deliberate norm-breaking and deviance on the one hand, and abnormality of psychiatric interest on the other. He spoke of "statistical" abnormality (which depends on the frequency distribution of the parameters that define the object of interest; e.g., in a population decimated by smallpox, persons without scars are the deviants) and "functional" abnormality, which is based on an assessment of how a given behavioral pattern figures in the total context of the personality—the psychodynamic purposes it serves. Does the behavior represent denial, repression, delusion, or any of a number of other psychodynamic defense mechanisms, and to what extent?

In commenting on the difference between deviance and psychiatric abnormality, Honigmann (1956) succinctly presents the generic conceptual and referential differences between these two approaches used to sort out the implications of the term *deviance:*

The deviant does not stand out because of his high level of anxiety, sensori-motor dysfunctions, or reality distortion. He is conspicuous through the fact that he underplays or overplays socially standardized behavior or innovates behavior. The policeman who becomes an authoritarian colossus overplays his role; the Crow Indian who holds back from battle because of the fear that he may be killed underplays a role. The purveyor of a new religion represents an innovator. All are deviants, but we cannot without further information classify them as also psychopathic. To classify the policeman, warrior, and prophet as psychiatrically abnormal, each must be judged by the criteria which we adopted from psychiatry—anxiety, regression and the others. (p. 442)

The operative question becomes, "What patterns of behavior in any given society are candidates for consideration as 'pathology'?" Along what must be considered as a continuum and not quantum steps, "What is 'normal' behavior as contrasted to 'abnormal'?" And in a cross-cultural framework, the operative question must be, "Whose criteria are being used to define abnormal behavior: those of the group itself (the emic categories) or those of an outside group (etic categories), such as the cultural constructs of Western psychiatry?" For example, the behavioral episodes often termed possession (in Western psychiatric terms, sometimes diagnosed as dissociation) are widely found in human societies of all times and places (cf. Ross, Joshi, and Currie 1990). There is a large literature dealing with such matters as ritualized healing cults, for example, and periods of out-of-awareness prescribed by various social and ceremonial occasions (Prince 1968; Crapanzano and Garrison 1977). Sometimes the behavior of persons in such situations is clearly of psychiatric relevance, but often it is simply the playing out of a public viewed and socially prescribed role. It is "normal" behavior appropriate to its situation of enactment. How does one begin to understand such behavior? Perhaps by applying the etic concepts of Western psychiatry?

In its approach to diagnosis—classification of patterns of pathologic interest—psychiatry adopts that of general medicine, formally labeled nosology, which has been characterized as an "eclectically assembled, chronologic polyglot of different terms and ideas that reflect every layer of nosologic thinking and technologic data from antiquity to the present" (Feinstein 1977:193). Much of the implicit focus in such a diagnostic approach has been based on the search for disease entities, an approach that suggests reification of pathological processes operating independent of context. Indeed, that dialectic continues today between alternative theoretical bases for viewing disease: on the one hand, the ontological approach (diseases are "real" entities) and on the other, a processual or physiological approach, in which the term *disease* serves simply as a useful construct that points to dysfunctional processes in a given context (cf. Temkin 1963; Engelhardt 1975).

As some modern commentaries on the metalogic of diagnosis suggest, an ontologic approach—looking for an autonomous entity, a "thing"—leads to quandaries in consideration of some of the major health issues in a society. The debilities of aging are a challenging example; dysfunctional, certainly, but is aging a disease? And in the domain of psychiatric or behavioral disorder, is grief a disease, as Engel (1977) asks? Explicitly modeling itself on the structure of the diagnostic system in medicine, where there may well be more utility in something of an ontological concept, how much more at risk of conceptual confusion may be psychiatry, when its objects of inquiry—behavioral and mental events—are not so amenable to sharp operational specification as are tissue-level pathologies, and which may be confounded further by local cultural definitions and justifications of "abnormality"?

The third edition (revised) of the American Psychiatric Association's *Diagnostic and Statistical Manual of Mental Disorders* (DSM III-R) (1987) attempted to ameliorate such confusions by urging use of standardized operational definitions in psychiatric conceptualizations, diagnoses, and clinical practice. Even so, in that diagnostic volume there are numerous areas in which attribution of pathology as contrasted simply to deviance may not have been warranted. There appears much of what Illich (1976) referred to as the "medicalization" of everyday life (which earlier, in a classic article, Ackerknecht had noted in his statement: "One of the characteristic mental traits of our culture is the labeling of phenomena with psychiatric diagnoses"; 1943:30). Another critic is uneasy about the inclusion in DSM III-R of such problems as "specific reading disorder" and "specific arithmetic disorder" being considered diagnoses of "developmental disorders" (1986:109), not to mention "pathological gambling," about which he pointedly comments:

Whether or not such a problem should be considered a form of psychiatric disorder or mental illness would seem to be debatable. Certainly, pathological gambling can have all sorts of negative and distressing consequences, but does it have to be labeled as psychiatric disorder? Many other problems in everyday life may have distressful effects, but they may be viewed as economic and social problems rather than psychiatric ones. (Garfield 1986:110)

The newest version of the American Psychiatric Association's diagnostic manual, DSM IV (1994), continues to include such behavior patterns as "specific arithmetic disorder" as a psychiatric diagnosis, a conceptualization of "disorder" that warrants reexamination in view of a number of considerations not the least of which are the cultural relativity of the behavior being analyzed and the possibility of ethnocentric projection of the analyst (Hughes 1993:27ff.).

THE "CULTURE-BOUND SYNDROMES"

The so-called culture-bound syndromes are a prime target for discussion in any chapter on ethnopsychiatry and represent an instructive focus for many of the issues already raised. Originally coined by the Chinese psychiatrist P. M. Yap (1962), for a generation or so the term has been found in the literature that deals with cross-cultural psychiatry (primarily that in medical anthropology and culture and personality studies, far less in psychiatry). The phenomena addressed by the conceptual construct take us directly into the middle of any analysis of deviance and the possible utility of etic Western psychiatric concepts for understanding such syndromes. Indeed, as noted in another place (Hughes 1985a: 3), the culture-bound syndromes can be interpreted as representing almost archetypical cases of deviant deviance; in other words, they are "abnormal" (to us) ways of being "crazy."

The term *culture-bound syndromes* is a catching designation, one creating an aura of exoticism and redolent of deep mysteries. It seems to fit well those episodes of wild, random, senseless killing called "amok"—periods of a person's being "out-of-mind"—or those theatrical displays of giggling and stereotyped imitation of gestures or sounds whose indigenous (Malay) term is *latah*.

But beyond such intriguing examples—and there are many; (for an extended discussion, see Simons and Hughes 1985)—what does (or may) the term *culture-bound syndrome* mean in conceptual and analytic terms? On the surface, it connotes some degree of determinative influence of the cultural context in fostering behavior patterns that are often (but not always) viewed by insiders as mental disorder and may or may not be so seen by outsiders as psychiatric conditions. The phrase has occasioned numerous articles, symposia, and books or book chapters dealing with its meaning and possible utility in determining the extent to which and in what ways—quite aside from any biologic predispositions or risk factors—the sociocultural context of the behavior of a given person is of major significance in the etiology, symptomatology, expression, course, and response to treatment (Simons and Hughes 1985, 1993; Littlewood and Lipsedge 1985). The conceptualization developed primarily out of Westerners' experience with non-western or "folk" societies, and the syndromes found have occasioned much discussion because they do not fit neatly into the Western diagnostic formulations.

It should also be noted, however, that aside from implications for research into the theoretical relationship between cultural factors and psychiatric disorders of this type, there are substantial questions raised regarding treatment and management of a reputed instance of a culture-bound syndrome when a Western-trained physician or health worker is confronted with such a case. That is possible not simply in the non-Western world but also in industrialized societies having minority groups of different ethnic backgrounds (such as Native Americans, blacks, Hispanics, or immigrant groups such as Vietnamese, Koreans, or numerous others in the contemporary United States).

Despite increased discussion of the culture-bound syndromes, it is clear that the semantic status of the term is by no means clear or precise; and among other sources of confusion, the phrase seems to be lodged in a twilight zone with respect to the etic categories of Western psychiatry (Hughes 1985a:3). The phrase almost seems to be a verbal Rorschach card, bringing forth a variety of interpretations and attributions. Perhaps one of the factors confounding its systematic incorporation into such psychiatric categorization is the extent to which the observed behaviors usually included under this rubric do not comprise a homogeneous class. While many of the symptoms found in the "culture-bound syndromes" are familiar to a Western psychiatrist, they are grouped together into "syndromes" in folk-labeled patterns that cross-cut Western psychiatry's diagnostic system.

In this respect it may be suggested that there are several alternative and at times conflicting metatheoretical assertions threading through the literature of culture-bound syndromes, and recognition of the semantic alternatives implied by such assertions should be the point of departure in any discussion of the term. These are:

1. The syndromes do not necessarily represent pathology, but rather (to the observer) are *simply different* culturally-patterned behavioral events;

2. Standard psychiatric diagnostic categories are *useful* and appropriate in sorting such syndromes;

3. Perhaps the standard psychiatric categories are *inadequate,* because they are the expression of such a unique cultural structuring of experience (Euro-American) that they are not universally generalizable.

4. The repeated use of the phrase *culture-bound syndromes*—it seems, to the point of reification—does not necessarily validate or legitimate the implied status of these assorted behavioral complexes as an **ontologically** *separate* *class* of psychiatric disorders, even if they can be shown to be "pathologic" behaviors; and

5. Perhaps there is such divergence in levels of abstraction and analysis to which the term *culture-bound syndrome* applies that the term itself should be abandoned if comparative discussion of structure, etiology, and social implications of these behavior patterns is to succeed (Hughes 1985a:3)

Regardless of the extent to which any given psychiatric disorder may be influenced in its etiology, symptomatic expression, course, and therapeutic potential by the cultural environment in which it occurs—and hence to that extent be "bound," as some assert that all such disorders are (Murphy 1977; Alarcon 1983; Marsella 1982; Hughes 1985a)—there is a much more problematic interpretation and use of the term *culture bound.* This is the implication that any psychiatric disorder so designated is unique to a particular society or at most to a narrow range of societies in which it is found. Such an interpretation often has been stimulated by reports of behavioral patterns found in other societies (especially traditional, non-Western societies) that were strikingly bizarre and exotic as compared to the familiar behavior of one's own society, so different that they seemed to be confined to a specific cultural-geographic locale. (Of course, every phenomenon is unique in the ultimate sense; it is only through use of conceptual constructs that we create degrees of similarity or sameness among diverse phenomena at varying levels of abstraction.)

However, when the observational evidence is closely examined, many disorders once thought to be localized to a given society (such as *latah,* presumably confined to Malaysian village societies) have been found in their generic symptomatic expression, though not their behavioral appearance and indigenous labeling, in other parts of the world as well (Simons 1985a). A glossary and synonymy that systematizes data on 185 such "culture-bound syndromes" (Hughes 1985b) clearly establishes the nonuniqueness of many of the major symptomatic constellations; and there have been several studies conducted of purportedly unique culture-bound syndromes found among the Zulus of southern Africa (Edwards et al. 1986), Pintupi of Australia (Morice 1978) and the Greenlandic Eskimos (Amering and Katschnig 1990) that show the possibility of translating a culture-bound syndrome into the symptomatic and syndromic language of Western psychiatry.

The central conceptual issue when the question is the uniqueness of a given syndrome is that of the level of abstraction used in such an analysis. Is it the emic level, the culturally specific label for a cluster of behaviors (which would make any given culture-bound syndrome unique in that respect); the level of similarity in observable behaviors (symptoms) characteristically demonstrated in such episodes in different cultural contexts; or a level of a sorting based on inferred neurologic or biologic mechanisms, as Simons has done (Simons 1985b)? It is important that the relevant semantic domain be specified.

Interpreting the term *culture-bound syndromes* in a psychodynamically informed manner, some authors have suggested that such syndromes are not confined to small-scale, underdeveloped societies but may also be found in industrialized social contexts as well. To cite but two examples, Helman (1987) discusses the "type A coronary-prone behavioral pattern" as a response to pervasive and particular value emphases in American society; and Ritenbaugh (1982) considers anorexia nervosa in the same fashion (see also Littlewood and Lipsedge 1985:122ff.). If the basic premise is accepted that salient values in the sociocultural environment of a given person have some degree of determinative relationship to personality dynamics—a point supported by a massive amount of research-based literature in "culture and personality" (in anthropology) and "character and social structure" (sociology)—then there is no a priori reason to exclude industrialized societies from being at risk in this respect.

How does the topic of culture-bound syndromes fare in the psychiatric diagnostic systems of the Western world? Not well (Hughes 1985a, 1989; Simons and Hughes 1993). The topic is rarely even mentioned in conventional psychiatric texts, and fitting the culture-bound syndromes into Western (etic) psychiatric nosological categories is a procrustean challenge. The standard diagnostic manuals are of no help in this regard. Consider, for example, that the term *culture* is missing from the indexes of DSM III and DSM III-R, and that the associated terms *cultural relativism* and *culture bound* are similarly absent. Further, the two features of the innovative multiaxial diagnostic system of the DSM III-R highly relevant for observing and recording behaviors presumptively infused with a "cultural" dimension—Axes IV (Psychosocial Stressors) and V (Highest Level of Adaptive Functioning in Last Year)—were apparently not systematically used by clinicians or researchers (Spitzer and Williams 1983:342–43; Rey et al. 1988), perhaps as much due to lack of appropriate formats for patient charting as to inherent reluctance to accept a new paradigm. Even in the DSM III-R, only two brief paragraphs touched explicitly on this issue. There it is stated, quite rightly, that

[caution] should be exercised in the application of DSM-III-R diagnostic criteria to assure that their use is culturally valid. It is important that the clinician not employ DSM-III-R in a mechanical fashion, insensitive to differences in language, values, behavioral-norms, and idiomatic expressions of distress. (1987:xxvi)

And in the clinically oriented volume of the *International Classification of Diseases* (ICD-9), in which one would expect to find an appropriate framework for such cross-cultural data, the situation is equally disappointing. The only references are to highly segmental uses of the term *culture* or related concepts—for example, *cultural deprivation* (1:880ff.), a subcategory of "social maladjustment." Neither of these terms, nor others that are prima facie psychosocial in nature (such as *family disruption*), are included as etiologic elements in the course and diagnosis of the disease process. The ICD-10, now in preparation, does include more references to the cultural dimension in various psychiatric disorders and symptom clusters. But even in the most recent edition of the American Psychiatric Association's diagnostic manual, DSM IV (1994), there is little systematic progress in incorporating the cultural dimension in data gathering and analysis with respect to assessing a patient's problems; and discussion of the "culture-bound syndromes" is confined to a brief appendix to the volume.

THE HEALING MODALITIES

Viewed cross-culturally, human societies have developed a wide variety of health care practitioners: herbalists, bonesetters, midwives, diviners, acupuncturists, magico-religious healers, and others. In some groups there are even folk healers specializing in mental disorder—"ethnopsychiatrists," one might say—who employ emically derived diagnostic systems relating to behavioral disorders (Lederer 1959; Leighton et al. 1963; Prince 1964). Usually the functions performed by such persons overlap; for example, the magico-religious healer also frequently prescribes herbal remedies, and non-Western folk medicines are rich in their indigenously developed pharmacopeia (Etkin 1986 and the chapter in this volume; Steiner 1986; Vogel 1973). In this respect it is important to note that people in most societies around the world continue to use such folk healers either exclusively or in conjunction with Western-type health care (for literature, see almost any issue of the journal *Social Science and Medicine*).

One type of magico-religious healer is usually taken as the focus—indeed, as the very prototype when discussion turns to "psychiatry" in non-Western societies. This is the shaman. Although the term *shaman* is not culturally authentic for universal use—the term actually coming from the name for such a healer in one of the Paleo-Siberian groups—it has come to be taken interchangeably with *native healer, medicine man* (or *woman*), and the like, and at this point its widespread adoption, however ambiguous ethnographically, should be accepted. The term will be used here in a general sense therefore to refer to the healer whose power and calling come from intimate contact with the spiritual world and whose healing activity includes elements of *materia medica* in the treatment process. (In anthropological discussions of religion, the other principal religious functionary, the priest, derives supernatural power from either oral or written sacred texts and instructions rather than from spiritual inspiration, although the distinction is not absolute.)

The role of shaman has been found in many societies throughout human history, and such personages have had numerous responsibilities, among the most important of which are to serve as a powerful resource for ensuring stability of the group through conducting a ritualistic response to threat. And "threat" does not mean merely sickness; it is also fear of famine from crop failure or poor hunting (depending on the society's subsistence base). The shaman also responds to the quandaries and puzzlement that come from trying to decide on a proper course of action in a problematic situation, either for the group as a whole or for families within that group—whether to make war or peace, where to find lost objects or missing persons, or how to resolve the multifarious other situations needing a firm and authoritative guide for action. Thus the shaman's role is wide ranging; indeed, one might suggest that it is an early exemplar of a social medicine perspective. As the medical historian Sigerist noted, "It is an insult to the medicine man [his term] to call him the ancestor of the modern physician. He is that, to be sure, but he is much more, namely the ancestor of most of our professions" (1967:161).

In 1936 Morris Opler published a classic article on shamanism among the Apache, the principal conclusions of which have stood the test of comparison and elaboration in subsequent interpretations of the powerful and emically omniscient role that particular type of healer has had in human society (for other examples, see Torrey 1973; Prince 1980; and relevant sections in a number of edited volumes in medical anthropology, such as Kiev 1964; Landy 1977; Romanucci-Ross et al. 1983; Gaines 1992; and, among others, the journals *Social Science and Medicine* and *Culture, Medicine and Psychiatry*).

Opler's central points (though not the culturally particularistic details, of course) are widely generalizable. These include such features as the involvement of the family and kinship group in both etiological explanations and therapy; use of empirical remedies; and setting off of the diagnostic and therapeutic encounter as a special situation that transfigures normal role relationships. Above all, informing all activities is a comprehensive conception of what shall be accepted as "disease"—indeed, it is *"dys-ease"* in its original etymologic sense rather than the more restrictive denotation, if not connotation, of "disease" in Western systems.

Some of the highlights of Opler's analysis may be taken as a model for shamanism and its sociopsychological context. The Apache shaman's power was believed to come from an all-encompassing nonempirical force pervading the world. But being privy to such power was not simply for the asking; rather, a signal must be given, an invitation offered to the aspirant. That signal took the form of a bird, an animal, a plant, or some other animate object that would give the shaman the script for a healing ceremony, such a program to include the details of proper offerings or sacrifices, prayers, songs, and behavior.

Although any group member (male or female) was a potential shaman, a subtle selection process occurred, and in practice the successful shaman turned out to have a number of behavioral characteristics that augured well for an ability to translate the putative supernatural basis of his or her healing power into the world of everyday events. For example, as Opler notes,

he [or she] is . . . not a credulous dupe of his own supernaturalistic claims and boastings, who undertakes to cure any ailment, no matter how hopeless. . . . The seasoned shaman was a shrewd and wary person who had witnessed enough suffering and death to recognize serious organic disturbances when he sees them, and was often reluctant to accept responsibility for curing these. (1936:1372–73)

In such a case he finds a convincing reason for referring to someone else or indicates that the patient should prepare himself or herself in particular ways before the attempted therapy could be undertaken (perhaps thereby giving natural healing processes a chance to take effect).

The reputation of a healer (shaman or otherwise) depended on success, and the Apache shaman was adept at understanding self-limiting disease processes, as well as in using herbal medication and harnessing the power of the patient's belief in his ability to bring about a cure or amelioration. Such a combination of knowledge and skill frequently resulted in a successful outcome; if that did not occur, there was always an explanation (such as the patient's or someone else's having "bad thoughts"; in this respect, one might compare this with noncompliance in Western medicine's etic terms, in which often the patient is blamed for not following the physician's orders strictly enough to effect the cure). Opler continues:

What I am suggesting is that the Apache shaman is far from an inspired automaton who enters upon his ritual without regard to the nature of the complaint, the circumstances and the probable outcome. He is a circumspect and careful worker more often, a good judge of his fellow men and of the ills to which humankind is heir. (pp. 1173–74)

The shaman would then actively take steps to encourage and foster the patient's belief in his powers to heal, such as directing the patient's family (kin were always extensively involved) to build a particular ceremonial structure for the ritual. When the arrangements were made, the first event was that of the shaman's once again reinforcing the belief of the patient and the patient's family in his curative powers. He would recount how he had obtained his skill and knowledge and how many people he had helped (an act perhaps comparable in its effect to the framed diplomas indicating past training and awards that decorate the modern physician's office wall?):

The insistence upon belief in the shaman and his "power" is one of the most dominant and omnipresent themes of Apache ritual life. There is no more common phrase in the ceremonial songs than the one which can be translated, "I believe it." It is assumed that the "power" will scarcely be inclined to extend itself or to expose its representative [the shaman] to danger on behalf of a patient who lacks the requisite degree of faith. (p. 1376)

Then the diagnostic process would begin, with the shaman trying to get at the root of the trouble. First he would set the background, reciting many events of the patient's life leading up to the appearance of the symptoms (which he would have gathered by listening to gossip, unobtrusive interviewing, and other data-gathering devices readily at hand in a small community). A competent shaman would have learned everything he possibly could about the patient before the ceremony; he would also urge the patient to contribute what might be useful information (to "give his own history") and remember things that might account for the sickness (analogous, perhaps, to the modern family physician's wide-ranging patient history?). Sometimes by this simple recitation, the symptom itself might even disappear, though the underlying disorder might well remain.

The event seized on for etiological significance would be presented in familiar emic Apache symbols—for example, the patient had come into contact with an owl, bear, snake, or other animal embodying evil or serving as the instrument of a sorcerer's malevolence. The shaman pointed out this contact or whatever else in the patient's history might seem to be the source of the trouble, and usually the patient eagerly accepted such an explanation. Against the background of the patient's belief in the shaman's powers and his or her commitment to the shaman's competence and power, one can infer that a substantial part of the therapeutic process consisted of suggestion and displacement of vague problems onto some concrete object or situation. (Indeed, the panhuman power of the word, especially as embodied in the diagnosis, is well represented in this process; how comforting it is, for example, to be told one has a "cryptogenic" disease—*cryptogenic* being a Latin-derived adjective meaning "hidden cause"—instead of being told by medical authority, "I just don't know what it is.")

But the shaman must go further; he must give a reason why the patient is ill, and he does so by consulting his spiritual helpers. Performing sacred songs and beseeching his powers to come to the aid of the patient, the shaman is told the reasons for the patient's illness—for example, a sorcerer had sent an "evil" animal such as a bear to frighten him or had "shot arrows" into the patient.

Then ensues the climax of this diagnostic-therapeutic process, a contest between the powers of the shaman and those of the sorcerer, spirits, or objects causing the distress.

In the place of his patient the shaman substitutes himself, and the battle between the malevolent power and the patient is transformed into warfare between the shaman and the sorcerer. As soon as the shaman has announced that the cause is sorcery, he declares against it. . . . He consults with his "power" on tactics. He relates how the sorcerer is trying to balk him and is desperately trying to hold his own. The theory is that a sorcerer, if bested, forfeits his power and his life. If the sorcerer cannot prevent the shaman from sucking the bone arrows and other evidences of his malice from the body of the victim, these objects "come back on himself." A sorcerer whose "power" is bested is shot by his own "arrows" and dies soon afterward. The strengthening psychological effect upon the patient of gaining a powerful ally can well be imagined. (Opler 1936:1382–83)

The setting for such a ceremony is a multimedia event: theatrics, suspense, and drama, with the family in attendance and as much involved as the sick person. Frank (1973) extensively discusses the varieties of group settings that ritually serve the therapeutic process:

Healing ceremonies are highly charged emotionally. . . . [Methods] of primitive healing involve an interplay between patient, healer, group, and the world of the supernatural; this serves to raise the patient's expectancy of cure, help him to harmonize his inner conflicts, reintegrate him with his group and the spiritual world, supply a conceptual framework to aid this, and stir him emotionally. The total process combats his demoralization and strengthens his sense of self-worth. (1973:66)

In a survey of "cultural psychiatry," Kennedy (1973:1170) presents an amalgam of commonly found elements in what he pointedly calls the "dramatic healing ritual":

Rather than being a private encounter of two individuals, the trance ritual is a semipublic event made up of at least three elements—patient, therapist, and audience, all of whom actively participate. Frequently there are auxiliary helpers such as assistants, musicians, and masters of ceremony; and in the audience are people who know the patient and curer in their daily life roles.

At the end of such a ceremony the shaman would impose special taboos upon the patient (a therapeutic regimen? "doctor's orders"?) and even family members. They may not eat a particular food, for example, must not perform certain acts, must avoid certain locations, and so forth. Such authoritative directives offer something concrete for the patient's troubled mind to focus on instead of remaining gripped by vague worry and anxiety. This is especially true when accompanied by requirements for the preparation and ingestion of particular kinds of empirical medicines.

Opler ends his article by discussing the extent to which the modern psychiatrist and the shaman are similar. Obviously details of pharmacopoeia differ, but many of the psychodynamics involved are congruent. Opler indicates (with apparent disapproval) that the shamanic healing process is conducive to—perhaps intended for—the creation of a high degree of dependence of the patient on the shaman—what Prince (1969:33) referred to as the patient's coming under the "cone of authority." Arguments will continue among professionals as to whether the gaining of insight and enhancement of a sense of autonomy, among other outcomes, should be the primary goal of psychotherapy in all cases, as contrasted to simply relief of symptoms. But what stands out clearly in discussions not only of shamanic healing in other societies but also as the effective ingredient in so much of the healing encounter in industrialized societies is that the sociopsychological and cultural context of the encounter may well be the most critical factor of all in bringing about a successful outcome for at least the functional types of disorders.

Such a psychologically induced outcome has been referred to as the "placebo effect": a powerful psychobiological process conducive to healing, or at least amelioration, fostered by an aura of compelling and emotion-triggering symbols, theatric reaffirmation of a system of belief, and, above all, a profound sense of confidence in the healer, all of which have been noted in all societies. Along with other commentators (e.g., Moerman 1983), Brody notes that

[Placebo] research suggests that the placebo response forms a part of virtually all healing encounters, and is not limited to circumstances in which a "dummy" pill is used. This suggests, in turn, that the placebo effect has been important in medicine throughout history, and that the modern physician has important elements in common with . . . "prescientific" predecessors. (Brody 1988a:149)

In this respect, in a memorable metaphor that well expresses the demonstrably powerful health protective effects of a supportive human relationship, Balint (1964) spoke of the "doctor as drug."

One theme has been background in this discussion: the artificiality of any ontologic distinction drawn between ethnomedicine and ethnopsychiatry and the embeddedness of both in a sociocultural context. Perhaps, therefore, drawing on earlier formulations, one may once again suggest that ''religion, medicine, and morality are frequently found together in the behavioral act or event, and 'folk medicine' becomes 'social medicine' to an extent not found in industrialized societies'' (Hughes 1968:88).

8

Ethnopharmacology: The Conjunction of Medical Ethnography and the Biology of Therapeutic Action

Nina L. Etkin

Ethnopharmacology is the study of indigenous medicines that connects the ethnography of health and healing to the physical composition of medicines and their physiologic actions. In biomedical inquiry, pharmacology is attentive to the sources, chemistry, and actions of drugs (pharmaceuticals). A hyphenated ethnopharmacology applies those principles to contexts in which the prevailing modes of treatment and prevention are other than pharmaceuticals and are principally botanical. Paradoxically—for a subfield that laid claim to a "mediating nexus between biological and cultural aspects of anthropology" (Landy 1977: 12)—a disproportionate amount of research in medical anthropology has been concerned with the cultural construction of therapeutics, the social relations of healing, and the political economy of health. Ethnopharmacologic investigations have begun to fill the void in a literature that lacks systematic investigations of how the physical attributes of medicines are interpreted in local contexts and whether the therapeutic modalities that anthropologists study directly influence the pathophysiology of illness. While they acknowledge that symbol and metaphor also are constituted in medicinal plants, ethnopharmacologists treat medicines as more than simply cultural objects. In this way, they illuminate an important set of criteria—physical action and taste, among others—that indigenous populations engage in the selection of medicines and the interpretation of therapeutic outcome. The methodology of ethnopharmacology combines established ethnographic inquiry with techniques adapted from botany and pharmacology. Attention to the specific circumstances of plant therapy and overlapping genres of use (medicine, food, religion, etc.) helps us to understand the extent to which people are exposed to pharmacologically active substances. By assimilating the evolutionary texture of anthropological inquiry, ethnopharmacology can be related to both archaeological and nonhuman primate studies. Where there is a coalescence of botanicals and pharmaceutical drugs, as occurs today in much of the "developing"—and even "developed"—world, ethnopharmacology offers insights that inform both the theoretical and the applied concerns of medical anthropology. Ethnopharmacology also is a key element in the multidisciplinary efforts that have been mounted in recent years to curb the erosion of biodiversity: anthropologists, especially, can help to distinguish some of the more important species by focusing attention on plants identified through local therapeutic models.

THE POSITION OF ETHNOPHARMACOLOGY IN MEDICAL ANTHROPOLOGY

Since its formal inception in the 1970s, chroniclers of medical anthropology have located its theoretical postulates in the intercalation of biological and behavioral aspects of health and healing. The intellectual message has been that the body is at once biologically and culturally constructed (Hahn and Kleinman 1983b; Scheper-Hughes and Lock 1987). Programmatic statements and prolegomena aside, most medical anthropologists have in fact been more interested to engage the epistemological and interpretive aspects of health, and issues of meaning (Browner, Ortiz de Montellano, and Rubel 1988). Only a small number champion an explicitly biocultural (or biobehavioral) perspective and also conduct empirical studies on the nature of the interrelations between biological and cultural variables (Etkin 1986, 1994a; Johns 1990; McElroy 1990; Ortiz de Montellano 1986).

Insofar as ethnopharmacology borrows some of the language and technique of bioscience, it has received tacit criticism in the recent spate of vitriolic "dialogue" (Singer 1989b) about biocultural approaches, in which these explanatory frames have been conflated with the reductionistic, narrow empiricism that characterizes some biomedical research. Wiley (1993), Morgan (1993a), and others have exposed the spurious nature of these arguments to demonstrate that a biocultural paradigm better represents the "dialectic of nature and culture" (Hahn and Kleinman 1983b) than the one once called for by the self-appointed visionaries of medical anthropology. One might argue that it elevates inquiry to an altogether different plane by embellishing medical ethnography with the corporeality of body, illness, and medicine. Plant medicines are viewed simultaneously as cultural objects and biodynamic substances. The pharmacologic potential of plants both contributes to and transcends their cultural meanings. This locates ethnopharmacology centrally among contemporary studies in medical anthropology that endeavor to comprehend the dynamics of human-environment relations and how these affect health.

In addition to explicitly anthropological studies of ethnomedicines, the literature of ethnopharmacology is broadly multidisciplinary and, fittingly, diverse. The academic and applied disciplines so represented include botany, pharmacognosy (drug discovery) and pharmacology, nutrition, and agroforestry. These other ethnopharmacologic studies are largely atheoretical, often based in field study of short duration and minimal cultural immersion. Much of this literature consists of compilations that list medicinal uses that have been reported by a small number of local specialists—compared, for example, with anthropological studies that focus on larger and more representative samples of respondents who instruct the researcher not only by responding to lists of plants but also through extensive interview and by their actions in the actual contexts in which plants are used. Simple lists of plants and their applications typically overlook some of the details that anthropologists regard as salient, such as preparation, combination, and intended outcome. In short, these other ethnopharmacologic studies are thin on "ethno-" and direct more attention to the pharmacologic and botanical aspects of the inquiry. In view of those disciplinary differences, such works are variably amenable to the level of cultural analysis and cross-population comparison that interests anthropologists.

Where pharmacologists tend to screen plants to discover pharmacologic potential, anthropologists' contributions to ethnopharmacology are framed by a suite of questions that interrelate cultural, botanical, and biological data. Pharmacologic investigations tend to be disengaged from the contexts of plant use, as they pursue certain activities—for example, antifertility (Lohiya et al. 1994) and antiviral actions (Beuscher et al. 1994); particular species, genera, and higher taxa (e.g., *Heimia salicifolia* [Malone and Rother 1994], genus *Kopsia* [Sévenet et al. 1994], and family Solanaceae [Dafni and Yaniv 1994]); specific phytochemical constituents, for example, verbasciside, an antimicrobial (Pardo et al. 1993); polyacetylenes (anti-inflammatory agents) (Redl et al. 1994); or geographic regions (e.g., Brazil [Souza Brito and Souza Brito 1993] or Turkey [Yesilada et al. 1993]). Often these provide the important details of chemistry and action from which anthropologists develop hypotheses about the outcome of treatment as it is related to indigenous explanatory models.

This shifts the intellectual compass from phytochemistry and pharmacologic action to the intersection of cultural and biological data. Browner and Ortiz de Montellano (1986) showed how the organoleptic qualities (smell, texture, taste) of plants both direct their selection and reflect their chemical makeup. Women in Colombia and Mexico identify "hot" and "irritating" plants to induce menses (the proximate goal), the larger or ultimate objective being to influence the timing and outcome of pregnancy. The oxytocic (labor-stimulating), emmenagogue (menstruation-promoting), and abortifacient actions that are revealed through pharmacologic study provide a deeper and more realistic comprehension of therapeutic objectives. Similarly, Heinrich, Rimpler, and Barrera (1992) demonstrated how a Mixe community uses chemosensation to identify medicinal plants: bitter or aromatic plants are selected for gastrointestinal disorders; "cooling" (aromatic) qualities signal efficacy for febrile disorders; sweet and sometimes sour qualities are valued for respiratory disorders; astringency identifies medicines for diarrhea and dysentery. Conversely, burning, itching, and salty are regarded as dangerous and are not used as medicines. The pharmacologic profiles of the species considered suggest efficacy consistent with intended outcome. Just as ethnographic data on medicinal plant use form the basis for constructing hypotheses regarding potential activity, the ordering of pharmacologic and botanical data by use, preparation, and so forth can illuminate the criteria applied by indigenous peoples to the organization of therapeutics.

METHODS IN ANTHROPOLOGICAL ETHNOPHARMACOLOGY

By its very nature, ethnopharmacology uses some of the methods of bioscience, but neither its methodology nor its theoretical underpinnings form the basis of anthropological studies in this area. Anthropologists are not concerned with plant chemistry to judge whether some indigenous peoples "got it right" (use pharmacologically active plants in a way that is consistent with the principles of biomedicine), but instead to ply the techniques of bioscience as one aspect of a broad-based inquiry into plant use.

Anthropological ethnopharmacology combines established ethnographic methods to investigate the cultural basis of health and therapeutics (including how that is informed by the biological characteristics of plants) and literature review and laboratory investigation to explore pharmacologic and other actions (Etkin 1993). The field methods discussed by Pelto and Pelto in Chapter 15 of this book all are relevant for ethnopharmacology and can be variably adapted for inquiry centering on how explanatory models of illness and health shape therapeutic strategies; selection criteria for plants and other medicines, including the interpretation of pharmacologic and other action; the combination of botanical medicines with pharmaceuticals; and so on. The depth of ethnographic inquiry especially distinguishes anthropological from other ethnopharmacologies. Intracultural diversity is revealed by engaging an array of respondents, not just medical and plant specialists. Although these latter individuals are valuable sources of (especially esoteric) knowledge, they represent more the unique experiences of individual lives, whereas the prevention and treatment of illness are community-wide processes that should be examined for diffuse (exoteric) sources of botanical and medical knowledge. These other individuals who are knowledgeable about plants include religious functionaries who use botanicals in sacred rites, food preparers, animal tenders, hunters who employ poisons and paralytics, and individuals who use plants for cosmetics, dyes, and other items of manufacture.

Using the ethnographic data as a guide to preparation and therapeutic application, some subset of plants that has been revealed in the course of study is collected in sufficient quantity for laboratory testing (about 5 kg minimum per species). Which subset becomes the focus of the extended study is dictated largely by the researcher's interests, the salience of a particular disease or plant type to the local community, and practical concerns regarding the availability of plants in sufficient volume for study and the technical expertise of the researchers to investigate certain actions (e.g., testing for anti-inflammatory or antimicrobial action is relatively easy; finding anticancer agents is not). The specific analyses undertaken for a given project are drawn from a great diversity of standardized pharmacologic techniques that test for particular action or constituents and may include animals (and rarely humans) as research subjects.

All plants for which data are collected are represented by voucher specimens: samples that are pressed flat to exhibit as many features as possible, dried, mounted on paper, and labeled with local names and collection site. These are later deposited at herbaria for identification by botanical taxonomists. Vouchers are the lingua franca of all ethnobotanical inquiry, providing the only irrefutable link between local and bioscientific knowledge. Previously published lists that correspond vernaculars to botanical names are not a substitute because common names change over time and place and may be applied to more than one botanical species. By identifying vouchers specific to a particular study, one can take advantage of published accounts of those plants, as well as design comparisons of the interpretation and use of particular species cross-culturally. Once the taxonomic identification has been determined, literature review is conducted using, for example, NAPRALERT (Natural Products Alert Data Base), a distillation of the world's literature on the ethnobotany, phytochemistry, and pharmacology of plants. Data on plant constituents and action embellish the medical ethnography and increase the number of hypotheses that can be entertained through the course of research. Significantly, in a biocultural framework, botanicals are marked both culturally and biodynamically; and plant chemistry and action can be both dependent and independent variables in the complex relationships that bear on health and healing.

CONTEXTS OF MEDICINAL PLANT USE

Careful attention to the contexts in which medicines are used distinguishes anthropological studies from other ethnopharmacologic inquiry.[1] Context of use is construed broadly to include interview, observation, and reflection.

Criteria in Plant Selection

Criteria that are applied in the selection of plants are complex and include physical characteristics such as texture, taste, color, and smell; age and maturity; growing location; and physiologic action. All of these are qualities that affect or are affected by the chemical composition of plants. For many medical cultures, plant selection overlaps cognitive principles based in binary oppositions such as sweet-sour, hot-cold, or yin-yang. These reside in explanatory models that emphasize balance and proportion—more typically in the symbolic realm than in the physical. Further, ethnobiologists have recorded indigenous taxonomies of plant appearance, action, and other characteristics that reflect people's experiences with their physical environment and their interpretation of it. This is reflected in some plant names—for example, wormwood (*Artemesia absinthium*, a powerful anthelminthic), the Hausa *madaci* ("most bitter") (*Khaya senegalensis*, a very bitter-tasting African mahogany), and birthwort (*Aristolochia clematitis*, efficacious in assisting childbirth). Culturological interpretations of these classificatory schemes that focus only on what plants mean miss essential elements of the therapeutic exercise, which is, at base, a deliberate conjunction of sign (texture or color, for example) with physiologic action (e.g., anti-inflammatory, hypotensive). Thus, the red color of plants used in American Indian medicine to treat wounds may well be a signature that identifies plants by the color of blood (redwood, *Sequoia sempervirens;* redbud, *Cercis canadensis*); but it also signifies that the red quinones that impart color to some of these plants are hemostatic and antimicrobial (Delaveau 1981)—properties that users of those plants could identify through their own experiences. Indeed, those physiologic actions may be the primary criteria for selection, with red color being simply the mnemonic tool for the identification of wound-healing plants.

Because pharmacologic action varies among individuals of a species and among plant parts, it is possible to manage the activity of medicinal preparations by specification to plant part (flower petal, leaf, seed); developmental stage of plant organ (new leaves, flower buds); and time of year and growing location (pharmacologic activity may vary with soil composition, rainfall, altitude, and other features of the local ecology). For example, market prices for qat (*Catha edulis*) in North Yemen fluctuate depending on time of day and source of harvest, reflecting that psychotropic activity diminishes over time and varies with growing location (Kennedy 1987).

Preparation

The way in which plant medicines are prepared is important, not only to understand the ritual or other signed elements of healing but also because this influences plant chemistry (Johns and Kubo 1988). For example the fibers of, especially raw, plants can interact with organic compounds, including some toxins, to reduce their availability and thus diminish their effects. Similarly, the concurrent consumption of medicinal plants and minerals or soils (geophagy), especially clay, results in the adsorption of some constituents, reducing their availability. Softening plant materials by soaking in water, heating, and the addition of sodium bicarbonate or lye (sodium or potassium hydroxide) extends the surface area on which digestive enzymes act and generally increases the availability of plant constituents. Potentially, this amplifies exposure to pharmacologically active substances, but this would be compromised by dilution of constituents with water, the interaction of lye and bicarbonates with organic materials, heat inactivation of some chemicals, and heat denaturation of the enzymes that would otherwise liberate active compounds. Other preparations that can affect the chemical composition of plant medicines include grating, crushing, and pounding; suspending or decocting in alcohol, water, or oil; dry-ing; or altering acid/base status (pH). These considerations distinguish anthropological studies of plant medicines and show how the pharmacologist's analysis of sterile extractions of single plants in acetone, methanol, and other solvents informs but is not an ethnopharmacologic study. This is demonstrated as well in the case of composite plant medicines.

Plant Interactions

As every plant comprises an array of constituents, the combination of plants in composite medicines presents a virtual chaos of pharmacologic potential. Interactions among these phytochemicals may be synergistic (when the action of one constituent is conspicuously increased by the other or others), additive (when the combined action of two or more constituents is summed), potentiating (when the effect is greater than additive), or antagonistic (when one or more constituents diminish the activity of one or more others). Where pharmacologists often regard the emphasis on composite preparation as a distraction, closer attention reveals interesting insights into the rationale of indigenous therapeutics. For example, while the three individual elements of the Ayurvedic *trikatu* demonstrate little activity against the various disorders for which this medicine is prescribed, *Zingiber officinale* (ginger), *Piper nigrum* (black pepper), and *P. longum* (long pepper) together significantly increase the bioavailability of constituents of the other plants to which they are added—such as sparteine (anti-inflammatory, diuretic, oxytocic: in Spanish broom, *Spartium junceum*) and vasicine (expectorant, oxytocic, and abortifacient: in adhatoda, *Justicia adhatoda*) (Atal, Zutchi, and Rao 1981). In other cases, the association of plants may diminish the toxicity of their individual constituents (such as tannins and saponins) (Freeland, Calcott, and Anderson 1985) while facilitating the low-concentration activities of those same constituents or the beneficial actions of other substances in the mixture. On the other hand, whereas an explicitly pharmacologic interpretation would predict antibiotic action for barberry (*Berberis vulgaris*) and anti-inflammatory activity for licorice (*Glycyrrhiza glabra*), when these plants are combined, berberine and glycyrrhizin precipitate, thus neutralizing the activities of both (Noguchi 1978).

Administration

How plant medicines are administered has pharmacologic implications as well. Biomedicine once dismissed the topical application of medicines for internal (nondermatologic) conditions as "theater" or "suggestive magic." Today, having "discovered" the principle of transdermal absorption of certain medicines, replaceable patches are used for drug administration (e.g., nicotine replacement in stop-smoking therapy and nitroglycerine for heart conditions). Hausa in Nigeria include on-skin medicines as one element of treatment for "spot diseases," such as measles. Topical application of bitter and astringent medicines (e.g., neem, *Azadirachta indica*) treats the external phase of measles; medicines consumed by mouth are directed at the internal phase of the illness, both to encourage egress of the internal sores through the skin with bitter and astringent medicines (e.g., *Entada africana, E. abyssinica*), and later to impart cold and aromatic qualities (e.g., *Citrus* spp., *Centaurea perrottetii*). Finally, astringent and emollient medicines (cassava, *Manihot esculenta*) are applied to resolve the rash.

Intended Outcome

Perhaps the most significant, and underexplored, element of context is the intended outcome of therapy. Whereas one could generalize that the objective of all medicines is to "get better," especially outside biomedicine this involves more than simply removing the agent of disease and resolving symptoms. Healing is not an event but a process in which the ultimate objective is preceded by a number of proximate goals: diagnosing etiology, transforming the body or its parts to prepare for healing, seeking evidence of disease egress, and the like (Etkin 1988a). The treatment of gastrointestinal disorders by Hausa in Nigeria is a case in point. Certain plants are taken to determine etiology: discomfort as reaction to consuming *Agelanthus dodoneifolius,* for example, confirms spirit-caused illness; other reactions variably invoke witchcraft or elements of the natural environment (dirt, cold). Vomiting, purging, and discolored stools are signs that disease agents leave the body and are achieved with *Ficus capensis* (bush fig) and *Cassia occidentalis* (coffee senna). Later in the therapeutic process, emollient and costive plants relieve symptoms of intestinal distress—such as locust bean (*Parkia filicoidea*) and tamarind (*Tamarindus indica*). This illustrates again that epistemological and interpretive studies in medical anthropology tell only part of the story of healing and that pharmacologic assessment outside of cultural context is not ethnopharmacology (albeit informative on another level).

MULTICONTEXTUAL PLANT USE

Just as the details of context are important, so too is documenting whether plants are used for more than one purpose. Where we are interested in the extent of exposure to pharmacologically active constituents, the potential health-mediating effects cannot be assessed unless one is mindful of all contexts of exposure. This suspends—but only temporarily—attention to the emic categories "eating," "doing medicine," and so on. In the evaluation of physiologic effects, those categories are important only to the extent that different genres of use designate different preparation and administration of the plants, which may affect phytochemical composition and activity.

Until recently single-use (single-context) studies dominated the literature of ethnopharmacology. Ethnomedical studies typically sought to correspond symptoms with treatments and neglected to elicit other circumstances of use; food surveys centered on plants consumed during "meals" proper, missing both non-meal consumption (e.g., snacks) and other uses of those "foods"; and plants used variously in cosmetics, manufacture, and so on, were not problematized beyond those applications to consider the physical and cultural implications of iterative use. Even though the "primary" application of a plant may indeed be as, say, medicine or cosmetic, one needs to comprehend the whole range of circumstances through which people are exposed to the active constituents of botanicals that they use. This more realistically depicts people's experience with plants and underscores the significance of individual species to which people are regularly exposed.

Today in anthropological ethnopharmacology, more and more attention is centered on multicontextual use, heeding the counsel of those who pioneered research on the overlapping dimensions of plant use (Etkin and Ross 1982b, 1991a, 1991b; Etkin 1986, 1994a, 1994b; Johns 1990). The most consequential impact that plants have on human physiology outside medicinal use is through diet (Etkin and Ross 1991a), since foods tend to be consumed both regularly and in relatively large amounts.[2] That said, one must appreciate also that these two circumstances of use are not always clearly distinguished from one another, especially when the discourse of healing includes such concepts as "tonics," "fortifying" and "healthy foods," "nourishing medicines," and the like. (The subjects of ethnopharmacologic study are aware of these blurred distinctions as well.) Opportunity for the prolonged contact of plants with body tissues is also provided by the use of botanicals as items of personal hygiene, cosmetics, adornment, and manufacture, especially of cordage, basketry, leather-working, and dyeing.

As illustration, consider these observations from our research among Hausa in northern Nigeria (Etkin 1994a). Significant overlap is revealed by addressing only four categories of use: medicine, food, cosmetics, and personal hygiene. Medicines overlap most prominently with foods: all but 5 of the 119 food plants identified by this population are subsumed within the 374 primary medicinals. Factoring cosmetics and items of personal hygiene into the equation emphasizes the point (Tables 8.1 and 8.2).

This intersection of just four categories is striking; expanding the number of use genres multiplies the intercategory junctions exponentially. This gives us an impression of how much people come into contact with plants in nonmedical (or metamedical) circumstances, but until we understand the physiologic significance of exposure to those botanicals, we cannot fully comprehend the health implications of overlapping categories of plant use. In view of the enormity of such a task, full pharmacologic evaluation of all plants for all illness categories exceeds the capacity of even the most ambitious projects. The task then becomes to problematize the inquiry first to a subset of plants, in this case plants used in at least three of the categories under consideration (Table 8.3).

Beyond limiting the number of plants for further scrutiny, inquiry needs to

Table 8.1
Hausa Cosmetic Plants: Overlapping Contexts of Use

Genus species	Hausa	Med	Food	Cos	Hyg
Acacia nilotica (L) Willd ex Del	GABARUWA	x		x	
Acacia nilotica (L) Willd ex Del var tomentosa (Benth) AF Hill	GABARUWA	x		x	
Anacardium occidentale L	KANJU	x	x	x	
Arachis hypogaea L	MAN GYADA	x	x	x	x
Argemone mexicana L	KWARKO	x		x	
Bombax buonopozense P Beauv	GURJIYA	x		x	
Cola nitida (Vent) Schott & Endl	GORO	x		x	
Cola acuminata (Pal) Schott & Endl	GORO	x		x	
Commiphora africana (A Rich) Engl	DASHI	x	x	x	x
Datura innoxia Mill	ZAKAMI	x		x	
Datura metel	ZAKAMI	x		x	
Diospyros mespiliformis Hochst	KANYA	x	x	x	
Feretia canthioides Hiern	KURUKURU	x		x	
Feretia apodanthera Del	KURUKURU	x		x	
Indigofera arrecta Hochst ex AR	BABA	x	x	x	x
Lawsonia inermis L	LALLE	x		x	
Nicotiana tabacum L	TABA	x		x	
Portulaca oleracea L	DABURIN SANIYA	x		x	
Thelepogon elegans Roth	LADANBALI	x		x	
Trianthema portulacastrum L	DABURIN SANIYA	x		x	

Source: Etkin (1994b, Table 3).

be narrowed to, for example, a specific symptom or illness, or a single class of activity. Our research strategy for Hausa plants problematizes a group of plants to single-activity categories, such as antimicrobial action (Etkin 1994a), allowing us to develop depth rather than only the breadth provided by lists of plants or their constituents. Similarly we have focused on single symptoms or disease complexes—such as gastrointestinal disorders (Etkin and Ross 1982b), disorders of the teeth and gums, and malaria (Etkin 1980, 1994a; Etkin and Ross 1991b). This links plant and activity to conditions that are likely to improve on treatment with this species. It also illustrates how that benefit might be amplified by further exposure as that plant is used in other contexts (see also Reinhard et al. 1985; Johns et al. 1990; Morgan 1981; Mathias-Mundy and McCorckle 1989). Inquiry can be further specified to categories of use that covary with, say, age, gender, or occupation; for Hausa, because leathercraft, weaving, farming, and exterior house construction are mostly the province of men, regular and prolonged contact with botanical dyes and insecticides carries a gendered pharmacologic potential. Similarly, the pharmacology of plants used in cleaning cooking utensils, some veterinary tasks,[3] the manufacture of plaited mats, and preparation of house floors is more germane for women.

Up to this point, I have configured the discussion to highlight apparently adaptive patterns of plant use: cases in which our knowledge of the composition and action of a particular species suggests that outcome is likely to be consistent with users' objectives.[4] For balance, ethnopharmacologic study should entertain as well the potential for untoward effects. The issue of toxicity has been ex-

Table 8.2

Hausa Plants Used for Personal Hygiene: Overlapping Contexts of Use

Genus species	Hausa	Med	Food	Cos	Hyg
Anogeissus leiocarpus (DC) Guill & Perr	MARKE	x			x
Arachis hypogaea L	MAN GYADA	x	x	x	x
Azadirachta indica A Juss	DARBEJIYA	x			x
Boerhavia diffusa L	GADON MACIJI	x			x
Boerhavia repens L	GADON MACIJI	x			x
Commiphora africana (A Rich) Engl	DASHI	x	x	x	x
Euphorbia lateriflora Schum & Thonn	BI DA SARTSE	x			x
Euphorbia balsamifera Aiton	AIYARA	x			x
Glossenema nubicum Decne	TATARIDA	x			x
Glossonema boveanum Decne	TATARIDA	x			x
Indigofera arrecta Hochst ex AR	BABA	x	x	x	x
Khaya senegalensis (Desr) A Juss	MADACI	x			x
Salvadora persica L	SHIWAKA	x	x		x
Vernonia colorata Drake	SHIWAKA	x	x		x
Vernonia amygdalina Del	SHIWAKA	x	x		x
(Unidentified)	SABULIN SALO	x			x

Source: Etkin (1994b, Table 4).

aggerated by those who wish to discredit ethnotherapeutics as lacking empirical basis. In fact there is more evidence that indigenous peoples are quite adroit at managing toxicity (Johns and Kubo 1988). And toxic and other unwanted effects in botanical therapy have been traced to improper use (including overdose) and adulterated products rather than an underlying flaw (de Smet 1991; Bye and Dutton 1991; Nyazema 1986; Qureshi, Shah, and Ageel 1992).[5] A guiding precept here for all medicines—animal, vegetable, and especially pharmaceuticals, which tend to be chemically more concentrated—is that the relationship between therapeutic and toxic dose is equivocal and is based as much in the specific circumstances of use as it is in chemical composition (Bisset 1991).

DIRECTIONS FOR FUTURE RESEARCH

Ethnopharmacology has applications to the various subdisciplines of anthropology beyond medical anthropology. By invoking the evolutionary perspective of anthropological inquiry, ethnopharmacology can be related to both archaeological and nonhuman primate studies. As archaeologists have relied on ethnographic analogy to project contemporary behaviors into the past, they have begun to transcend the conventional paradigm through which evidence of edible plants is interpreted to reflect past foodways. A handful of researchers has drawn attention to both potential medicinal species and their overlapping use as food: Pyramarn (1989) interpreting late Stone Age sites in Thailand and Reinhard, Hamilton, and Hevly (1991), Sobolik and Gerick (1992), and Trigg et al. (1994) inferring from coprolite analysis in the U.S. Southwest. This can be projected to a more distant hypothetical past through consideration of the varied uses of

Table 8.3
Hausa Plants Used in at Least Three Contexts

Genus species	Hausa	Med	Food	Cos	Hyg
Anacardium occidentale L	KANJU	x	x	x	
Arachis hypogaea L	MAN GYADA	x	x	x	x
Commiphora africana (A Rich) Engl	DASHI	x	x	x	x
Diospyros mespiliformis Hochst	KANYA	x	x	x	
Indigofera arrecta Hochst ex AR	BABA	x	x	x	x
Salvadora persica L	SHIWAKA	x	x		x
Vernonia colorata Drake	SHIWAKA	x	x		x
Vernonia amygdalina Del	SHIWAKA	x	x		x

Source: Etkin (1994b, Table 5).

plants by other animals. Increasingly, researchers in nonhuman primate behavior question whether what they record in the field as feeding behaviors are just that. For example, howler monkeys taste and smell plants to discern different qualities, some apparently to influence birth spacing, and they teach these behaviors intergenerationally (Glander 1994). Chimpanzees also manipulate plants in idiosyncratic ways[6] and consume at different times of day,[7] depending on whether they are feeding or doing "medicine," presumably to affect the availability and action of pharmacologically active constituents. These behaviors have analogues in the human use of these plants in preventive and therapeutic medicine, and the pharmacologic profiles of the plants in question (revealing antimicrobial, anthelminthic, and other actions) suggest that these are not serendipitous associations but the result of the evolution (including cultural transmission) of "feeding" techniques by which individuals avail themselves of pharmacologic action and avoid toxic doses. The accumulating evidence (much still anecdotal) suggest that this phenomenon can be generalized beyond primates to mammals, birds, insects, and other taxa (P. Newton 1991). This introduces novel interpretations of primate-plant interactions—including primate social organization and ranging—and offers insights into our prehominid past. These expanded perspectives in archaeology and primate studies will benefit from additional, more systematic study to reveal the role of active plant constituents through the course of human evolution.

Striking a note of irony, the pharmacologic study of indigenous medicines is helping us to understand the global proliferation of pharmaceuticals. Most of the "developing" world currently is witness to a coalescence of botanicals and pharmaceuticals: people accept and experiment with this imported medical technology while they continue using familiar plants and other medicines. One could argue that the mirror image of this occurs in the "developed" West where people, once more or less content with pharmaceuticals, now factor "herbal medicines" and other "alternatives" into the therapeutic mix. The concurrent or serial use of plants and drugs is an extension of people's interactions with both the pharmacologically active and the signed attributes of medicinal plants. This involves the integration of pharmaceuticals into existing therapeutic models rather than the wholesale, or even gradual, disaffection with the "old ways" that health "developers" and the pharmaceutical industry expected. Through an "indigenization of pharmaceuticals" (Etkin, Ross, and Muazzamu 1990), drugs are evaluated by the same criteria that are applied to botanicals: physiologic action, taste, color, texture, and so forth. Commonly this results in pharmaceuticals' being taken for conditions other than what manufacturers intend, most clearly when pharmaceuticals are used for what their manufacturers regard as side rather than primary effects (Etkin 1994b). This application of ethnopharmacology to the study of medical systems instructs us in the cultural construction and transformation of therapeutic knowledge and in this way contributes to theory in medical anthropology. On a more applied level, ethnopharmacology can reveal how the combination of active plants and drugs creates a potential for adverse (and to a lesser extent beneficial) reactions between these two classes of pharmacologically active medicine. This highlights in the practical domain the merits of enriching medical ethnography with pharmacologic study.

Ethnopharmacologic studies should become a key element in addressing the problem of eroding biodiversity. At present, the rate and extent to which genetic resources are being depleted worldwide threatens species extinction to an extent never before experienced in human history. This issue has become increasingly politicized as resources, largely of the "developing" world, are deliberated from a variety of Western postures, predominantly economics (Morowitz 1991). "Important" or "interesting" species tend to be defined by polities that are culturally and politically not engaged with the threatened environments and the people who inhabit them. Thus, the value of particular taxa has not been adequately assessed in the local contexts of their use. Instead, conservation efforts generally focus on food crops, ignoring "wild" foods and other resources—notably medicines and other plants whose salience does not bear directly on the expertise and interest of outsiders. Some recent efforts to address biodiversity issues through focus on medicinal plants (e.g., Farnsworth and Soejarto 1991) still betray a Western bias that values knowledge of plants for potential development by the pharmaceutical industry—a selfish enterprise, by their own admission (Huxtable 1992). Closer attention to the social and cultural matrix in which those plants are embedded, including the various contexts of their use, will identify "important" species. Ethnopharmacology can bring to bear its extensive knowledge not only of which plants are valued in a particular microecology and why, but also the physiologic implications of diminishing diversity or otherwise changing the configuration of species present.

NOTES

1. Portions of this discussion are based on an entry written for *The Encyclopedia of Cultural Anthropology* (Etkin in press).

2. Important as pharmacologic assessment is, one must not lose sight of the fact that the subjects of ethnopharmacologic study are not ambivalent about how they use botanicals: in a dietary context, a plant is unequivocally "nonmedicine" and is regarded instead for its nutritive value and eaten by all household members who "eat from the same pot." The same plant in preventive and therapeutic contexts is clearly "not food" and may be ingested alone or in a composite preparation by the ailing individual, by the healer and patient, or even by whole groups who consume therapeutic meals that are communal (although meant to benefit a particular person).

3. The relation of ethnoveterinary to human therapeutics and its currently understudied status are reflected in the view that ethnoveterinary medicine is a "peninsula on the shore of local knowledge systems" (Nolan 1989:v).

4. Although anthropologists are assured that therapeutic models will be revealed in sufficient detail through "thick ethnography," we echo the concern of pharmacologists that one cannot extrapolate with confidence from the analysis of plant chemistry to the human experience (Etkin 1988b; Romanucci-Ross and Moerman 1988). Pharmacologic potential is confounded at least by the social and cultural constructions of therapeutics, including "placebo effects."

5. Potentially toxic nonbotanical ethnomedicines have been recorded, the lead tetroxide salt *azarcon* (*greta, liga, rueda,* etc.) being perhaps the most familiar (Yáñez et al. 1994; Trotter 1985); but the physiologic implications of human consumption, especially in what volume and with what regularity, have not been established.

6. Chimpanzees select the young leaves of various plants (*Aspilia* spp., *Lippia plicata, Ficus exasperata,* and *Commelina* spp.), rub them between the buccal (inner cheek) and tongue surfaces, and swallow them whole. Absorption through the buccal mucosa leads to rapid absorption into the systemic circulation to reach target organs directly and protects pharmacologically active constituents from inactivation in the low pH (acidic) environment of the stomach and degradation by hepatic enzymes (Newton and Nishida 1990). Buccal administration of drugs finds parallels in many indigenous therapeutic systems (e.g., for coca and tobacco), including in biomedicine the buccal or sublingual administration of apomorphine (for Parkinson's disease), bromfenac and buprenophrine (for pain), diazepam (Valium) and triazolam (sedative, antianxiety), and nifedipine (for hypertension).

7. Early morning ingestion for "medicinal" purposes may reflect higher pharmacologic activity at that time and/or that after overnight fasting, chimpanzees need to replenish blood levels of the active plant constituents.

9
Studying Biomedicine as a Cultural System

Lorna Amarasingham Rhodes

Western biomedicine and medical anthropology are intimately connected.[1] Many medical anthropologists work in biomedical settings or study problems that have been defined in biomedical terms. Medical anthropologists also study biomedicine itself, exploring the ways in which it is socially, culturally, and historically constructed and showing how its perspectives influence the lives of its patients. In addition, most medical anthropologists are members of societies in which biomedicine provides the dominant forms of explanation and treatment for illness and are thus participants in as well as observers of the culture of biomedicine.

In this chapter I explore some of the implications and paradoxes of this relationship. My focus is on the ways medical anthropologists and others in related fields (mainly history and sociology) approach biomedicine as an object of study. My emphasis is on biomedicine as it is understood by these writers; discussing the diversity, internal complexity, and changing conditions of current biomedical practice in the United States is beyond my scope here.

Recently a good deal of discussion and controversy has arisen within medical anthropology about its relationship to biomedicine. Often the issue is phrased as a difference between ''clinically applied'' and ''critical'' medical anthropology. Clinically applied medical anthropology has been described as ''serving to clarify specific issues in health maintenance and response to sickness'' (Chrisman and Maretzki 1982b:2). Its orientation is the application of anthropological perspectives to particular clinical situations and problems. Critical medical anthropology, on the other hand, defines itself in terms of a concern with the macrolevel of political and economic forces that shape medicine and determine the nature and extent of its interventions. Margaret Lock describes the critical approach as one that pays attention to ''macro-structural questions, the role of

power in social life, and the way in which biomedicine is culturally constructed"
(Lock 1986a:110; see also Singer 1995). Biomedical theory and practice is problematic not simply when it fails to address cultural and social issues involved
in individual patient care but because of its embeddedness and (often) sustaining
role in dominant political and economic systems.[2]

The precise nature of the division between clinically applied and critical medical anthropology is by no means a matter of agreement among medical anthropologists, and there are numerous variations on these definitions.[3] Morsy (1989a)
points out that critical analysis is common in other disciplines and objects to
using a label that sets it apart as special. On the other hand, M. Singer, Lani
Davison, and Gina Gerdis (1988:373) make a case for separating "critical"
analyses that "explicate culture in non-cultural terms" from "culturalist" approaches that avoid economic or political forms of explanation. In fact, many
studies in medical anthropology are not easily assigned to particular camps.
Nevertheless, the argument between clinically applied and critical medical anthropology reveals a central problematic issue: How is biomedicine understood
and described from within medical anthropology?

I begin the exploration of this question by considering the anthropological
concept of the cultural system, showing how several recent works illuminate
biomedicine's cultural construction and the ways it functions as a system for
producing and expressing cultural meanings. I then turn briefly to clinically
applied approaches, showing how they deal with the cultural dichotomies contained in clinical practice. Finally, I explore some of the premises of the critical
perspective as it touches on the issue of biomedical knowledge and practice. I
end by discussing some of the research strategies implied by each of these
orientations and suggest some directions for future work.

BIOMEDICINE AS A CULTURAL SYSTEM

In a series of classic articles, Clifford Geertz (1973c:108) suggests that cultural systems can best be understood in terms of their capacity to express the
nature of the world and to shape that world to their dimensions. Thus, for
example, religion "formulates, by means of symbols, an image of a genuine
order of the world." This simultaneous shaping and expression produces a congruence between culture and experience that provides an "aura of factuality"
within which cultural systems "make sense" and seem "uniquely real" to their
participants. For our purposes, the crucial phrase here is "aura of factuality."
The implication of Geertz's analysis is that cultural systems achieve a feeling
of factuality, of realness, that is, in part or whole, a by-product of their symbolic
forms.

In Western society biomedicine is generally believed to operate in a realm of
"facts"; many people experience their most intimate contact with science
through the biomedical description of the facts of bodily function and disease.
This realm of bodily fact is often perceived to be quite separate from other

cultural and social domains. "To a degree perhaps unique to segmented Western society, the participants of this ethnomedicine [biomedicine] emphatically distinguish their medicine from other aspects of institutions of their society. Illness is thought of as a 'natural' occurrence" (Hahn and Kleinman 1983b:312). Given this assumption that nature and the body exist in a directly apprehendable realm of fact, the problem for a cultural analysis of biomedicine is the delineation of the "aura" in the "aura of factuality" that it promotes. The issue is not simply the description of biomedicine but the discovery of strategies that will make visible its nature as a cultural system. As Emily Martin points out (1987:52), it takes a "jolt" to see the "contingent nature" of biomedical description.

Several recent explorations of biomedicine undertake specific and deliberate strategies to provide this jolt by making visible the culture of biomedicine. One strategy is historical contextualization; biomedicine is shown as the historically embedded product of particular cultural and social assumptions, thereby highlighting the "arbitrariness of institutions" (Foucault 1988:11). Another strategy is to uncover, through analysis of metaphor and other forms of speech, ways in which social meaning is embedded in biomedical categories. Attending to the life worlds of clinicians is a third strategy; the daily practice of clinicians is revealing of biomedicine's theoretical and pragmatic foundations. All of these forms of analysis aim to recover from the domain of the "natural" and the "given" those aspects of biomedicine that are cultural and constructed.

Most historical discussions of biomedicine emphasize its origin in an elaboration of the Cartesian dichotomy between mind and body.[4] Biomedical theory developed out of the possibility, following René Descartes, of a separation of the physical body from the mental and social. The body, as part of the natural world, becomes knowable as a bounded material entity; diseases similarly are physical entities occurring in specific locations within the body. Robert Hahn and Arthur Kleinman (1983b:313) describe the consequence: physical reductionism is a central tenet of biomedicine. This medicine also radically separates body from nonbody; the body is thought to be knowable and treatable in isolation.

As Nancy Scheper-Hughes and Margaret Lock (1987:10) point out, even those who try to take an integrated perspective on illness "find themselves trapped by the Cartesian legacy. We lack a precise vocabulary with which to deal with mind-body-society interaction and so are left suspended in hyphens." This is not just a matter of vocabulary but of epistemology; biomedicine participates in deep-seated cultural assumptions about what it means to know the body.

The particularity of this way of knowing the body can be seen in biomedical texts and practices that provide a mechanistic and desocialized imagery of bodily processes.[5] For example, in a section of *The Woman in the Body* (1987) entitled "Science as a Cultural System," Martin examines the images of women's bodies found in medical textbooks and suggests that several metaphors of the body permeate their seemingly "scientific" (that is, in this context, neutral or value-free) descriptions of physical processes. Thus, the processes of menstruation and menopause are described in terms of production and control. The female reproductive system is geared to "production" and is organized as a hierarchical system of communication among hormones, cells, and the brain. This imagery corresponds to that of our economic system. In menopause, "what is being described is the breakdown of a system of authority . . . at every point in this system, functions 'fail' and 'falter.' Follicles 'fail to muster strength' to reach ovulation. As functions fail, so do the members of the system decline" (p. 42). The key to this metaphor, Martin says, is functionlessness: "these images frighten us in part because in our stage of advanced capitalism, they are close to a reality we find difficult to see clearly: broken down hierarchy and organizational members who no longer play their designated parts" (p. 44). In these images, the "natural" functioning of the body is described in a way that fits a wider social view of women as defined by their reproductive function.

A similarly circular relationship between social and medical imagery can be seen in Rayna Rapp's (1988a:149) description of the process of genetic counseling. She points out that "statistics and medical terminology are genres of communication, not simply neutral vocabularies. . . . Much of the scientific information that counselors want to convey is technical and invisible." The visual aids used by counselors, such as charts and graphs, have an effect in "shaping the perceptions of the client" and thus, for some clients, redefining what is known in terms congruent with the biomedical definition of the "natural." The "codes, genres and assumptions construct the conversations genetic counselors may have with their patients" (p. 151), producing as natural a particular way of seeing the body and its reproductive life.

A revealing account of the historical embeddedness of biomedical knowledge is provided by Michel Foucault. For Foucault, medicine is one of a number of related disciplines that have shaped the body as a vulnerable site for the articulation of social relationships. In *The Birth of the Clinic* (1975) Foucault argues that modern medicine had its birth in the period around 1800 when medicine became clinically based and concerned with both the inside of the body and the control of the health of populations. Foucault's thought is complex, and my discussion here limited, but two examples can perhaps give some idea of the sense in which he perceives that medicine both shapes and expresses its historical context.

Foucault describes the period around 1800 as one in which medicine shifted not from a less to a more accurate understanding of the body but from one kind of knowledge to another. Before 1800 Europe had a "medicine of species" that depended on classification; diseases were organized into families and species and related more to one another than to the body of the patient. Medicine after 1800 was dominated by what Foucault calls "the gaze," a new way of seeing that looked into the body and focused on what was individual and abnormal.

Suddenly doctors were able to see and to describe what for centuries had been beneath the level of the visible. It was not so much that doctors suddenly opened their eyes; rather the old codes of knowledge had determined what was seen (Sheridan 1980:39). A new way of seeing produced a new kind of knowledge: "clinical experience sees a new space opening up before it; the tangible space of the body . . . the medicine of organs, sites, causes, a clinic wholly ordered in accordance with pathological anatomy" (Foucault 1975:122). For Foucault the historical context, and particularly its shaping of what is possible, of what can be seen, determines what at any time is considered to be true. Practitioners of the early nineteenth century did not suddenly become better observers and therefore better able to discover the truth about the body; rather, there was a fundamental change in what constituted observation. This change brought about profound changes in medicine, and these in turn shape the body we perceive. In this argument, the issue of shaping goes deeper than what is said. Foucault is interested in what *can* be said and in the mutual shaping of perception and possibility that gives rise to a particular medicine at a particular historical moment.

Foucault later extends this argument to show that in the nineteenth century, the body became an object of social control in a new sense. Minutely observed in clinics, prisons, and hospitals, bodies could be made into docile instruments of and for the exercise of power. One tactic of discipline is the dossier—the collection of documents that locates, describes, and accounts for each prisoner, patient, or child. As Foucault (1979:192) puts it, "The turning of real lives into writing functions as a procedure of objectification and subjection." Thus, for Foucault, neither "objective" description nor the case format in which such description is often framed constitutes value-neutral aspects of medicine. Rather than functioning to delineate a reality that exists independent of its description, they are techniques for the shaping of reality that create patients as individuals susceptible to a particular kind of judgment. Thus, people are profoundly shaped by disciplinary mechanisms that permeate our society, with medicine primary among them.

Issues of the relationship between mind and body, questions about what is knowable, and integration into the discipline of institutional life are enacted in the daily practice of clinicians. An example of a study that explores the lived world of a practitioner is Robert Hahn's "Portrait of an Internist" (1995). Hahn portrays the symbolic world of a clinician; the internist uses and reflects on biomedicine's categories, and his practice is revealing of how these categories exist in the larger culture. Hahn's strategy is to explore the interface between the personal and social that is provided by the world of work, showing the "goals, assumptions and uncertainties of medical logic" (1985:53). His internist enacts in work the production, of both self and society.

The internist described in Hahn's portrait engages directly the questions of realism and nominalism inherent in biomedicine's Cartesian origins. Thus, the internist "refers to his conception of the patient's problem, most often a physiological one, as 'a picture' . . . a 'thing' "; sometimes "pictures" "make sense," and sometimes he "makes sense of" them. As Hahn points out, "If

purported facts fail to make sense, the anomaly must inhere in the facts; but, if
Barry (the internist) is unable to make sense of the facts, it may be . . . that the
difficulty lies in Barry's sense-making activity. . . . These are respectively metaphors of realism and nominalism, of naturalism and constructionism'' (1995:
140). Thus, this physician enacts, through work and in relation to the bodies of
his patients, some of the fundamental issues embedded in the history of medicine
itself.

The assumption behind Geertz's definition of a cultural system is that "culture
can be explained primarily in terms of itself" (Singer, Davison, and Gerdes
1988:370; Good and Good 1981; Fabrega 1979). However, these examples suggest that the culture of biomedicine does not lend itself to explanation in terms
of itself. One problem is the same as that of Hahn's internist in the passage
quoted: the relationship between constructed and natural fact. Hahn points out
that social science observers in biomedical settings have often paid insufficient
attention to its materiality. Biomedical practice depends on the assumption of
an objectified nature subject to scientifically formulated "reality testing," and
although, as Hahn points out (1984), reality testing is fundamental to all healing
traditions, we find our particular brand especially compelling. Thus, from the
perspective of patients, practitioners, social scientists, and laypeople in our society and despite much evidence of limitations or confusion, nature as it is
understood by biomedicine demands to be taken seriously (that is, not questioned) in studies of biomedicine. This paradox, usually not in evidence in studies of other medical systems—for example, most studies of Ayurveda do not
generally consider its disease categories as descriptive of actual diseases but of
socially constructed ones (see, for example, Obeyesekere 1978)—means that the
categories of the culture under study are also the categories used to study it.

A second difficulty arises not so much in connection with factuality as with
its aura. The closed circle of belief and expression suggested by the notion of
cultural system appears flawed, even fragile, in several of these accounts. This
may result in part from the way illness itself threatens the cultural order with
chaos and loss of meaning and thus "calls into question particular socio-cultural
resolutions" of the dilemmas of human existence (Comaroff 1982:51). Paradox
and doubt may be intrinsic to the experience of the body; "physical form . . .
generates, from its own internal contradictions, the potential basis for critical
awareness" (Comaroff 1982:51).

In addition, however, biomedicine participates in a cultural separation of mind
and body, nature and culture, in ways that may produce a sense of dissonance
expressed in increasing criticism and doubt. Martin, for example, found that
women she interviewed expressed diverse images of their bodily processes, contradicting and resisting biomedical formulations (1987). Similarly, Rapp's work
suggests a complex interplay between social context and the expression of medical "information," with some counseling recipients unwilling to accept the
language of risk in which advice was proffered and with that language itself
constantly modified in interaction (1988a). Thus, as Jean Comaroff puts it,

"there has been an awareness that 'factual' knowledge might imply social values, that medicine has bequeathed us powerful metaphors along with its 'natural' truths and that these might . . . reinforce the deep-seated paradoxes raised by illness" (1982:56). The examples given here suggest that critical perspectives tend to emerge out of the cultural analysis of biomedicine.

BRACKETING BIOMEDICINE

One solution to the problem posed by medicine's grounding in "fact" is to segregate biomedical and social science ways of knowing. Most of clinically applied anthroplogy, and much research in medical anthroplogy as a whole, is based on a bracketing of biomedical expertise as referring to areas of knowledge not within the purview of the anthropologist.

This bracketing is the basis for the well-known distinction between disease and illness proposed by Leon Eisenberg (1977) and Arthur Kleinman (1980) (see also Young 1982; Hahn and Kleinman 1984). This distinction is created by dividing up the field of "sickness" into a domain of disease, considered to be pathology as biomedically defined, and illness, which encompasses the cultural meaning and social relationships experienced by the patient. Allan Young sums it up thus: "Disease refers to abnormalities in the structure and/or function of organs, pathological states whether or not they are culturally recognized." This is the "arena of the biomedical model." Illness, on the other hand, "refers to a person's perceptions and experiences of certain socially disvalued states including, but not limited to, disease" (1982:264). Thus illness includes the experiences and beliefs of individuals; disease is what biomedicine discovers "in" the person regardless of his or her (personal or cultural) awareness.[6]

The disease-illness distinction has provided the basis for much work in medical anthropology on the explanatory models and semantic illness networks of patients and, to some extent, of practitioners. These studies set aside the disease half of the distinction and concentrate on understanding the illness experiences and behavior of individuals and cultural groups. By "setting aside," I do not mean that disease itself is not considered problematic for those who experience it but that the definition of disease—its status as a real, natural phenomenon— is considered nonproblematic. This has allowed medical anthropologists to study culture (beliefs, issues of meaning, experience of illness) in medical settings without dealing with questions of the cultural construction of medicine itself. It also allows for the defining of research problems (for example, the study of groups of patients suffering from a particular disease or the study of the relationship between cultural and physical aspects of causation in a particular disorder) in ways that are relevant to the social context supporting the research. As Noel Chrisman and Thomas Maretzki say, "In our research, anthropologists have explicitly or implicitly drawn on clinical medicine as the standard for judging the 'real' world of sickness" (1982b:22).

One consequence is that medical anthropologists have been able to do research and teaching in medical settings, finding ways to incorporate anthropology into practice while respecting the orientation and commitments of clinicians. For the anthropologist who is, as Chrisman and Maretzki describe, bicultural in anthropology and medicine, the ideal is a translation of perspectives, enabling clinicians to make use of anthropological insights. Often these insights have to do with negotiation among perspectives (as in, for example, Kleinman's use of explanatory models, 1980); at other times they have to do with patient advocacy (as in, for example, obstetrics) or with the clarification of ways that the biomedical perspective influences the cultural interpretations of patients.

On the other hand, the disease-illness distinction is a variant of the mind-body and culture-nature dichotomies (Hahn 1984a). By using it to separate natural facts from cultural constructions, medical anthropology runs the risk of taking on characteristics of biomedicine itself. Instead of offering a perspective that comes from a position of stranger (Chrisman and Maretzki 1982b), the anthropologist may be a kissing cousin in disguise. For example, the emphasis on case studies reproduces in anthropology the individual-centered and "objective" approach of the medical case study (but see Hunter 1991 for a discussion of narrative in medicine). Similarly, the use of scientific language to describe disease reproduces the position "from the outside looking over or into a space" (Pratt 1986) that is fundamental to the medical gaze. The anthropologist is also influenced by the premise of biomedicine that "it is *the* medicine, real medicine; only other ethnomedicines are specially denominated, 'osteopathic medicine,' 'Chinese medicine' " (Hahn and Kleinman 1983:312). In both biomedical settings and the study of other kinds of medicine, it is hard to avoid the assumption that what needs to be explained are the "alternatives," the "other" perspectives, the "misunderstandings" or "misuses" of biomedicine rather than biomedicine itself.

An interesting recent development is that as biomedicine expands its definitions of physical disorder, incorporating problems with recognizably large social components (as in, for example, alcoholism and posttraumatic stress disorder), the position of the anthropologist becomes problematic. These conditions, with their roots in problematic social environments, seem to be ripe for anthropological analysis and understanding. However, attempts to bring social and cultural considerations to bear on biological phenomena tend to participate, often unwittingly, in a process of naturalization that turns them into things comparable to diseases. The bringing of chronic or behavioral conditions into the domain of biomedical treatment (the very thing that brings them to the attention of the biomedically based medical anthropologist) tends to result in their naturalization and "reinterpretation as events requiring medical intervention." Thus, the more they are translated into the reified, concrete terminology of "disorders," the less room there is for the anthropologist's perspective on the cultural shaping of both the symptoms and their interpretation. As Young has shown for posttraumatic stress disorder, the production of "knowledge" about such disorders is itself a cultural process (1988).

CRITICAL PERSPECTIVES

Much work in anthropology has explored the positive aspects of cultural systems in providing and sustaining meaning in human social life. But there is another perspective from which the congruence between the shaping and expressive aspects of culture can be seen as perverse. Religion, for example, appears in this view as an "opiate," preventing people from recognizing the truth of their situation. Medicine, in its powerful mediation of human physical and emotional frailty, can similarly be understood in terms of its relationship to a larger social (political and economic) system in which it serves to conceal sources of injustice and suffering. From this point of view, medicine cannot be described apart from the relations of power that constitute its social context. As Howard Waitzkin puts it: "Major problems in medicine are also problems of society; the health system is so intimately tied to the broader society that attempts to study one without the other are misleading. Difficulties in health and medical care emerge from social contradictions and rarely can be separated from those contradictions" (1983:41).

There are two aspects to this relationship. One is that health problems themselves may be socially caused, creating what Waitzkin calls the "second sickness" (1983). The other, related, aspect is that medicine may function to conceal the social origins of sickness and to suppress the possibility of protest.

When biomedicine is seen in this light, clinical knowledge itself becomes problematic; its connections to the larger system mean that it "cannot be either evaluated or transformed in any simple, decontextualized manner" (Comaroff and Maguire 1981:121). Nor can it be seen merely as a "web of significance" (following Geertz) approachable through understanding; it must also (or perhaps, instead) be considered as a "web of mystification" (Singer, Davison and Gerdes 1988).

Critical analyses of biomedicine are attempts at demystification. One strategy aims to uncover the incidence and causes of the "second sickness" by exploring ways in which medical care fails to reach, recognize, or correct socially created problems. Many analyses stress the relationship between capitalist production (and the profit motive inherent in it) and the failure to protect workers and others from its effects (e.g., Waitzkin 1983; Michaels 1988; Taussig 1978). Others focus on the maldistribution of medical care and the effects on the health of populations created by the dominance of complex technology (Young 1978; Navarro 1976).

A second strategy aims to uncover how biomedicine mystifies sickness through its participation in the nature-culture dichotomy. Medicine, because of its bias toward the uncovering of natural facts, represents the body in ways that are powerfully suggestive of a natural reality separate from the social. The effect, if not the intention, is to make the social invisible and to place sickness, as a natural process or entity, inside the individual.

Martin's point in her argument about menopause is that the "shriveling" of the ovaries is a metaphor that rests on and reinforces the social representation of the "shriveling" of production in the older woman. Because medicine has clothed the social representation in scientific language, it is difficult to discover its origins (1987). Similarly, Michael Taussig (1980a) describes the way a hospitalized patient is convinced of her own helplessness in the face of disease. She minimizes her own strength because she has been taught to rely on experts who function to invalidate her intuitive understanding of the social origin of her problem. Her disease is treated as a thing, part of a natural world separate from the social world that oppresses her. Thus Taussig considers medicine to express a hidden ideology, one that reifies the social and separates it into a natural domain where it cannot be understood for what it is.

By placing the body and bodily experience in the realm of nature, biomedicine conceals both the social causes of sickness and the social embeddedness of the experience of sickness. Thus, for example, the diagnostic category of premenstrual syndrome (PMS) creates a "disorder" that may serve to obscure the social relations that are the context of women's suffering (Martin 1987; Johnson 1987a). Similarly, the processes of childbirth and dying may be isolated from their social contexts and treated in largely technical terms that prevent those involved from taking care of themselves and each other (Illich 1976; Osherson and Amarasingham 1981; Comaroff 1982).

Recent cross-cultural and historical studies suggest that these tendencies toward reification and mystification are widely associated with biomedical practice. Lock's work on school refusal and on menopause in Japan shows that Japanese biomedicine similarly describes social problems as "syndromes" to be treated (Lock 1986a). In northeast Brazil, medical treatment, especially in the form of tranquilizers, serves to conceal the economic and social origin of starvation (Scheper-Hughes 1992). An example from the history of psychiatry comes from Andrew Scull (1979), who shows that asylums in nineteenth-century England had the effect of isolating and controlling those in the population who could not survive under the conditions of early industrialization. Asylums maintained a distinction between the mad and the able-bodied, who could not be given relief for fear of undermining their value as surplus labor. Medical definitions of insanity contributed to and perpetuated the separation of "useless" from "useful" individuals. Scull sees the current move toward deinstitutionalization to be similarly motivated by economic policy; welfare and disability payments make it cheaper for the state to maintain disabled people outside asylums (Scull 1977).

Other areas of medicine have also been seen as fostering dependence in order to conceal and support class and gender interests. E. Richard Brown (1979), for example, shows that late-nineteenth-century capitalism in the United States deliberately fostered biomedical definitions of problems that might otherwise have been seen as related to industrial development. The notion of the body as a mechanism that could be repaired corresponded in important ways to factory production (Scull 1979). Similarly, nineteenth-century medical theories about the fragility and emotionality of women served to bolster male dominance and the creation of the home as a domain separate from the workplace (Ehrenreich and English 1978).

These analyses regard biomedicine's aura of factuality as precisely its source of power. Medicine can describe events in a value-neutral language that makes them appear to be part of the natural world and thus neutralizes what are, in reality, social problems. In the nineteenth century, villagers whose ability to support aging relatives had been undermined by social change were convinced that asylum care was provided by "experts" (doctors) and thus superior to their own; women who rebelled against restrictive conditions could be persuaded that bed rest was the only remedy for their restless female organs. Similarly, today, Brazilian peasants believe tranquilizers to be "medicine" for starvation (Scheper-Hughes 1992), and women angry over the unfair distribution of domestic work regard their anger as a "symptom" of PMS (Martin 1987).

For some writers this analysis of the embeddedness of biomedical categories in social life (and their tendency to perpetuate sickness-causing aspects of social life) is not enough. Additionally, it is important to recognize the ways in which biomedicine also gives rise to resistance. Martin attempts to make visible, through the analysis of women's speech, the way ordinary women resist the biomedical description of women's bodily life. For example, women may refuse to go to the hospital for childbirth, or they create original metaphors to describe bodily processes. Brigitte Jordan, in an analysis of the medical "training" given to Maya midwives (1989), shows that the midwives ignore much of what is presented to them and instead use medical supplies (masks, birth control pills) as props and symbols. They are resistant to changes in their way of delivering babies, preferring their own situated knowledge. Foucault suggests that this kind of "subjugated," situated knowledge, arising out of practice at a local level, forms the basis for a potential resistance to biomedical domination (1980b); however, he refuses to speculate about the ultimate shape that any change might take, insisting that while we can critique our system, we cannot be programmatic in our approach to change (1984).

Those who emphasize the misuse of medicine are more prescriptive. If the problem is the creation of sickness under capitalism and the maldistribution and misappropriation of biomedicine, then the solution does not lie so much with changes in biomedicine itself or with pockets of resistance among patients or practitioners as in larger-scale changes in the system. Hans Baer, Merrill Singer, and John Johnsen issue this challenge: "Attention to the influence of class-interests as well as to the workings of power in large-scale organizations is vital for a truly critical medical anthropology. . . . An approach that is sensitive to these issues will not cater to the furtherance of 'medical cultural hegemony' of the capitalist world system, but will help create a *new medical system*" (1986: 97; emphasis in original; see also Singer 1995 for a more contextualized approach).

Criticism of biomedicine—regardless of whether the stress is on discovering resistance or creating a new system—often seems to involve a paradox. On the one hand, biomedicine as part of society (the "medical establishment") is seen as failing to serve the real best interests of that society. On the other hand, the techniques of biomedicine (its science) are seen as one means for discovering these real best interests. In some instances, biomedical categories themselves are employed to critique the use of biomedicine. For instance, Nancy Scheper-Hughes uses biomedical definitions of starvation to challenge the misuse of biomedicine to conceal it. This sidesteps the question, raised by those who consistently question biomedical categories (for example, Foucault), as to whether the science of biomedicine itself does not contain intrinsic assumptions about society and about the nature of reality that are, at best, disempowering and, at worst, harmful to body and society (as in, for example, Illich's 1976 critique of medicine's iatrogenic effects).

As an example of the complexity of this problem, consider Jordan's account of the training of Mayan midwives (1989). Jordan suggests that these midwives are competent in their own right, rarely losing a mother or baby; she also suggests a few areas in which their management of labor and delivery is questionable by modern obstetrical standards. Is there a way to take what is "good" (useful? relevant?) from biomedicine and incorporate it into their practice? Who should decide what that usefulness or relevance is, especially as medical standards themselves change rapidly? Is it not possible that a few seemingly benign changes might undermine the midwives' entire practice? On the other hand, can Jordan, who knows, for example, that encouraging pushing too soon may damage the mother or baby, simply consider this aspect of the midwives' practice a part of their "culture," thereby refusing to acknowledge the possible benefits of medical training? In a situation like this, it becomes clear that we are torn between our own belief that the body can be considered part of the natural world, with at least part of its truth discoverable by biomedicine, and our (often also strong) belief that biomedical intervention can be either oppressive or outright wrong.

CONCLUSION

When I teach medical anthropology I often point out that illness entails an intensity and vulnerability that reveal the most basic attitudes of the society in which it occurs. This is what makes medical anthropology particularly interesting. The study of life-and-death situations often throws into relief issues and contradictions that are less visible when there is less at stake. In this chapter I have been concerned with what happens when we turn our gaze on our own medical system. Not surprisingly, we find that fundamental attitudes of our society and, in fact, our very epistemology, emerge as problematic. At the same time, the vulnerability of self, body, and society to illness engages us, to a greater or lesser extent depending on context and inclination, in the same problem faced by clinicians: the need to act, to provide useful understanding or in some other way to contribute to the alleviation of suffering.

How one thinks of biomedicine makes a difference in medical anthropology, influencing research, teaching, and one's orientation in one's own society. When biomedicine is contextualized and regarded as a cultural system, what Scheper-Hughes and Lock call the "as-ifness" of our "ethnoepistemology" is revealed (1987:30). A researcher oriented to this perspective is likely to be interested in how medicine's aura of factuality is achieved, focusing on historical, social, or linguistic contexts. She or he is likely to adopt a questioning stance toward the biomedical definitions of health problems. Thus Young (1988), for example, takes posttraumatic stress disorder as his object of study, not as the definition of what he should study. Similarly, Howard Stein (1982b) questions not "cultural influences" on alcoholism but how "alcoholism" is a socially constructed category. Emily Martin (1994) addresses "immunity" as a contemporary discourse rather than (merely) as a scientific discovery "about" the body. Comparative work is particularly congenial to this perspective because movement through time or space reveals the arbitrary and culturally constructed nature of medical categories. On the other hand, it may be difficult to persuade those engaged in direct care of the usefulness of epistemological doubt; nor do problems framed in terms that "explain culture in terms of culture" always make sense to those accustomed to a biological bottom line for research.

The second approach takes the environment created by biomedicine—clinics and professional schools—as given and tries to contribute an anthropological understanding that will improve the treatment of patients. Often this understanding is in the form of analyses of the meanings patients attribute to illness and of the process of care seeking; more rarely, understanding extends to the meanings clinicians attribute to their work. A medical anthropologist working within this framework is likely to do research on a "medical problem"—a disease or diseaselike entity or a clinically defined issue like doctor-patient relationships. The aim may be to discover certain facts about the problem or to show how cultural and social factors contribute to it. Conclusions are likely to point to useful changes or interventions. The point here is not that these steps do not result in criticism of biomedical practice—they often do—but that they rarely lead to an examination of biomedical knowledge itself as culturally constructed. What is made visible are likely to be problems within medicine, not medicine itself.

Finally, the third approach I have outlined attempts to shift the focus of attention to larger (macro) social problems such as class and gender inequality, corporate domination, and the health-destroying features of capitalism. The starting point is different; the clinic is no longer a bounded site for research but part of a larger system of domination or mystification. The improvement of the doctor-patient relationship is not the issue; rather, the question is how it reflects and augments relationships of power in the larger society. The medical anthropologist with this perspective is likely to focus on an area of social injustice and suffering and show how medicine contributes to mystifying the social forces involved. This perspective seems to require Gramsci's "pessimism of intellect, optimism of will" (Frankenberg 1988b:331) in the face of resistance to change at the macrosocial level. Or, as Taussig (1980a:7) puts it, "It is essential to pose the challenge [of developing a critique] but it is utopian to believe we can imagine our way out of our culture without acting on it in practical ways that alter its social infrastructure."

Since the contradictions in medical anthropology's relationship to biomedicine are reflective of contradictions in the society in which we work, they are unlikely to be resolved through any sort of agreed-upon theoretical framework for the discipline. In fact, it would probably be to the detriment of the liveliness and self-reflection evident in current medical anthropology were there easy solutions to the differences between clinical and critical approaches. Nor can we avoid the discomfort of "suspension in hyphens" when we consider the ways in which our epistemology mires us in the time-worn dilemmas of our culture. However, there are several fruitful directions for research that address some of the problems raised in this chapter.

The first is to press on with the study of biomedicine. The studies I have described here suggest the enormous richness of biomedical practice and history as areas for research in medical anthropology. Others, such as Charles Bosk's study of error on a surgical ward (1979), Donna Haraway's work on the immune system (1988), and Good's discussion of the construction of medical objects (1994) point to areas (the less "social" medical specialties, the imagery of biological science, the production of knowledge within medicine) that have barely been touched on by medical anthropology.

One promising direction is the close examination of practitioners. Their world of work, their formation of professional identity, and their situated knowledge provide a counterpoint to our already extensive study of patients (see, for example, Hahn 1995). The practice of biomedicine often differs significantly from the standard descriptions of biomedicine as a system of knowledge, and these differences need to be explored (see, for example, Gordon 1988). In addition, such a close reading of practice is likely to discover seeds (if not a full-blown flowering) of criticism within biomedical practice itself and, perhaps, the basis for a critical analysis arising from below.

Second, we need to shift our perception of boundaries. We can seek out ways to define our object of study that avoid some of the more obvious contradictions in our own culture. This is what Scheper-Hughes and Lock suggest in their article, "The Mindful Body: A Prolegomenon to Future Work in Medical Anthropology" (1987). They propose that we make the body our object; by including its capacity to express and reflect emotional, social, and political life, we may be able to escape the "mind/body, nature/culture, individual/society epistemological muddle" (1987:28). Hahn makes a similar suggestion, proposing that we give our attention to "suffering" rather than "disease" or "illness." This, he says, creates a framework based on a "pan-human phenomenon" that can encompass various kinds of medical knowledge as "accounts for suffering" (1984a:22, 1995). These proposals aim to shift our vision, to create a larger framework within which problems of society and problems of individuals can be seen as mutually illuminating.

Third, we must experiment with mixed forms of analysis. Often we present our work in ways that reflect the epistemological muddles we are trying to escape. Medical anthropology might benefit from closer attention to recent work on reflexivity and experimental ethnography that explores the roots and implications of writing styles in anthropology (for example, Clifford and Marcus 1986; Marcus and Fischer 1986). Another possibility is to experiment with combining close phenomenological analysis of individual situations with a "reading out" of the social criticism embedded in such situations. In a study of stroke patients, for example, Kaufman shows how their situations reflect medical and societal limitations (1988). Scheper-Hughes approaches the suffering of northeast Brazilians by combining intimate portraits with a critical analysis. These approaches require a shifting of attention back and forth from the close-up involvement required to understand the details of individual lives to the more distanced view necessary to see the social forces expressed and reflected in them. This leap may be hard to make because of the difficulty of showing precisely how the microlevel and macrolevel are connected; there is also the difficulty of knowing how far to go beyond the interpretations offered by those involved (see, for example, Csordas 1988b). Nevertheless, the attempt is worth making if it allows us to be specific about the complexities of the body-person-society connection.

Medical anthropology speaks of, and speaks from within, the complex intersection of social institutions and the bodies and selves of individuals. Our concern with the connections among person, culture, and society places us squarely in the midst of fundamental anthropological debates about the nature of culture and the construction of social reality. At the same time, our involvement in illness and care leads to a concern with criticism and social action. These issues are likely to impinge, whether recognized or not, on theory and practice in the field of medical anthropology.

NOTES

1. All the terms we have for our medicine—*biomedicine, allopathic* medicine, *Western* medicine—are limited and inadequate. *Biomedicine* seems the best choice, though it implies, as Frankenberg points out, "an unjustifiable identity of biological (itself far from unitary) thinking and the medical gaze" (1988c:455). In this chapter I use *medicine* interchangeably with *biomedicine*.

2. The fact that "criticism" is an issue in medical anthropology—named, defined, argued over—may reflect the association between medical anthropology and biomedicine. There seems to be a sensitivity and defensiveness about "criticism" of a medicine with which we (as individuals and as a field) are, to varying degrees, intimate.

3. It is not my intention to provide a classification of medical anthropologists by type. In fact, there is variation within many individuals' work in terms of their alignment with one or another of these perspectives.

4. Many older studies of medicine do not make visible its aspect as a system of knowledge. For example, earlier studies of medical settings (e.g., Fox 1959; Caudill 1958b), while illuminating social relationships and issues of meaning within the clinic, do not examine the theoretical premises on which the clinical practice itself is based.

5. Interestingly Sontag (1978), who has given us a rich description of the metaphors associated with illness, exempts biomedicine itself (as theory) from her analysis. She replicates the cultural assumption that only patients and wrong-headed clinicians have "beliefs"; true science is metaphor free.

6. Kleinman's views of the relationship between disease and illness have changed (e.g., 1983) to reflect an increasing emphasis on the ways in which illness is converted to disease by biomedical practitioners.

Part III

Health Issues in Human Populations

10

Disease, Ecology, and Human Behavior

Peter J. Brown, Marcia C. Inhorn, and Daniel J. Smith

Disease is an inevitable part of life, and coping with disease is a universal aspect of the human experience. All humans, during the course of their lives, harbor infections by disease organisms and suffer the consequences of those infections. The experience of disease, by individuals or whole populations, is as inescapable as death itself. Yet the particular diseases that afflict people, as well as the way in which symptoms are interpreted and acted upon, vary greatly by culture. Understanding the nature of interactions between disease and culture can be a productive way of understanding humanity and is therefore an important topic in medical anthropology. Because of its biocultural, evolutionary, and cross-cultural perspectives, anthropology has much to offer to the understanding of the causes and consequences of disease. From an anthropological perspective, diseases cannot be explained as purely ''things in themselves''; they must be analyzed and understood within a human context—that is, in relation to ecology and culture.

The distribution of disease in a population is neither constant nor random. The diseases that characteristically afflict members of a population vary significantly among societies because of differences in culture, ecological setting, and historical period. More important, within a single society, there may be striking variations in the kind and severity of diseases that afflict individuals of different ages, sexes, social classes, and ethnic groups. Understanding the descriptive epidemiological distribution of disease morbidity and mortality is important to medical anthropologists particularly because the social patterning of disease distribution often reflects the cultural coding of behaviors. Understanding the role of culture in disease distribution is also necessary for the implementation of successful disease control programs

Culture plays a major role in determining the patterns of disease and death in a population for two reasons. First, culture may shape important behaviors (with respect to diet, activity patterns, water use, sexual practices, etc.) that predispose individuals to acquire certain diseases. Second, through culture, people actively change the nature of their environment, often in ways that affect their health. The archaeological and historical record clearly demonstrates that the environmental changes caused by humans can have profound effects, both positive and negative, on disease rates. Although humans have a dual system of inheritance through both genes and culture, culture is the primary mechanism for survival. Culture is a mechanism of adaptation to environmental threats, such as diseases, which act as agents of natural selection in the evolution of both human biology and culture. Cultural practices, however, can also be maladaptive when they exacerbate health problems.

Ecology is the study of the relationship of organisms in an environment. Human societies coinhabit their environment with many other organisms, including those producing disease. An ecological approach to human health and illness emphasizes the fact that the environment and its health risks are, to a significant extent, created by the culture. In many cultures, people think of themselves as masters of their environment, because they exploit so many plants and animals within the food chain as sources of energy and nutrients. Yet at the same time, humans are being exploited by microorganisms, including those that cause disease, as a source of food and shelter. Disease ecology primarily focuses on the multiplex interactions of the pathogen, the environment, and the human host. The nutritional, physiological, genetic, and mental condition of the human individual host all play significant, if still incompletely understood, roles in both infectious and noninfectious disease states. The current international health problems called "emerging infections" provide a good example of the mutability of these ecologic interactions.

The study of disease and human behavior in an ecological setting is a fundamental task for medical anthropology. The approach contributes to basic and applied research in the field by providing a strategy for answering some of the major questions raised by both general anthropology and epidemiology. For example, it can be applied to anthropological questions concerning the interaction of biology and culture in human evolution or to questions of why particular cultural behaviors may "make sense" and be retained in an ecological setting. This type of research strategy is truly biocultural and can therefore help to bridge the gap between biological and cultural anthropology. In epidemiology, the contribution of an anthropological focus on human behavioral patterns can help unravel fundamental questions of disease causality. The study of disease, ecology, and behavior also has important implications for public health programs. Through the study of behavioral patterns related to the social epidemiology of disease, it is possible to design health programs that are both effective and culturally acceptable. Moreover, the ecological approach can help to anticipate the health implications of technological change or new political-economic policies.

This chapter discusses basic concepts and methods in the study of disease, ecology, and behavior; it is not an exhaustive review of the literature. Instead, we summarize many illustrative examples of research that focuses on particular diseases in particular cultural settings. These examples emphasize infectious diseases for several reasons: first, the etiology (causation) of these diseases is the best understood; second, the ecological approach described here is most applicable to this category of disease, (although it is also applicable to the study of chronic diseases with complex etiologies, which are characteristic of industrialized societies, as well as nutritional deficiency diseases, which are characteristic of the poor in economically developing societies); and, finally, infectious diseases still represent the major cause of morbidity and mortality in nonindustrialized societies, which anthropologists have traditionally studied.

THE THEORETICAL ORIENTATION OF DISEASE ECOLOGY

What Is Disease?

In the enormous literature of biomedicine, there is no universally accepted definition of disease. Like many theoretically important concepts, "disease" is essentially left undefined and is used in ambiguous ways. For example, it is often defined by what it is not. Disease is generally seen as a failure of normal physiological activities and a departure from a state of health. But such a definition is uninformative. The problem is that within this definition is a concept of "normal." Yet it is clear that normality must be considered as culturally constructed; for example, conditions that have been considered as normal in particular populations include persistent diarrhea (Desowitz 1981), malaria (Ackerknecht 1945), the bloody urine of schistosomiasis (Heyneman 1979), and the skin discolorations of pinta (Ackerknecht 1943). "Health," of course, is so notoriously difficult to define that the World Health Organization's (WHO) utopian phrase, "a state of complete physical, mental, and social well-being," has little use for those who wish to measure health.

Medical social scientists have often made the distinction between disease and illness. In this case, disease refers to a set of objective, clinically identifiable symptoms, while illness refers to an individual's perception of those symptoms. This perception is what motivates the individual to seek medical care or to assume the sick role (Mechanic 1968). A persistent paradox in modern medical systems is the fact that many patients seeking medical care (i.e., who have an illness) do not have any identifiable disease, while at the same time, many people with disease do not define themselves as ill and thus do not seek medical help (Zola 1972). Although the distinction between disease and illness is useful, it assumes that the biomedical definition of disease is objective and culture free. But this is clearly not the case. Biomedicine is a cultural system in which certain kinds of information are privileged and certain cultural values are used to in-terpret symptoms (Hahn 1995).

When defining disease, it is useful to compare the conceptions of the layper-son, the biomedical specialist, and the disease ecologist. Most people, even in complex societies, conceive of diseases as invisible entities "out there," that can attack victims and cause sickness, pain, loss of vitality, and even death. Although diseases are usually named, they generally cannot be controlled by ordinary individuals. From the emic perspective of the lay patient, there is little difference between a disease caused by a "germ" and one caused by evil spirits or other supernatural agents. In either case, the sick person may be a completely innocent victim of the disease (as in most pediatric cases) or may have partly encouraged it to attack by way of irresponsible behavior (e.g., breaking post-partum taboos, smoking cigarettes). For most people, the large number of un-known diseases "out there" makes the world a dangerous place. People can attempt to prevent "catching" a disease by avoiding contexts where they are exposed to pathogenic agents or by avoiding conditions where they might be more likely to have diseases "sent" to them.

For the practitioner of biomedicine, disease is the expression of pathology alone. One textbook begins, "Pathology is the study of disease by scientific methods. Disease may, in turn, be defined as an abnormal variation in the struc-ture or function of any part of the body" (Anderson 1985:1). Diseases can be identified by discrete sets of signs and symptoms or by diagnostic tests. Diseases can be categorized, within the taxonomy of biomedicine, primarily in terms of the biological characteristics of the etiological agents. The standard categoriza-tion system is the *International Classification of Disease* (ICD), currently in its ninth edition and the analogous system for psychiatric disorders is the *Diag-nostic and Statistical Manual,* currently in its fourth edition. These listings form an authoritative text linking diagnostic labels, clinical findings, and patients' symptoms, and therefore they suggest a uniformity of biomedical practice that only theoretically exists. In reality, both the taxonomic and diagnostic systems of biomedicine, however, are based on certain cultural assumptions about cau-sality and normality; the practice of biomedicine varies according to local traditions. The use of particular diagnostic categories or the prescription of par-ticular therapies or procedures also varies significantly according to cultural geography (Payer 1988; Konner 1993). Furthermore, it has been argued that in clinical settings the disease is treated rather than the patient; from the viewpoint of the practitioner, the disease often takes on an existence quite apart from the patient. A more patient-centered approach focusing on the experience of "sick-ness" has recently been advocated by Hahn (1995). The idea that biomedicine is itself a cultural construction is a basic insight of critical medical anthropology. Nevertheless, the ICD classification system remains useful for organizing en-cyclopedic volumes like the invaluable *Cambridge World History of Infectious Disease* (Kiple 1993).

In contrast, from an ecological perspective, disease does not exist as a thing in and of itself. Disease is a process triggered by an interaction between a host and an environmental insult, often a pathogenic organism or "germ." Disease is one possible outcome of the relationship between the host and the potential pathogen. Since the advent of bacteriology and germ theory, it has been recognized that infection is a necessary but not sufficient condition for disease to occur. For tuberculosis, for example, this principle has been recognized since the work of the turn-of-the-century bacteriologist, Koch.[1] Normal, healthy individuals typically harbor many different colonies of viruses and bacteria that are not pathogenic (i.e., disease producing), primarily because these agents are held in check by the human immune system. Indeed, individuals are constantly being challenged by microorganisms in their environment (Burnet and White 1978). Disease occurs only when the host's immunological system is unable to keep pace with the reproduction of the pathogen, a process that is affected by age and can be accelerated through malnutrition, coinfection, or immunosuppression (Scrimshaw, Taylot, and Gordon 1976).

According to Jacques May in his classic volume, *The Ecology of Human Disease,* disease is "very simply that alteration of living tissues that jeopardizes their survival in their environment" (1958:1). This means that disease is the temporary expression of maladjustment of an individual trying to cope with the challenges of his or her environment. In this model the most common eventual outcome of this maladjustment is, on the level of the population, a mutual accommodation between host and pathogen. This is most often a relationship of dynamic tension, wherein a change in the host (e.g., the use of an antibiotic) can necessitate a corresponding change in the pathogen (e.g., the evolution of antibiotic resistance).

What Is Ecology?

Ecology is the study of the relationship between a species and its total environment. Most often considered a subfield of biology, ecology deals with the interactions between organisms and their environment on the population, community, and ecosystem levels of organization (Ehrlich, Ehrlich, and Holdren 1973; Orlove 1980; Moran 1990). Integral to most ecological studies is the idea that the complex set of interactions between organisms in an ecological niche (territory) makes up a system (Odum 1971). This "ecosystem" includes not only natural resources (e.g., water, minerals) but also plants, animals, and humans. Two of the assumptions of this model are that the ecosystem is maintained through mutually dependent interactions between members of the system and that the common goal of the various species in the system is homeostasis. The primary benefit of homeostatic balance is the prevention of environmental degradation and thus the mutual survival of species in that environment.

In this view, human activities such as agriculture create imbalances in natural ecosystems. Humans are not capable of ecological change but also ecological destruction. There is no doubt that humans have often been responsible for radical changes in their environment and that such ecological changes have had negative effects on health. The impact of the construction of dams on the prevalence of schistosomiasis is a good example. Archaeologists and paleopathologists have shown that humans have systematically changed their environment all the way back to the paleolithic past (Swedlund and Armelagos 1990). But the ecological perspective does not require the assumption of a cooperative, mutually dependent "system" in nature, which would maintain itself if not for human disruption. Modern evolutionary theorists, in fact, question whether community ecosystems are a biological reality at all (Ayala 1983). With few exceptions, the apparent "system" may be nothing more than the sum total of individual behaviors aimed at the maximization of reproductive success.

In the social sciences, particularly in sociology, the term *ecology* is sometimes used to refer to studies of certain behavior traits, mapped from a central (usually urban) locale. This is not what anthropologists and biologists mean by the term. Medical geography, on the other hand, emphasizes the study of the distribution of disease in regard to place, using the mapping techniques of cartography as its basic tool (Learmonth 1988). The ecological approach in medical anthropology has been a standard paradigm, primarily because of the successful textbook by McElroy and Townsend (1989), who use the label "medical ecology" (McElroy 1990). This approach has been criticized for ignoring the political-economic dimensions of health and illness and therefore "blaming the victims" of disease (Singer 1989b). Such criticisms have a certain validity, just as traditional cultural ecological studies have been criticized for underemphasizing history and power relations (e.g., the "revisionist" studies of !Kung history; [Wilmsen 1989; Lee 1992]). Nevertheless, these criticisms have touched off an important debate, spearheaded by Wiley (1992), about the value of biocultural approaches and the concept of adaptation in medical anthropology. One consequence of this debate, we believe, has been a recognition by many biologically oriented medical anthropologists and biological anthropologists of the need to incorporate macrosociological political-economic variables into their ecological models (Goodman and Leatherman 1996).

We find the distinction between cultural ecology and political ecology to be useful in this regard. These refer, in large measure, to different levels of analysis: cultural ecology to the level of individuals or human groups interacting with other species (plants, animals, pathogens) in the environment and requiring a microsociological analysis; political ecology referring to historical interactions between human groups (ethnic groups, classes, nations) that affect the ecology through population movements, land use, or differential access to resources and requiring a macrosociological perspective. These approaches are complementary, as we will demonstrate. However, it is important to note here that adding the dimension of political ecology to microsociological studies reveals the "unnatural history" of many diseases (Turshen 1984).

What Is Disease Ecology?

Disease ecology focuses on the interactions between two organisms: the pathogen and the host. Unlike the more general ecological approach, however, the emphasis is not on the harmonic cooperation between humans and agents of disease (Armelagos et al. 1978). This is because diseases are most often viewed as serious threats to human health. Humans are, from the viewpoint of a disease organism, the "environment" in which the disease organism lives and reproduces and to which it must adapt. The disease ecologist tries, metaphorically, to understand the disease organism's "worldview" and its adaptive strategies for survival and reproduction. The ecological model is much more easily applied to diseases caused by infectious agents and often exacerbated by malnutrition than the "diseases of lifestyle" that characterize modern affluent populations. Furthermore, a basic understanding of the biology of disease is a prerequisite for this type of research.

The notion of adaptation is a fundamental principle of disease ecology— adaptation from the perspective of both the disease agent and the host. As Lieban states, "Health and disease are measures of the effectiveness with which human groups, combining cultural and biological resources, adapt to their environments" (1973:1031). This notion is valid only if our understanding of the concept of environment is broad enough to include the ways in which other human groups with superior political or economic power impinge on the environment, forcing accommodation.

As such, studies in disease ecology must include at least three levels of causation: (1) a microbiological level, in which agents of disease act within the human body; (2) a cultural ecological (or microsociological) level, in which individual behaviors, encouraged or constrained by sociocultural context, put people at risk for contracting particular diseases; and (3) a political ecological (or macrosociological) level, in which historical factors involving interactions between human groups shape people's (often differential) access to resources and their relationship with the physical environment.

Disease ecology is one of the foundations of medical anthropology and is, by definition, a biocultural enterprise, as are the closely related disciplines of medical geography and epidemiology. The study of disease ecology both allows and requires a bridging of the biological and cultural paradigms in anthropology. This approach in medical anthropology owes much to the pioneering work of Alland, whose book, *Adaptation in Cultural Evolution* (1970), first used evolutionary theory to examine how cultural behaviors enhance hygiene, health, and reproductive fitness. Although this early book suffered from some of the weakness of a group-selectionist argument, its underlying ecological and evolutionary approach for understanding human-pathogen interaction is still valid.

DISEASE AND BIOCULTURAL EVOLUTION

Evolution refers simply to the process of change over time. Human evolution includes changes in both biology, through modification of gene frequencies, and cultural forms. It is the latter, cultural change, that accounts for the tremendous success of our species. In fact, human evolution has never been a purely biological process. Evidence from paleoanthropology suggests a cultural dimension to hominid existence, as well as an ongoing interplay of genes and culture, which affected the survival and reproduction of early ancestors (Durham 1982, 1991). Furthermore, it is important to remember that evolutionary change does not imply progress; evolution, whether biological or cultural, does not necessarily mean that things get "better."

Evolutionary change occurs only in relation to a particular environment. For example, the evolution of the gene for the sickle cell trait was context dependent on an environment characterized by *Plasmodium falciparum* malaria. The gene codes for an abnormal structure of the hemoglobin molecule in the red blood cell. In moderate amounts, the abnormal hemoglobin can protect individuals from death from malaria and is therefore considered to be an evolutionary adaptation to the disease. Outside the malarial context, however, this genetic adaptation does not confer an advantage; in fact, homozygous carriers of the sickle cell allele are at the most extreme disadvantage, because they will die from sickle cell anemia. The threat of malaria continues to be an enormous and increasing problem throughout the world, with estimates of around 100 million clinical cases and 2 million deaths per year (Oaks et al. 1991). As such, the genetic "disorders" of the hemoglobinopathies, despite their relatively high costs, continue to protect millions of people from malaria-related death today, especially in sub-Saharan Africa.

Natural selection is the primary driving force for evolutionary change in both biological and cultural systems. This means that, in general, traits that improve the chance of survival and reproduction in an environment will be maintained or increase in frequency. Conversely, traits that result in premature death or lower fertility will, in the long run, become very rare or disappear. This does not mean that biological or cultural traits are always able to solve environmental problems. It is also important to remember that selection occurs only upon pre-existing variations of genetic or cultural forms; it is not the case of necessity's being the mother of invention. The conditions of natural selection also depend on local ecological conditions: competition from other species, the availability of food and water, climatic conditions, and so forth. In both biological and cultural evolution, traits are selected that enhance reproductive fitness. However, there are important differences between these two processes, because biological and cultural evolution differ in terms of units of variation, sources of variation, and measurement of adaptive value (for an extended discussion of these differences, see Brown 1986).

Although the actual agents of natural selection are seldom specified in studies of biocultural evolution, these are generally factors that affect differential mortality, of which there are five major sources: (1) diseases, (2) food shortages, (3) trauma and accidents, (4) predation and competition with conspecifics, and (5) climate and thermoregulation. The geneticist Haldane (1949) was one of the first theoreticians to emphasize the importance of the first source, disease, in evolution. Disease is important in human biocultural evolution for the simple fact that it causes death—or, to put it in Darwinian terms, it results in differential rates of mortality and fertility. In other words, throughout human history, disease has been a significant force of natural selection, shaping both human biology and culture. In recent years, evolutionary biologists have come to focus on human-pathogen interactions in an area called "Darwinian medicine." Ewald (1994) has emphasized the evolution of virulence in pathogens, while Nesse and Williams (1994) have analyzed the evolution of host responses to infections and their symptomatology. While much of this recent work is reminiscent of Dubos's classic *Man Adapting* (1965), current work in Darwinian medicine has the advantage of more advanced evolutionary paradigms and a concern with practical medical questions such as the advisability of treatment for fevers or the origin of allergies.

Disease and Evolution: Three Mechanisms

There are three main mechanisms through which disease affects human biological and cultural evolution: (1) large-scale mortality from epidemics, (2) excess mortality from endemic diseases, and (3) parasitism (Brown 1987).

The primary way in which disease affects the process of natural selection has been through the massive mortality caused by epidemics. In the context of the enormously strong selective pressure of an epidemic, evolution can occur very rapidly; in other words, epidemic diseases play an important evolutionary role simply because they can cause extinction (Haldane 1949). A well-studied example of this phenomenon involves myxomatosis, a viral disease of rabbits that was introduced in 1950 to the wild rabbit population of Australia as a means of controlling overpopulation (Fenner and Ratcliffe 1965). In the first year after introduction, the die-off of the rabbit population was 99.8 percent; in the second year, it was 90 percent; and, by the seventh year, it was only 25 percent. Fifteen years following the introduction of the disease, the rabbit population was only one-fifth its original size, but the mortality due to myxomatosis was nearly zero. This change was the result of powerful selection of both the rabbit population and the virus. If rabbits had been eradicated in Australia, then the virus would have become extinct there too; thus, mutual adaptation was to the advantage of both species. The myxomatosis example illustrates an important process in which virulent epidemic diseases eventually become benign endemic diseases in a population through the process of mutual accommodation.

The massive mortality associated with epidemic diseases has also had an important effect on human cultural history. The most comprehensive treatment of this theme is in McNeill's landmark volume, *Plagues and Peoples* (1976), in which he demonstrates the active role that epidemics have played in the expansion of empires throughout history. Such expansion was facilitated, McNeill argues, by the "confluence of disease pools"; that is, infectious diseases were unwittingly spread from state-level societies with a complex repertoire of endemic childhood diseases to smaller and simpler societies, for which the introduction of these new diseases brought massive population losses and socioeconomic disorganization.

McNeill's general model of the active historical role of epidemic disease is significantly different from the earlier work of historians, who viewed diseases as minor and exceptional events that "spoiled" political plans (Zinssner 1943; Hopkins 1983). McNeill concludes that disease played a crucial role in accelerating the conquest, subjugation, and acculturation of tribes and chiefdoms. This process depended on the historical transition of introduced epidemic diseases into local endemic diseases characteristic of childhood. In addition to diseases of obvious historical importance, like plague, smallpox, and syphilis, McNeill suggests that less dramatic agents such as measles, chicken pox, diptheria, as well as unnamed respiratory and gastrointestinal disorders (which he generally calls "microparasites"), followed this pattern. The well-known example of infectious epidemics and the depopulation of North American Indian groups (sometimes before actual face-to-face contact with Europeans) is a case in point: disease played an important role in the saga of "how the West was won" (see Krech 1978). Recently, Kunitz (1994) has reconsidered the demographic impact of the initial contact of indigenous populations in Polynesia, Australia, and other parts of the world. He shows that the pattern McNeill described may not be generalizable as an overall theory of world history because of local conditions of population density and disease ecology.

The second mechanism by which disease affects the processes of natural and cultural selection is through gradual population losses from the chronically high mortality caused by endemic diseases. Endemic diseases can have important demographic effects that are often not recognized by the population itself. High infant mortality rates, for example, may be considered an uncontrollable fact of life and may be compensated for through high birthrates and associated cultural beliefs regarding child spacing and ideal family size. The negative demographic and socioeconomic effects of endemic childhood diseases are often hidden and therefore insidious. For example, endemic malaria in a tropical environment usually has a low case-fatality ratio (approximately 1 death per 100 cases), and mortality is even rarer in adults (Bruce-Chwatt 1980). However, because malarial infections are so widespread, debilitating victims who eventually succumb to other diseases, the demographic impact of endemic malaria can be remarkably strong. This can be seen in "natural experiments" of malaria eradication, in which health improvements have resulted in sudden and unprecedented increases in population growth rates. Such effects have been seen following malaria control programs in Sri Lanka (where malaria control appears to have accounted for 26 percent of the increase in population growth rates [Gray 1974]) and in Sardinia (Brown 1986). In a different type of study, conducted in communities with endemic malaria along the northern shore of Lake Victoria, Kenya, the single health intervention of insecticide spraying resulted in a 50 percent overall reduction in child and infant mortality rates in four years (Payne et al. 1976; Oaks et al. 1991).

The third mechanism through which disease can affect the process of natural selection is parasitism, a concept that has generally been neglected by medical anthropologists (Brown 1987). Parasitism refers to an evolutionary strategy in the struggle for life in which the underlying problems are eating and being eaten. The relationship of hosts and parasites is usually one of mutual adaptation through interactions, which produce a state of equilibrium. McNeill (1976) suggested that a distinction between microparasites and macroparasites, based on whether the parasite can be seen by the host, is useful, because humans are much better able to design adaptations to visible macroparasites than microparasites. Using this distinction, Brown (1987) compared the relative energy drain from malaria parasites in comparison to the energy drain required by traditional landlord-tenant contracts in Sardinia; although neither parasite killed the host, the macroparasites represented a much larger energy drain. It is disadvantageous for a parasite to kill its host, although most parasites cause some degree of real damage to their hosts, manifested through diseases that may affect the growth rate of the host population (Anderson and May 1978). Parasitic species drain nurients and energy from their hosts, thereby affecting the host's fitness. There is a substantial literature on the economic costs of parasitic disease demonstrating lower agricultural productivity in populations suffering from guinea worm, schistosomiasis, or malaria (Basch 1990).

In the simplest sense, parasitism affects culture in three ways: (1) by consuming food energy produced by individuals, (2) by producing disease symptoms, and (3) by limiting population growth. It has often been assumed, particularly in the literature of public health, that parasitic diseases sap the energy of individuals and therefore limit the possibility of cultural advancement. This "vicious circle" argument—that "people are sick because they are poor and they get poorer because they are sick" (Winslow 1951)—is an underlying tenet of international health policy. There is much research yet to be done by medical anthropologists to understand better the effects of parasitism on human behavior. There has been more research on the role of human behavior on parasitic disease transmission (Dunn 1979; Holland 1989; Inhorn and Brown 1990).

Disease and Cultural Evolution

Cultural systems have evolved from the original human lifestyle of food foraging to modern industrialized states. Anthropologists have long recognized a general pattern of cultural evolution from simple to complex societies and from low-energy to high-energy-harnessing economies (Sahlins and Service 1960).

This is simply a pattern of general historical change from prehistory to the present that has been characterized by four processes: (1) increased population size, (2) expansion of technology, (3) increased social inequality, and (4) greater transformation of the environment.

Disease ecology and epidemiological patterns are correlated with stages in cultural evolution (Armelagos and Dewey 1970; McElroy and Townsend 1989; Cohen 1989). In general, food-foraging populations throughout history had relatively low rates of infectious diseases, due to their small population size and mobility, although the total morbidity and mortality from disease varied with ecological setting (Dunn 1968). Diseases that require larger contiguous populations in order to be transmitted (e.g., measles, mumps, smallpox, influenza) were probably nonexistent until the introduction of agriculture and preindustrial cities. Paleopathological studies of the health implications surrounding the introduction of agriculture have demonstrated that in virtually every society on record, the new economic form was associated with increases in malnutrition and infectious disease (Brothwell and Sandison 1967; Cohen and Armelagos 1984; Cohen 1989). The high prevalence of infectious diseases in the preindustrial cities of ancient civilization resulted in consistent labor shortages and population decline (McNeill 1976; Knauft 1987). Today, despite advances of biomedical science since the eighteenth century, modern complex societies are characterized by a new epidemiological pattern: the "Western diseases" of obesity, hypertension, cardiovascular disease, and so forth (Trowell and Burkitt 1981; Brown and Konner 1987). In short, new cultural lifestyles have brought new disease problems throughout history.

Biological and Cultural Adaptations to Disease

The concept of adaptation refers to a fundamental process of evolution in which particular traits are selected in a given environment because they increase an organism's chances for survival and reproduction. Adaptation implies that the environment poses certain "problems," which organisms in the environment must "solve." Natural selection is the mechanism by which such solutions are found (Lewontin 1978, 1984). The concept does not imply that the resulting biological or cultural traits are the only or optimal solutions to environmental problems. Most important, it does not mean that adaptations exist for every environmental problem (or disease). Indeed, the fact that cultural behaviors play a direct role in disease transmission and can hinder disease control programs is an important theme.

Although primarily used in evolutionary biology, the concept of adaptation has been central to discussions in both medical anthropology and cultural ecology (Alland 1966, 1970; Alland and McCay 1973; Brown 1986; Ellen 1982; Landy 1983a; McElroy and Townsend 1990; Netting 1965; Rappaport 1976, 1979; Wiley 1992). Anthropologists have been concerned with describing examples of the successful outcome of adaptations on a genetic or cultural level.

In terms of genetic adaptation to disease, the most comprehensive work focuses on polymorphisms of the hemoglobin system, such as sickle cell trait and other hereditary disorders of the blood, which are most likely the result of natural selection by malaria.

Similarly, the human immune system can be viewed as the product of genetic adaptation to disease pressures. A primary biological characteristic of the immune system is its adaptability; in other words, it is a generalized mechanism capable of providing protection against potential (i.e., yet-to-evolve) pathogens (Baker 1984). The evolution of the immune system is the product of human adaptation to disease; at the same time, the immune system has required that disease organisms adapt to their host-victims. This pattern of mutual adaptation is an important feature of the relationship between humans and disease (Dubos 1965). From this perspective, agents of acute, lethal infectious diseases are less well adapted to their human environment than the agents of endemic or chronic infections. Thus, more lethal forms of a disease, such as AIDS, are probably younger and have had a shorter history of contact and mutual adaptation.

Cultural adaptations to diseases include behaviors and beliefs that function to limit morbidity and mortality in two general ways. First, there are behaviors and beliefs that have preventive functions, by reducing exposure to disease organisms for certain segments of society. Second, there are beliefs and behaviors about appropriate therapy for diseases, generally termed *ethnomedicine*.

Particular patterns of social organization and behavior may have latent functions in preventing the spread of disease, even though their conscious purpose may be unrelated to health. Examples of such preventive adaptations include settlement patterns in elevated locations removed from malaria-endemic lowlands (Brown 1981); storage of night soil before its use as fertilizer (Alland 1970); and traditional laundry soaps with molluscicidal properties in schistosomiasis-endemic areas (Kloos and Lemma 1977). Another way of looking at this, however, is to consider the ways in which the presence of disease in various ecological settings has limited economic or productive possibilities. For example, the presence of endemic malaria may make lowland areas unsuitable for human habitation, thereby restricting subsistence strategies that are too costly in terms of health.

In contrast, the cultural behaviors related to curative medicine are usually the result of conscious attempts to control sickness and death. Yet there is little evidence to suggest that either traditional curative medicine or even modern scientific medicine has had any significant impact on general health or fecundity. McKeown (1976a, 1976b) has conclusively demonstrated that changes in lifestyle (better sanitation, nutrition, and birth control), not the advancement of medicine, best account for improvements in health over the past two centuries.

It is interesting to note that behaviors with disease-preventive functions may be a feature of nonhuman primate societies. Freeland (1976) suggests that many aspects of the social organization of terrestrial Old World monkeys may minimize the probability of acquiring new pathogens or the impact of a disease already harbored by an individual in the group. He argues that the composition of a primate group itself and sexual fidelity of individual primates to other members of the group is the result of selection for the avoidance of new diseases. Similarly, the maintenance of home ranges for groups and the patterns of movement within territories may be effective disease-avoidance mechanisms. Finally, the movement of groups between sleeping sites may reduce exposure to contamination from fecal material and thus limit the spread of a disease already harbored by a group member.

Examples of Cultural Adaptations to Disease: Malaria

Anthropologists interested in cultural adaptations to disease have paid particular attention to the problem of malaria. This may be due to the fact that malaria has reportedly killed more people than any other single disease (Livingstone 1971) and that genetic adaptations to this disease have been well studied. The importance of human behavioral factors in malaria control has long been recognized by malariologists (see bibliography by Sotiroff-Junker 1978). The identification of culturally adaptive behaviors requires knowledge of the biological etiology of the disease, the social distribution of the disease, and local variation in the ecology of insect vectors of the disease.

The medical anthropological literature includes five examples of cultural adaptations to malaria. May (1960), for one, has suggested that the traditional house type of the hill tribes of Vietnam—where cooking and sleeping platforms are elevated on stilts—reduced exposure of the population to the mosquito vector *Anopheles minimus,* which has a flight ceiling of about ten feet.

Brown in his analysis of traditional Sardinian culture (1981), argues that the nucleated settlement pattern, particularly the pastoral pattern of inverse transhumance (flock movement to high elevations in summer), reduces exposure to malaria. In the ecological context of a nondomestic vector (*A. labranchiae*), social groups that are expected to stay within the confines of the nucleated settlement have the lowest rates of the disease. In addition, traditional behaviors based on the folk etiology of miasma also have a preventive effect (Brown 1986).

MacCormack (1984, 1985) has studied cultural traditions and behavioral factors related to malaria control in Tanzania. This work has led to further explorations of preventive adaptations, which reduce exposure to the vector. In Sierra Leone, for example, individuals envelop themselves at night (the prime mosquito feeding period) in a thick cotton cloth, which is inpenetrable by the local malaria vector (*A. albimanus*). Similarly, in many parts of Africa, people traditionally sleep under locally woven bed nets that can be impregnated with mosquito repellent.

In a different vein, Katz and Schall (1979) have examined the practice of fava bean consumption and its relationship to malaria in the circum-Mediterranean region, where populations have high gene frequencies of glucose-6-

phosphate-dehydrogenase (G6PD) deficiency. This dietary staple appears to have antimalarial qualities. However, for males with the G6PD deficiency trait, fava bean consumption can trigger a potentially fatal hemolytic crisis. G6PD deficiency is a widespread sex-linked genetic trait that limits the production of an important red blood cell enzyme; understanding the evolution of this trait may help identify new pathways for the development of antimalarial drugs. Through an analysis of the biochemistry of the gene-bean interaction, Katz and Schall argue that the combination of nonexpressed gene and fava bean consumption provides significant protection from malaria death in females.

A final example is the herbal medicines of the Hausa of Nigeria. Etkin and Ross (1982a, 1982b) have identified thirty-one "antimalarial plant medicines" used by either herbal specialists or the general population in response to the general symptoms of malaria. Some of these medicinal plants have been shown to change the oxidation-reduction status of red blood cells, a physiological condition known to impede the development of the malaria parasite (Eaton et al. 1976). Empirical tests of the traditional medicines, using an animal model of malaria, also demonstrate that three of these substances were highly effective cures. More recently, Etkin (1986, 1994) has shown that ethnomedical and dietary preparations using *artemesium,* especially as used in traditional Chinese medicine, have clear antimalarial properties.

These five examples of disease-limiting cultural behaviors illustrate the general principles suggested by the current theory of biocultural evolution. However, this discussion should not imply that cultural behaviors always or regularly improve health. There are many examples, from both the historical and ethnographic record in which cultural behaviors function to increase the prevalence of diseases. A conpendium of such maladaptive behaviors can be found in Edgerton's recent book, *Sick Societies* (1992). Such cases represent a challenge to both theoretical and applied medical anthropology. Finally, the current worldwide resurgence of malaria, particularly choloroquine-resistant strains of the disease, represents the classic example of a reemerging infection caused, in large measure, by human behaviors (including overuse of certain insecticides and incomplete use of antimalarial chemoprophlyaxis) that have exacerbated the problems of insecticide-resistant strains of anopheles mosquitoes and chemotherapeutic-resistant strains of the parasite.

DISEASE AND HUMAN BEHAVIORAL PATTERNS

As the field of epidemiology has made clear since its inception in the late 1800s, diseases are not distributed randomly in human populations. Some individuals—and some groups of individuals—are at increased risk from various diseases, for reasons that are often unclear. Epidemiologists not only describe patterns of disease occurrence through space and through time, but they attempt to elucidate disease etiology through the search for risk factors that appear to be significantly associated with disease outcome.

Disease risk factors are of two major types. *Endogenous risk factors* are those that are biologically intrinsic to the human host. For example, genetic diseases, such as sickle cell anemia or hemophilia, have, by definition, an endogenous etiology. More commonly, however, genetic inheritance implies a predisposition to a disease that requires other variables or cofactors for expression to occur. *Exogenous risk factors* are those that are extrinsic to the body of the human host. Some of these may be biotic, such as microorganisms that cause infectious diseases; others are nonbiotic substances present in the environment, such as toxic chemicals in the workplace. In most cases of disease, both endogenous and exogenous factors are involved—hence, the notion of "multiple causation," or "multifactorial etiology" (Dunn and Janes 1986).

Humans may unwittingly increase the likelihood of disease by exposing themselves or others to risk factors of both the exogenous and endogenous variety. In many cases, this enhanced exposure potential occurs through disruption of existing ecological relationships between the host, the agent(s) of disease, and the environment. In this way, human behavior itself may be said to be a risk factor for disease, in that human activity may be a necessary component in the chain of events leading to a disease outcome.

Anthropologists, as professional observers and interpreters of human behavior, have an obvious and crucial role to play in the understanding of disease etiology: they can facilitate risk factor identification by describing distinctive patterns of human behavior related to the social distribution of disease. In this capacity, anthropologists may contribute directly to the generation of causal hypotheses, as they did in the case of kuru and cannibalism in New Guinea (Hunt 1978). In addition, anthropological descriptions of risk factor exposure based on long-term ethnographic observation may be more valid than those normally obtained through the standard epidemiological technique of questionnaire surveys (Inhorn and Buss 1993, 1994).

Perhaps most important, anthropologists are especially equipped to understand disease-promoting human behaviors in sociocultural context. This includes the distribution of these behaviors through space and time, as well as the ideological and political-economic factors that serve to legitimate these behaviors. It is in this latter capacity—as interpreters of human behavior who elucidate how and why people act the way they do—that anthropologists may contribute directly to medical anthropological theory building and indirectly to disease prevention and control.

DISEASE ETIOLOGY: CATEGORIES AND CASE EXAMPLES

The endogenous and exogenous factors that contribute to the development of disease in humans are numerous and have yet to be fully delineated. In fact, the etiological causal web remains to be untangled for many diseases, especially those of a chronic nature (e.g., coronary heart disease, hypertension, diabetes mellitus, cancer). Understanding the multifactorial nature of disease causality is the primary task of analytical epidemiology, which, in recent years, has acknowledged the contributory role of human behavioral factors and their social and cultural determinants.

Indeed, human behavioral factors play a role in every major category of disease causation, although their role is sometimes subtle or indirect. In Western medical textbooks, six major etiological categories of disease are generally described, but rarely the behavioral components in their etiological causal webs or the ways in which anthropologists have contributed to their understanding, highlighted. Here, we briefly describe these categories, providing examples of anthropological interest to support the notion of a crucial disease-behavior link.

Genetic

Genetic abnormalities that are heritable or occur as a result of mutation may be responsible for disease if they interfere with the normal functioning of the affected individual. So-called genetic diseases must be distinguished from congenital diseases, which, although appearing at birth, may be due to factors in the intrauterine environment that act upon the fetus (Sheldon 1984).

Among the most thoroughly understood of the genetic diseases is a group of conditions called hemoglobinopathies, including the sickle cell trait (Hb^s), glucose-6-phosphate-dehydrogenase (G6PD) deficiency, thalassemia, and hemoglobins Hb^c and Hb^f (Livingstone 1985). These hemoglobin defects have received the most attention from anthropologists, who have been interested in their potentially protective effects against *Plasmodium falciparum* malaria.

In the 1950s, researchers began to suspect that various heritable human biochemical polymorphisms conferred protection on affected individuals against specific infectious diseases. Through descriptive epidemiology, Allison (1954) was the first to hypothesize that the heterozygous condition known as sickle cell trait appeared with greater frequency in areas of Africa in which potentially lethal *P. falciparum* malaria was present. This association led Allison to hypothesize that hemoglobin S, when present in the heterozygous condition, conferred protection from death by malaria; this association has only recently been systematically confirmed (Durham 1983, 1991).

In a now classic anthropological work that followed, Livingstone (1958) related the widespread distribution of the sickle cell trait in West Africa to the history of human behavior, technological transfer, and ecological disruption in that region. He suggested that falciparum malaria did not spread widely in West Africa until the introduction of iron tools and, subsequently, swidden agriculture. The diffusion of the new technology, leading to changes in production capacity and the alteration of the forest habitat, effectively increased the available breeding grounds for *A. gambiae,* the major mosquito vector of *P. falciparum,* as well as the density of sedentary human populations. This, in turn, allowed falciparum malaria to become established as an endemic disease among agricultural groups in West Africa and as a significant selective agent for the sickle cell allele. In short, human behavior (swidden agriculture), through its effect on the environment (destruction of forest habitats and creation of *A. gambiae* breeding sites), affected the distribution and incidence of not only one but two endemic diseases in West Africa (falciparum malaria and sickle cell anemia), as well as the structure of the gene pool in this region. (See Livingstone, 1976 for an historical reconstruction.)

In a refinement of Livingstone's work, Wiesenfeld (1967) demonstrated that the particular type of agricultural system utilized significantly affected the rates of both sickle cell trait and falciparum malaria. Specifically, societies heavily reliant on root and tree crops (the Malaysian agricultural complex) created a more malarious environment, leading to a selective advantage for individuals with the heterozygous condition in those societies.

Nutritional

Disease may result from malnutrition—from either dietary deficiency or excessive (or otherwise harmful) consumption patterns. The most common worldwide cause of disease attributable to nutrition is malnutrition due to inadequate caloric intake (protein-energy malnutrition) (Sheldon 1984). However, protein-energy malnutrition must be understood not only as a biomedical "disease," but as a reflection of social inequality and consequent hunger (Cassidy 1982).

In addition, nutrition plays a major role in most of the "diseases of civilization," including diabetes mellitus, coronary heart disease, hypertension, and even some forms of cancer. Yet because of the etiological complexity of these conditions, the magnitude of the contribution of nutritional risk factors has yet to be fully delineated. Furthermore, the nutritional component in, for example, coronary heart disease may vary from one population to the next and even between individuals.

Despite the current uncertainty surrounding nutritional factors in these First World diseases, it is clear that a number of specific vitamin- and mineral-deficiency diseases, largely eliminated in the industrialized world, continue to plague populations in poorer nations. These include the five major vitamin-deficiency diseases: beriberi (lack of thiamin), pellagra (lack of niacin), scurvy (lack of vitamin C), rickets (lack of vitamin D), and keratomalacia (lack of vitamin A). In addition, two of the mineral-deficiency diseases, anemia and goiter (from inadequate intake of iron and iodine, respectively), are found widely throughout the Third World.

In a study of nutritional deficiency and its effects on social organization in the Andean region of Ecuador, Greene (1973, 1977, 1980) has shown how the neurobiological consequences of nutritional deficiency diseases are related to the development and continuation of a highly stratified social system. In this context, adequately nourished landowners exploit the malnourished rural populace (*indigenas* and *mestizos*) for cheap labor. Indigenous diets low in iodine and protein have led to high rates of goiter and protein-energy malnutrition, the latter being exacerbated in this case by the early weaning of children to low-protein diets. The problem of endemic goiter is serious because of its association with cretinism and deaf-mutism. As Greene explains, the large number of mentally deficient individuals in this population has led to a redefinition of normalcy to markedly lower levels of cognitive functioning and an attempt by society to integrate behaviorally impaired individuals into the community (see also Buchbinder 1977).

Environmental

Agents occurring naturally or as a result of human intervention in the external environment may cause disease. Physical agents, including unusual temperatures, electrical hazards, and irradiation, as well as trauma, may produce pathology (Sheldon 1984). In addition, contaminants in the air and water, especially in urban, industrial areas, may place the general public at increased risk of disease, although, as of now, the long-term health effects of environmental pollution remain speculative.

Of great interest to epidemiologists in the past twenty years has been the effect of exposure to various substances, especially toxic chemicals, in the workplace. For example, occupational epidemiologists have shown that exposure to the dust of asbestos, a substance once commonly used in construction, is a primary causal factor in the development of mesothelioma, an otherwise rare tumor of the mesothelium (Selikoff 1968). Moreover, exposure to asbestos appears to exacerbate the carcinogenic effects of cigarette smoking in the development of lung cancer (Hammond, Selikoff, and Seidman 1979). In another major occupational study of Pennsylvania steelworkers, investigators have shown that men who work on the coke (liquefied coal) ovens and are exposed to coke oven fumes over an extended period of time suffer significantly higher rates of mortality from respiratory cancers (Lloyd et al. 1970; Lloyd 1971). As with the previous example, coke oven workers who also smoke appear to be at increased risk.

Numerous other occupational groups have been shown to be at higher risk of various diseases because of workplace exposures. These include miners, agricultural laborers exposed to various pesticides, and workers in cotton mills, dry cleaners, and the reinforced plastics industry, to name only a few. In addition to the risk of toxic exposure, workers may suffer the physical trauma of manual labor that is repetitive and unceasing. For example, anthropologists in Australia (Reid and Reynolds 1990) have documented the 1980s ''epidemic'' of repetition strain injury (RSI), an occupational illness involving musculoskeletal pain of uncertain etiology. In their study, they seek to understand the diverse and contradictory explanatory models (EMs) of RSI forwarded by state agencies, industrial managers, clinicians, lawyers, and workers themselves, arguing that these disparate EMs reveal many of the structural tensions inherent in the Australian workplace and in Australian society at large.

Psychogenic

It is now recognized that "psychogenic" factors may cause organic disease. "Psychosomatic illness" is the broad rubric under which somatic complaints of unknown etiology with a presumed psychological component are often placed. Medical anthropologists have made major contributions to understanding the process of somatization, or the physical manifestation of psychological distress (e.g., Kleinman 1980). Unfortunately, however, etiological explanations for these conditions have tended to be reductionistic—involving either mental models or biological models but rarely synthetic models. Recent developments in the field of psychoneuroimmunology appear very promising in this regard (Sapolsky 1994).

In fact, anthropologists have perpetuated this dualism through an ongoing debate about the nature and etiology of "voodoo death." Some anthropologists have argued that voodoo death occurs when the psychosocially traumatized victim gives up the will to live, thereby experiencing a form of "social" death (Thompson 1939; Warner 1958; Lewis 1977); others have concluded that voodoo death occurs as the result of demonstrable biological mechanisms, such as dysfunction of the automatic nervous system (Cannon 1942), surgical shock from terror (Yap 1974, 1977), difficulty in swallowing (Lex 1974), or dehydration (Eastwell 1982). Although the cause of voodoo death probably involves some combination of biological, psychological, and culturally determined behavioral factors, such a synthetic model has yet to be fully developed.

Iatrogenic

With the expansion of medicine, iatrogenic factors, or the deleterious effects of medical interventions, have been recognized as a growing cause of disease (Illich 1975). Perhaps the most common type of clinical iatrogenesis involves the negative "side" effects of medications (e.g., stroke following the administration of oral contraceptives, congenital limb-reduction defects following the administration of the tranquilizer thalidomide to pregnant women, blindness following the administration of antiparasitic medications, involuntary facial and other body movements following the administration of antipsychotic drugs). However, nondrug therapies, and even diagnostic procedures, may be iatrogenic. For example, the common therapeutic practice during the first half of this century of irradiating the head and neck region for the treatment of, among other things, adolescent acne was later found to be a cause of thyroid cancer in individuals who had undergone this procedure ten to thirty-five years earlier (Jackson 1984).

Criticism of the iatrogenic nature of medical practice has been directed most vociferously at Western biomedicine (Illich 1975). Yet evidence from the ethnographic and clinical literature suggests that iatrogenesis is not an exclusively Western phenomenon. For example, on the Guinea coast of West Africa, where infection with the subcutaneous tissue-dwelling "guinea worm" (*Dracunculus medinensis*) is endemic, traditional healers' practices, which include piercing the guinea worm ulcer with a red-hot metal rod, are partly responsible for the high rates of secondary infection and considerable morbidity accompanying this helminthic parasitic disease (Edungbola and Watts 1985). Trotter (1987) has also shown that the Mexican-American folk remedies for empacho, azaron and greta, contain about 90 percent lead oxide and are a significant cause of lead poisoning. Anthropologists have recently been involved in alerting the local and medical communities to the dangers of these two folk remedies.

Similarly, in Egypt, where the chlamydial eye disease trachoma is endemic and leads to visual impairment and blindness in rural populations, traditional healers' practices may lead to futher ocular injury (Lane and Millar 1987; Millar and Lane 1988). These "ethno-ophthalmological" practices include, among other things, scraping the inner surface of the eyelid with an unsterilized shaving blade or "slicing" open an infant's eyes with the blood-drenched tip of a goose or pigeon feather, in order to ensure that the child's eyes are "big and beautiful." In addition, in Egypt, outdated biomedical practices maintained by physicians and "copied" by traditional healers may lead to significant iatrogenesis. This has been particularly well documented in the area of Egyptian gynecology, in which obsolete and irrational invasive procedures may cause or exacerbate infertility problems in patients being treated by gynecologists (Inhorn 1994; Inhorn and Buss 1993, 1994).

Infectious

Biologic agents, ranging in complexity from microscopic, obligate intracellular viruses to large and structurally complex helminthic parasites, are the cause of infectious diseases in humans. Disease occurs when the interaction between the human host and the infectious agent, or the "host-parasite relationship," is no longer symbiotic, shifting in favor of the agent. However, the most successful agents are not those that overcome and kill the host quickly, thus preventing their own reproduction. Rather, all the infectious agents, including viruses, bacteria, fungi, parasites, and several classes of intermediate forms, are more successful as either symbionts or commensals—as agents infecting the human host without causing disease (Sheldon 1984).

Whether infection with a specific microorganism results in disease depends on a number of intervening variables, the most important of which are the pathogenicity of the agent (i.e., its inherent ability to cause disease); the route of transmission of the agent to the host; and the nature and strength of host defense mechanisms (Brachman 1985b). All of these factors, in turn, are affected by the environment. Environmental factors, including such "natural" factors as temperature, moisture, altitude, and indigenous plants and animals, as well as such "artificial" factors as dams and irrigation schemes, human dwellings, and domesticated animals, may serve to promote the transmission of an infectious disease or, conversely, to limit or prevent its occurrence.

Typically, the infectious diseases are categorized into two major types: acute and chronic, according to the ways in which they affect susceptible populations through space and through time. *Acute* infectious diseases, like measles or influenza, are generally characterized by sudden onset, marked symptomatology, and, most important, rapid resolution, either through death of affected individuals or the self-limiting nature of the illness. In many cases, natural immunity to subsequent infection is acquired following recovery. When this occurs on a community-wide level, it is known as *herd immunity*. In so-called virgin-soil populations (those without herd immunity), acute infectious diseases tend to occur in epidemics, which are said to exist when an unusual number of cases of the disease occurs in a given time period and geographic area as compared with the previous experience with the disease in the same area (Evans 1982a). The classic diagnostic features of an epidemic are (1) an index case (i.e., the primary case of an illness that may serve as a source of infection to others), (2) an incubation period (i.e., the definable interval between exposure and the appearance of the first detectable sign or symptom of the illness), (3) an attack or case ratio (i.e., the incidence rate in the affected population during the outbreak), and (4) an epidemic curve (i.e., the temporal pattern of the epidemic as illustrated by a histogram plotting number of cases against time interval) (Evans 1986).

For diseases already present at some identifiable level in the community, it is necessary to know the total number of existing cases (prevalence), as well as the total number of new cases in the population still at risk (incidence), in order to determine whether an increase over normal levels of disease (i.e., an epidemic) has occurred. When such increases occur over a widespread area (e.g., a region, a continent, or globally), the term *pandemic* is used to designate the widespread geographic distribution of the epidemic.

Chronic infectious diseases, on the other hand, pose more difficult problems in definition, because their course of occurrence and diffusion in susceptible populations must be viewed over years rather than days, weeks, or months (Evans 1982b). Chronic infectious diseases, such as schistosomiasis, tuberculosis, or AIDS, not only lack the short course of the acute infections, but they typically—although not invariably—lack the classic diagnostic features of an epidemic as described above. In general, chronic infectious diseases are *endemic,* a term denoting the constant or usual presence of an infection or a disease in a community (Evans 1982a).

From the standpoint of disease and human behavioral studies, the chronic infectious diseases are of greatest inherent interest because of their crippling effect on societies. Although acute, epidemic infectious diseases are potentially devastating, they tend to burn themselves out quickly in human populations, before behavioral and ideological responses on the part of the affected population are typically called into play. Chronic infectious diseases, on the other hand, are often associated with high morbidity, which may result in the incapacitation of members of affected populations. Because of their morbidity and their continual presence in the community, chronic infectious diseases may trigger adaptive responses, including culturally conditioned behavioral changes that may reduce, intentionally or unintentionally, disease transmission.

Such behavioral change may be more likely to occur when affected populations are aware of the nature of the infectious agent, its route of transmission, and human behavioral factors involved in this transmission cycle (Alland 1970). Information of this sort, usually the domain of Western biomedicine, is not regularly or effectively communicated to those most in need of understanding. Moreover, health education programs designed to prevent infectious diseases through behavioral change have had a limited impact, because of a variety of complex problems, ranging from lack of voluntary community participation in prevention efforts (e.g., Phillips 1955; Barnes and Jenkins 1972) to health educators' lack of understanding of local channels of communication and authority (e.g., Hanks and Hanks 1955). These problems are apparent in the case of schistosomiasis and AIDS.

TWO PERSPECTIVES ON DISEASE AND HUMAN BEHAVIOR: SCHISTOSOMIASIS AND AIDS

So far, human behavioral factors in disease causation have been viewed largely from a cultural ecological (microsociological) perspective. That is, the individual manifestations of culturally prescribed behavioral patterns are seen as risk factors for individual contraction of disease.

Certainly, understanding human behavior, one of the most fundamental goals of sociocultural anthropology, is even more important in the context of a disease threat. However, the danger of viewing disease and human behavior on a solely microsociological level is that individuals may be incorrectly considered responsible, even culpable, for their own diseases. Even worse, entire societies may be blamed for maintaining unhealthful practices in their cultural repertoires.

To avoid such victim blaming and to truly understand disease causation, adoption of a political-ecological (macrosociological) perspective is also necessary. From this standpoint, disease is viewed on the level of the population, and disease rates are seen as the result of sociopolitical and economic forces, operating through time and in some cases on a worldwide level. The macrosociological perspective emphasizes larger social forces and not the cumulative effects of individual behaviors per se as the ultimate causes of poor health.

Any medical anthropological study that hopes to shed light on the disease-behavior connection must ultimately adopt these complementary perspectives. Unfortunately, the social scientific literature contains many examples of studies undertaken from one perspective or the other, but synthetic studies, which attempt to evaluate behavioral patterns and to place these patterns in macrostructural context, are rare. Furthermore, the current tendency within medical anthropology is to blame the overarching social-political-economic system for the health problems experienced at the local level without first describing in detail what those local health problems are and how behavioral risk factors may or may not be involved.

Human Behavior in Political-Economic Context: Shistosomiasis and Water Resources

The social scientific literature on the parasitic disease schistosomiasis is a particularly useful illustration of this problematic dualism. Furthermore, the rapid spread of schistosomiasis on the African continent today is largely due to the interaction of human behavioral and ecological factors, which must be viewed within a larger political-economic context.

Schistosomiasis (bilharzia) is a life-threatening blood fluke infection of humans. Like malaria and a number of other parasitic diseases, schistosomiasis is "water based" in that the three major species of schistosomes (*Schistosoma haematobium, S. mansoni,* and *S. japonicum*) share a developmental life cycle in which water plays a major role (Katz, Despommier, and Gwadz, 1982). Briefly, infected humans pass the eggs of the parasite, which are contained in their urine (*S. haematobium*) or feces (*S. mansoni* and *S. japonicum*), into the water, particularly in areas lacking modern sanitation. The eggs develop in the water, hatch, and release larval forms of the parasite. If the appropriate form of snail is present, these larvae penetrate the snail tissue, where they continue development. After several weeks, infective larvae (cercariae) are released from the snail into the water, where they live independently for up to forty-eight hours. These motile larvae seek out and penetrate human skin; once inside the human circulatory system, they mature into adult worms, mate, and pass to the veins of the bladder (*S. haematobium*) or mesenteric venules (*S. mansoni* and *S. japonicum*). Attached by their suckers to the walls of the veins, the adult worms, coupled for life, mate continuously during their five- to ten-year life span and produce hundreds to thousands of eggs each day. These eggs cause morbidity in humans, adhering to the vessel walls and causing damage to the bladder or intestine. After they are eliminated in human waste, these eggs allow the parasitic life cycle to continue.

Because of the obvious human role in the perpetuation of the schistosomal life cycle, numerous studies of human water-contact behavior and schistosomiasis transmission have been undertaken within the past thirty years. These studies, advocated and supported by the World Health Organization (WHO 1979b), can be characterized as macrosociological in nature, because of their primary focus on human behavioral factors in schistosomiasis transmission.

The first studies of this type were undertaken in the 1960s, in locations ranging from Surinam (Van der Kuyp 1961) and Puerto Rico (Jobin and Ruiz-Tiben 1968) to Rhodesia (Husting 1970; 1983) and Egypt (Farooq 1966; Farooq et al. 1966; Farooq and Mallah 1966; Farooq and Samaan 1967). The most extensive investigations were carried out in Egypt, where Farooq and his colleagues performed elaborate observational studies of the daily social, occupational, and religious uses of water in a Nile Delta village. Their most striking finding was that Muslims had higher schistosomiasis prevalence rates than Christians, due to the frequent practice of *wudu,* or ritual ablution before prayer, among the Muslims. Furthermore, the researchers concluded that swimming, a popular summertime activity for children, was responsible for the high rates of infection in the younger age groups.

Following a decade-long gap in research activity, a "new generation" of schistosomiasis investigators began to undertake water-contact studies in Africa (Kloos et al. 1977, 1980–1981, 1983; Dalton and Pole 1978; Polderman 1979; Edungbola 1980; Fenwick et al. 1982). As with the earlier studies, most of these more recent works examined the ways in which individuals became infected through water contact rather than the ways in which individuals infected water through urination and defecation in waterways. A notable exception was provided by an anthropologist, Ann Cheesmond, who along with a colleague, studied human excretory behavior in a schistosomiasis-endemic area of the Gezira, Sudan (Cheesmond and Fenwick 1981). From the standpoint of schistosomiasis transmission and control, Cheesmond's findings were heartening: 70 percent of the urination episodes and 93 percent of the defecation episodes observed occurred in sites far removed from any body of water, privacy being a more important consideration than proximity to water for the purposes of ablution. In fact, only 31 percent of those observed washed themselves after excretion, despite Islamic prescriptions to do so.

Despite the large number of water-contact studies undertaken and the recent major impetus for future water-contact studies from WHO, such studies are limited by their reliance on observation alone. As anthropologist Frederick Dunn aptly noted in "Behavioural Aspects of the Control of Parasitic Diseases":

Let us consider human water contact, as one important element in the epidemiology of schistosomiasis. Any study of water contact must take into account at least the following: consumption of water (drinking, cooking, etc.); excretion and postexcretory ablutions in the water; bathing for hygienic reasons and laundering; swimming and other play in the water; ritual bathing; health education efforts to minimize water contact through changes in behaviour; technical efforts to minimize water contact by providing alternatives, e.g., bridges, safe laundry sites, and latrines; fishing; agricultural practices involving water use and contact; washing and watering of domestic animals; and travel practices, especially stream-crossing and boating, that require contact with water. . . . In so far as the programme may require change in human behaviour it will not suffice to have only this detailed description. A further series of studies, essentially anthropological and psychological, will be needed in each situation to specify why people behave as they do, where and when. . . . Any effort to change human behaviour must rest on such studies. (1979: 503)

Unfortunately, few of the behavioral studies surrounding schistosomiasis have assessed the underlying cultural logic of water-contact patterns or, for that matter, whether groups affected by schistosomiasis associate this condition with water and water-related activities. In three studies in which community members were actually questioned about their knowledge of schistosomiasis and its transmission, investigators found high levels of awareness of the disease and its symptoms but varying levels of knowledge about transmission or ways in which individuals could protect themselves from infection (Kloos et al. 1980–1981; Tiglao 1982; Zumstein 1983). Furthermore, as Kloos and colleagues noted, villagers in rural Ethiopia perceived schistosomiasis, with its vague symptoms, to be a relatively minor health problem, considering their struggle with more readily apparent helminthic infections, such as ascaris (giant roundworm).

Most of these schistosomiasis studies have attempted to quantify behavior and correlate disease-promoting behavior and disease prevalence. However, few are truly anthropological, because they fail to place the behavioral patterns observed in sociocultural context. Moreover, none of the studies successfully bridges the micro-to-macro gap, by contextualizing water-contact patterns in terms of political, economic or ecological origins of unsafe water itself.

This last issue can be raised in terms of water resource development projects and their effect on the spread of schistosomiasis. Research on this issue can be characterized as macrosociological, because it focuses on the ecological disruption and health hazards engendered by politically and economically motivated development schemes. As Hughes and Hunter (1970) note in their review of disease and development in Africa, few of the economic development projects initiated on that continent over the past two centuries have been undertaken within a preconceived, ecological framework. This lack of ecological foresight has resulted in the escalation of ''developopogenic'' diseases, including schistosomiasis, onchocerciasis, trypanosomiasis, and malaria.

Of these diseases, schistosomiasis is the most rapidly spreading (Heyneman 1983)—a spread that is attributable almost entirely to the construction of high dams for hydroelectric power, artificial lakes for fish breeding, reservoirs for water storage, and irrigation systems for agriculture (Heyneman 1971, 1979, 1983; Scudder 1973; Kloos and Thompson 1979). The expansion of old waterways and the creation of new ones has provided an ecological ''free zone'' for snails, the intermediate hosts. As the snail population has spread into new aquatic environments, so have schistosomal parasites and human infections.

The spread of schistosomiasis has been the most severe in Africa, and particularly in Egypt. This is largely due to the construction over the past century of the Aswan Dam–Lake Nasser complex (designed to provide hydroelectric power and perennial irrigation to the country). In a cross-sectional survey carried out in the 1950s in four selected sites in Egypt, schistosomiasis prevalence rates increased an average of 51 percent in three years (Lanoix 1958). Although the Egyptian government has made efforts over the past two decades to control the schistosomiasis problem among the rural population through mass treatment campaigns and mollusciciding (chemical extermination of the snail population), a report by Egyptian scholars has suggested that few, if any, real gains in schistosomiasis control have been made (Abdel-Salam et al., 1986).

Egypt is not alone in its predicament. The schistosomal upsurge witnessed in that country has been repeated over and over again in other parts of Africa, following the construction of virtually every major dam and reservoir complex, irrigation system, and artificial lake (Desowitz 1981). For example, in studies undertaken in the Awash Valley of Ethiopia, Kloos and his colleagues have described the expanding distribution of schistosome-transmitting snail populations and escalating rates of human infection following government-sponsored creation of large, irrigated farming estates (Kloos 1977, 1985; Kloos and Lemma 1977; Kloos, Lemma, and De Sole 1978; Kloos and Thompson 1979). In Sudan, the disease cycle was established within a few years of the start of the Gezira scheme, a large-scale, irrigated cotton project south of Khartoum (Kloos and Thompson 1979; Fenwick, Cheesmond, and Amin 1981; Gruenbaum 1983). In this case, the change in irrigation methods from seasonal flooding to the use of pump irrigation created more extensive and stable snail habitats and intensified human water contact during periods of crop irrigation. In Nigeria, *S. haematobium* prevalence rates soared following construction of a low earth dam and perennial access to a large body of infective water (Pugh and Gilles 1978). This increase was likely to continue, researchers predicted, given government plans to build more dams in the area.

Culture as Ecological Context: The AIDS Epidemic in Sub-Saharan Africa

Over the past decade, Western biomedicine has become less sanguine about its ability to control infectious diseases. Parasite resistance to antibiotics (Institute of Medicine 1992), a resurgence in the West of diseases such as tuberculosis (Ryan 1993), and the dramatic human consequences of the AIDS pandemic have reminded biomedicine that the relationship between human populations and disease parasites continues to evolve. Perhaps more than any other disease in modern history, AIDS demonstrates the complex interactions between a disease agent and human behavior within varying ecological contexts. More pointedly, the AIDS pandemic underlines the need to understand ecological context as social, political and economic—that is, as cultural as well as biological.

The AIDS pandemic has spurred a vast literature in medical anthropology and related social and biological sciences (Bolton and Orozco 1994). Here we review briefly some of the recent anthropological literature on AIDS in sub-Saharan Africa in order to demonstrate the productivity of an ecological perspective that includes human culture as a central component of the environment. Given that no vaccine or cure for AIDS appears to be on the horizon and given that HIV transmission is potentially controllable through modifications in human behavior, understanding the dynamic relationship of culture, behavior, and disease is crucial if efforts to limit the tragedy of HIV/AIDS are to succeed.

Already the dimensions of the AIDS epidemic in sub-Saharan Africa are staggering. While about 10 percent of the world's population resides in the region, it is estimated that more than half of persons infected with HIV live in sub-Saharan Africa (Merson 1993). With more than 8 million Africans already infected and the numbers continuing to grow, the degree of human suffering is and will continue to be immense, even without taking into account dire projections about wider social, economic, and demographic consequences (Danzinger 1994). In addition, up to 80 percent of women with HIV live in sub-Saharan Africa (Caldwell, Orubuloye, and Caldwell 1992), and given rates of perinatal transmission (Ryder et al. 1989), the proportion of children with HIV is also high relative to other regions of the world.

The anthropological literature on HIV/AIDS in sub-Saharan Africa has uncovered some of the assumptions and blinders that shape and restrict efforts to control the transmission of HIV. The studies reviewed here represent only a small fraction of the anthropological contribution and have been selected because they raise issues about the relationship between macro- and microsociological parameters that shape human behavior and pose problems for what kind of definition of "culture" is appropriate. These are questions that must be addressed by an ecologically oriented medical anthropology if an ecological approach is to be wide enough to account for the complex interaction of disease, ecology, and human behavior. Because the culture concept has been misused to blame the victims of AIDS in ways similar to those with regard to schistosomiasis, we must emphasize that cultural issues are no less relevant for understanding the AIDS pandemic in other parts of the world than they are in sub-Saharan Africa.

Three overlapping areas of research demonstrate the importance of understanding both macrosociological and microsociological contexts in order to address more effectively and control the AIDS epidemic in Africa. These areas of research include: (1) examination and deconstruction of epidemiological categories, particularly so-called high-risk groups; (2) ethnographic study of the dynamics of sexual decision making and sexual networking; and (3) critical assessments of the promotion of condoms to stem HIV transmission.

High-Risk Groups

The early anthropological literature on AIDS in Africa focused on identifying cultural practices that might contribute to the transmission of HIV. Identified cultural practices included: "promiscuity"; blood rituals; ritual/medical enemas; female circumcision/infibulation; shared instruments for injections, ritual scarification, group circumcision, tattooing and shaving; and contact with nonhuman primates (Hrdy 1987). Epidemiologists identified patterns of HIV transmission that seemed to predominate in different regions of the world, with sub-Saharan Africa classified as "Pattern II," meaning that heterosexual relations were believed to be the principal means of transmission. "Pattern I" regions included the United States, where homosexual relations and intravenous drug use were believed to be the main modes of transmission. The usefulness and veracity of these epidemiological categories have been questioned by cross-cultural and historical research (Parker 1987, 1992; Packard and Epstein 1991; Farmer 1992). Nonetheless, there remains a wide consensus among both epidemiologists and anthropologists that heterosexual transmission accounts for about 80 percent of HIV transmission in sub-Saharan Africa.

The epidemiological categorization of high-risk groups has been criticized by some anthropologists as oversimplified constructions that deny variation and mask the underlying social influences on individual behavior (Carovano 1991, Schoepf et al. 1991; Schoepf 1992b; Schiller, Crystal, and Lewellen 1994). Membership in such groups, like sexual behavior more generally, has been treated as if it were an independent variable rather than as itself subject to complex economic, political and cultural constraints (de Zalduondo 1991; Seidel 1993). In sub-Saharan Africa, identified high-risk groups have included truck drivers, long-distance traders, mobile military personnel, and, most prominently, "prostitutes." Anthropologically oriented research in Africa has contributed much to deconstructing the category of "prostitute" and contextualizing the heterogeneous practices and settings of commercial sex work.

A number of studies have commented on the difficulty of defining prostitution without accounting for local social and historical contexts (Day 1988; Caldwell, Caldwell, and Quigger 1989; Larson 1989). Larson (1989) used historical and anthropological data to show significant differences in commercial sex patterns between African cities characterized as indigenous and those created by colonial powers. The structure of colonially created urban centers with large male populations and few females produced social and economic consequences that affected the dynamics and networks of sexual relations. Comparing Kampala, Uganda, and Nairobi, Kenya, she demonstrates that patterns of sexual relations in general and commercial sex in particular were determined by a complex interplay between social and economic forces, such as colonial labor migration policies and traditional marriage norms of dominant ethnic groups.

Women engaged in commercial sex work have been depicted as reservoirs of HIV infection rather than as links in broader networks of HIV transmission. Interventions aimed at prostitutes have been criticized as constructed to protect men from women, ignoring the role of male clients in the transmission of HIV (de Zalduondo 1991). Anthropologist Brooke Schoepf (1988, 1992a, 1992b) and historian Luise White (1986, 1990) have shown that prostitution involves much more than the sale of a commodity. Relationships between commercial sex workers and their clients sometimes involve long-term social investments and significant emotional ties. In addition, commercial sex workers maintain other important social ties, including relationships with noncommercial lovers and families in both urban and rural areas (de Zalduondo 1991). Such ties complicate the messages for condom use targeted at this high-risk group. Women in prostitution may find it difficult to negotiate condom use with more intimate partners because of its implications for the emotional and reproductive aspects of the relationship. In more economic relationships, women may not have the power to insist on safer sex because commercial sex work is in most instances primarily an economic survival strategy (Schoepf 1988, 1992b).

The use of the category of high-risk group, particularly of "prostitute," has hampered prevention efforts by homogenizing rather dissimilar relationships and practices, depersonalizing women, and decontextualizing the sexual encounter. Much evidence on sexual networking has shown that simple constructions of risk groups are not appropriate for understanding situations of risk, particularly for women who are not prostitutes (Orubuloye, Caldwell, and Caldwell, 1991, 1992; Obbo 1993; McGrath et al. 1993). Interventions aimed at commercial sex workers must necessarily take into account the economic, political, and gendered context of the sexual behavior, acknowledging the constraints on women's behavior imposed by economic necessity and culturally defined sexual norms. "Prostitution" is not a behavior to be modified but a catch-all category that masks a complex web of social forces and diverse practices that must be addressed with local specificity if the reduction of risk is to be realistic.

Sexual Networking and Decision Making

To some extent the focus on high-risk groups such as commercial sex workers has obscured the wider risks to women in Africa who are not prostitutes (Schoepf 1992b; McGrath et al. 1993). Studies of sexual networking have shown that men and women are at risk through a wide range of "normal" sexual practices (Orubuloye, Caldwell, and Caldwell 1991, 1993; Ulin 1992; Schoepf 1992b; Obbo 1993; McGrath et al. 1993; Orubuloye et al. 1993). In Uganda, Obbo has shown that HIV transmission in local urban and rural settings occurs through small circles of lovers who are connected by common school, workplace, or residence affiliations. In such relationships interpersonal and emotional ties are strong, and these ties color perceptions of risk. Messages aimed at promiscuity will not be effective in situations where sexual relationships are not perceived as promiscuous.

Studies in Nigeria (Orubuloye, Caldwell, and Caldwell 1991, 1992) and Uganda (McGrath et al. 1993) have shown that women's sexual networking has three principal motivations: (1) economic survival, (2) sexual satisfaction, and (3) revenge against the sexual adventures of husbands or partners. As part of a long-term study of sexuality and fertility among a Yoruba population in southwestern Nigeria, Orubuloye and the Caldwells have shown that high levels of sexual networking exist in both rural and urban settings. While their research suggests that levels of sexual networking are slightly higher among men than women and in urban as opposed to rural settings, it also shows that frequent migration back and forth between rural and urban areas makes simple dichotomous characterizations erroneous. Similar evidence of high rural-urban interdependence (sexual as well as economic) has been demonstrated throughout the continent (e.g., Larson 1989; Obbo 1993).

The Nigeria studies suggest that Yoruba women's sexual networking is most frequently associated with economic need and among married women occurs most often among the younger wives in polygynous marriages, who feel economically insecure. Sexual networking by married men is most common among men in monogamous unions. Orubuloye, Caldwell, and Caldwell (1991) suggest that nonmarital male sexuality (both pre- and extramarital) is shaped by social structural factors such as the late age of marriage and the maintenance of long postpartum sexual prohibitions for lactating women, as well as by cultural beliefs in men's polygynous rights. Orubuloye and the Caldwells are somewhat exceptional in exploring men's sexual beliefs and practices, as well as women's. The literature is dominated by explorations of women's sexuality, a phenomenon perhaps partly explained by efforts to help empower women (Schoepf 1988, 1992b) but also perhaps by age-old associations of women's bodies with sexuality and reproduction (Douglas 1966; Ortner 1974; MacCormack and Strathern 1980).

Efforts to prevent the spread of HIV in Africa have focused on two messages for behavior change: limit sexual partners and use condoms. While data on sexual networking are useful for understanding HIV transmission and for targeting preventive interventions, designing effective prevention strategies depends on understanding the dynamics of sexual decision making. Women may find it difficult, if not impossible, to limit their sexual partners when sex is used as a means for economic survival. Guyer (1988) has shown that some Nigerian women use a strategy of lateral fertility (having children with several men) as opposed to lineal fertility (many children with one man) to expand economic support and reduce the risks of poverty. Many women in the commercial sex industry rely on multiple partners as a matter of sheer survival (de Zalduondo 1991; Schoepf 1992b). To such people the risk of AIDS somewhere down the line may not be perceived as nearly as risky as the economic consequences of partner reduction.

In addition, even women who limit sex to exclusive relations with their husband often perceive themselves to be at risk because they cannot control their spouses' sexual behavior. McGrath et al. (1993) have shown that women in Kampala, Uganda, feel unable to control their risk for HIV because they lack the power to negotiate conjugal sexual decision making. Because of poverty and cultural constructions of women's status, many African women are unable to control their sexual relationships with men (de Zalduondo 1991; Bledsoe 1990; Schoepf 1988, 1992b). Men's behavior has been influenced by the AIDS epidemic but not always in ways that reduce risk. For example, Schoepf (1992c) has shown that in Zaire men believe they can reduce risk by being more selective in choosing partners, including: (1) very young girls, who because of their youth are believed to have had fewer sexual contacts; (2) plump women, as stoutness is perceived as a sign of health; (3) women from rural areas, as AIDS is perceived to be an urban disease; and (4) women whom one already knows, as such women are perceived as less dangerous. In addition, traditional beliefs about disease therapy sometimes lead men to believe that they can rid themselves of AIDS by having sex with another women (thereby passing sickness out of themselves and onto another) or by having sex with a virgin. Needless to say, these strategies are unlikely to decrease risk and may lead to greater infection among school girls and rural women.

Women are often in no position to refuse sex, as they are economically dependent on men for child support, jobs, school fees, and commodities to which they have no other means of access (Bledsoe 1990). Orubuloye, Caldwell, and Caldwell (1993) have shown that Yoruba women in Nigeria can say ''no'' to sex in some culturally defined situations, such as during menstruation, during traditional periods of postpartum abstinence, at latter stages of pregnancy, after achieving grandmotherhood, and after menopause. But within marriage, or even within other stable informal sexual relationships, women have only a limited ability to refuse sex, and then only for a short period of time. Refusal over a matter of weeks or months becomes a threat to the conjugal union. Women are usually economically and socially disinclined to end marriage and other stable sexual relationships.

That Yoruba women have difficulty refusing their men sex is particularly interesting for understanding women's power in sexual decision making, because women's status among the Yoruba is considered high and their autonomy relatively great in comparison to groups in eastern and central Africa, where the AIDS epidemic is worst. Yoruba women have a tradition of economic independence as traders who maintain separate household budgets from their husbands. In addition, Yoruba women maintain close ties with their patrilineage and are much more easily accepted back to their natal communities after divorce than women in many societies in eastern and central Africa, where marriage more dramatically reduces a woman's affiliation with her natal family. Yet despite this relative autonomy, Orubuloye, Caldwell, and Caldwell (1993) found that Yoruba women face considerable constraints in refusing men sex. The lesson for AIDS prevention programs is that efforts to promote behavior change need to understand what is culturally permissive behavior change (McGrath et al. 1993). Knowledge of risk, and even the desire of individual actors to reduce risk, is not necessarily sufficient to enable individuals to alter their behavior.

Condom Promotion

African interpretations of condoms and the apparent reluctance of many people to use condoms during sex as a method of HIV-AIDS prevention illustrates the complex relationship between social and economic structures, cultural beliefs, sexuality, and HIV. While AIDS-prevention programs tend to view condoms as a simple technology designed to reduce risk, African responses to condoms and condom promotion programs are not necessarily those predicted by public health planners (Bledsoe 1990). For Africans the introduction of condoms can be more than a simple transfer of technology. A rich tradition in anthropology has demonstrated that bodily substances are replete with symbolic meaning and cosmic importance (Douglas 1966, 1970; Buckley and Gottlieb 1988; Schoepf et al. 1991).

Chris Taylor (1990) has examined the low use of condoms in Rwanda, despite high awareness of AIDS and its sexual transmission and widespread availability of condoms. Taylor shows that Rwandan concepts of personhood are closely tied to notions of shared body fluids. Individual physiology and the exchange of bodily fluids during sex are related symbolically to collective health and fertility. Explanations of pathology often include notions of blockage in the natural and reciprocal flow of body fluids. "The person" in Rwanda is defined and completed relationally. Conception is believed to result from the cumulative admixture of male semen and female blood. Condoms represent blockage and therefore pose a threat to fertility, health, and collective well-being. In such a cosmological setting condoms may be perceived as a greater risk than HIV-AIDS.

Condoms impede fertility, a central value in many African societies. Using evidence from the local print media in a number of African countries, Caroline Bledsoe (1990) has examined the cultural logic that underlies Africans' views of AIDS and condoms. She identifies the following constellation of perceptions that inhibit condom use, particularly condom use initiated by women: (1) condoms deny the man and his lineage children; (2) women who ask for condoms are promiscuous or prostitutes; (3) condom use signals a desire to end a relationship; (4) women who use condoms keep outside lovers; (5) women who request condoms suspect their male partners of harboring HIV infection; and (6) women who request condoms are HIV infected. Given such perceptions, women are unlikely to use condoms with partners with whom they want a relationship. Ethnographic reports from a variety of African countries and populations have reinforced the conclusion that condom use in intimate noncommercial relationships is highly problematic (Irwin et al. 1991; Orubuloye, Caldwell, and Caldwell 1991; Schoepf 1992c; McGrath et al. 1993). Priscilla Ulin (1992) has correctly noted that "to provide women exclusively with HIV prevention methods that contradict most societies' fertility norms is to provide many women no options at all" (p. 136). For commercial sex workers, who may not be concerned with issues of fertility, trust, and intimacy in their sexual encounters, often the ability to negotiate condom use is prohibited by more immediate economic concerns.

Clearly efforts to promote behavior change to prevent HIV-AIDS transmission require an understanding of the complex relationship between individual decision making and action and larger social, economic, and cultural constraints that shape the actual and perceived boundaries of possibility. Increasingly, ecologically oriented anthropologists have recognized the need for integrating larger sociocultural and political-economic influences and constraints into models of the relationship between disease and human behavior (McGrath 1990; Armelagos, Ryan, and Anderson 1990). We are only beginning to understand the complex relationship between HIV and human behavior. Efforts to prevent the spread of HIV-AIDS will depend on integrated, interdisciplinary biocultural research that recognizes human culture as a key component of ecology.

CONCLUSION: DIRECTIONS FOR FUTURE RESEARCH

The study of disease and human behavior from an ecological perspective has contributed, and should continue to contribute, to the solution of both theoretical questions in general and medical anthropology and practical problems in public health. The research strategy described in this chapter has two complementary dimensions: (1) analysis of the social and ecological distribution of disease as it affects human culture and biology and (2) analysis of human behavior, and its sociocultural and political-economic determinants, as it affects the changing distribution of disease. Both of these approaches require the crossing of the subdisciplinary boundaries that currently divide anthropology, for they examine the interaction of cultural and biological phenomena from both a diachronic and synchronic perspective. We believe that this biocultural orientation, stemming from an earlier, holistic tradition in anthropology, continues to be theoretically attractive and is directly applicable to the improvement of health, particularly in less-"developed" countries. Furthermore, because this biocultural approach to problems of disease and human behavior concerns all of the subdisciplines of anthropology (as well as epidemiology and medical geography), it has the potential to provide a synthesizing theoretical framework and, in so doing, to unify the now fragmented discipline itself.

This chapter on the study of disease and human behavior from an ecological perspective has emphasized five major themes:

1. Diseases occur within ecological settings and thus are context dependent and the diseases themselves are subject to evolutionary pressures.
2. Cultural practices can directly alter ecological relationships between hosts and agents of disease and can thereby influence, either positively or negatively, human health.
3. Biological and cultural traits with adaptive value against disease will generally be selected for and maintained in a population, according to evolutionary theory, because they enhance reproductive fitness.
4. Human behavior plays a significant role in the etiology of every major category of disease, and particularly the infectious diseases.
5. The understanding of the influence of human behavior on disease rates requires a synthesis of micro- and macrosociological perspectives.

Although a significant amount of exemplary research on the interaction of disease and human behavior in ecological context has already been conducted, the opportunities for future medical anthropological research in this field are great. Of the numerous diseases that now plague populations and individuals around the world, an inordinately small number of them has ever been studied by anthropologists, despite the fact that many of these diseases are significant causes of morbidity and mortality and are recognized as such by those afflicted, who may view the disease with great alarm. Moreover, many of the anthropological studies of disease that have been conducted to date have not been undertaken for their own sake; rather, they have been part and parcel of biomedical initiatives to elucidate the causes of diseases or to eliminate them in a "culturally appropriate" manner. Finally, both diseases themselves, as well as the culturally determined behaviors influencing them, are constantly changing, and new diseases, such as HIV-AIDS, Ebola virus, and other emerging infections, continue to appear (Garrett 1994; Morse 1994). In fact, the recognition of new diseases, many of them evolving in the environments of modern hospitals, is very impressive: the Institute of Medicine's analysis recognized seventeen emergent bacteria, twenty-seven emergent viruses, and eleven examples of emergent protozoa, helminths, and fungi (Lederberg, Shope, and Oaks, 1992). The introduction of new diseases and the appearance of new twists on old ones present major challenges to anthropologists interested in biological and cultural adaptations to disease threats.

Given this scenario, three research priorities stand out as being particularly important at this time. First, bioculturally oriented medical anthropologists must attempt to refine the definition of disease so that it is no longer defined by what it is not (the absence of "health") or by juxtaposing it as the objective counterpart to the more subjective concept of illness. If bioculturally oriented medical anthropologists are to study diseases without being labeled handmaidens of the biomedical establishment by so-called critical medical anthropologists, then disease models that acknowledge and incorporate the fundamental differences in culturally constructed notions of disease (including, necessarily, the Western biomedical construction) must be formulated.

Second, studies of cultural adaptations to disease threats must progress beyond the level of description to quantitatively rigorous analyses of the effects of particular behaviors on disease morbidity and mortality. However, quantitative research on the impact of human behavior, including traditional ethnomedical practices, on disease rates has yet to be undertaken for almost any disease category.

Finally, future studies of the disease-culture interaction must begin to combine the cultural, ecological (microsociological) and political ecological (macrosociological) levels of analysis. There is a paucity of, and hence a pressing need for, synthetic models to describe disease problems. Most research today tends to focus on either individual behavioral risk factors for various diseases (often based on observational or questionnaire survey data alone) or the overarching political-economic system that allows such diseases to be maintained (often in the absence of supportive ethnographic data). Unfortunately, such either-or research often leads to victim blaming—if not by the researchers themselves (who may never have intended to assign culpability for the disease problems under study), then by those who use the research to justify their own political and economic biases and objectives. Synthetic models, which attempt to examine in detail the interaction of disease and culture on a local level and then frame this interaction in terms of the regional, national, and global forces impinging on it, are desperately needed if disease problems are to be fully understood. Only with such full understanding will the utopian goal of disease control and the elimination of unnecessary human suffering be possible.

NOTE

1. In fact, infection with *Mycobacterium tubcerulosis* itself is not a necessary cause of tuberculosis, since the disease can be caused by other species of mycobacteria (see Harris and McClement 1983, cited by Hahn 1995).

11

Anthropology and Studies of Human Reproduction

Carole H. Browner and Carolyn F. Sargent

Human reproduction is never entirely a biological affair; all societies shape their members' reproductive behavior. This cultural patterning of reproduction includes the beliefs and practices surrounding menstruation; proscriptions on the circumstances under which pregnancy may occur and who may legitimately reproduce; the prenatal and postpartum practices that mothers-to-be and their significant others observe; the management of labor, the circumstances under which interventions occur, and the form such interventions may take; and comparative study of the significance of the menopause.

Despite the fact that the way a society structures human reproductive behavior inevitably draws upon and reflects that society's core values and structural principles, such links have seldom been explicated in the anthropological literature. There is instead a sense that anthropological studies of human reproduction are isolated from the broader currents that shape social and medical anthropological research. In contrast, we hope to show that reproductive studies can provide a particularly powerful lens through which to view broader social processes. Not only does the domain bridge the biological and the cultural, as does much other medical anthropological research, but it inevitably articulates with a society's patterns of gender role organization and their associated ideological and sociopolitical dynamics. In the following account, we describe how anthropological studies of human reproduction can inform larger medical and social anthropological concerns and how, in turn, insights from medical and social anthropology have influenced analyses of human reproductive behavior. We will draw on examples from our own work and that of colleagues who employ similar theoretical perspectives. This chapter, then, is not a comprehensive review of the anthropological literature, which instead can be found in McClain's (1982) and Ginsburg and Rapp's (1991) excellent accounts.

We first consider the concept of reproduction in its diverse meanings, in order to contextualize the discussion that follows. This concept has been inconsistently used in the literature, and its varied meanings are often conflated (Edholm, Harris, and Young 1977). Moreover, the nature of the relationships among different types of reproductive and productive processes has not been distinctly detailed. Nevertheless, the reproduction-production distinction continues to appeal to social scientists because, Collier and Yanagisako suggest, "it represents a symbolically meaningful and institutionally experienced opposition that our own culture draws between the production of people and the production of things" (Collier and Yanagisako 1987:24).

REPRODUCTION AS BIOLOGICAL PROCESS

Biological reproduction is the production of human beings; it is a necessary condition for the perpetuation of society. The term refers to the physiology of human reproductive processes, including menstruation, coitus, conception, gestation, pregnancy, parturition, infertility, abortion, and menopause. Yet these species-wide physiological processes are not invariant but rather are experienced through cultural filters. Biological reproduction is inevitably a social activity, determined by changing material conditions and social relations (Petchesky 1984:8).

Research on biological reproduction has been dominated by medical and health-related concerns, such as identifying the nature of normal and abnormal gestational processes (Annis 1978). There has also been extensive research on the physiological and psychological correlates of reproductive disorders such as infertility (Edelmann and Connolly 1986; Leader, Taylor, and Daniluk 1984; Muller 1990), spontaneous abortion (LaRoche et al. 1984; Llewellyn-Jones 1986), and prematurity (Fuchs and Stubblefield 1984; Elder and Hendrix 1981). Recent attention has been devoted to uncovering the psychological, social, or cultural factors that may contribute to "aberrant" reproductive behavior such as teenage pregnancy (Hofferth and Hayes 1987; Phipps-Syonas 1980; Jones et al. 1986; Ooms 1981; Ward 1990) or repeat therapeutic abortion (Gibb 1984; Lewin 1985). An additional large body of literature beyond the scope of this chapter concerns demography and the macrolevel factors that shape population processes (Greenhalgh 1990; Handwerker, 1990).

REPRODUCTION AS SOCIOCULTURAL PROCESS

Reproduction also refers to the activities and relationships involved in the perpetuation of social systems. Following Marx, the term is used to describe the progressive continuity of production itself, that is, the perpetual processes of production-circulation-consumption-production that account for the ability of social systems to endure over time (Harris and Young 1981:114). In a separate but related sense, the term also refers to the relationships and activities involved in feeding, socializing, and otherwise sustaining the members of a society who carry out its productive activities (Edholm, Harris, and Young 1977). More recently feminist scholars have broadened the concept of reproduction to include the entire set of social relationships associated with the maintenance of a society's political and ideological structures and the sustenance of its nonproducing members (Beneria and Roldon 1987; Gailey 1987; Stephen 1991).

Recent controversies concerning use of the reproduction concept underscore the need for continued exploration as to how its distinct dimensions are interrelated and determined culturally and socially. Such studies could profitably elucidate the relationship between a society's structural and symbolic principles and its paradigms of maternity, that is, the socially and culturally constructed forces that shape maternal roles, childbirth, and related reproductive activities and that link culturally constituted notions of femininity and maternal behavior.

HOW STUDIES OF REPRODUCTION INFORM ANTHROPOLOGY

Early Ethnographies and Surveys

When the goals of many anthropologists were primarily ethnographic, research on reproduction also took on a strong ethnographic cast. Most of the data early researchers collected on reproduction are contained within comprehensive ethnographies rather than in works devoted exclusively to the subject. Notable exceptions are Montagu's (1949) detailed analysis of Australian aboriginal concepts of conception and fetal development and Malinowski's (1932) account of Trobriand Islanders' understandings and practices regarding human reproduction.

Prior to 1970, several comparative surveys of the world ethnographic literature on reproduction appeared (Engelmann 1883; Ford 1945; Lorimer 1954; Mead and Newton 1967; Nag 1966; Spencer 1949–1950). They ranged in quality from carefully detailed efforts by Ford and Nag that demonstrate broad theoretical principles (such as how particular birth practices might be biologically or socially adaptive) to superficial accounts like Spencer's that primarily provide a laundry list of reproductive customs around the world.

More recent surveys by Newton and Newton (1972) and Oakley (1977), while also employing a cross-cultural comparative approach, sought to demonstrate how insight into reproductive behavior in preindustrial societies might contribute to the solution of maternity care problems in the industrialized world. While providing much valuable information on the management of reproduction crossculturally, none of this work linked the domain of reproduction to broadly determined sociocultural or political-economic processes.

Paradigms of Maternity

The proliferation of international public health efforts devoted to maternal and child health following World War II and the second wave of feminism that began in the 1960s drew attention to the reproductive domain as a neglected area of investigation. The best research produced during this period documents how cross-cultural constructions of gender articulate with maternity. Kitzinger's work offers the first extended discourse on how the experience of motherhood is structured by broader sociocultural dynamics. She observes, for instance, that many ritual dances in preindustrial societies are not primarily expressions of the power of sexuality per se but rather of the power of fertility; successful performance of the female role in such societies is inexorably tied to a woman's reproductive behavior. She writes, "In such cultures young girls learn that pregnancy is fruition and that they will become more, not less, beautiful when pregnant" (Kitzinger 1978:36).

Ann Oakley's extensive writings (Oakley 1972, 1976, 1979a, 1979b, 1980) on the ways that motherhood is socially and culturally shaped have had an enormous impact on the field. Using twentieth-century Great Britain as an example, she describes the multitude of ways men idealize motherhood while simultaneously manifesting hostility toward women and female culture (Oakley 1980:284). Other important recent feminist scholarship on the topic has similarly been concerned with the relationship between women's status and motherhood in industrial and preindustrial societies. Some of these studies draw on the cross-cultural literature to argue that women's universal oppression is explicitly rooted in constraints that maternity and child rearing impose (Beneria 1979; Brown 1974; Ortner 1974; Rosaldo 1974, 1980a; Rosaldo and Lamphere 1974). Others use cross-cultural data to offer alternate constructions to our own society's version of appropriate maternal role behavior (Jordan 1993; Kitzinger 1978).

The nature of the relationship between women's status and maternity is evident in the vast majority of the world's societies, where a woman's worth is measured by the number of children she bears; her status may be further enhanced if she prolifically produces male offspring. Throughout the Middle East, for example, a woman is

raised for marriage and procreation, [she] acquires her own social status only by fecundity. . . . The young woman [is inevitably]. . . . taken to be responsible for the sterility of the couple, [and] will do everything to change her state: pilgrimages, magic practices . . . and so forth. If she does not succeed, she will have only a diminished status. (Vieille 1978:456–57)

Similarly, Paulme observes, "an African woman sets greater store by her children than by her husband, for it is only by becoming a mother that she feels truly fulfilled" (Paulme 1960:14).

Accounts such as these blur the distinction between the prestige a mother accrues by virtue of successfully bearing and rearing live offspring and the feelings of satisfaction she may experience as a result of these accomplishments. A growing literature documents, however, that women may derive important self-esteem from performing the maternal role, while responding to powerful societal or community-based pronatalist pressures. In pre–World War II Japan, for instance, childbearing was considered woman's most important function, as reflected in the aphorism, "A woman is a borrowed womb" (Bernstein and Kidd 1982:101–112). Similarly, writing of Jamaica, Clarke reports that the "childless woman is an object of pity, contempt or derision," (Clarke 1957: 95), while in Egypt, Morsy found that women who do not become mothers are considered "useless" (Morsy 1982:150).

The pressures to be prolific that are imposed upon women throughout the world take both positive and negative forms. Analysis of their intent can cast important light on the differential value societies place on children (Cain 1988; Handwerker 1990). In agrarian societies, for instance, pressures on women to reproduce are overt and relentless, as a consequence of those societies' enormous need for labor (Caldwell 1981; Nag, White, and Peet 1978). These pressures are reflected in paradigms of maternity that glorify fertility, childbearing, and maternal role. But it is not only agrarian societies that manifest pronatalist pressures. In industrial societies, says Blake, "people make their 'voluntary' reproductive choices in an institutional context that severely constrains them not to choose non-marriage, not to choose childlessness, not to choose only one child" (Blake 1974:30).

But not all societies value women primarily for their reproductive potential. Collier and Rosaldo show that in many hunter-gatherer and hunter-horticultural societies, themes of motherhood and biological reproduction are far less central to cultural conceptions of the female role than are women as sexual beings. They write, "Contrary to our expectation that motherhood provides women everywhere with a natural source of emotional satisfaction and cultural value, we found that neither women nor men in very simple societies celebrate women as nurturers or women's unique capacity to give life" (Collier and Rosaldo 1981:275; see also Nolte and Hastings 1991).

In more technologically complex societies, women may not be valued primarily for their reproductive potential either. For example, land for cultivation was already in short supply throughout Western Europe by the mid-eighteenth century, and impartible inheritance became the rule. Demographers argue that this inheritance pattern helped lower fertility rates and generated cultural norms mandating fertility limitation. In Hungary, for example, if a married women remained sterile, she was sympathized with; if she had no living children, it was said, "It is her concern"; but if she had more than two children, she was ridiculed, despised, condemned—"Can she not take care?" or "I would be ashamed if I littered as much" (Andorka 1978:95, quoted in Simonelli 1990: 102).

Analysis of the cultural construction of pregnancy can illuminate not only the myriad of ways women are pressured to become mothers but also the broader contexts within which women perform the maternal role. Working in a Colombian city, for instance, Browner found pregnancy to be a time of increased anxiety and vulnerability, for many pregnancies women are abandoned by their conjugal partners and they lack ready access to alternative sources of income. After interviewing over one hundred pregnant women, Browner found that those who were socially isolated were much more likely than those who were not to perceive their partner's minor health disturbances as ''caused'' by the woman's pregnancy, that is, as an empathic response that symbolized to the women their partner's willingness to assume paternal responsibility. She concluded that women with very few of their own kin or friends in their active social networks were much more likely than the rest to perceive their partner's health problems as ''pregnancy'' symptoms, presumably because these women experienced greater economic and social dependency (Browner 1983).

Analyzing conjugal behavior during pregnancy can also cast light on tensions between the sexes seen in parts of the Caribbean. As in the Colombian case, most Caribbean women regard pregnancy as a time of heightened vulnerability. This is because men, who may father children with several mates, are not impelled to support them all regularly. In the absence of a sustained financial commitment from their male partners, women forge extended social networks, often maintaining exceptionally strong bonds with kin, particularly female relatives (Moses 1977:152; also Powell 1982; Prior 1993; Roberts and Sinclair 1978; Sobo 1993). While providing important sources of reassurance and other emotional support, such networks also serve as a dependable source of financial assistance.

Paradigms of maternity may also influence cultural constructions of female virtue. Sargent (1982), for instance, shows that in Bariba society, female virtue is displayed during parturition through stoicism and thereafter through self-sacrifice for one's children. Elsewhere women gain important prestige from maternal self-sacrifice as well (Lewin 1974). ''Stories of mothers' deaths aptly illustrate this, as they usually focus on the lifelong suffering of the mother, the martyrdom of her last days, and the never-ending admiration such behavior gained for her in the eyes of those who knew her'' (Browner and Lewin 1982: 68).

Clearly members of societies do not always share reproductive goals. Kin, neighbors, and members of other social collectivities may have reproductive goals that conflict with one another—and with the goals of women themselves. There have been surprisingly few studies of conflicts between the reproductive desires of a society's fecund women and other individuals, groups, or larger entities (Browner 1986; Ginsburg 1989; Simonelli 1990). In her review of the subject, Petchesky observes that, ''utterly lacking is any sense that the methods and goals of reproduction, and control over them, may themselves be a contested area within [a] culture—particularly between women and men'' (Petchesky 1984:10). Also absent is an awareness that differential access to a society's sources of power and prestige will determine how conflicts over reproduction are conducted—and even whether resolution ever occurs.

Recent research has shown that analyzing a society's attitudes toward and management of menstruation and menopause can also illuminate the social position of women. Accounts by Buckley (1988), Powers (1980), Underhill, (1965), and Wright (1982) of menstrual taboos in diverse Native American societies reveal an important new perspective. Ethnocentrism led early Western researchers to interpret Native American menstrual taboos erroneously as signs of female defilement and degradation (Buckley and Gottlieb 1988). In reality, the female reproductive role was highly valued in those societies; a menstruating woman was considered to be at the height of her creative powers. Said one of Powers's male informants, "During their monthly time women separate themselves from men. Men must . . . [take a sweat bath] once a month while women are naturally purifying themselves to keep their medicine effective" (Powers 1980:57). Buckley's reanalysis of Yurok data and Wright's of data from the Navajo show that menstrual blood is a generative substance, which, when not occupied for reproduction, was considered dangerous to other things with creative potential (Buckley 1982; Wright 1982). Secluding menstruating women, then, is not necessarily a mark of their defilement; it can also express women's power.

Similarly, literature on the menopause reveals the importance of reproduction in its broadest sense for structuring the social position of women. Accounts by Brown and Kerns (1985), for instance, show that once women are menopausal, roles previously closed to them, such as midwife or healer, become open. The postmenopausal women Barnett interviewed in rural Peru indicated that they were satisfied with their present lives because of the enhanced status their society granted adults over forty and because menopause signaled the end of women's responsibilities for child care (Barnett 1988:40–41). Bariba women in Africa also experience positive status changes with the onset of menopause. Bariba women of reproductive age are prohibited from contact with medicines and other activities associated with healing. But postmenopausal women can serve as healers and thereby attain status and power outside their own households (Sargent 1982:61; cf. Beyene 1989).

The status changes that accompany menopause in industrial societies are typically less positive. In such societies, menopause often represents not only a loss of fertility but a commensurate loss of life's meaning (Kaufert 1985; Lock 1993b). The reasons for these differences in the postmenopausal statuses of women in traditional and industrial societies are not entirely clear. Research is needed on how menopause is affected by interactions among such biocultural factors as diet, fertility, and levels of physical activity. Comparative studies of women in industrial and preindustrial societies would lead to a better understanding of the relative significance of these diverse factors (Beyene 1989:139).

Various studies have consistently found that the diminished status seen in postmenopausal women in industrial societies reflects the negative attitude toward biological aging that both sexes experience in those societies (Secunda 1984; Friedan 1993). But while the loss of status that accompanies biological aging for men may be compensated for by the prestige they may accrue by virtue of occupational achievements, women are denied equivalent treatment. This large group of studies, then, demonstrates that paradigms of maternity have an impact both narrowly on women, in societal expectations of maternal role performance, and broadly, because women's social position is explicitly tied to the significance of children in their society.

THE MANAGEMENT OF OBSTETRICAL EVENTS

Considerable research has been devoted to the cultural patterning of childbirth. Some scholars have addressed the epistemological status of childbirth and the degree to which the birth process is physiological event or cultural production (Jordan 1993; Oakley 1980; Romalis, ed. 1981). Others have elucidated the beliefs and behaviors characteristic of pregnancy, labor, and the puerperium (Mead and Newton 1967; Newton and Newton 1972). These works demonstrate that human reproductive behavior is as highly patterned culturally as is any other societal domain. "The act of giving birth to a child is never simply a physiological act but rather a performance defined by and enacted within a cultural context" (Romalis 1981:6). The increasing medicalization of childbirth in industrial societies has attracted the attention of such authors as William Ray Arney (1982), Rita Arditti, Renate Klein, and Shelley Minden (1984), Carole Browner and Nancy Press (1995), Susan Irwin and Brigitte Jordan (1987), Judith Walzer Leavitt (1986, 1987), Ann Oakley (1986), Emily Martin (1987), Karen Michaelson et al. (1988), and Carolyn Sargent and Nancy Stark (1989). These authors show that childbirth experiences even in advanced industrial societies are shaped by broad sociocultural, political, and economic processes (Davis-Floyd 1992; Whiteford and Poland 1989).

As a cultural and social event, childbirth has consequences not only for the new mother but for others in her social milieu. This fact has received proportionately less research attention than has the significance of reproduction for the mother herself.

In the discussion that follows, we consider how analyses of the cultural patterning of obstetrical events can deepen our understanding of such broader anthropological issues as how gender roles and relations are organized cross-culturally, the nature of domestic power relations, the forces that shape ritual behavior, and the components of ethnomedical systems. To do so we offer two extended case studies of childbirth.

A Case of Protracted Labor in Rural Benin

Adama, having recently remarried, was pregnant for the twelfth time.[1] Because all but one of her previous children had died soon after birth, she was worried about this pregnancy. She and her new husband had no living children; thus she feared that loss of her current pregnancy would jeopardize their marriage. Labor began when she was only eight months pregnant. This frightened Adama, in part because eight-month babies are considered likely to be witches.

When her labor failed to progress, Adama sought advice from her older brother's wife and two of her husband's elderly female relatives. In an effort to accelerate labor, they gave her aromatic herbs to smell. This treatment proved ineffective, and a renowned local midwife was summoned. She administered additional aromatic herbs and massaged Adama's back and abdomen. A healthy baby was born soon after, but the placenta did not closely follow. Aware of the danger of this condition, the midwife and other birth attendants quickly began a series of interventions. These included gagging Adama with a porridge stick, massaging her abdomen with a straw broom, pulling on the umbilical cord, and having her squat over burning herbs. When none of these treatments brought forth the placenta, the midwife filled a gourd with water and threw a needle into its skin while reciting incantations. She then instructed Adama to drink the water from the gourd and dropped the gourd onto the baby. The placenta was then promptly delivered (Sargent 1982:111–14).

This case contains several themes of anthropological interest. Adama's desire to bear a healthy child for her husband stems in part from her recognition of the relationship between female adult status and successful childbearing. It also derives from the fact that a respected position as a wife in a polygynous household is dependent on that woman's ability to bear healthy children.

Adama's fears of a witch birth resulted from the fact that witches are primary agents of misfortune in Bariba cosmology. Because they are believed to present themselves at birth, any problematic birth, including an eight-month pregnancy, can be a potential witch baby. Since witches are thought to kill their patrilineal kin, any witch birth is of concern to a baby's patrilineage. Although in principle witch births are viewed as acts of God, the women who produce them are likely to be blamed by their husband's kin. Because her union was recent and in the light of her unfortunate reproductive history, Adama felt particularly vulnerable to such accusation.

Among the Bariba, a midwife is not usually summoned unless complications occur. Should a birth attendant be needed (for many Bariba women deliver alone), elderly female kin from either side of the family may be called. When they have exhausted their own knowledge, they recommend whether, when, and who to call for help. However, these relatives lack authority to compel the parturient to comply with their advice. In Adama's case, a midwife from her husband's ethnic group and social network group was called. That choice illustrated the importance of ethnic loyalty in the selection of a health care specialist. It also illuminated the nature of more general Bariba principles of community alliance and organization.

The obstetrical procedures followed during Bariba childbirth are consistent with more general therapeutic principles. For instance, aromatic herbs are often burned to treat a variety of afflictions, especially those characterized by protrusions from the body, such as hemorrhoids or hernia. In the case of Adama's labor, aromatic herbs were burned to accelerate delivery of the baby and the placenta. Among the Bariba, incantations are recited not only during labor and delivery but at other times when spiritual assistance is needed, such as during illness or other uncertain times. Among the Bariba, as well as elsewhere in West Africa, words themselves carry power that may be instrumental in eliciting good fortune. Thus " 'the doctor's 'word' is more powerful than the medicine itself' " (Kiteme in Sargent 1982:60).

A Case of Birth and Death in Rural Malaysia

Asmah, a healthy woman in her early twenties, was pregnant with her first child. As is usually the case, a village midwife was called when labor began. When her labor failed to progress, Asmah's husband called a government-trained midwife. The government midwife examined Asmah, listened for the fetal heartbeat, and declared that if the birth were to occur that day, it would take place within the next hour. Asmah asked the village midwife to tie a wrapped sarong around her waist to encourage the baby to descend. Meanwhile, the village midwife recited prayers and massaged Asmah's abdomen. The government midwife then reexamined Asmah, said delivery was not, in fact, imminent, and promised to return later.

When the government midwife returned, she found Asmah's contractions still irregular and weak. Upon physical examination, she noticed meconium escaping from Asmah's vagina, a sign of fetal distress. She communicated her concern to Asmah and her husband and recommended that the woman be hospitalized. The couple refused. The village midwife then left, telling the family to call her again when the pains became stronger.

When the government midwife was called again several hours later, a ritual specialist in difficult labors was already there. He recited Koranic verses, but to no avail. A second ritual specialist, who recited native incantations and threw rice to repel noxious spiritual presences, was then called.

Eventually Asmah delivered an underdeveloped dead infant whose umbilical cord was looped three times around its neck. Relatives in attendance consoled one another saying, "It's nothing, it's all right." No visible signs of emotion were displayed by anyone at the sight of the dead child, nor did Asmah express pain, discomfort, or distress during her entire twenty-two-hour labor (Laderman 1983:159–66).

This case illustrates principles fundamental to Malay culture and social organization. Two of the most prominent concern the importance of female modesty and emotional restraint. "The Malay womanly ideal is circumspect, modest, and deferent, and those who deviate too far from the norm run the risk of divorce" (Laderman 1987:295). During parturition, Asmah's attendants respected her modesty by keeping the doors and windows shut and putting mats against the walls so that outsiders could not see in. It was only as the labor grew unusually protracted that the midwife suggested opening the windows and doors to expel possibly harmful spirits. This was because considerations of feminine modesty "outweigh the possible benefits that a magical correspondence between open windows and open wombs might confer," except in the case of especially threatening circumstances (Laderman 1983:165).

Display of strong emotions is strongly discouraged throughout rural Malaysia (Laderman 1983:166). During one labor that Laderman observed, a young woman about to deliver her first child was slapped lightly on the face when she cried out. Those in attendance admonished her, asking rhetorically if she had no shame, to cry out in that manner. Laderman subsequently sought to determine whether the villagers with whom she worked believed that strong emotional expression could negatively affect physical health. "I never have any strong emotions," she was almost invariably told. Emotional restraint was plainly evident in both Asmah's behavior and that of all others present during delivery.

The treatment practices used during Asmah's parturition are consistent with the larger body of Malay ritual practice, in which sympathetic magic is a key therapeutic principle. Loosening the hair of the laboring woman and opening the cupboards, windows, and doors are two strategies most commonly employed. Recitation of incantations is another prominent therapeutic intervention, used during childbirth to enhance the safety of mother and child. These interventions are designed to evoke a more harmonious relationship between the laboring woman and the universe and to distract the woman from her pain (Laderman 1987a:296).

In the preceding cases, we illustrate how analyses of the management of obstetrical events can illuminate our understanding of broader cultural and social principles. There are additional principles that can also be elucidated through interpretations of obstetrical events. For example, analyzing the roles and activities of obstetrical care providers can cast light on the nature of occupational specializations in a society (Browner 1989a; Cosminsky 1976; Jordan 1989; McClain 1989; Paul 1975; Sargent 1982:44–46). Similarly, examining the allocation of responsibility and authority during labor and delivery can provide insight into a society's broader patterns of stratification. The differential involvement of women and men during parturition and, if men are involved, the point at which their assistance is sought can illuminate gender relations and the distribution of gender-based power within domestic groups and in societies. Similarly, analyses of the hierarchy of authority in the obstetrical domain can provide unique insight into how legitimate decision-making power is distributed in societies and how the domain of authoritative knowledge is constituted. Authoritative knowledge encompasses ideas that are privileged either because they have more persuasive power than others or because they are associated with a stronger base of power (Jordan 1993:154; Davis-Floyd and Sargent n.d.).

DECISION MODELS AND COGNITION

There are two bodies of literature pertaining to the anthropology of reproduction that have illuminated the comparative study of belief and cognition. The
first concerns folk concepts of ethnophysiology and their relationship to reproductive, therapeutic, and ritual practice. The second deals with the structure of
decision making and the considerations that inform reproductive choices.

Some of the earliest ethnological research sought to articulate ethnophysiological understandings of human reproductive processes. While beliefs about
conception are well represented in that literature, far less attention has been paid
to menstruation, perceptions of pregnancy (cf. Jordan 1977; Browner 1980),
gestation and fetal development, and menopause.

Most early ethnographers devoted only a sentence or two to the ethnophysiology of reproduction. Montagu's (1949) classic description of the embryol-
ogical beliefs of primitive peoples and ancient societies through the eighteenth
century is a rare exception, in the remarkable detail it provides about emic
understandings of conception, fetal development, and embryology. Margaret
Mead's work is another rare exception. Even Montagu and Mead, however, fail
to provide the depth of detail seen in subsequent research on the subject.

Works by Margarita Kay (1977a), Arthur Rubel, Carl O'Nell, and Rolando
Ardon (1975), Michele Shedlin and Paula Hollerbach (1978), Clarissa Scott
(1975), Loudell Snow (1974), Gisele Tucker (1986), and Carol McClain (1975),
among others, demonstrate that many cultures possess well-developed understandings about conception, gestation, and parturition. To date, little of this work
has considered the relationship between ethnophysiological understandings and
those of biomedicine (Browner, Ortiz de Montellano, and Rubel 1988; Sobo
1993). Instead, however, some anthropologists have shown that folk concepts
of reproduction can have important practical applications for reproductive behavior. McClain, for example, found that many of the Mexican women with
whom she worked refused to accept injections during pregnancy because they
understood that injections cause the cervix to close. Those women believed that
the fetus breathes through its mother's cervix so declined injections rather than
jeopardize the well-being of their fetus (McClain 1975). A comparative study
of indigenous fertility regulating practices in seven societies (Newman 1985)
details relationships between ethnophysiological concepts and fertility-regulating
behavior (see also MacCormack 1982; MacCormack and Draper 1987). Interestingly, many of the herbal remedies women use for the management of
pregnancy and the treatment of female reproductive health problems appear in
several societies, with similar ethnophysiological rationales often provided for
the selection of those particular substances.

Research on the ethnophysiology of reproduction holds the potential for illuminating more general ethnomedical principles, but to date little work has
elucidated the connections. Instead, researchers have shown how folk concepts
of reproduction are informed by the broader ethnomedical systems of which

they are part (Kay 1982; Newman 1985). One exception is Browner's (1985a) article on the criteria used in an indigenous Mexican village for selecting herbal remedies for reproduction and reproductive health. She shows that within the domain of reproduction, the hot-cold theory is subsumed by a broader set of therapeutic practices intended to help the body expel or retain certain substances.[2] She suggests that these more comprehensive folk principles of expulsion and retention may also be fundamental to health care concepts and practices beyond the reproductive domain.

Laderman's account of Malay ethnophysiology of pregnancy, childbirth, and the postpartum period is valuable for the insight it provides not only into general Malay therapeutic understandings but also into core concepts of Malaysian culture.

The birth of a baby is much more than just a physiological event. . . . It is also the most important rite of passage, requiring spiritual prophylaxis and ritual expertise. . . . Cultural signposts furnish [Malay women] and their husbands with information about the advantages and risks of following subsidiary paths, or even leaving the highroad altogether. . . . Some of these signposts are phrased in humoral terms and others are not; theirs is a metalanguage, the language of Malay adat, custom in its widest and deepest sense, embodying all the shared norms, values, beliefs and traditions of the society. (1987b:359)

The second body of literature that has informed cognitive research focuses on reproductive decision making and the considerations that shape fertility-related behavior. There has been extensive research by anthropologists and researchers from other disciplines designed to investigate the social, psychological, and cultural dimensions of population growth and the reasons poor women throughout the world often seem reluctant to use modern contraceptives.

Much of this work consists of cross-cultural surveys designed to determine women's (and occasionally men's) knowledge, attitudes, and practices with regard to modern birth control techniques (Berelson 1966). There have also been a few in-depth studies that have looked at the relationship between birth control methods or the organization of contraceptive clinics and women's decisions about whether to use contraceptives (Coleman 1983; Marshall 1977; Polgar 1971; Polgar and Marshall 1976; Scrimshaw 1980). Additional research has focused on the considerations women take into account in deciding whether to terminate a pregnancy (Browner 1976, 1979; Friedlander, Ksul, and Stimel 1984; Luker 1975). Other aspects of reproductive decision making have been less fully studied by anthropologists, although demographers have developed a considerable literature on the subject (Handwerker 1990).

Given the extensive ethnographic literature on medical choice (see Sargent 1982, 1989), the scant anthropological contribution to the study of reproductive decision making is surprising. One interesting study that does address this issue is Nardi's analysis of reproductive decision making in western Samoa. In it, Nardi articulates how the value of child labor, old age security, husband's ap-

proval, and the intrinsic desirability of children influence women's fertility decision-making behavior (Nardi 1983).

Other recent cross-cultural research has been devoted to analyzing factors that
influence women's decisions about the use of obstetrical services. McClain
(1985), for example, investigated how a group of California women decided
whether to attempt trial of labor instead of elective repeat cesarean section. She
found that the women did not assess their potential delivery outcomes in strict
probabilistic terms. Instead, they based their decisions on their previous childbirth experiences and their expectations concerning the two types of delivery.
Goforth's (1988) research on women's choice of birth attendants in a Yucatec
Maya community demonstrated that access to economic resources was the best
predictor of pregnant women's decisions to use traditional or biomedical obstetrical practitioners. Sargent's (1989) study of obstetrical decision making in
rural and urban Benin describes how Bariba women's diverse objectives and
goals, most of which are nonmedical in nature, lead them to make particular
obstetrical choices.

One strength these studies share is that their implications extend beyond the
reproductive domain. Each author has explicitly delineated her study's larger
significance, for either decision theory or social organization more generally.
We are encouraged by this trend and hope that it stimulates additional research
linking reproductive behavior to broader social processes.

DIRECTIONS FOR FUTURE RESEARCH

There are several directions that anthropological research on the patterning of
reproduction could profitably take. Still urgently needed is a fuller understanding
of how ethnicity and social class mold women's wishes, expectations, and behavior within the reproductive domain. This will move us toward more accurately articulating the multiple paradigms of maternity held by different groups
of women within heterogeneous societies. Until now, where paradigms of maternity have been detailed, researchers have described unitary models rather than
ones that reflect the diversity of women's experiences, attitudes, and values. It
will be through rich ethnographic data of the sort we have discussed in this
chapter that we will come to understand how ethnographic research can com-
pellingly elucidate diverse paradigms of maternity and their relationships to
broader societal principles and structural processes.

To their detriment, the early ethnographic studies generally ignored reproductive issues or failed to provide detailed accounts of women's roles, activities,
and attitudes within the reproductive domain. In contrast, most recent analyses
of reproduction totally neglect men. Exceptions such as C. Romalis's (1981)
description of a father's role in labor and delivery, Ebin's (1994) work on the
activities of male reproductive specialists, and two recent studies of men's ad-

aptation to the paternal role (Briesemeister and Haines 1988; Whiteford and Sharinus 1988) illustrate an encouraging trend.

Human reproductive behavior is socially constructed and formed by political and economic processes. Many anthropologists, and others who study human reproductive behavior, are therefore concerned about the development and dissemination of new technologies for prenatal testing, fertility enhancement, and selective reproduction. In many parts of America, ultrasonography is now a routine part of prenatal care; other forms of prenatal screening are also quickly becoming the norm (Browner and Press 1995). Since most genetic disorders have neither treatment nor cure, selective abortion is the only means to reduce their impact. This has made the technology controversial, particularly for Catholics and others who advocate the fetus's "right to life" (Lawler 1988; Peel 1985) Feminist scholars and advocates for the disabled are also concerned about technologies that can be used selectively to abort fetuses by sex or for other reasons (Arditti, Klein, and Minden 1984; Callahan 1986; Corea et al. 1987; Overall 1987; Spallone and Steinberg 1987; Stanworth 1987). Meanwhile, progress in developing new techniques to treat infertility holds the potential for dramatically redefining American paradigms of maternity (Becker 1990; Blank 1984; Franklin 1990; Overall 1987; Ragoné 1994; Sandelowski 1993).

But despite these technologies' actual or potential impact, there are still very few firsthand data on what users think and feel about them and the associated issues their widespread use will inevitably entail. Rapp's (1987, 1988b, 1993) work on amniocentesis is an important exception in its analysis of the meaning of the procedure to women who choose it and in its consideration of how race and social class help to shape that experience. Rothman (1986, 1988) deals with related issues in her penetrating comparative study of women who accepted and refused the amniocentesis procedure. But as both the historical and cross-cultural literature unequivocally show, neither the use of technology to influence reproductive outcomes nor concern about the meanings of such interventions is new (Devereux 1976; Himes 1970; Lorimer 1958; McLaren 1984). What is new are the implications for totally reshaping human society that these particular types of technology hold.

Throughout contemporary society, these wide-ranging technological developments and pressing debates will have profound implications for the future of motherhood and the status, role, and experience of all women. The insight anthropologists could contribute by virtue of their cross-cultural knowledge and relativistic perspective can be crucial in charting these debates' future course. Exciting new research by Morgan (1989) on cross-cultural perceptions of when human life begins and Tsing (1990) on the cultural meanings of infanticide are examples of directions such work could profitably take.

We began this chapter by showing that analyzing patterns of human reproductive behavior revealed latent dimensions of broader cultural and sociopolitical dynamics. Similarly, studying the characteristics and shape of reproductive activities will cast important light on gender politics and social organization.

NOTES

1. All proper names are pseudonyms.

2. This theory, common in many parts of the world, holds that the essence of good health is somatic equilibrium, which is achieved by balancing intakes of heat and coldness that enter the body. Hot and cold refer to substances' metaphorical qualities; they are not necessarily equivalent to physical temperature.

12

Alcohol and Drug Studies

Linda A. Bennett and Paul W. Cook, Jr.

OVERVIEW OF THE ANTHROPOLOGICAL PERSPECTIVE

Anthropological work on alcohol and other drugs often challenges conventional assumptions about substance use and abuse (Agar et al. 1981; Douglas 1987; Dreher 1984c; Heath 1987b; Leland 1976; MacAndrew and Edgerton 1969; Bennett 1994; McDonald 1994; Singer et al. 1992; Wilbert 1987; Singer 1986a). In this chapter, we delineate this theme by highlighting areas where the uniqueness of anthropological contributions to understanding drug use and abuse is clearly seen. We have not reviewed the entire field of anthropological research in the area; given the enormous body of literature, especially in alcohol studies, such a review would constitute a project beyond the scope of this book. Furthermore, several excellent reviews have been published on specific topics within this research domain.

Anthropologists tend to take a different tack in approaching studies of substance use and abuse; consequently, their work is often controversial to policymakers and treatment providers. Controversy—and sometimes skepticism—frequently surround the approach and methods applied (Bennett 1988; Heath 1985; Room 1984; Stall 1985), interpretation of data (Fisher 1987; Schaefer 1981), and recommendations for policy (Dreher 1984c; Levy and Kunitz 1981). This controversy has been recognized within this discipline itself (Marshall 1990a). In certain instances, their orientation is congruent with that of colleagues in other disciplines. In recent years, in fact, some anthropologists have created or joined interdisciplinary research groups and are working as team researchers (Marshall 1982, 1983:11; True 1984:95; Bennett et al. 1987; Brown et al. 1988; Hall et al. 1983; Lex et al. 1984; Marshall 1982; Ratner 1993; Delaney and Ames 1993).

Anthropological interest in studies of drug use and abuse has been apparent for several decades (Heath 1976; Marshall 1987). Until the 1970s, however, most of this research was a by-product of broader ethnographic studies of small societies in Latin America, Africa, Oceania, and the North American Indian and Eskimo tribes. In this tradition, data collected on the use of mind-altering substances formed one component of an overall study, such as noting the use of plants for medicinal purposes or describing curing ceremonies where sacred plants were employed.

Cross-cultural research on substances has been conducted through the use of data housed in the Human Relations Area Files (Barry 1982; Horton 1943; Narroll 1983; Schaefer 1976), by in-depth analysis of available ethnographic data (MacAndrew and Edgerton 1969), through special conferences in which drug use data were presented for a variety of societies, communities, or ethnic groups (Bennett and Ames 1985; Everett et al. 1976; Marshall 1982), or through projects in which the anthropologists conducted a controlled comparison or contrasted different drug use traditions cross-culturally (Bunzel 1940, 1976; Levy and Kunitz 1974; Bennett et al. 1993).

Thus, it is fair to conclude that as of the early 1970s, anthropology had not yet developed an explicit drug research tradition, especially with respect to abuse of drugs (Heath 1976, 1987b). With increased funding available for such studies and with the expansion of applied anthropology, the situation has changed dramatically over the past two decades.

In response to the AIDS epidemic, anthropologists have become central participants in a major research agenda on the sociocultural context of risk behaviors in an effort to develop effective prevention programs. In fact, anthropologists have been quite successful in obtaining funding for AIDS- and HIV-related projects in large part because of the need to conduct qualitative studies in this area. Increased risk for HIV infection as related to alcohol and drug use has been an important aspect of this research (e.g., Carlson et al. 1994; Finlinson et al. 1993; Page et al. 1990; Singer et al. 1991; Singer 1993; Stall et al. 1990; Trotter et al. 1995). The field of drug studies has developed into several subspecializations among anthropologists concerned with family, AIDS, treatment, and special populations (such as North American Indians, Hispanic groups, black Americans, the working class, and women).

Up to the present, anthropological discussions of substance use and abuse are almost always treated separately with respect to alcohol and other drugs. This tendency reflects wider patterns in national and international policy and research, as well as treatment of substance abuse. For example, the National Institute on Alcohol Abuse and Alcoholism was established in 1970 separate from the National Institute on Drug Abuse, and the World Health Organization continues to separate alcohol from the ''illicit'' drugs in most of its working conferences and publications. In anthropology, it is relatively rare for more than one drug to be encompassed in anthropological studies and publications (Agar et al. 1981;

Douglas 1987; Lex et al. 1984, 1986, 1988; Marshall 1987; Strug et al. 1985; Lebot et al. 1992; Kennedy 1987).

Anthropologists in the substance use-abuse field have focused primarily on studies of alcohol, reflecting, in part, the relative order of usage of particular drugs throughout the world: first, ethanol; second, nicotine; third, caffeine; fourth, betel; and fifth, marijuana (Marshall 1987:38). Over the past twenty years, however, a substantial tradition has developed in cannabis research, mainly conducted in the Caribbean and Latin America (Carter 1980; Rubin 1975a; Rubin and Comitas 1975). Similarly, there has been an increasing interest in tobacco studies, and trends in publications and symposia at anthropology meetings seem to indicate that this line of research is gathering momentum. Some research has focused on the role tobacco plays in social relationships (Black 1984). Another theme has been the interaction of transnational tobacco companies seeking new markets in Third World countries (Stebbins 1987). Several researchers with roots in early studies of religious experience and hallucinogens (Wallace 1959) have specialized in the cultural context of the ingestion of hallucinogens such as peyote and mescaline in the past two decades (Dobkin de Rios 1975, 1977, 1984, 1989; Furst 1972, 1976; Hill 1988; La Barre 1970, 1980).

Due in part to American society's definition of heroin, opium, marijuana, and cocaine use as clearly deviant behavior, and in part to demand for legal and/or clinical intervention, studies on such drugs by anthropologists have attracted considerable attention. The street culture around the use of heroin and the use of methadone in the treatment of heroin addiction has, for example, drawn a kind of interest that is perhaps more curious than serious. While such anthropological research tended to focus on heroin in the 1970s, it shifted to an interest in crack-cocaine in the 1980s and 1990s, as use patterns and the wider society's concern about the use and abuse of certain substances changed. The typical anthropologist's emic focus on the drug user's cognitive and social worlds is often at odds with the clinician's and policymaker's perception of the problem. The clinical and policy domains of our society take a more etic stance with respect to use of these "illicit" drugs and thus express impatience, at the very least, with arguments that suggest the use of these substances is not necessarily deviant from the user's perspective (Agar et al. 1981; Dreher 1984c). This perspective has characterized much of the anthropological research on alcohol and drugs during the 1990s.

Regardless of the position taken regarding the deviance of such drug use, it is becoming apparent that prevention and treatment programs must do more than remove the drug in order to be lastingly effective. Drug use fits into a cluster of behaviors and beliefs, and treatment agendas must deal with that reality in proposing alternative ways of life to a recovering addict. Thus, a lucid understanding of the cognitive and social worlds of drug users is highly pertinent to preventive and intervention efforts.

In addition to twenty years of research on heroin addicts (e.g., Agar 1973;

1977; Carlson 1977; Preble and Casey 1969; Smits 1980), anthropologists have more recently undertaken studies on cocaine, as cocaine has gained popularity as the drug of choice for many Americans. One such study examines the ways in which cocaine users interpret their environment, and the resultant influences of the user subculture on drug use patterns (Morningstar and Chitwood 1984). Another combines interest in issues of multiple drug use by investigating cocaine use among methadone clients (Strug et al. 1985). Thus far, a small body of research on cocaine exists in anthropology (Ratner 1993; Sterk-Elifson and Elifson 1993). Because of the relatively widespread indigenous use of kava and betel in Oceania, anthropologists working there have in the course of ethnographic research reported on the use of these substances (e.g., Brunton 1989; Lebot et al. 1992); Iamo 1987; Lindstrom 1987b; Marshall 1987).

Anthropologists approach research in drug use and abuse by illuminating the cultural context in which they take place. For example, while American society has dramatically moved in an antitobacco direction, some anthropologists have recently called attention to the functional role of tobacco use (Robbins and Kline 1988). Consequently, anthropologists at times have been seen as rabble-rousers and troublemakers who rock the boat of cherished assumptions about the pathology or deviancy of drug use (Heath 1987b). For example, anthropologists have been taken to task for overstressing the functional role of alcohol in culture and ignoring its dysfunctional use (Room 1984). Three decades ago, David Mandelbaum clearly articulated the anthropological slant on functional and dysfunctional use of alcohol: "Drunkenness cannot be understood apart from drinking in general, and drinking cannot be understood apart from the characteristic features of social relations of which it is part and which are reflected and expressed in the act of drinking" (1965). More recently, Mac Marshall has similarly stressed the essential value in examining deviant drug use within the context of normal patterns: "All the ethnographic accounts . . . show the necessity of understanding the variety of normal drinking styles in any social setting before attempting to deal with abnormal (or addictive) drinking" (1979a:10).

As colleagues in other disciplines have taken a greater interest in the role of culture in drug use and abuse, they have understood and applied the concept of culture in ways that are sometimes discrepant with the concept in anthropology (Bennett 1988, 1989; Heath 1986; Marshall 1990a). Specifically, in the minds of many scholars outside anthropology, "culture" has become synonymous with presumed membership in a particular ethnic group, nationality, racial group, religious affiliation, class, and so forth as related to particular drug use and abuse patterns. This perspective stands in contrast to the more traditional anthropological view of culture as a dynamic process through which individuals and societies learn the sum total of their society's behaviors and associated belief systems, including those encompassing drug use practices and beliefs.

CEREMONIAL ROLES OF MIND-ALTERING PLANTS IN TRADITIONAL SOCIETIES

Fieldwork focusing on the magicoreligious use of hallucinogenic plants is perhaps the (nonalcohol) drug field's best representative of traditional academic anthropology, as distinct from the growing applied area of the discipline. In the case of the sacred plant hallucinogens—such as peyote, mescaline, and mushrooms—traditional ethnographic research is not typically undertaken to improve treatment or to inform policy. Its aim is to broaden the understanding of the human experience by illuminating the perspectives and experience of others. The vantage point of cultural relativism has especially influenced this line of anthropological research. While this influence has helped provide fresh insight into the cross-cultural use of hallucinogens, it has also reinforced the controversial posture of much anthropological research on drug use.

Cross-cultural assessments of the role of hallucinogen use illustrate how controversy may take form. While most people in Western society typically believe that the use of hallucinogenic drugs is dysfunctional, ethnographies of tribal cultures have often shown that these substances have been used for generations without disruptive effects to the society. In Western and some non-Western societies, drug users have divergent experiences apparently related to wider cultural differences. Comments from Marlene Dobkin de Rios illustrate this point: "Lacking specific cultural traditions of drug use which program their experience, Westerners often report idiosyncratic patterns. . . . There seems to be good evidence that in a society where plant hallucinogens are used, each individual builds up a certain expectation of drug use which, in fact, permits the evocation of particular types of visions" (1984:9, 197).

Other ethnographers have written similar accounts of the user experience in traditional societies, noting the power of culture to shape the drug encounter, to "determine the nature and intensity of the ecstatic experience and how that experience is interpreted and assimilated" (Furst 1976:10). Both Dobkin de Rios (1984) and Peter Furst (1976) find such elements as ritual preparation for and ritual control of the drug experience common to societies with magicoreligious traditions of hallucinogen use. In these societies, the substances are used to evoke visions or stir insight; as sacred plants, they rate a level of regard not accorded recreational drugs in complex societies.

In comparing mainstream American and North American Indian societies, Weston La Barre (1980:65) observes that in some tribal groups, American Indian adolescents receive drugs and guidance in their use from adults through socially established and respectable channels. This procedure differs considerably in intent from that of many other American adolescents who are resisting the influences of the dominant culture. In the former case, the adult order is reinforced; in the latter, it is assailed.

La Barre (1980:82–83) draws on a body of anthropological knowledge about hallucinogens to connect "altered states of consciousness," including dreams, hallucination, and similar states with the origins of religion. He finds such altered states to be genuine human universals and asserts that the experience of shamans while in such states, often induced by hallucinogens, shapes the revelations on which religions are based.

DYSFUNCTIONAL OR FUNCTIONAL DRUG USE:
THE EXAMPLE OF CANNABIS

Cannabis is a widespread drug of ancient vintage, usually classified as a hallucinogen based on its effects on mood and perception (Brill 1981). Anthropologists have studied its use and its role in social structure in a number of cultures. Jamaica, for example, has a high rate of regular users of cannabis, making it an excellent place to study the issues that unfold around the use and abuse of this drug, known to Jamaicans as *ganja*.

> In Jamaica, *ganja* use is integrally linked to all aspects of working-class social structure: cultivation, cash crops, marketing, economics, consumer-cultivator-dealer networks; interclass relationships and processes of avoidance or cooperation; parent-child, peer and mate relationships; folk medicine; folk religious doctrines; . . . gossip sanctions; personality and culture; interclass stereotypes; legal and church sanctions; perceived requisites of behavioral changes for social mobility; and adaptive strategies. (Rubin and Comitas 1975:161)

Ganja figures strongly in the economic realm. On the lowest rung of the Jamaican socioeconomic ladder, poor families with few marketable skills make their living however they can, often engaging in several diverse economic activities. One of these activities may be the cultivation of cannabis. Vera Rubin and Lambros Comitas point out that vendors of cannabis typically lead a stable family life and are otherwise law abiding and conservative.

Working-class Jamaicans often believe that use of *ganja* makes work go more pleasantly and allows them to work harder; however, the middle and upper classes, who employ the lower classes and supervise their work, believe the drug is detrimental to work performance. Melanie Dreher (1983) has investigated the interplay of these differing views in the setting of a Jamaican sugar estate. Three farms were contrasted, all having different proportions of cannabis smokers to nonsmokers. Dreher examined productivity figures by categories of smokers and nonsmokers and found no significant differences in the work performance of smokers and nonsmokers. The results support neither the views of the workers nor the managers (1983:4).

Dreher's study illustrates the increasing use of quantitative data in anthropological work on drug use, but it also points to the levels of subtlety and sophistication that can be added to research by the inclusion of qualitative material. This dimension of research is one of anthropology's strongest assets; it allows for deeper and more accurate understanding of complex questions and helps restrain impulses to hasty generalization (Agar 1980).

Dreher has also studied the use of cannabis among Jamaican women (1984a, 1987). She examined the different patterns of *ganja* use among women in two similar Jamaican villages, where women in one village seemed more inclined to smoke cannabis than in the other. At the time of this study, smoking was contrary to norms for Jamaican women, although they routinely made cannabis teas for medicinal purposes. In the village with the higher rate of smokers, women were found to have more economic opportunity and thus more independence. Women in the village with fewer smokers found it adaptive to conform to the norms, so that they would not alienate men who were potential husbands and sources of support.

By taking a cross-cultural look at what is considered to be a growing problem in the United States, Dreher has undertaken applied research to shed light on an important policy question. A common conceptual framework for the behavior of drug users whose conduct is outside society's usual limits is the social-psychological notion of deviance. Dreher argues that the behavior of the women she studied is better understood anthropologically in terms of intracultural variation. Again, we see a contextual focus, a perspective that, instead of looking solely at individual action, allows for the connecting of individual action to sociocultural structure. Currently more tolerance for *ganja* smoking has developed among lower-class Jamaican women. Use of the substance fits into a constellation of personal characteristics to which the term "roots daughter" has been given. Connected to the ideas generated by the Rastafarian religion about what is "natural" and African, a "roots daughter" is dignified, independent, and intelligent (Dreher 1987). Findings of this later research indicate changing attitudes and thereby remind us of culture's dynamic nature.

Anthropological research often probes the role of ritual in human action, as in the case of the Colombian work of William Partridge (1977). He found that smoking of cannabis was associated with work life through the action of ritual. An important part of worker comradeship is sharing cannabis when one can afford it; those who have it share it with whomever may not have it at that time. Workers who use but do not provide cannabis for sharing at work breaks are considered undependable and isolate themselves from the social networks from which work gangs are developed in the agricultural economy. In this fashion, meaning is shifted from one social context to another. In a domain similar to ritual, Rubin (1975b) has looked at the first experience of smokers as a rite of passage, an experience that strongly influences whether boys become regular smokers. If their first experience is a good one, they will probably become regular smokers; if not, they tend not to become users.

The practice of learning about the cultural intricacies of studied groups makes the anthropological enterprise often more time-consuming than other research approaches. In the Costa Rican work of J. Bryan Page, for example, a command of "proper" Spanish was not adequate to the task of following conversations in the argot of the drug culture on the street (1977). The arcane vernacular was found to be useful to the speakers; one use was the concealment of illegal economic activity, economic activity again motivated by need. Research in Costa Rica involved life histories, participant observation, and ethnographic interviews and subdivided smokers into different categories whose members found their smoking experiences to be shaped considerably by conditioned expectations and socioeconomic factors. Users who enjoyed economic stability and good social support found the smoking of cannabis to enhance activity; those users with less secure lives did not have universally pleasing experiences (Carter 1980; Page et al. 1988; True et al. 1980).

In a keynote address to the Alcohol and Drug Study Group, Dreher documented several theoretical and methodological contributions from anthropology, especially as distinct from the research forthcoming from sociology and social psychology. Not surprisingly, the use of cannabis in modern society is viewed by anthropologists as a "sociocultural phenomenon rather than an individual characteristic" (1984c:7). The holistic and comparative approach, the use of society or community as the unit of analysis, the reliance upon ethnohistorical and ethnographic studies, and the combination of qualitative and quantitative methods make anthropological research on cannabis unique.

The cannabis question is obviously a loaded issue in American society at the present, and therefore it is not surprising that there is resistance to accepting the results of these "controversial" anthropological findings. However, the same skepticism regarding these conclusions about the potential functional role of *ganja* use in certain cultural contexts is remarkably familiar to some of the resistance alcohol researchers in anthropology have encountered when they call into question certain widespread assumptions about the etiology and diagnosis of alcoholism. The question of where to draw the line between acceptable usage—if usage of a particular drug is thought ever to be acceptable—and dysfunctional-pathological usage is extremely complicated. This message is probably one of the most important ones that anthropology offers, especially on controversial drugs such as cannabis.

SOCIOCULTURAL CONTEXT OF ALCOHOL USE

In 1940 Ruth Bunzel pioneered the way for anthropological research on alcohol through the publication of the results of a controlled comparison of the role of drinking in two different Central American societies where she had conducted in-depth ethnographic fieldwork. She had not set out to study drinking or alcoholism specifically. Applying psychoanalytic concepts, Bunzel connected drinking behavior to its wider sociocultural context. By identifying positive functions within these drinking patterns as well as explicating drunken behavior, Bunzel found that drinking seemed to help lubricate social relations in the village of Chamula in Mexico. In comparison, in the Guatemalan village of Chichicastenango, alcohol provided a release from anxieties related to a stressful environment (Bunzel 1976:22).

In the late 1950s Dwight B. Heath took up the gauntlet of this genre of research in his study of culture change following the Bolivian revolution of 1952 (Heath 1958). One area of investigation was change in drinking behavior as an indication of shifting interethnic social relations between the peasants and the mestizos: "drinking is a useful index, being both highly visible and an integral part of the etiquette of relations between men" (1971:180). With this work and an earlier study among the Navajo Indians, Heath began the first sustained effort in anthropology to advance alcohol studies.

The number of ethnographies concerned with drinking practices and beliefs has proliferated since the 1950s. In Peru alone, three publications during the late 1960s and early 1970s focus on alcohol. In one example, Ozzie Simmons offers a description of the sociocultural integration of alcohol use within Lunahuana, a Spanish-speaking coastal village in Peru: "the meshing of drinking with a configuration of culture and social structure [gives] alcohol positive symbolic and functional roles" within the society (1968:168). Similarly, Paul Doughty found that "the use of alcoholic drinks was highly patterned and integral to normal social interaction" within the mestizo community of Huaylas in highland Peru (1971:187). Allan Holmberg summarizes that for the agricultural peasant village of Viru on the north coast of Peru, "traditional patterns of drinking are such an integral part of the value structure of Viru that they are not likely to change in the near future" (1971:198).

A more recent example of basic ethnographic research out of which alcohol data developed but was not the central theme or intent of the research is Ndolamb Ngokwey's fieldwork among the Lele of Kasai in the Republic of Zaire (1987) in which he analyzes the drinking of palm wine: when it is drunk and within what contexts, types of wine drunk, drinking manners, and its connection with health and illness. By concluding that "Lele rules and practices concerning palm wine reproduce cultural values, notions, and categories" (1987:119), Ngokwey clearly articulates the sociocultural integration theme. He also raises another issue, which runs through much of the literature on alcohol (as well as other drugs): gender differences in consumption.

Gerald Mars, an anthropologist focusing on occupational issues, is another recent researcher whose studies uncovered distinctive patterns in drinking styles. Among longshoremen in Newfoundland, Canada, two distinct groups emerged: the "regular men" and the "outside men." The regular men were regularly hired and rehired to work on the docks at the port of St. John's, where one of the requirements to be a "regular man" was to learn the proper drinking behavior for members of the group. These patterns were so fundamental to the continuities between nonwork and work roles that in Mars's research the men rarely mentioned the importance of drinking roles without explicit questions because "I didn't think you counted drinking! *Everyone* always drinks with their buddies!" (1987:93).

The consumption of alcohol is always subject to rules and regulations, and breaching those rules arouses strong emotional response (Heath 1976:43). Currently we see such intense emotionality expressed through the Mothers Against Drunk Driving (MADD) campaign. MADD has garnered phenomenal support in American society, to the point of strongly influencing such formal legal controls as blood alcohol levels permissible for drivers, and the penalties for exceeding those levels.

Gender issues and alcohol and drug use and abuse have garnered considerable attention recently (Heath 1991). Two edited books, for example, address differences between men and women with respect to the proper and improper use of alcohol (Gefou-Madianou 1992) and alcohol and drugs (McDonald 1994) in different cultural settings. This genre of research offers much promise regarding its relevance to gender studies generally and, more particularly, regarding an explicit concern that women's drinking and drug use patterns be better documented and understood. Typically the province of sociologists in the past, workplace-based research on alcohol consumption and abuse has been studied by anthropologists at the Prevention Research Center (e.g., Ames and Janes 1992; Ames 1993).

Acculturation and Culture Change Studies

By the 1960s, anthropologists had developed an increased interest in applying their ethnographic and often emic approach in order better to understand the problematic use of alcohol. This was particularly the case with respect to American Indians. As part of the interdisciplinary team at the Tri-Ethnic Research Project at the University of Colorado, Theodore Graves contrasted Spanish-American, Anglo-American, and Ute Indian groups living in the same area as a means for addressing the question: "Under what conditions is acculturation accompanied by symptoms of social and psychological disorganization, and under what conditions it is not?" (1967:306). Stark differences in drinking practices and problems with alcohol as well as other types of social problems existed among these three cultural groups.

Graves and his colleagues combined ethnographic observations with structured and unstructured interviews conducted with a randomly selected sample from the three groups. He found that the relatively unacculturated Spanish-Americans and Indians evidence patterns of alcohol use and abuse distinct from each other. While the Spanish-Americans retained strong controls socially and psychologically, the Indians were weak on this dimension. Furthermore, while the unacculturated Indian groups displayed excessive drinking patterns and problems associated with heavy drinking, the Spanish as a group did not (1967:317).

With this study, a long tradition in acculturation studies of American Indians and other ethnic groups in the United States was well underway (Bennett and Ames 1985). Paradoxically, acculturation is sometimes hypothesized to be a protective factor against dysfunctional drinking practices and at other times a risk factor. As Graves pointed out in 1967,

> Acculturation is obviously not the unqualified evil that some observers regard it. When traditional cultural strategies for personal satisfaction have become inapplicable, a reorientation toward a set of new and potentially attainable goals appears to be a promising path to mental health. Furthermore, where traditional social and personal control systems are weak, . . . acculturation may also serve to promote the development of new controls, and thereby make the group better able to prevent disruptive individual behavior. (1967: 319)

Change in drinking patterns under conditions of culture change and/or acculturation has been an ongoing theme of alcohol research in the past three decades. The Institute of Applied Social and Economic Research (ISAER) Alcohol Project in Papua New Guinea is an example of an ambitious two-year research project directed by anthropologist Mac Marshall and undertaken to address a growing problem with alcohol there (1982, 1988). A notable feature of the resulting conference and monograph is the fact that most presentations were made by scholars—including many anthropologists—who had conducted in-depth ethnographic research at a particular field site on Papua New Guinea. While none of these researchers had intentionally undertaken a study of alcohol and culture, each discovered that alcohol consumption was important enough to collect data on the topic (Marshall 1982:xxiii). In 1982 Marshall edited a monograph on changes in drinking patterns in highland and coastal villages and urban areas of Papua New Guinea and problems associated with drinking. The significance of this project is seen in the fact that it constitutes "the first time anywhere that such a large body of ethnographic information has been assembled specifically in the service of public policy decisions on alcohol" (Marshall 1982:xxiii).

Drunken Comportment

Two issues—the extent to which alcohol consumption poses serious social problems and the extent to which available alcohol control policies help to stem the tide of those perceived problems—have historical reference in anthropology in the "drunken comportment" concept. In their 1969 book, psychologist Craig MacAndrew and anthropologist Robert Edgerton examine the phenomenon of drunkenness cross-culturally using ethnographic and ethnohistorical data to evaluate several assumptions held about behavior under the influence of alcohol. First, drawing upon ethnographic data reported from five societies, they evaluate evidence for the "disinhibiting" effects of alcohol. They found that "even during periods of extreme intoxication, the inhibitions that are normally in effect *remain* in effect. Drunken persons in these societies . . . may stagger, speak thickly, and become stuporous, without any corresponding display of changes-for-the-worse. . . . In a word, if alcohol were a 'superego solvent' for one group of people due to its toxic action, then the same disinhibiting effect *ought* to be evident in *all* people. In point of fact, however, *it is not*'' (1969:36). In short, MacAndrew and Edgerton call into question the common assumption held by many people in American society that alcohol serves as an disinhibitor, a point of view often perpetuated by medical science (Marshall 1985:68). Thus, even in the midst of increasing cross-disciplinary cooperation, anthropologists continue to find themselves in a position to question seemingly entrenched viewpoints about alcohol and alcohol-related behaviors. Unfortunately, noncritical thinking about alcohol and alcoholism also characterizes some of the research on alcohol. As Heath has succinctly put it, ''polemic masquerades as science in much of what is written on alcoholism'' (Bennett 1988:110).

The Disease Concept of Alcoholism

In understanding alcohol abuse—how it develops, how it is diagnosed, and how to prevent it or intervene in it—alcohologists tend to rely upon simplistic oppositions such as the nature-nurture or genetic-environment contrasts. Similarly the disease concept is often contrasted with the moral model concept in which alcoholism is seen to stem from weaknesses of individuals, which keep them from controlling their drinking. Historically, American society experienced a long period in which the moral model reigned supreme—during the 150 years of strong temperance and prohibition movements (beginning in the late 1700s with the rum trade, and continuing through the repeal of prohibition in 1933) (Ames 1985b).

With the founding of the Yale Center for Alcohol Studies after World War II under the leadership of E. M. Jellinek, the disease or biomedical model was developed as a counter to the moral model. The disease model, according to Jellinek, explains alcoholism as a progressive disease with clear symptoms and certain recognizable, inevitable phases (1960). The insistence on fidelity to the disease concept in the treatment of alcoholism, however, is a more convenient, established theory than scientific understanding based upon scholarly work. In reality, American society has superimposed the disease model upon the moral weaknesses model in popular understanding of the etiology and nature of alcoholism (Ames 1985b). Thus, alcoholics can be held responsible for their addiction based on personality features while at the same time be excused based on a presumed physiological predisposition.

In addition to the confusion around the moral-medical distinction, many well-meaning professionals, as well as the general public, operate with a vague idea of what is really meant by the disease concept and assume that whatever it is is clearly supported by scientific evidence. Contrary to some popular beliefs, the same symptoms are not always present in all alcoholics or in those seeking treatment for alcoholism. The course of alcoholism varies widely. Also, from a disease point of view, we might expect that biomedical criteria would be used to diagnose alcoholism. In fact, however, mainly behavioral criteria are applied. Drinking patterns and behavior under the influence of alcohol figure more prominently in diagnostic criteria established to distinguish moderate, heavy, and alcoholic drinking than do strict biomedical indicators such as organ damage and withdrawal signs (Levy 1984:182).

We recently surveyed a group of anthropologists as to their points of view about the disease concept of alcoholism. This is far from a neutral topic—some respondents commented on its sensitivity—but responses were frank. David Strug noted that he had never "felt comfortable . . . with the disease concept of alcoholism based on a biomedical model. . . . The cultural component will always remain a contextual constant that must be considered" (Bennett 1988: 115). In connecting the idea of alcoholism with disease, Merrill Singer concludes that it reflects "broader patterns of medicalization, privatization of suffering and politically-endorsed individualized problem-solving patterns" (Bennett 1988: 116). While virtually all respondents expressed skepticism about the disease concept, Dwight Heath was the most clearly dubious among these reports: "If alcoholism is a disease, it is a most unusual one inasmuch as an individual can often bring an end to it by modifying his/her behavior even in the absence of any other intervention. Most of the reasons commonly given for calling it a disease are fallacious" (1988:117).

Interestingly, these opinions are generally consistent with the World Health Organization's (1980) position that alcohol problems do not necessarily follow a coherent pattern throughout the general population and do not necessarily have to do with a physiological dependence on alcohol. Anthropologists insist, as do some other alcohologists (Room 1983), that alcoholism is a complex phenomenon, perhaps having predisposing factors (genetic and physiological) in combination with a series of precipitating factors (including psychological, social, and cultural) contributing to etiology. The need for a biocultural synthesis of studies of individual and cultural variation is compelling (Bennett 1988).

The "Firewater Myth"

The "firewater myth" is a major arena where the genetic versus environment debate with respect to population-level differences has been waged for decades and continues to attract the attention of anthropologists and others concerned with these issues. Here conventional wisdom states categorically that North American Indians cannot handle alcohol because of their physical constitution, an idea going back to the nineteenth century. Joy Leland has traced the history of the argument and examined the available published data as of the mid-1970s (Leland 1976).

One explanation for widespread disagreement as to the extent of alcohol addiction among American Indians is the lack of a set of agreed-upon symptoms of alcohol abuse. Leland points out that we are far from having such a list of symptoms for the "dominant society," let alone distinctive cultural groups such as American Indians. In her review, Leland tabulates the presence or absence of forty-four symptoms of alcohol addiction proposed by E. M. Jellinek (1952) that are documented in the available literature on North American Indian groups. Using the symptoms checklist, it was not possible to confirm the firewater hypothesis. On the other hand, the reverse of that hypothesis cannot be decisively supported or discredited (Leland 1976:104, 123). Much more scrutiny is necessary before any firm conclusions can be drawn about the extent of alcohol addiction among American Indian groups, let alone the potential biocultural basis for such addiction.

The term *firewater myth* uses the word *myth* in the sense meaning "misconception," or a notion based on something other than fact. Myths of this kind can mold attitudes, and thus actions, as can myths of a more traditional stripe, such as creation myths: "Myths are powerful influences in human affairs: they condition situations, their preconceptions create consequences" (Leland 1976: 123).

EMERGING DIRECTIONS FOR THE FUTURE

In addition to maintaining its well-established course of explicating the cultural context of drug use and abuse, anthropology might target three areas for special attention: culturally focused treatment and research, biocultural studies of alcoholism, and broadening anthropology's impact on the alcohol and drug field.

Culturally Focused Treatment and Research

Anthropologists have argued that knowledge about cultural variation in drug use and abuse patterns—as well as the wider cultural context—is important for planning effective prevention, intervention, and treatment strategies (Ames 1982; Gilbert and Cervantes 1987; Hall 1986; Heggenhougen 1984; Trotter and Chavira 1978; Weibel-Orlando 1984, 1987, 1988; Westermeyer 1982). In fact, Joan Weibel-Orlando asserts that "we accept, as a disciplinary mission, the role of revealer/advocate. We advocate the right of a people to heal themselves in any manner they see fit. . . . [To do so is a] noble cause consistent with long-established anthropological ethics and belief in the cultural relativity of all institutions including those that attempt to heal and bring people back into 'balance' " (1988:11, 13).

What is the evidence for the efficacy of treatment programs designed with the cultural background of the clients in mind? H. K. Heggenhougen (1984:3–5) points out that traditional systems of healing have been applied to addiction for some time. In Hong Kong, for example, acupuncture has been used to treat withdrawal. He also notes that conventional treatment programs do not have outstanding success in treating addiction and that they are not available to all who need them. Although the efficacy of alternative treatment for addiction is still uncertain, he argues that treatment provided through traditional or indigenous medical system is a needed resource.

Joseph Westermeyer (1982) has made a similar point. He studied Laotian opium addicts in voluntary treatment at a Buddhist monastery in Thailand. Alternatively, treatment at a medical center was available, where patients were slowly withdrawn from opium through methadone therapy. Clients of the monastery's program underwent "cold turkey" withdrawal, yet many addicts continued to seek it out because of its "traditional and reassuring location" (1982: 217). Some difficulties arose at the monastery due to language barriers between the Thai monks and some of the Laotian tribal people: clients at the medical facility complained of the same problems. Both groups, however (monastery and medical center), had good overall feelings about their treatment experiences (1982:222–23). Both have similar long-term outcomes in client abstention. The monastery had a substantial cost advantage over the medical facility but lost favor because of the mortality among older addicts in the withdrawal (1982: 249–50). A combination of the best features of both might be optimal.

Many anthropologists have posited the increased efficacy of treatment programs that take into account the cultural milieu of patients. This hypothesis, however, has not been solidly tested. Weibel-Orlando—after acknowledging her own strong support of this position, especially with respect to treatment programs for North American Indian groups—then calls into question the research base for the argument: "Most of our enthusiasm for indigenous curing strategies as viable contemporary alcohol and drug interventions is based on anecdotal materials. . . . More systematic and observational investigations of the efficacy of such interventions are needed" (1988:16).

Biocultural Synthesis of Alcoholism Etiology

Discussion of the firewater myth debate leads directly to the question of why anthropologists have not led the way in studies combining biological and cultural factors in presumed population-level differences in the incidence and prevalence of alcoholism. On an individual and family level, a biocultural synthesis might help unravel some of the thorny questions around the interplay between predisposing (genetic) and precipitating (personal, social, and cultural) factors in alcoholism etiology. With its integrative approach, anthropology would seem to be in a particularly good position to design and conduct such studies.

James Schaefer proposes two types of studies that would address these issues (1981). He points out the need for both general population and large family pedigree studies. If both were to be conducted in a well-conceptualized manner, together they could provide fresh insights into the "biophysiological or sociopsychological predispositions to alcoholism" (1981:106).

With respect to existing data about differences between North American Indian groups and other ethnic groups, Schaefer strongly contends that "we are a long way from having conclusive evidence of differences in ethanol metabolism by racial group'' (1981:106). In addition to the methodological problems with existing studies, he highlights the basic point—too often overlooked in these discussions—that hypothesized physiological differences between groups in ethanol metabolism cannot be automatically presumed to place the group at increased or decreased risk for alcoholism; certain questions must first be addressed. For example, what are the consequences of relatively greater physical discomfort after drinking, and what are the likely consequences of more rapid metabolism of ethanol upon actual drinking patterns for a group? Do these differences provide increased or decreased protection from possible addiction? ''A paradox thus emerges. Biophysiologically based hypersensitivity reactions may be 'protective'; however, in some cases social, psychological and cultural factors may transcend the 'protection.' Indeed, a wide spectrum of behavioral evidence points to increased amounts of cultural stress, powerlessness and anxiety as conditions which exacerbate alcohol use'' (1981:109). The family pedigree study approach would be a fruitful direction in attempting a biocultural investigation of alcoholism etiology. To date such studies have focused on biophysiological measures, drug use histories, and social-demographic variables. The cultural orientation of anthropology should be a core component of such studies.

Increasing Anthropology's Impact

Much anthropological evidence has *not* been incorporated into professional and lay understanding of alcohol and drug use and abuse. A major gap exists between research findings and the application of results. Why might that be the case?

One, the issues are complex, and it is truly difficult to sustain the attention of a reader or listener long enough so that he or she can make an informed decision. The more that anthropologists—and other scientists—clearly present the evidence for and against a position and the more that it can be interpreted in real-life terms, the better the chances are to make changes in public opinion. Second, conclusions from anthropology often seem to go against the grain of common sense, making the business of influencing people's thinking an uphill struggle. An open acknowledgement of those differences is perhaps more constructive than assuming audiences will be swayed by a solid argument.

Third, anthropologists may not be placing enough importance on presenting their arguments to the right audiences. It is essential that anthropologists *not* limit their written and oral presentations to other researchers. Courses and workshops in the area of alcohol and drug studies can, for example, draw students who are hungering to explore the relationship between culture and biology in the development of drug-related problems. They also provide a good forum for expanding the dialogue between researchers and clinicians. Publication in popular contexts and delivering public talks are also critical to advancing the general understanding of alcohol and drug use and abuse. Anthropology can and should be an active force in expanding informed discourse on alcohol and drugs, leaving its distinctive imprint on the process of inquiry.

13

Culture, Stress, and Disease

William W. Dressler

The literature on stress and disease grew at a geometric rate over the 1980s (Vingerhoets and Marcelissen 1988) and shows no signs of slowing. Research on stress and disease focuses on those social and psychological factors that are related to health outcomes, independent of behavioral factors that mechanically increase individual exposure to physical or chemical insults (e.g., smoking, poor diet). It is well established that a portion of the risk associated with the development of diseases such as depression, hypertension, and coronary heart disease is due to the social and cultural circumstances in which a person lives, as well as the beliefs and attitudes held by that person. The research issue now is not to demonstrate merely that this is so but rather to work out in a refined and systematic way the process involved. This includes identifying the variables of greatest relevance to the prediction of disease, determining the interactions among those variables, and examining how relationships are modified by the social and cultural contexts in which they occur.

Quite a bit of work has been done with respect to identifying relevant variables and pursuing the interactions among those variables, but very little has been done with respect to examining in a systematic way how those relationships vary across different social and cultural contexts. For many researchers, the effects of "cultural factors" are thought to be those demonstrated by the classic work of Cassel and his colleagues (Cassel, Patrick, and Jenkins 1960; Henry and Cassel 1969), who showed how rates of essential hypertension and related health problems increased with culture change or "modernization." In this research, "culture change" is synonymous with "stress"; extending the model involves breaking down the imperfect indicator of stress into smaller and more discrete pieces, which in turn can be related to disease. Precisely the same, and essentially reductionist, strategy can be seen in the sociological literature on stress and disease; the aim has been to break down the concept into discrete psychological-behavioral elements that are more directly related to disease (Pearlin 1982).

These research strategies have resulted in what Young (1980) refers to as an "asocial" stress model. Little or no consideration is given to how psychosocial risks and resistance resources are embedded in contexts of different social relationships, or in how specific historical circumstances have generated specific configurations of stress, adaptation, and disease. A small amount of work has been devoted to the content of the stress model across cultures (Fairbank and Hough 1981). By this I mean the cultural contribution to differences in the perception of what is stressful or what is helpful in coping with stressful circumstances. But there has been relatively little work done on how the social and contextual nature of stress and disease can alter the actual relationships between various factors in the model. If there is to be serious cross-cultural study of stress, then the central problems to be solved must involve both how the content of stressors and adaptive factors varies by cultural context and how the relationships of stress, disease, and adaptation are modified by the social and cultural contexts in which these occur.

The contribution of such a research program to an understanding of disease in human populations should not be underestimated. The study of stress and disease is generally thought to be an excellent example of Engel's (1977) biopsychosocial model, which has been proposed as an alternative to the reductionist biomedical model. However, much of the research on stress and disease fits quite comfortably into the confines of the biomedical model, because psychosocial factors are treated as if they were independent of social and historical contexts. What is currently thought important is, for example, whether there has been a recent life crisis for an individual, not the significance of that particular crisis in the larger cultural context of the community or the meaning of the crisis in the context of the recent social or economic trends in the community. A more explicit focus on these issues would indeed lead to a serious consideration of the broad range of influences on disease. My aim in this chapter is to review the literature on stress and disease from this vantage point, both to clarify what is or is not known about psychosocial and behavioral risk factors and to understand better needed future directions in research.

THE CONCEPT OF STRESS

Discussions of the concept of stress sometimes engender in participants in such discussions the very phenomena of interest; in other words, some people find the concept of stress frustrating, upsetting, and worrisome. Mostly this stems from the inconsistent and uncritical use of the idea in many areas of research. Some persons use the term to refer to outside pressures brought to bear on an individual. Sometimes the stress is very specific, such as particular occupational arrangements, while at other times it is very vague, as in the "stress of modern society.'' Other persons use the term to refer to a response of the individual to some environmental stimulus. This was the sense in which the concept was originally defined by Selye (1975): to refer to a generalized physiologic pattern in laboratory animals in response to a wide variety of environmental stimuli.

In reviewing the concept of stress, Mason (1975) pointed out two things. First, over the years the concept has gained a decidedly psychological connotation and lost much of its physiological utility. Second, research has progressed to a sufficient degree to classify or categorize different stimuli and responses more precisely, rather than lumping them together all under the rubric of stress. This latter observation has been amplified by a number of writers. Cobb (1976) and Cassel (1976) led the way in pointing out that what gets lumped under stress actually involves two linked sets of factors related to health in different ways. On the one hand are events and circumstances that occur and increase the probability that an individual will become ill. There are risk factors or stressors. On the other hand are social relationships and beliefs and values that, when present or possessed by an individual, lower the risk of falling ill. These are resistance resources. The point is that the concept of stress per se becomes less useful in describing actual variables of interest or relationships, and becomes instead a broad term descriptive of an entire process. It was this trend in research and theoretical development that led Mason (1975) to suggest that the term *stress* be thought of analogously to the concept of pathogen in infectious disease. When one speaks of pathogens in infectious disease, everyone is generally aware of what is being referred to but is very clear that there are many specifics left unstated. Similarly, when one speaks of stress, or perhaps more accurately, the stress process, it should be clear that these descriptions just orient one's thinking toward a type of process leading to disease, and these terms do not refer to any concrete entity. ''Stress'' is not an ''it'' (see also Lazarus and Folkman 1986).

What, then, is the stress process? Scott and Howard (1970) provided an excellent description of a formal model of the stress process. Every organism, every individual human being, lives in an environmental context that includes both physical and social facets. Human life is a continuing transaction between the individual and these environments. The individual seeks to maintain a preferred state of existence, balancing energy intake and discharge and involving a preferred activity level, both physiologically and psychobehaviorally. This preferred state can be referred to as homeostasis, although the precise homeostatic state, which people think of as normal daily activities, can change.

Difficulties can arise from a variety of sources in this process. The environment, whether physical or social, can change. If this change involves something salient to the maintenance of the individual's preferred adjustment, such as the loss of his or her job, that individual must intensify his or her activity in that area in order to return to a preferred state. In order to deal with this threatened loss of adjustment, a person must be able to recognize it, accurately identify a solution, and, above all, have resources in the environment that can be brought to bear on the problem (e.g., live in a community where there are other jobs available). When a person can successfully meet an environmental challenge, then adjustment has occurred and "normal" life is maintained. Where a person cannot—if environmental challenges are too great or resources too meager—adjustment cannot occur, and some sort of breakdown of the system—the individual—occurs. Often, but not necessarily, this breakdown is what we refer to as disease. If any single event or circumstance could accurately be termed stress, it should be the simultaneous confluence of environmental demands and inadequate resources for adaptation.

Two things should be made explicit about this theoretical orientation. First, it is highly abstract. Clearly, demands and resources can be found in many levels of human life, including human biology, psychology, social relationships, and culture. It becomes the task of the researcher to analyze specific situations and determine what specific factors are involved in the process. Second, there is a great emphasis in this abstract model on the environment. Commonsense thinking about stress carries with it a strong mentalistic bias. By that I mean a bias toward thinking of stress as a metaphor for psychological upset, worry, anxiety, and frustration. Also implicit in this bias is the notion that what is stressful depends on what individuals perceive as stressful (i.e., "one person's meat is another person's poison"). Carried to an extreme, this bias can lead us to ignore the social environment. The mentalistic bias in conceptualizing stress amounts to saying that appropriate variables cannot be identified, except insofar as factors are consciously perceived by the individual. The emphasis on the environment in the theoretical perspective applied here is essential because social, cultural, and historical processes generate the stressors that place individuals at risk of disease. Individual beliefs, values, and perceptions may (and do) modify the impact of those stressors, but the stressors, arising from environmental constraints, exist and exert influences, often quite apart from what individuals think about them.

The task of research is one of providing substance for this abstract theoretical sketch. Already various schools (to use the term loosely) of thought have developed in stress research, including theories emphasizing person-environment fit (French, Rodgers, and Cobb 1974), person-environment transactions (Lazarus and Folkman 1986), transition models (Jacobson 1986; Parkes 1988), social readjustment models (Dohrenwend and Dohrenwend 1981), and models derived from social role theory (Pearlin 1982). These various models are not mutually exclusive, and all are compatible with Scott and Howard's (1970) systems theory formulation; indeed, as Colby (1987) has shown, models of stress are one part of a larger theory of human adaptation. Rather than be detained by the details of any of these middle-range theories, my concern will be with empirical results, and especially with results that bear on the fundamental questions of the social and cultural definition of stressors and resistance resources and on the contextual modification of relationships among stressors, adaptation, and disease. This is also in keeping with Caudill's (1958a) observation that these stress factors operate at different phenomenal levels and will spill over (in his terms) and have different effects at different levels.

ACUTE STRESSORS AND DISEASE

Two broad categories of stressors have been investigated: acute stressors and chronic stressors. Acute stressors include natural disasters such as tornadoes (Wallace 1956) and life events that are part of the normal life cycle (Holmes and Rahe 1967). Probably three-quarters of all research on stress and mental health since the publication of the famous Holmes-Rahe article has focused on these factors. These life events include both major points of crisis or transition in the life cycle, such as death of a spouse or child, divorce, and loss of a job, as well as fairly minor events, such as Christmas and getting a parking ticket. The number of events studied for etiologic significance varies in different studies, ranging from as low as fifteen to over one hundred. The key to the inventory, whatever the size, is that these events place new adaptive demands on the individual experiencing them. The person whose spouse dies is faced with readjustments in many spheres of life. The individual who loses his or her job must change normal daily activities and begin to search for new employment, which may mean a complete alteration of regular life. Even something seemingly positive and small-scale like a holiday means changes in habit and social interaction (such as reunions with family members) that can have profound social psychological implications. As the amount of social readjustment required increases, either through the accumulation of many small events or the occurrence of one or two major events, the risk of mental illness increases. This risk increases because the likelihood that an individual's adaptive capacities will be overwhelmed is correspondingly increased.

The predictive efficacy of life events has been demonstrated in many studies (Dohrenwend and Dohrenwend 1974, 1981; Barrett 1979). This relationship has been replicated in both retrospective and prospective studies, so there can be little doubt about the role of life events in the etiology of mental illness. What has been disappointing about life events research, however, has been the relatively small magnitude of the effects and the small amount of research on the definition of significant events. Studies have confirmed that the correlation of life events and symptoms is only about .20 (Tausig 1982). A great deal of research effort has been expended to define the psychosocial parameters of life events that may improve this strength of association. Parameters such as the perceived predictability, controllability, desirability, and subjective impact of life events have been investigated (Thoits 1981). None of these dimensions has been shown markedly to improve the predictive efficacy of simple counts of life events.

There is some intriguing evidence that using a brief inventory of events that are culturally regarded as undesirable accounts for most of the association of life events and depression. In research with American samples, using a brief inventory (about twenty events) of life events that includes truly major events in the adult life cycle, such as deaths of relatives, divorce or other marital separations, or unemployment, accounts for essentially all of the effect of life events on depression (Tausig 1982).

Research investigating the variation in the definition of stressful events in different societies has not been extensive, although a few examples can be found. Dressler (1991) found that unemployment could not be treated simply as another in an inventory of life events in an African-American community in the rural southern United States, because of the cultural salience of work; unemployment was found to have an effect on depression in that community independent of other life events. Scheder (1988) observed life events to occur more frequently among diabetic Mexican-American migrant farmworkers than among nondiabetics. The simple count of the number of life events was related to disease status more strongly than individual perceptions of the "stressfulness" of the migrant way of life.

Another, more dramatic, example comes from a study by Quirk and Casco (1994) in Honduras. They compared individuals who had lost family members with a control group who had not experienced such loss; individuals experiencing social loss were further subdivided into those whose family members had died of natural causes and those whose family members disappeared during civil war. Symptoms of anxiety and somatization were twice as prevalent among families of the disappeared than in either other group.

An extensive cross-national study of stressful life events and schizophrenia has been carried out within the World Health Organization's larger studies of psychiatric disorder (Day et al. 1987). Samples of patients were drawn from India, Colombia, Denmark, Nigeria, Japan, Czechoslovakia, and the United States and were diagnosed as schizophrenic using standardized criteria. A standardized methodology for identifying and evaluating the impact of stressful life events, modeled on the work of Brown and Harris (1978) was employed:

The conceptual approach embodied in the WHO life event schedule . . . was "objective" (or "sociological") in orientation; that is to say, it assumed that the influence of life events on episodes of illness could be defined and measured without taking into account the patient's idiosyncratic (i.e. "subjective") perception of the significance of things occurring in his/her life world. Instead, "life events" were defined to be changes that would have been considered stress provoking by an average member of the patient's group. (Day et al. 1987)

It was found that life events could be reliably assessed across these diverse contexts using this methodology, especially with respect to events likely to have a large impact on patients. Consistent with hypothesis that life events play a triggering role in the onset of florid schizophrenic symptoms, in each of the societies studied, life events clustered in a two- to three-week period before the onset of symptoms.

There is some evidence that the risk produced by the occurrence of life events is a function of the social class context in which they occur. In a community study in an American city, Kessler and Cleary (1980) found that the effect of life events on depression was concentrated among lower-class respondents; there was no effect in the middle-class group. Similarly, in research in an African-American community, the effect of unemployment and noneconomic life events on depression was concentrated among low-income persons (Dressler 1991). These studies point to the importance of social context and social meanings as determinants of the etiologic significance of life events, determinants more important than idiosyncratic perceptions of life events.

CHRONIC STRESSORS AND DISEASE

Rahe and Arthur (1978) explicitly note that life events are only one category of stressors—acute stressors. Chronic social stressors are risk factors that do not have the discrete and identifiable onset as do life events but rather persist in the structure of everyday social roles and circumstances. The social disorganization hypothesis (Leighton et al. 1963) and the life stress hypothesis (Langer and Michael 1963) are classic examples of chronic and ongoing stressful circumstances.

More explicit attempts to study chronic social stressors have been made by Leonard Pearlin and his associates (Pearlin and Schooler 1978; Ilfeld 1977; Pearlin 1982). These investigators have examined the ways in which the basic social roles of spouse, parent, worker, provider, and neighbor are perceived as difficult by individuals. Where conflict, worry, and upset are seen as enduring in these roles, the risk of depression is greater. Lazarus and his colleagues (Kanner et al. 1980) have also investigated common and seemingly mundane persistent concerns, which they call "hassles," and have found them to be related to depression. Dressler (1991) examined chronic social role stressors in an African-American community in the rural southern United States. He found some interesting differences in the content of the chronic social role stressors, in that social role problems associated with racism and discrimination were a part of the definition of chronic difficulties. These chronic stressors were found to be related to more depressive symptoms. Furthermore, in Pearlin's largely Euro-American sample, marital stressors were most strongly related to depression (Ilfeld 1977); in the black community, economic stressors were the strongest correlate (Dressler 1991), in keeping with the general cultural salience of economic adjustment.

Graves and Graves (1985) examined the impact of a kind of hybrid stressor measured in their study of Polynesian migrants to New Zealand. This measure included some life events (e.g., death of a close family member), as well as chronic role difficulties, such as work and family problems. The correlation of stressors with more reported psychosomatic symptoms was about the same ($r = .37$) for migrants from Samoa, the Cook Islands, and European New Zealanders.

A chronic stressor that has been investigated cross-culturally is lifestyle incongruity (Dressler 1993a). Drawing on earlier work by Chance (1965) and Graves (1967), this factor is defined as the degree to which lifestyle exceeds occupational class. Operationally, lifestyle is measured by the ownership of material culture and the adoption of "cosmopolitan" behaviors, and occupational class is measured with standard occupational rankings. Lifestyle incongruity is related to higher blood pressure in St. Lucia, Brazil, Mexico, and Alabama (Dressler 1993a); higher depressive symptoms in Alabama (Dressler 1991); and higher serum lipids in Brazil (Dressler, Santos, and Viteri 1993) and England (Dressler, Evans, and Gray 1992). One of the most intriguing aspects of this factor is that it is related to disease independent of individual perceptions of stressful events, feelings of relative economic deprivation, or perceptions of chronic economic stressors.

Similar inconsistencies have been investigated elsewhere. Chance (1965) found a similar discrepancy to be related to emotional symptoms among Alaskan Eskimo, and Graves (1987) found this discrepancy predicted problem drinking among Native Americans and Mexican Americans. McGarvey and Schendel (1986) found blood pressures among Samoans to be higher among those persons with inconsistencies in education and occupation. Beiser et al. (1976) found blood pressure among women in Senegal to be higher if they were oriented toward urban, Western culture but did not have the language skills (in French) to participate in that culture.

Janes (1990) examined status inconsistency in his study of Samoan migrants to northern California. He was able to distinguish between a type of inconsistency stemming from norms and expectations in American society generally (a disparity between education and occupation) and a type of inconsistency stemming from Samoan culture (a disparity between household income and leadership position in the extended family). Both forms of inconsistency were related to higher blood pressure for males; for females, higher blood pressure was related to chronic economic stresses within the household.

When the effects of acute and chronic stressors have been compared, it has generally been found that they have independent effects on depression (Aneschensel and Stone 1982). Similarly, different kinds of chronic stressors have independent effects as well (Dressler 1991). These latter studies are especially intriguing, since lifestyle incongruity has been measured "objectively," in the sense that there is no verbal report from the respondent of the stressfulness in any sense of lifestyle, and chronic social role stressors have been measured "subjectively," in the sense that this measurement relies explicitly on verbal reports by the respondent of problems or difficulties. These appear to be two distinct phenomena with parallel effects on depression and blood pressure. Furthermore, the effects of lifestyle incongruity are invariant across communities. The implications of these observations will be explored more fully in the discussion section.

RESISTANCE RESOURCES

Since the mid-1970s, with the publication of two very influential review papers (Cassel 1976; Cobb 1976), a focus of research has become those factors that directly reduce or moderate the risk of disease. The topic of most interest has been social support (Cohen and Syme 1985; Henderson 1984b; Cohen and Wills 1985; Orth-Gomer and Unden 1987), with considerable interest given also to personal coping resources (Folkman 1984; Gore 1985). These two factors fall under the general rubric of resistance resources (Antonovsky 1979), and interest in these factors derives from theoretical perspectives and from common sense. With respect to the latter, it is clear that everyone who experiences some kind of stressful event or circumstance does not necessarily fall ill, just as some peoples exposed to an infectious disease agent fail to become sick. On a more theoretical level, since the publication of Durkheim's (1951; original 1897) classic study of suicide, it has been clear that the sense of social solidarity, of mutual support and aid within a social group, is a fundamental dimension of social interaction that contributes to better functioning and the health of individuals. Since Durkheim, modern life, with its social centrifugal forces, has been seen as a threat to this sense, or as contributing to anomie, a feeling of the loss of this integrative system and attendant sentiments. In a sense, this classic model sees the stress process as unidimensional, with positive and healthy individual functioning occurring under conditions of high social solidarity, and negative and unhealthy functioning occurring under the loss of that social solidarity. Contemporary models of the stress process simply make this a two-dimensional, as opposed to one-dimensional, process. The first dimension is, of course, the risk or stressor dimension; the second and counterbalancing dimension is the resistance resource dimension, including both social supports and personal coping resources.

A further emphasis in contemporary models is the buffering hypothesis: in terms of the prediction of mental illness, the availability of social support or personal coping resources per se, has no particular effect on mental illness; however, the effect of stressors on mental illness is dependent on the level of available resistance resources. Persons with high resources will be unaffected by stressors, whereas persons with low resources will experience a considerable impact of stressors. Put differently, persons with meager resources for coping with demands are most vulnerable.

Social Support

What are these resources? Social support may be defined as the perceived availability of help or assistance from other persons during times of felt need. A few additional definitions are in order for putting this in the proper context. Social structure is a set of norms and values that define the range of behaviors and kinds of interactions permissible within a culture for specified classes of individuals. Social organization is the observable and statistically quantifiable manifestation of these norms. Social networks are the concrete relationships among a defined set of individuals. A social support system is a subset of an individual's ego-centered social network, upon whom that individual relies for social support (Dressler 1994).

As in any other fresh area of inquiry, social support has been assessed in a bewildering variety of ways; programmatic reviews recommend the best approaches to the concept (Orth-Gomer and Unden 1987; Sarason and Sarason 1994), although these programs are not necessarily in agreement. Cohen and Wills (1985) distinguish studies that examine structural measures of social support (those describing the existence/or quantity of relationships) from functional measures of social support (those describing the kinds of supportive transactions occurring). In my terminology these two alternatives are *network measures* versus *support measures*.

Earlier studies relied heavily on network or structural measures of support, finding that individuals who are married or who live with other persons are at lower risk of depression if a life event occurs (Eaton 1978). Attention has shifted to the perception of support available within a network; this research consistently demonstrates a buffering effect of the perceived availability of support on stressors (Brown and Harris 1978; Dressler 1991). Some (e.g., Jacobson 1987) have argued that the actual support received in a social transaction must be taken into account to understand the stress-buffering effect of support, reasoning that if support perceived to be available was not forthcoming, this would negate any beneficial effect. Surprisingly, available research (Wethington and Kessler 1986) indicates this is not the case; the perception that support is available reduces the impact of stressors regardless of actual support received.

Dressler (1994) has reviewed the literature on cross-cultural research on social support. The form that a system of social support assumes and the ways in which effects are manifest are highly variable across societies. For example, in a study from a village in Mexico, it was found that, for males, the strongest effect of social support on blood pressure was for the level of support perceived from *compadres*. For females, level of support perceived from family members was most important, primarily for older women (ibid.). In St. Lucia (a West Indian island), support systems develop through the distinctive evolution of the household (Dressler 1982). In the African-American community in the rural South, salient social supports are organized within specific contexts of intracultural diversity. For younger persons, nonkin systems of support are most important, while for older persons the traditional support system of extended kin is most important (Dressler 1991, 1993).

Janes (1990) provides an example of a different organization of social support. He notes the dilemma experienced by Samoan migrants to the United States. Their involvement in the extended kin group is important for mutual support; at the same time, such involvement can drain scarce resources. The solution to this dilemma is a kind of core support system, derived from the affectively close relationship maintained by siblings throughout their lives. He found that individuals who had more adult siblings living close by had lower blood pressures.

These contextual modifications of the social support–disease relationship have also been observed in research in Polynesia. In traditional villages in Polynesia, greater involvement in the salient social groups (primarily large kindreds) of the community is associated with lower secretion of stress hormones (Hanna, James, and Martz 1986), and with fewer reported psychosomatic symptoms (Graves and Graves 1979). Graves and Graves (1980) argue that the adaptation to urban settings places different demands on individuals, which in turn alters the nature of support systems. These hypotheses were supported in a study of migrants to New Zealand; Samoans reported more symptoms in association with reports of more relatives in the community (Graves and Graves 1985).

Research on social support and health indicates that the definition of social support systems and the relationship of support and disease are more variable across social and cultural contexts than are the definitions or effects of stressors, although the recent work of Palinkas and his associates (Palinkas, Russell, Downs, and Petterson 1992; Palinkas, Downs, Petterson, and Russell 1993) offers a slightly different perspective on this issue. They examined the impact of the *Exxon Valdez* oil spill on Alaskan Natives and European-Americans. They found that while exposure to the spill had similar effects on the two ethnic groups, the effects associated with depressive symptoms were different within each group. For European-Americans, the direct economic impact of the spill was more likely to be associated with depression, while for Alaskan Natives, negative changes in the quality of social relationships were associated with depression.

Personal Coping Resources

Resistance resources also include the beliefs, attitudes, and behavioral strategies individuals use in coping with stressful events and circumstances. The study of coping is most often associated with Lazarus and his cognitive appraisal model of the coping process (Lazarus and Folkman 1986). Coping, in this model, consists of attempts through cognitive restructuring and behavioral changes to alter the impact of a stressful circumstance. The recent work of this group has shown that an active and intentional approach to problem solving and a redefinition of stressful events as less threatening are both related to lower negative emotional reactions (Folkman and Lazarus 1988; see also Pearlin and Schooler 1978).

A number of studies have examined the cultural context of these coping styles. These styles are often distinguished as an "active" or "problem-focused" style, characterized by problem solving, versus a "passive" or "defensive" or "emotion-focused" style, characterized by attempts to control negative emotional reactions. Some cross-cultural research is consistent with the hypothesis that an active coping style is related to better health status (Colby et al. 1985). In certain contexts, however, it has been found that an active coping style can compromise health. For example, James and his associates (James, Hainett, and Kalsbeet 1983; James 1994) have observed that an active coping style, when coupled with few economic resources in an African-American community in the rural South, was related to higher blood pressure. These studies suggest that there are particular social environmental circumstances in which the anticipated effects of a particular coping style can change, depending on available resources and thus the meaning of coping.

Several studies of more specialized institutional resources deserve mention here. Ness (1980) found that faith-healing activities in a fundamentalist church in Newfoundland could have beneficial mental health effects. Similarly, Garrison (1977a) and Finkler (1981), in studies of spiritualist healing centers in Hispanic cultures in the United States and Costa Rica, provide evidence that these provide emotionally supportive environments for individuals coping with chronic stressors. Brown and Gary (1987) found religiosity to moderate the impact of stressful life events on the depressive symptoms of black Americans in a southern city. And Murphy (1982a), reviewing cross-cultural evidence on hypertension, speculates that societies in which blood pressure levels are low may have compensatory mechanisms, including ritual activities, which help to discharge autonomic nervous system arousal that might otherwise result in peripheral vascular resistance. All of these studies help to emphasize that a diversity of personal and institutional resources may prove to be important in accounting for disease resistance cross-culturally.

INTEGRATIVE STUDIES

Finally, a few more comprehensive studies need to be mentioned within the specific rubric of stress research. No review of social and cultural components of the stress process would be complete without noting the seminal contributions of George Brown and his associates (Brown and Harris 1978). Brown set out to understand how life events, chronic stressors, social supports, and other vulnerability factors interact to precipitate major depression. This work cannot be easily summarized, but in it he has demonstrated that stressors and supports interact to predict depression (the so-called buffering model) and that these factors are embedded in the context of individual lives. Brown's concept of embeddedness, and especially his approach to the perception of stress and support, varies considerably from received wisdom. He argues that individual perceptions of stress or support are necessarily distorted and of little utility for understanding the etiologic significance of those factors. What is important is the socially patterned meaning of those factors, a meaning embedded in a symbolic network that the individual subject is in little position to apprehend. Therefore, Brown exploits the shared culture of subject and observer to define what is a stressor or support and goes on to demonstrate the considerable empirical value of doing so. Brown also challenges current notions of endogenous versus reactive depressions, suggesting instead that the contextual vulnerability factors distinguishing the two have been overlooked. These contextual factors can be delineated with a replicable method developed by these investigators, and anyone interested in this area should explore Brown's work.

Bruhn and Wolf (1979) describe the exploration of the epidemiologic puzzle of a remarkably low cardiovascular disease mortality rate among Italian-Americans in a Pennsylvania community, a group that by conventional (mainly dietary) measures of risk should have had a much higher mortality rate. These investigators attribute the findings to the highly integrated social organization of the community and show that as that organization has changed over time, heart disease has increased.

Kleinman (1986) provides a detailed analysis of neurasthenia and depression in the context of profound social change in the People's Republic of China. He finds that an understanding of the development of depression requires an understanding of how social change, and especially the Cultural Revolution, generated specific kinds of stressful experiences, and altered the nature of traditional social support systems for many individuals. Notable in this work is the combination of social scientific theory and detailed psychiatric case analysis to generate a comprehensive model of depression in a specific cultural context.

Dressler has examined blood pressure in the West Indies (1982) and depression in a southern African-American community (1991) with the aim of developing comprehensive quantitative models of the phenomena that are embedded in enthnography and precise historical processes. In each case, he focuses on how social structural change generated by economic and political processes leads to a specific pattern of stressors and resistance resources within a community and on how cultural influences shape the social production of disease.

Jane's (1990) research among Samoan migrants is a model of a study integrating the variety of factors involved in the stress process, as well as a model of sound anthropological methods integrated with epidemiologic techniques.

SPECIAL TOPICS AND PUZZLES

There are a number of directions in the cultural study of stress and disease that cannot fit neatly into the categories of the stress model outline or that form a separate literature. Cross-cultural research has also generated some specific puzzles that call into question some of the received wisdom of social and behavioral epidemiology. One special topic is the study of the adaption of migrants to their host culture. A number of studies have demonstrated that following migration, individuals are in poorer health than in their premigrant status or compared to nonmigrants (Salmond et al. 1985; Hackenberg et al. 1983; Baker 1986).

In one sense migration could be treated as a stressful life event or acute stressor, but a variety of studies have shown that the stressful effects of migration can persist for years if an effective adaptive strategy within the host culture is not established (Graves and Graves 1980, 1985). Much of this research has looked at immigrants to the United States. Westermeyer, Neider, and Vang (1984) found that increasing length of residence in the host culture was related to more symptoms of emotional maladjustment if individuals did not have either personal or social resources to assist in coping with the novel environment.

Premigration experiences also influence adjustment. In a study of Southeast Asian immigrants, August and Gianola (1987) found that these migrants exhibited posttraumatic stress disorder, much as Vietnam War veterans do. Chung and Singer (1993), in a study of Southeast Asian migrants, found premigration traumatic experiences to be associated with anxiety and depression five years or more after migration. Vega, Kolody, and Valle (1987), emphasizing a quite different premigration experience, found that Mexican migrant women were better adjusted in the United States if they had stronger premigration support and if they were able to maintain some contact with their premigration support network.

Tran (1987), McSpadden (1987), and Walsh and Walsh (1987) all explored the importance of social relationships in facilitating immigrant adjustment. In a study of Vietnamese refugees, Tran (1987) found that participation in ethnic organizations and the availability of close confidants of similar ethnicity were related to better mental health. Other resources, such as English-language ability and education, were found to be important primarily through the indirect effect of increasing income. Walsh and Walsh (1987), in a study of blood pressure among a diverse group of immigrants, found generalized perceptions of the availability of social support to be related to lower blood pressure, independent from a variety of other variables. Finally, McSpadden (1987) found that Ethiopian refugees who were assisted in their settlement in the United States through a voluntary association (such as a church congregation) exhibited better mental health status than those who were assisted by individual caseworkers.

Studies of acculturation are complementary to studies of migrants, often being carried out on groups of migrants to a new cultural setting. What distinguishes acculturation from migration studies is the emphasis on a precise set of measurements of ''acculturation'' in the former studies as opposed to the group-level comparisons in the latter studies. Also, acculturative processes may be occurring in situations of political and economic change, such as when marginal and minority populations are gradually drawn into increased participation in larger national social structures.

Richman et al. (1987) and Berry et al. (1987) review studies of acculturation, drawing on the classic statement of Redfield, Linton, and Herskovits (1936) to define the process. Berry et al. (1987) also review a whole series of studies conducted by a group of cross-cultural psychologists, led by J. W. Berry, of acculturation as a predictor of symptoms of emotional stress. What ties all of these studies together is mainly the operational definition of acculturation. It is defined as the adoption of a new language, new material lifestyles, exposure to new information through the media, and, sometimes, the adoption of new forms of employment. The new forms of these behaviors are those of the dominant culture, and the adopters are members of a subordinant group, whether they be migrants, members of an ethnic minority, or members of a peripheral and dominated community.

In the studies reviewed by Berry et al. (1987), higher education predicts lower symptom levels, as does an attitude that traditional cultural identity can be maintained in the context of the dominant culture. Furthermore, when the variables listed above were combined into a single index, it was related to lower symptoms. As the authors note, this finding runs counter to traditional wisdom, since more behavioral acculturation is thought to be related to more symptoms; however, these authors note that a combined index is dominated by measured years of formal education, which is related to access to the larger culture, and hence fewer symptoms.

Studies of acculturation and cardiovascular disease provide a different picture. Studies of coronary heart disease among Japanese Americans in California (Marmot and Syme 1976) and Hawaii (Reed et al. 1982) show that those who are more acculturated (i.e., more Western education, more English-language use, more participation in Western institutions) have higher rates of cardiovascular disease. Similarly, in a study of elderly Navajo, Kunitz and Levy (1986) found a greater prevalence of hypertension among the more acculturated, especially for women.

Burnam et al. (1987) examined acculturation in relation to diagnostic categories of psychiatric disorder among Mexican Americans in Los Angeles. Using an acculturation scale, they found that the more acculturated had higher rates of a variety of disorders, until migrant status was controlled for. All of the predictive strength of acculturation was accounted for by the fact that U.S.-born Mexican Americans had a higher prevalence of mental disorders than immigrant Mexican Americans.

If studies of migration and acculturation represent special topics in the cultural study of stress and disease, the study of social class and disease presents a special puzzle. It is widely accepted that nearly all forms of disease, but especially various forms of cardiovascular disease and mental illness, are inversely related to social class, whether that is assessed on the basis of occupation, income, education, or some combination of these variables (Macintyre 1986). Most would agree with Fabrega's (1974:56) observation that social class is an abstract category that masks more precise psychosocial factors more closely related to disease. This leads to the attempt to reduce the social class–disease effect to more precise, and usually individual-level, variables.

But the historical and cross-cultural evidence presents a different picture. I have referred to studies (Kessler and Cleary 1980; Dressler 1991) showing that more precise measurements of stressful events and circumstances do not supersede the effects of social class, but rather their effects are contingent on social class. Rose and Marmot (1981) and Morgenstern (1980) found in Britain and the United States that the inverse effect of social class on cardiovascular disease mortality has emerged only within the past thirty years; prior to about 1950, higher mortality rates were found in the highest social classes. The current inverse pattern in Britain is found only among Britons and Irish immigrants; mortality is higher among higher-class Caribbean immigrants (Marmot and Theorell 1988).

The historical pattern observed for Britain and the United States appears to be repeating itself in developing societies. Research is accumulating to show that in such societies, there is a direct, rather than inverse, association of social class and risk of cardiovascular disease (Dressler 1993a). It would appear that at some point in the process of social change, the patterning of disease and disease risk changes from a direct to an inverse relationship. What the parameters and determinants of this process are remains to be determined.

Another factor worth mentioning here but unfortunately on which there has been little sociocultural research, is the so-called type A behavior pattern, characterized by a chronic struggle to achieve, a heightened sense of time urgency, and chronic hostility. It is probably the single most well-researched behavioral predictor of coronary heart disease, having been confirmed as a risk factor in numerous prospective studies (Friedman and Booth-Kewley 1988). A. Young (1980) and Helman (1987) offered excellent theoretical analyses of the Western cultural principles underlying the behavior pattern, suggesting that if it appears in other cultural contexts, it ought to be manifest in quite different ways. Dressler (1993b) examined the type A behavior pattern in an African-American community in the rural U.S. South, finding in fact that the specific dimensions of the pattern were manifest differently, and were associated with blood pressure differently than among middle-class whites.

DISCUSSION

My aim here is to explore more fully some of the implications of the results of the research I have reviewed and to point out some places of potential convergence in separate traditions of research, with the goal of outlining a future direction for empirical work. A striking pattern in these findings is the relatively small amount of cross-cultural variability in the definitions and effects of stressors. Whether stressful life events, chronic social role stressor, or structural imbalances like lifestyle incongruity are examined, there is a fair agreement among researchers working in disparate settings that these are important risk factors for disease. Of course, the precise definition of particular stressors does vary, as, for example, when problems associated with racism are emphasized as chronically stressful circumstances in an African-American community. But it is striking that once these definitional matters are taken into account, there is a consistent and replicable effect of stressors on disease.

A common denominator to all this research, whether it has been carried out among women in London (Brown and Harris 1978), Polynesian migrants to New Zealand (Graves and Graves 1985), or African Americans (Dressler 1991), is that Western, industrial, "modern" society provides the macrolevel historical context in which these studies are conducted. Fundamental to the definition of this context is the differentiation of systems of social stratification and the changing values emphasis described so well by Worsley (1981). What I am suggesting is that this particular pattern of development, as described by world systems theory, carries within it specific structural relationships that generate stressful events and circumstances that vary only a little depending on the setting in which they occur.

The effects of stressful events are one example of this. Consistently across studies, it is the occurrence of these life events, regardless of respondents' idiosyncratic reports of the "stressfulness" of those events, that increases disease risk. In studies in developed countries, the important events are the truly major, disruptive transitions involving the loss of valued statuses. As the WHO international study found, these truly major events can be reliably identified, and predict disease onset, in both developed and developing countries. It seems likely that these events come to be socially and culturally defined as transitions to valued statuses in the process of economic change and development and that the occurrence of an event signifying the loss of a valued status results in increased risk of disease.

This can perhaps be seen more clearly in the example of lifestyle incongruity. Mass consumption of material culture is a pattern that has diffused widely throughout the Western world in the linked process of development and dependency. It is also well known that productive capacities that can absorb labor are outstripped by consumption values in the process of development, thus virtually ensuring the structural imbalance described by lifestyle incongruity. The only things that change from setting to setting are the precise items consumed and the degree of socioeconomic differentiation (see Dressler 1993). More important than these local variations is the general pattern that the imbalance between the valued status defined by material consumption and the valued status defined by occupational class reliably predicts disease risk across these settings.

These same arguments extend as well to chronic social stressors. These stressors are defined as perceived problems in major social role areas such as spouse, worker, and economic provider. As occupational and domestic roles organized within an industrial mode of production supplant the more culturally variable social roles of traditional cultures, it is the perceived difficulties associated with these "modern" roles that generalize across settings as predictors of disease. Two points are important here. First, there is evidence that conventional notions of stress are important to disease risk. These perceived difficulties are precisely what people usually mean by the term, and there is consistent evidence that they are important. Second, it is striking that these perceptions themselves generalize across cultural settings and are consistently associated with disease (Graves and Graves 1985). This implies that these individual perceptions are a function of the socially patterned meanings of major social roles in an industrial mode of production. All of this evidence—for events, role stressors, and structural imbalance—suggests that the sociocultural risk of disease is more importantly a function of the socially defined rather than idiosyncratically defined impact of events and circumstances. While these observations may seem heretical to a conventional understanding of stress and disease, not to mention to the particular variant of cultural determinism in current vogue in anthropology, it nevertheless is consistent with the available empirical evidence, as well as a historical materialist theoretical orientation. What would be useful now is a well-designed program of cross-cultural studies to examine these ideas with greater specificity, including societies not within the Western sphere of development.

The payoff of such a program of research, as well as a note of caution with respect to the theoretical perspective just offered, is the recent superb work by Lawrence Palinkas and his associates (Palinkas et al. 1992, 1993) on the *Exxon Valdez* disaster. In a controlled comparison of ethnic groups affected by the disaster, they found that social and economic stressors could be reliably measured the same way within each group but that the same stressors had distinct effects within each group. Only through such systematic research can these sorts of issues be systematically examined.

Where the definition of variables, and the relationships of those variables to disease outcomes, appears to vary most dramatically across cultural contexts is in the study of resistance resources. This is especially true in the study of social support systems. Assuming for the moment that the perception of social support is the most important feature of support systems, and this can be only a tentative assumption, those relationships defined as supportive vary considerably within and between cultures. The available evidence suggests that an important factor in this regard is the kin-nonkin distinction, although even within categories of kin, a kind of distance function can assume prominence (Dressler 1994).

Even more remarkable is the cross-cultural variability in the effects of social support (Graves and Graves 1985). As we have seen, in some settings social support is related to a lower disease risk and buffers the effects of stressors; in other settings social "support" is related to a higher disease risk. It would be convenient to redefine some forms of social "support" as social "stress," but this replaces empirical analysis with semantic juggling that will not extend our understanding. If in particular circumstances an individual states that he or she believes support to be available, and that belief in turn is related to a greater likelihood of disease, we must accept that statement and search for the contextual circumstances that determine why it is risk enhancing rather than risk reducing.

Some (e.g., Jacobson 1986, 1987) have argued that what is important in the study of social support is the specific timing of that support in relation to different stages of the onset and unfolding of a stressful transition and that this process is best investigated phenomenologically. This hypothesis provides a useful starting point for the investigation of social support and specific kinds of risk factors, such as migration, where there is a definite onset and unfolding of the stressor. It fails to provide a useful model for investigating either the direct effects of social support or the other kinds of moderating effects that support might have with respect to chronic or structural stressors, nor can a phenomenological study of support stand alone without careful epidemiologic studies that relate support factors to measured disease outcomes.

Everything said thus far about the study of social support applies equally, or perhaps more heavily, to the study of personal coping resources. At least with respect to social support, there is a preliminary taxonomy of what variables are relevant to the investigation. With respect to personal coping resources, a wide range of factors could potentially be important, as Lazarus (1966) argued in his seminal work on the topic. The most interesting lead in this respect is Colby's (1987) work on the adaptive potential of a particular structure of beliefs and values regarding personal efficacy, creativity, and altruism. Not only does Colby ground his perspective in a theory with enough generality to be of considerable utility for the cross-cultural study of disease, he has taken important initial steps in defining adaptive potential in operational terms and has tested it in several preliminary studies. Cross-cultural researchers in stress and disease should follow this lead.

Overall, research using an explicit model of stress has progressed well beyond a simplistic reductionist model in which all of the impact of the social and cultural setting on disease risk can be condensed to what individuals can consciously report as their perceptions (a model that, as Young 1980 shows, primarily recapitulates Western notions of personhood). Rather, social and individual meanings combine in complex interactions between stressors on the one hand and resistance resources on the other. Elsewhere I have argued that social constraints and individual beliefs and values ultimately are resolved, and bridge the gap between society and human biology, through the definition of social identities (Dressler 1991). More theoretical work in refining the stress model needs to be done to understand this process better.

Research on migration, acculturation, and other factors such as the type A behavior pattern need to be incorporated into more comprehensive models of stress and disease. These have so far represented a separate literature with respect to stress and disease. A better approach would be to develop more complex models; for example, migration could be contrasted with the occurrence of other stressful events or chronic stressors in the prediction of disease outcomes. Similarly, is acculturation per se a stressful experience, or does it influence access to valued rewards within a society, thus making this process one component of larger social class processes? The epidemiologic puzzle of the cross-cultural variability of the social class–disease relationship can also be worked out only if more complex models are developed, requiring a cumulative empiricism all too rare in anthropological research.

One topic that has not been addressed at all in this review has been the nature of the outcome variable studied. I have freely assumed a definition of disease following Kleinman, Eisenberg, and Good (1978), further assuming that outcome variables such as depression and high blood pressure could be equally unambiguously defined. This is clearly not the case, as shown in a variety of ways (Good and Kleinman 1985). Good, Good, and Moradi (1985) make the problem explicit in the study of depressive disorders. In a carefully combined interpretive and quantitative analysis of depression among Iranian migrants, they show that symptoms associated with a Western definition of depressive disorder can be distinguished from symptoms that serve an expressive-interpretive role in Iranian culture. Only the former show a patterned association with migration experience. This raises the possibility that stress factors predict "disease" but perhaps not "illness." Other studies (Kleinman 1986) suggest that both disease and illness are related to stressors and resistance resources, but that additional factors distinguish the epidemiology of the two outcomes. More research is required.

Finally, future research should follow the lead established by Kleinman (1986) and others, in which the relationship of stress and disease is investigated within a context of solid ethnography. By grounding the study of stress and disease in a larger understanding of historical change, unequal relations of power and status, and a refined definition of social organization, the intersection of human behavior and human biology in the process of evolutionary change can be better explained.

14
Nutrition in Medical Anthropology

Sara A. Quandt

THE SCOPE AND HISTORY OF NUTRITIONAL ANTHROPOLOGY

Within the field of medical anthropology, cultural and physical anthropology perspectives collaborate on and complement the study of nutrition. The very nature of eating calls for such a merger of theory and method. On one hand, food is culturally defined: what is edible in one culture (e.g., insects among the Tukanoan Indians of Colombia [Dufour 1987]) is shunned in another, and the reasons can be interpreted using a variety of the theoretical approaches of cultural anthropology. On the other hand, once food is consumed, it becomes part of nutrition, the process by which the body uses exogenously obtained chemicals (nutrients) for the maintenance of body functions, health, and growth. This process can be explained and variations in it interpreted within the theoretical framework of physical anthropology. Thus, the field of nutritional anthropology attempts to integrate studies of human behavior and social organization with those of nutritional status, nutrient requirements, and growth, and in so doing, it draws on a wide array of anthropological approaches.

Nutrition in medical anthropology is often traced back to the pioneering work of Audrey Richards, first among the southern Bantu (1932) and later among the Bemba (1939) of Rhodesia. A student of Malinowski, Richards applied a functionalist framework to relate food consumption and production to the lives and health of individuals in African cultures. This and subsequent work in the 1940s by both European and American (e.g., Mead 1943) anthropologists is frequently labeled "foodways research" (see Montgomery and Bennett 1979; Camp 1979). It was, from its inception, applied anthropology, assessing needs and proposing policies to ameliorate human problems in both colonial and wartime situations.

After a period of quiescence in the 1950s and 1960s, such research reemerged in the 1970s under the label of "nutritional anthropology," with a concern for both food usage and contemporary problems in nutritional status. Examples of this reemergence are found in Fitzgerald (1976) and Jerome, Kandel, and Pelto (1980).

This chapter will focus on contemporary nutritional anthropology and its place in medical anthropology. After identifying its theoretical foundations and guiding orientations, the chapter will review work in several substantive areas of interest to medical anthropology. It will then provide an overview of methods of nutritional anthropology and suggest areas for future research.

THEORETICAL FOUNDATIONS OF NUTRITIONAL ANTHROPOLOGY

Nutritional anthropology can be distinguished by its theoretical foundations from both nutritional science and studies within cultural anthropology usually focusing on symbolic or structural rather than materialist analyses of food. The latter are frequently referred to as the anthropology of food; Douglas (1966, 1972, 1984) and Levi-Strauss (1965) are examples. In contrast to the anthropology of food, nutritional anthropology is based on ecological theory. This means that human dietary behavior and requirements are considered within the environmental context, including the physical and social environments. While such an ecological framework is not the exclusive domain of nutritional anthropology (see Kolasa 1981 for a discussion of the history of ecology in nutritional science), anthropology, far more than nutritional science, applies this ecological approach from an explicitly cross-cultural, comparative stance (Raphael and Davis 1985). By comparing apparent adaptations to similar environments, it is possible to begin sorting out what may be the result of adaptation and what is the product of history.

Nutritional anthropology is made unique by the coupling of ecological theory with evolutionary theory and by integrating both biology and culture into the evolution model. This sets humans into the perspective of long-term change and adaptation through natural selection, predicting that variations in morphology and physiology related to food consumption or production will have been selected for in terms of prevailing selective pressures. However, because humans have the unique ability to produce culture to buffer themselves from the environment, culture can also be subject to selection. Thus, Katz (1982, 1987) has proposed "biocultural evolution" as an appropriate label for the theory underlying nutritional anthropology. Human populations have a body of biological variation in DNA, the "genetic information pool," as well as a body of cultural variation in language, beliefs, and material culture, the "cultural information pool." These information pools provide the raw material for biocultural selection and, over time, for biocultural evolution and adaptation. Recently, Durham (1991) has developed a more detailed model of what he calls *coevolution,* identifying five major patterns in which genes and culture interact in predictable ways to produce culture change. Durham's work is an important theoretical advance for nutritional anthropology, providing an explanation of cultural change that, although borrowing from biological evolution, highlights the considerable differences between biological and cultural reproduction.

The first hominids, the Australopithecines, evolved in Africa at least 4 million years ago. They consumed a largely vegetable diet that in some cases required considerable amounts of oral processing. While there is debate about whether they procured meat by scavenging or hunting, there is general agreement that these hominids managed to obtain and consume at least some meat and therefore consumed a mixed diet of both vegetable matter and meat despite the limitations of the savanna environment (Gordon 1987). Proficiency at obtaining meat increased over time, so that by the Middle Pleistocene, about 700,000 years ago (Butzer 1975), hunting was clearly a significant subsistence strategy. Meat provided a concentrated source of high-quality protein and appears to be linked to the social cohesion of groups and the occupation of home base camps. Thus, dietary behavior, nutrient intake, and social organization were linked even among the earliest humans.

From then until about 12,000 years ago, hominids moved into virtually the whole range of habitable environments but maintained a foraging lifestyle. With the transition to food production around 12,000 years ago, social organization and dietary behavior changed dramatically; as humans became more sedentary, groups became larger and more stratified, and the diet gradually became concentrated on a smaller number of staple foods.

As this summary of human evolution suggests, humans have spent most of their existence living in small, nomadic groups consuming diets highly dependent on seasonally available wild plant and animal foods. A sedentary lifestyle with dependence on food production is a relatively recent development. One would expect that biocultural adaptations to the earlier pattern might include nutrient requirements, metabolic pathways, taste preferences, and dietary patterns. Thus, nutritional anthropology views humans today in terms of this evolutionary record.

GUIDING CONCEPTS OF NUTRITIONAL ANTHROPOLOGY

Two concepts basic to nutritional anthropology derived from its theoretical foundations deserve fuller explanation: foodways and nutritional thriftiness.

The concept of foodways is critical to nutritional anthropology. Foodways characterize populations and consist of all information surrounding the ways food is obtained, distributed, processed, and consumed by a particular population (Harris and Ross 1987b; Ritenbaugh 1978).

Nutritional anthropologists have a set of premises or assumptions concerning human foodways that derive from ecology and biocultural evolution. These premises guide research design as well as analysis and combine to produce the following argument. An adequate foodway—that is, one providing appropriate types and amounts of nutrients to population members—is necessary for the survival and growth of any population, including a species. Any population whose foodway, for whatever reason, is inadequate or inappropriate to its environment will be less likely to survive than one whose foodway is adequate. Because the species *Homo sapiens* has been surviving and increasing in number for a considerable time, it can be assumed that, in general, its foodways have been successful. Foodways with great time depth are probably adaptive. That is, they are the result of the coevolution of a set of coherent behaviors that facilitate (if not optimize) the ability of the population to survive. Whenever widespread malnutrition occurs in a population, the foodway is clearly inadequate.

The utility of the foodways concept has been demonstrated in the analysis of food systems centered on particular food-processing techniques. Katz, Hediger, and Valleroy (1974) have studied maize processing techniques in the New World. They argue that dependence on maize occurs only with alkali processing, a technique that alters the nutrient composition of the maize so that it better fits human nutrient requirements. Similar arguments can be formulated for other food-processing techniques (Katz 1982). In situations where one component of the food way is lost (e.g., the loss of alkali processing in the adoption of a maize-dependent diet in the southeast United States), the inadequacy of the resulting foodway can be measured in terms of morbidity and mortality.

Dietary patterns also lend themselves to foodways analysis. The nonrandom pattern of consumption of different types of dairy products and its association with lactose malabsorption has been analyzed by a number of scientists (McCracken 1971; Harrison 1975). Simoons (1978) has compiled data to show that the genetic variant for lactose absorption is associated with a long history of dairying and the consumption of raw milk. He proposes that a foodway characterized by high rates of milk consumption in populations able to digest and absorb lactose evolved as a biocultural adaptation to general dietary stress and suggests that other such links between food use and human evolution may exist.

While many foodways appear to be adequate, others clearly are not. The existence of an inadequate foodway can mean one of four things. First, the foodway may be relatively recent and not yet subject to biological or cultural selection. Second, the environment, whether social or physical, may have changed, making a previously adequate foodway maladaptive. Third, other positive factors may neutralize negative effects and maintain the foodway. Or fourth, the negative impact of the foodway is so slight that cultural selection against it is not likely to occur.

The concept of nutritional thriftiness also guides research in nutritional anthropology. This is the idea that energy and other nutrients must be extracted from the environment and therefore can be factors limiting the survival of individual humans and *Homo sapiens* as a species. Thus, any physiological, morphological, or behavioral variants that favor survival in the most nutrient-efficient way will be selected for (Quandt 1984).

Stini (1969, 1975) has claimed nutritional thriftiness in populations from highland Peru who consume a diet deficient in protein. He found that sexual dimorphism in lean body mass was reduced in adulthood. This reduction is not accompanied by a substantial reduction in work performance, making males, in effect, more efficient because they require less energy to do approximately the same work. The apparent buffering of females from the effects of nutritional stress thus maintains tissue reserves important for reproduction. This physiological plasticity reflects a nutritionally thrifty adaptation, which maintains work capacity as well as reproductive capacity.[1]

Other examples of nutritional thriftiness come from metabolic studies of cold response and anthropometric analyses of the secular trend. In both the San of the Kalahari and Australian aborigines (Frisancho 1993; James and Trayhurn 1976), individuals respond to cold temperatures at night with a reduced cold response. That is, their core temperatures drop, reducing the rate of heat dissipation. Whether such energy-saving adaptations are genetic and the result of natural selection in these populations or physiological adaptations acquired during development and possible in any human population is unknown. The response of height to nutritional stress during the growth phase has been recorded in a variety of populations (Komlos 1994). This plasticity conveys an advantage of quick response to changing environmental circumstances.

Perhaps the most widely accepted nutritionally thrifty adaptations involve the relationship between fat reserves in females and fecundity. Frisch and coworkers (Frisch and Revelle 1971; Frisch et al. 1973) have argued that there is a minimum level of body fat necessary for attaining menarche, maintaining menstrual cycles, and resuming ovulation postpartum. While their data and methods have been criticized (Johnston et al. 1975; Trussell 1980; Huffman, Chowdhury, and Mosley 1978), the underlying idea that reproductive capacity (fecundity) will be conserved and used only where nutritional status adequate to support a pregnancy and lactation (Quandt 1984) continues to guide research in nutritional anthropology and demography (Howell 1979). It has also been linked to the high incidence of obesity and diabetes among Native Americans (Weiss, Ferrel, and Hanis 1984), making it a relevant concept in studying the epidemiology of chronic disease.

SUBSTANTIVE ISSUES IN NUTRITIONAL ANTHROPOLOGY

Nutrition and Reproduction

For any species, including *Homo sapiens,* to survive and evolve, reproduction must be successful. While much of biological reproduction is outside individual and societal control, nutrition, a major factor in every step of the process, is not. This linkage of nutrition and reproduction is, then, a natural focus for nutritional anthropologists.

From the standpoint of demography, a woman's reproductive career spans the time from menarche to menopause (Bongaarts and Potter 1983). Within this span are conception, pregnancy, and birth, followed by periods of lactation-induced postpartum infecundibility and then, once ovulation has returned, the wait to conceive again. While the length of pregnancy is fixed within rather narrow biological limits, the other components of the birth interval are largely under biobehavioral control, as is the number of reproductive cycles and completed fertility of a woman.

In terms of possible nutritional influences, the onset of the period of reproduction is even earlier. Winikoff (1988) points out that there is a continuous, circular relationship between mothers and daughters such that good or poor health and nutritional status can be perpetuated over generations. Poor nutritional status during pregnancy will lead to a smaller, less healthy baby at birth, as well as lower reserves of energy and other nutrients in the mother for lactation and child care. The result will be a mother who enters her next reproductive cycle with nutrient stores depleted, as well as (if the infant is a female) a young girl who goes through her periods of growth and maturation impaired and begins her own first pregnancy in suboptimal nutritional status.

Evidence for the components of this model is found in many societies. Selective nutritional discrimination against girls has been noted by researchers for decades, often in cultures with a pronounced preference for males. Jelliffe (1957) reports that the Hindu ceremony after which breast feeding is supplemented is held at six months for boys and seven months for girls. Girls in India tend to be weaned earlier, as the interbirth interval is shorter following the birth of a girl than that of a boy (Gordon, Wylon, and Ascoli 1967). Lindenbaum (1977) reports that in Bangladesh, girls receive less food and care than boys as toddlers. Similar patterns of neglect or discrimination are noted in West Africa (Gessain 1963), Jordan (Pharaon et al. 1965), and elsewhere. More recent research has sought to expand on these observations (Levine 1987; Johansson and Nygren 1991).

Older girls often follow the same eating patterns as their mothers, serving males first and then eating what is left, often with less nutrient-dense food like meat than goes to males (Gittelsohn 1991). As maternal height and prepregnancy weight are some of the best predictors of infant size and nutritional status at birth, cultural practices that deprive women and growing girls of nutritious foods can have far-reaching effects.

Although the relationship between a pregnant woman and her fetus was formerly characterized as one in which the fetus was an active parasite and the mother a passive source of nutrients, this relationship is now better understood by medical scientists as one in which the mother is active as a filter of environmental effects, while the fetus is the more passive recipient. This change in orientation is crucial for understanding that the food behaviors of pregnant women are important for the birth outcome of their infants.

In general, biological needs of the fetus appear to be at odds with the behavioral and cultural practices of women during pregnancy. While pregnancy is a time of increased nutrient needs, it is also a time in which women report a change in food behavior due to cravings and aversions. In a study of American women, 76 percent of women reported at least one craving during pregnancy and 85 percent at least one aversion; actual food consumption followed these changes in attitude toward food (Tierson, Olsen, and Hook 1985). Geophagy (earth eating) and other forms of pica have been the subject of considerable interest (Crosby 1971; Hunter 1973; Vermeer 1971). Hunter presents a "culture-nutrition" hypothesis for clay consumption, seeing it as the institutionalization of cravings based on real physiological needs.

In addition to idiosyncratic changes in diet, many cultures impose food taboos during pregnancy (e.g., Ferro-Luzzi 1980; O'Laughlin 1974). Taken at face value, these taboos appear to potentiate maternal undernutrition. However, as Laderman (1984) demonstrates, drawing such conclusions requires data about actual dietary intake and compliance to taboos. She cautions that food taboos reported by Malaysian women are often for foods unimportant in the diet and that rules exist by which women can break the taboos. Moreover, some investigators point to the protective nature of taboos. Hook (1978, 1980) argues that some natural food aversions exist for foods such as coffee and alcoholic beverages that can be teratogenic. Laderman (1984) notes that several of the fish proscribed during pregnancy can have toxic effects.

After parturition, the infant's nutritional needs can be met in several ways, and nutritional anthropologists have conducted research on a variety of topics related to infant feeding practices. If the child is breast-fed, there is a transitional period during which the infant gradually breaks from the total nutritional dependence on the mother of gestation (Mead and Newton 1967). If breast feeding does not occur, the transition occurs abruptly at birth.

As one would expect from humans' mammalian heritage, humans have specific adaptations to facilitate lactation. Maternal fat deposition takes place during pregnancy, providing an energy source for lactation, which buffers the infant from fluctuations in the mother's postpartum dietary intake. Data from maternal supplementation experiments conducted during pregnancy indicate just how strong this adaptation is. Beaton (1983) calculates that an intervention that gives the mother 34,000 supplemental kilocalories during pregnancy will produce only a 100-gram increase in infant birthweight; but it will increase the maternal pregnancy weight gain by 6.8 pounds, representing a caloric storage for lactation of 23,000 kilocalories. This preferential storage of energy may indicate that humans evolved in conditions of an undependable food supply.

Other aspects of the lactation process can be used to reconstruct biologic breast feeding, the way in which early humans probably breast-fed. Human milk is relatively low in fat and high in carbohydrate. As fat has the greater satiety value, biologic breast feeding probably consisted of frequent short feeding bouts, requiring that the infant and mother not be separated. This is in contrast with the practice of leaving infants cached in nests practiced by insectivores (humans' closest nonprimate relatives), which produce a milk much higher in fat. Frequent feeding bouts has two quite different effects on the mother, both of which directly benefit the nursing infant (Quandt 1984). First, the hormonal changes produced by frequent feeding change the way maternal fat cells function. Those fat cells in the breast actively take up lipids from the blood and transfer them to milk; peripheral fat cells turn off the mechanism of uptake, thereby shunting lipids from dietary sources to the breast and milk production. Second, the hormonal changes of frequent feeding suppress ovulation, delaying pregnancy and the arrival of another infant who would compete for maternal care and breast milk.

While these aspects of lactation physiology allow reconstruction of biologic breastfeeding, cross-cultural differences in breast-feeding practices indicate the biocultural nature of this infant feeding modality. Current medical recommendations call for exclusive breast feeding for the first three to six months of life, with semisoft foods added to the diet at that point as breast milk supplements. Breast feeding should continue at least to a year; however, few populations practice this form of feeding.

Data from developing countries over the past several decades reveal a tremendous variety of practices, many quite different from the recommended diet. This includes widespread use of commercial formula and other breast milk substitutes, early introduction of nonmilk foods in some places, and very late introduction of such food in others. In general, artificial feeding rather than breast feeding is associated with higher maternal education and socioeconomic status in developing countries. While the opposite is true in the United States and other Western countries today, this represents a change over the past two decades (Institute of Medicine 1991).

There has been considerable research by nutritional anthropologists on the social, economic, and cultural foundations of such practices. Gussler (1987) summarizes the patterns as due to (1) changes in social patterns, particularly loss of support from the extended family; (2) changes in women's economic roles, especially new labor patterns incompatible with breast feeding and traditional child care; (3) an increase in lactation problems caused by psychosocial stress; (4) the use of modern rather than traditional health care practitioners and facilities, particularly for childbirth; (5) changes in attitudes and values about sexuality and the body; and (6) the availability of commercial infant foods and feeding devices.

The influence of changing patterns of mothers' work has been the subject of considerable interest. In countries like the United States, an increasingly large percentage of mothers work outside the home while their children are infants. In urban areas of developing countries, this same pattern of wage labor participation exists. In rural areas, women's roles and responsibilities also change, often as the result of planned or unplanned development activities (Spring 1986). Many of the recent changes in women's work have resulted in physical separation of mothers and infants, with consequent problems in maintaining breast milk production and breast feeding.

Nerlove (1974) and Gussler (1987) stress the importance of the concept of discretionary versus nondiscretionary activities for understanding how infant care and economic roles interact. Activities are classified according to prevailing values and beliefs. If breast feeding is considered nondiscretionary, it will be accommodated even if extrahousehold work is also considered nondiscretionary. Conversely, if infant care activities are considered discretionary, they will give way to changing demands of nondiscretionary work activities. Marshall (1985) and colleagues show variation in how both traditional and modern work patterns interact to affect infant feeding in the South Pacific. This collection is particularly valuable because contributors show the variety of ways in which cultures sort out competing demands for women's time and energy, even within a single culture area. They demonstrate the role of recent culture change, as a combination of modern hospital practices (e.g., scheduled feedings and separation of mothers and infants), changes in the economy, and changing values (e.g., standards of modesty) that act together to erode breast-feeding practices.

Not all such feeding practices are the result of recent culture change. Anthropologists working in the Caribbean (Marchione 1980; Gussler and Mock 1983; Quandt 1988) have noted the prevalence of extremely early use of paps and porridges as breast milk substitutes. King and Ashworth (1987) point out that at least in the English-speaking Caribbean, this pattern can be traced to the plantation system and women's economic roles as either slaves or free laborers. Early supplementation was encouraged as a way to get women back to work as soon as possible. The norm for this type of feeding was certainly present among the upper classes of England at the time. Some of the recipes found today for these breast milk substitutes (Quandt 1988) are remarkably similar to those found in historical sources from Europe during the eighteenth and nineteenth centuries (Fildes 1986).

The potential impact on breast feeding of women's activities that separate mother and child is shown by Quandt's work on the duration of exclusive breast feeding (1985, 1986b). She showed that among middle-class American mothers, number of feedings per day at one and two months as well as the maximum time between feedings predicted duration. More than seven feedings per day and shorter maximum time between feeding interval was associated with longer exclusive breastfeeding. She hypothesized that this is due to the more intensive breast-feeding style's promoting the hormone levels necessary for milk production, a conclusion supported by evidence of differences in patterns of maternal fat store change during breast feeding by breast-feeding style (Quandt 1983). She also proposes that even among U.S. mothers, variation in environmental factors such as dwelling size or configuration may contribute to separation of mother and child and therefore to variation in breast-feeding styles and in duration of exclusive breast feeding. Applying these findings to women's work, this research suggests that even when intention to breast-feed exclusively is strong, extrahousehold work that separates mother and child for long periods of time may make carrying out these intentions quite difficult.

Although there are direct biological controls over breast feeding, there are also indirect biological regulators of this and other infant feeding modalities. Quandt (1985) has shown that smaller infants tend to be supplemented sooner, probably due to maternal concern over small body size. Bryant (1982) has found differences among Cubans, Puerto Ricans, and Anglos in feeding practices governed by mothers' assessment of infant body size (often strongly influenced by members of social networks) and cultural values and beliefs about body size. Graver (1988) found compliance to recommended dietary changes for obese infants was compromised by mothers' pride, especially for boys, in their infants' large size. Certainly not all cultures value large infants and promote infant growth through feeding practices. Nichter and Nichter (1986) note that their baby was considered unattractive and unhealthy by South Asian informants at least in part because he was large by local standards. Margaret Mead (1977) and, more recently, Katherine Dettwyler (1994) have pointed out that when endemic malnutrition produces a population of small children, such body size may be perceived as normal. Feeding practices that tend to produce children of "abnormal" size may therefore be resisted. However, there has been very little research focused directly on parental expectations for and interpretations of infant growth and its ramifications for infant feeding and other child-rearing practices (Pelto 1987).

In sum, the area of reproduction, spanning pregnancy, parturition, and lactation, has been a major focus for medical anthropology. The fact that all of these aspects of reproduction are biologically affected by nutrition yet experienced by women within a cultural context makes the nutritional anthropologist particularly qualified to add insight to such research.

Malnutrition

As the term *malnutrition* implies, it refers to nutrition significantly different from some optimal standard. As such, it can be either under- or overnutrition. Because the causes and consequences of both forms of malnutrition are both biological and cultural, nutritional anthropologists have made important contributions to research in this area.

The value of a biocultural approach can be demonstrated by comparing conceptual models of social and nutritional sciences of the determinants of malnutrition. The social sciences traditionally have analyzed the association of socioeconomic factors, and to some extent beliefs and values, with malnutrition. These have included variables such as household income, maternal education, paternal occupation, social class, and values placed on body size. Many of the associations found have been strong and consistent cross-culturally. Nutritional sciences, in contrast, have focused on patterns of dietary intake and activity levels, as well as (in the case of undernutrition) environmental contamination and associated infectious disease. Again, strong and consistent associations have been found. However, because social scientists have traditionally not sought to link their findings to specific proximate, biological causes of malnutrition and nutritional scientists have tended to be superficial in their treatment of the ultimate causes of biological precursors to malnutrition, a critical gap exists in the model for malnutrition causation. A biocultural approach, by eliminating the unknowns in the model, reduces the compartmentalization of knowledge and facilitates interventions. As the following discussions of under- and overnutrition will show, this biocultural approach has been much more fully developed for the study and development of interventions for undernutrition than for overnutrition.

Undernutrition

Undernutrition was first labeled as a deficiency disease by Cecily Williams in the 1930s. She described the symptoms of the deficiency—flaking skin, depigmentation of hair and skin, weight loss, and irritability—as well as its epidemiology and attributed it to protein deficiency (1933). Subsequently, she proposed the name *kwashiorkor* for the deficiency, from the name used by the Ga, the African tribe among whom she first recognized the problem (1935). Later Trowell, Davies, and Dean (1954) differentiated marasmus from kwashiorkor. Over the next twenty years, medical and nutritional scientists debated the limiting factor in these conditions (protein or energy?) and whether they had separate and distinct etiologies (see Cassidy 1982). Today, energy deficiency is generally considered the primary problem, producing secondary protein deficiency. However, it is clear that biologically the issue is far more complicated than simply energy. For example, vitamin A deficiency or supplementation seems to exacerbate or ameliorate the symptoms of undernutrition.

Whatever the label applied, general undernutrition tends to follow the same patterns of distribution in many populations. It is most commonly found among lower socioeconomic groups in both developing and developed countries. It usually appears first among weanlings, children from about one to four years of age, and is most likely to lead to increased mortality at these ages.

Anthropologists studying both living people and skeletal populations have noted that childhood undernutrition is more prevalent among agriculturalists than among hunter-gatherers. Cassidy, for example, compares skeletal populations from two archaeological sites in Kentucky (1980b). One, Indian Knoll, was inhabited by hunter-gatherers approximately 4,000 years ago; the second, Hardin Village, was inhabited by agriculturalists between A.D. 1500 and 1675. Mortality profiles constructed for the two populations show that significantly more children died before the age of seventeen in Hardin Village than at Indian Knoll, with the most pronounced difference between the ages of one and three years.

The distribution of undernutrition within and between populations has been linked to a variety of factors. Infectious diseases are more common in settled populations (Armelagos and Dewey 1970), and toddlers are susceptible due to declining effects of breast feeding–transmitted immune factors and increasing exposure to environmental pathogens. The synergistic effects of infection and undernutrition are well documented (Ulijaszek 1990). Mata (1978; Mata, Urrutia, and Lechtig 1971) presents longitudinal data for individual children demonstrating that diarrhea, respiratory infections, and diseases such as measles after the introduction of solid food can virtually halt growth.

The low-energy density of weaning foods and foods fed to young children has also been implicated in toddler undernutrition. Applied nutritional anthropologists have explored the development and introduction of higher-density preparations. They have identified issues such as maternal acceptance of new foods and economic availability of ingredients as barriers to acceptance. While such barriers can be overcome with education, social marketing, and programs of income assistance, nutritional anthropologists have identified others less amenable to solution. Cassidy has written extensively on cross-cultural differences in the recognition of undernutrition (1980a, 1982, 1987). She argues that "protein energy malnutrition" is a culture-bound syndrome of Western origin that lacks salience in many cultures. She notes that concepts of individuality and when a child achieves full group membership are culturally defined and may account for food-related behaviors labeled by cultural outsiders as neglect. Dettwyler (1994) notes similar barriers to improved childhood nutrition in Mali.

Seasonality of foods, of infection, and of work have been linked to annual cycles of undernutrition. Long-term field research in the Gambia, for example, has shown how the seasonal effects of energy imbalance are linked to seasonal patterns of birthweight and breast milk production (Prentice et al. 1983a, 1983b). Anthropologists have identified a number of culture-specific techniques for moderating seasonal effects. Migratory groups ranging from the San (Lee 1979) to the Eskimo (Mauss and Beuchat 1904, cited by De Garine and Koppert 1990) move to accommodate the spatial and temporal distribution of available resources. Other groups, such as the Serer of Senegal, have cultural institutions that extend scarce resources (De Garine and Koppert 1990). The Serer impose progressive restrictions on food consumption and energy expenditure during the hot months preceding harvest. This culturally controlled period of scarcity allows them to store food in granaries for the subsequent period of intensive labor required to harvest and replant crops.

Over the past two decades, nutritional anthropologists have been instrumental in shifting the research focus on undernutrition to the level of the household. It is in the household where demographic and socioeconomic constraints translate into the specific behaviors that determine which individual will be undernourished and which will not. This research focus has been termed the "household production of nutrition" (Bentley and Pelto 1991).

Although there is a long history in nutrition of using the household as a unit for the production and consumption of food, only recently has the complexity of using households as a focal point for nutrition been appreciated. Anthropologists have been instrumental in identifying the difficulties in establishing boundaries for households. In Africa, for example, polygynous households comprise residential compounds. While the individual "kitchen" is frequently the unit for consumption and production, there are exceptions (Krieger 1994). Even in the United States, household boundaries blur. Groger (1992), for example, found rural African-American elders parceling off land to accommodate children, who then reciprocated with instrumental social support. Quandt and associates (1994, n.d.) found intergenerational food exchange occurring on a regular basis.

Nutritional anthropologists have exposed the dynamics of the household in food acquisition, distribution, and consumption. Examples of the variety of approaches used are found in a recent edited volume (Sharman et al. 1991). The concept of nutritional strategy developed by DeWalt (1981) has been key to understanding interhousehold variation. Nutritional strategies are sets of decisions about food made in households in the course of meeting the biological requirements for food. DeWalt (1983) was able to show how differences between households in the patterns of decisions about food purchase or production resulted in variations in nutritional status that might not have been predicted from economic data.

Current anthropological interest in gender dynamics, power relations, household income distribution, and division of labor have been linked to explain intrahousehold variation in nutritional status. Leonard (1991) showed that young children in Andean households were preferentially fed in periods of food scarcity and therefore experienced less seasonal fluctuation in nutritional status. In contrast, Cassidy (1987) noted that adults in Belize take better food rather than feed their children, reasoning that the children "are doing nothing" and therefore cannot be hungry. Gittelsohn (1991) found age and gender differences in such specific food behaviors as taking second helpings and eating meat at household meals, which resulted in less adequate dietary intake for females, particularly younger wives. Such studies make it clear that household dynamics play a large part in determining who is fed what and that intra- and interpopulation variation in nutritional status may be tied to such nonbiological factors.

Overnutrition

The characterization of overnutrition as malnutrition is a relatively recent phenomenon. It reflects the natural history and epidemiology of overnutrition, as well as advances in research on chronic disease for which it is now considered a risk factor. These, in turn, suggest a biocultural basis for obesity, which can be studied from several anthropological perspectives.

Evolutionary theory and the concept of nutritional thriftiness have been useful for understanding the ability of humans to store excess energy intake in the form of fat, a condition with considerable negative health implications. Reviews of mammalian body composition show that humans are relatively fat mammals.

What is more, *Homo sapiens* has the ability both to increase the size of fat cells and produce new fat cells for accumulation of massive amounts of adipose tissue. Fat stores in humans are energy reserves, rather than for insulation against the cold, as is the usual mammalian condition (Pond 1978). This has led anthropologists to consider the role of food scarcity as a selective pressure favoring energy storage capabilities. A review of food insecurity throughout human history indicates that periods of shortage and scarcity have been common. Foraging provided food for most of the human past, a mode of food acquisition that was apparently exceedingly successful at providing for day-to-day needs but was not consistent with accumulation and storage of surplus food. Indeed the material culture for food storage is a hallmark of later food strategies. Under nomadic foraging conditions, the ability to store surplus energy in fat cells would have had the same selective advantage that filling granaries has for food producers.

Although preindustrial food producers had the material culture to store excess food, they were not immune from food shortages. Both the ethnographic and archaeological records indicate that hungry seasons are a regular component of the food production cycle. Like foragers, food producers often undergo annual cycles of weight gain and loss. Thus, the constancy of food shortages provides a strong selective pressure for the energy efficiency that today produces obesity.

The strong association of obesity with modernization (Brown and Konner 1987) supports the contention that the ability to store excess energy as fat is a pan-human characteristic. The appearance of widespread obesity seems to have occurred only about 200 years ago in Europe, when societal affluence began to approach the point at which even the poor had access to sufficient food to become obese (Trowell 1975). As the transition to high prevalence of obesity has now occurred in a variety of modernizing populations, it has become clear that it is not just abundance that encourages obesity but a change in the composition of the diet to one with a high percentage of calories from fat, a low ratio of polyunsaturated to saturated fatty acids, and a low level of fiber (Popkin 1994).

Weiss, Ferrell, and Harris (1984) have distinguished the obesity observed in Native Americans from that noted elsewhere in the world. They point out that among Native Americans, obesity is part of a complex of diseases including non–insulin dependent diabetes mellitus and disorders of the gall bladder, but excluding coronary disease, which appear with particular intensity in females at reproductive age. They argue that the strong selective pressures of food shortages operating on a small population moving from Asia to the Americas favored fat storage and fat metabolism, particularly for females of reproductive age. This nutritional thriftiness would have conveyed a strong advantage for nomadic hunter-gatherers in a cold climate.

The biological ability to store energy as fat is supported by cultural proscriptions for plumpness. Ritenbaugh (1982) and Brown and Konner (1987) review the ethnographic literature, which contains widespread examples of plumpness, but not morbid obesity, carrying social meanings of good health, prosperity, fertility, sexuality, and other positive connotations. Even within contemporary U.S. society, some groups consider larger body sizes as ideal (Stevens, Kumanyika, and Keil 1994; Massara 1980). Indeed, considered in cross-cultural perspective, the current American value on thinness in women is highly anomalous.

With both selective pressures and cultural values supporting obesity, it appears paradoxical that obesity is linked so strongly to a variety of chronic and degenerative diseases. The linkage is sufficiently ubiquitous for Popkin (1994) to propose it as a nutritional transition akin to the demographic and epidemiologic transitions used to explain changes in fertility, mortality, and morbidity across modernizing societies.

While epidemiological analyses have found numerous associations between obesity and chronic disease, anthropologists and others have helped focus attention on the complexity of the association. Ritenbaugh (1882), for example, has demonstrated that cultural appraisals of obesity have led reference standards, rather than vice versa. Micozzi and others (Cornoni-Huntley et al. 1991) have shown excess mortality in older adults associated with *both* the highest and lowest percentiles of body weight and body mass index. In addition, they have identified weight loss as a predictor of mortality, independent of smoking and disease status.

METHODS FOR NUTRITIONAL ANTHROPOLOGY

Nutritional anthropologists use the full range of anthropological methods, from paleopathology techniques of biological anthropology to ethnoscience methods of cognitive anthropology, to textual analysis of critical or interpretive anthropology. In addition, many rely heavily on the collection of dietary intake data. While tools for such data collection are readily available from the nutritional sciences, it is necessary to understand their strengths and limitations, particularly because anthropological research conditions and objectives are often quite different from those of nutritionists.

Generally the purpose of collecting dietary intake data is to obtain an accurate estimate of the dietary intake and nutritional status of individuals and groups by applying a valid and reliable technique. The most accurate dietary methods are employed in balance studies and require weighed food and food aliquot analysis (Burke 1947; Hunscher and Macy 1951). Such methods are costly, time inefficient, and impractical when the dietary intake of large groups of subjects must be addressed, and they fail to capture usual dietary intake.

Although no totally satisfactory method exists for assessing the dietary practices of free-living individuals within a population, the twenty-four-hour dietary recall, food records, and food frequency questionnaire have been successfully used in epidemiologic and clinical studies. More recently, semiquantitative food frequency instruments have been developed for use in such studies (e.g., Block et al. 1994). Shorter methods have also been tested in community studies (e.g., Kristal et al. 1990). Each method has inherent advantages and disadvantages, and the final choice must balance the scientific objectives of the study with practical concerns (Quandt 1987a). Thompson and Byers (1994) have produced a useful compendium of dietary assessment methods, which evaluates the strengths and weaknesses of each and provides data on studies of reliability and validity.

It is important to differentiate methods from the research design or strategy in which methods are used (Quandt 1986a). In most cases, an overall design, including plans for data analysis, should be chosen first. Then the specific methods for data collection can be selected. There is no single ideal research strategy or method. For any study, it is best to choose the simplest, fastest, and least expensive method that will meet the study objectives. This is especially true for anthropologists, who are frequently collecting data on a broad range of topics in addition to dietary intake.

Several factors should be taken into account. First, should the study document consumption of foods or intake of nutrients? If the former, is it necessary to document all foods, or are there specific foods of interest? If the latter, the research design must take into account food preparation techniques that alter the nutrient composition of foods, as well as differences in nutrient distribution across different types of food. For example, techniques to measure calcium intake (which is concentrated in a relatively small number of foods) could be quite different from those to measure energy intake. Second, are data needed on usual intake or on the precise diet within a finite and specified time period? Usual diet is a statistically defined concept, and probabilistic research designs can be employed to measure it (e.g., Beaton et al. 1983; Liu et al. 1978; Nelson et al. 1989; Quandt 1987b). Third, how variable is the population of interest? Age, gender, and ethnicity are a few of many dimensions on which diet may vary, and dietary assessment methods and research strategies must take this into account. Many of the existing methods have been validated on only very specific populations. The choice of methods therefore must include a careful review of the demonstrated success with which a given method captures the data on interest for a population similar to the study focus. If such data are not available, it is frequently necessary to build in a validation study. A final consideration is the type of analysis proposed for the dietary data. When using statistical techniques that compute a measure of association between diet and other variables on an individual basis (e.g., correlation or regression), data for individuals must be highly reliable. If a classification analysis that assigned individuals to groups such as quintiles is used, the reliability requirements can be less stringent. When group statistics will be computed, even greater error in individual measurements can be tolerated if group sizes are large.

Because the research questions and field setting of anthropological research often differ substantially from those of other nutritionists, nutritional anthropologists have been instrumental in the study of field methods. Quandt and Ritenbaugh (1986) and Pelto, Pelto, and Messer (1989) provide reviews oriented to anthropologists. In addition, Scrimshaw and Hurtado (1987) have produced a set of rapid assessment procedures for use in nutrition and primary health care program development. Future anthropological contributions to the development of dietary methods could include two areas: First, there is a need to develop a dietary life history. As epidemiologic studies focus increasingly on diet as a risk factor for the development of chronic disease, there is more of a need to gather precise information on earlier food consumption. Willett (1990) has reviewed studies of remote diet and found them to be relatively rare. Several anthropologists have begun to experiment with using a combination of qualitative and quantitative techniques to reconstruct lifetime diet. Quandt and colleagues have gathered dietary data in the context of a project to document the oral histories of farm families (Roos, Quandt, and DeWalt 1993). Ritenbaugh and colleagues (personal communication 1994) worked with military veterans to reconstruct past eating and drinking behavior, using tours of duty and marital histories as contexts for recall. Second, anthropologists can be instrumental in extending the coverage of dietary collection methods to non-Western populations and eating situations. Intrahousehold distribution of food, eating from a common pot, and the use of nonstandard measures are a few of the challenges that anthropologists have dealt with successfully.

CONCLUSIONS: DIRECTIONS FOR FUTURE RESEARCH

Nutritional anthropology has provided important insights into why contemporary humans eat what they eat. By analyzing nutrient requirements and metabolic physiology through the life cycle from an evolutionary perspective, it has been possible to understand the health and disease sequelae of food consumption and to identify widespread patterns across human populations. The contributions of anthropology were so widely and rapidly accepted that it is hard to comprehend that less than three decades ago the idea of widespread lactase deficiency was virtually unknown. International food aid was often based on milk, and the failure of recipients to consume it was considered evidence of ignorance or lack of gratitude rather than of biological or cultural inappropriateness.

Other anthropological ideas have had equally far-reaching effects. Focusing on the household as the unit of production for the nutritional status of its members has been of critical importance in highlighting the inter- and intrahousehold differences in nutrition-related behaviors and has been the basis for both theoretical insights into the distribution of nutritional status and applied projects to ameliorate the pressing problems of undernutrition.

The role of nutritional anthropology in both the domestic and international health care arenas continues. As populations undergo the nutritional transition (Popkin 1994), increasing efforts worldwide are being placed on the prevention of chronic disease through dietary change. At present, many of the efforts to change diet are oriented toward individuals and use behavior change models based in psychology (e.g., Prochaska and DiClemente 1984; Rosenstock 1990). For the most part, these models were developed for behaviors related to smoking, alcohol use, and unsafe sex, with the goal of extinguishing the behavior. The application of these models to dietary change has frequently failed to consider that eating is conceptually quite different. One cannot "just say no" to food in the same way that one can quit smoking, and nutritional strategies of households are frequently beyond the control of individuals targeted for behavior change. Anthropologists can play a major role in developing more appropriate models for food behavior, particularly ones that can be applied to community behavior change.

Current efforts in epidemiology and public health nutrition to understand food consumption behavior in the United States and elsewhere have focused on ethnicity, gender, and social class as sources of variation. While this emphasis on diversity is a positive step toward accommodating the heterogeneity of populations in food and health policy, anthropologists need to take a more active role in forcing the discussion of what these demographic labels mean and how they translate into food behavior. It will only be with the focus shifted from these immutable characteristics to behavior that the determinants of food consumption and constraints on change to more positive behaviors can be understood. Currently, labels such as "race" and "ethnicity" are used uncritically in many studies, with little attention to where there are biological differences between categories and where differences reflect behavioral or cultural factors. The current focus on overnutrition in relation to diabetes, heart disease, and cancer provides ample opportunities for anthropological contributions.

NOTE

1. While this buffering of female reproductive capacity is important from a long-term evolutionary perspective, there are clear short-term costs to individuals and populations in quality of life and possibly in cognitive performance, which cannot be ignored. Thus, despite the concept's utility for understanding human variation in nutritional status in relation to population adaptation, anthropologists have urged caution in assuming the existence of nutritionally thrifty adaptations without adequate consideration of competing hypotheses (Pelto and Pelto 1989).

Part IV

Methods in Medical
Anthropology

15

Research Designs in Medical Anthropology

Pertti J. Pelto and Gretel H. Pelto

Medical anthropology is primarily an applied subdiscipline, as should be apparent from the materials covered in this book. The roots of the subdiscipline reach back to an intellectual, academic interest in describing and understanding the ways in which various non-Western peoples have explained illness and given treatment to the sick; but the preponderance of research in the 1980s and 1990s has centered on pragmatic issues of improving the health and health care situations of contemporary people, both ''Western'' or ''non-Western.''

Health problems throughout the world constitute a sector of applied research that is by nature interdisciplinary; most health issues require data from the biological sciences, clinical medical practice, and the social-behavioral sciences. Research in health problems often involves other types of expertise as well; for example, the role of entomology is very important to understanding various vector-borne diseases such as malaria, typhoid, and dengue fevers, and the growing interest in research on health care systems requires information from economics and political science. Although there are many instances of research in which individual anthropologists, medical doctors, or biologists ''did it on their own,'' such solo performances are increasingly suspect, given the complex data involved in health issues.

The interdisciplinary nature of the illness and health care sector is partly responsible for the fact that methodological issues are strongly affected by national and international agencies and other organizations that sponsor research. In the United States a very large share of health-related research is funded by the National Institute for Mental Health, National Institute for Drug and Alcohol, National Cancer Institute, National Institute on Aging, and other federal agencies. On the international health scene, the World Health Organization (WHO), the U.N. International Children's Emergency Fund (UNICEF), the U.S. Agency for International Development (USAID), and a variety of other organizations sponsor health-related research.

Proposals for research in any of these national and international agencies are judged by interdisciplinary review panels, often (but not always) dominated by biomedical scientists. These factors have had considerable influence in shaping the directions of research methodology in medical anthropology. Also, increasing numbers of medical anthropologists are based in medical schools, schools of public health, and other health agencies, in which collegial relations are strongly interdisciplinary.

On the other hand, a substantial portion of research in medical anthropology continues to be funded by the anthropology division in the National Science Foundation, the Wenner-Gren Foundation, and other sources in which the review panels are primarily anthropologists. These anthropology-oriented sources are especially likely to be tapped for funding by medical anthropologists whose primary affiliations are in anthropology departments. In such cases the research designs and other methodological features are somewhat less affected by the interdisciplinary (particularly the biomedical) realm of discourse. It is probably fair to suggest that such "anthropology-oriented" medical anthropology is less often applied in nature. However, one can find many exceptions to these patterns.

The growth of medical anthropology over the past two decades has been especially evident in the applied, interdisciplinary realm. In applied research, the solutions to specific practical questions about health and illness are the central concern, and development of theory plays a secondary role. Theoretical concerns are not totally ignored, but the areas of theoretical interest are often in "theories of the middle range," where conceptual issues are strongly intermingled with methodological strategies. Medical anthropologists often pay lip-service to aspects of grand theory, but the research is usually at a considerable remove from broader theoretical abstractions.

In any case it is possible to examine a great many issues in the methodology of medical anthropology without direct commitment to a particular theoretical position. In fact, much of anthropological method is essentially theory-less, in the sense that the basic methods of data gathering are the same regardless of the theoretical system adopted by the investigator (Bernard et al. 1986; Plattner et al. 1989). In field research it appears that practically all anthropologists use a mixture of interviewing (both structured and unstructured) plus direct observation (again, both structured and unstructured). Specific questions asked and specific targets for observation differ, depending on theoretical interests, but the processes of data gathering are broadly similar regardless of theoretical orientation. It is in the language of theoretical discourse that anthropologists differ markedly, even when discussing basically similar data. This is not to say that two different theoretical discourses necessarily disagree with one another; quite often the different theoretical vocabularies are in some sort of complementary, noncontrastive relationship.

Our examination of field methodologies in medical anthropology will be presented in a generally nontheoretical, or theory-neutral, manner. However, certain methodological tools and techniques will be presented with reference to particular research examples, which may include some of the theoretical language of the authors of the research.

BASIC RESEARCH QUESTIONS IN MEDICAL ANTHROPOLOGY

Research design becomes specific when we address specific questions. In much of the research in health care, as carried out by medical anthropologists and others, the basic questions very often consist of variations on three main (applied) thematic areas:

1. *Descriptive questions.* What do people believe about illnesses—their causes and treatments? What do they do (e.g., behaviors that increase or decrease risks of illness; specific treatment-seeking behaviors)? What are the characteristics of the health services and systems in which these actions occur?

2. *Analytic questions.* What factors and systems explain variations in beliefs, actions, and outcomes?

3. *Intervention-oriented questions.* What are the ways to change and improve the health of particular populations, in terms of system changes, changes in knowledge and actions, and prevention of illness-causing conditions?

These are not the only types of basic questions in medical anthropology, but a very large share of research is focused on specific issues related to these fundamental concerns. In a great many instances of research, then, the *dependent variable* of interest centers on a particular illness or condition—often the actual frequency of the illness. A great deal of medical and health care research, after all, is directed to lessening the frequency (incidence or prevalence) of specific illnesses. Just as frequently, however, the dependent variables center on people's choices of forms of treatment. Who uses "indigenous" treatments versus "cosmopolitan" resources to "do something" about a particular health problem?

The *independent variables* are much more varied, and they are by nature more directly reflective of basic theoretical approaches. The following hypotheses concerning "causes" or "factors" affecting treatment choices are all in the same grammatical form and can be examined with basically similar methodology, but they reflect different theoretical assumptions and language:

1. People [in community *x*] avoid cosmopolitan health care because of their traditional health beliefs.

2. People [in community *x*] choose indigenous versus cosmopolitan health care depending on their assessment of the severity of the illness and their ability to meet the costs of the specific health care.

3. People [in community x] will go to cosmopolitan health providers and will follow the medical advice to the extent that the information fits with their explanatory models of a specific illness.

4. People [in community x] see health care as a political expression, and they choose or reject cosmopolitan health care on political and ideological grounds.

5. People [in community x] are likely to be more accepting of the newly introduced primary health care (cosmopolitan) if they have the opportunity to participate actively in the planning of the health service system.

Although these are only a small fragment from all possible research statements, generalizations, or hypotheses, they are useful in illustrating ways in which different researchers, with different theoretical approaches, often have the same implicit or explicit dependent variable (a behavioral outcome) in mind, and they will use basically similar methodological approaches to gather the relevant data. In the five hypothetical cases, each researcher would presumably collect data on people's choices of health care alternatives, through direct observation or interviewing, and would also collect information about the network of independent variables specified in their particular theoretical model. Some researchers may adopt a strategy of direct observation plus unstructured interviews; others might rely mainly on quite structured interviews; still others will opt for various mixtures of quantified and qualitative data gathering.

CONCEPTS AND DEFINITIONS

Before exploring the wide-ranging inventory of research designs in medical anthropology it will be useful to present some basic definitions of terms that are central to methodological discussions. These terms play a central role in the structure of research proposals, so they constitute a key element in the vocabulary of "grantsmanship," as well as in the analysis of different approaches to theory building and problem solving in medical anthropology.

Data

Data are the recorded results of empirical observations in fieldwork, both quantitative and qualitative. All field notes are data; the recorded responses on structured interviews, and their transformations into computerized data sets, are data. Photographs, documents, and other physical materials also constitute data. Note that we use the term *data* to refer to both the physical materials (including tape recordings) and the variables or "themes" or other attributes extracted from the primary materials. Sometimes we use the term *raw data* to refer to the actual physical materials, including unprocessed field notes.

Variables

A *dependent variable* is an outcome or condition or phenomenon that is to be explained or accounted for or predicted, by, reference to presumed "causal factors," "prior conditions," "determinants," "disposing features," or other conceptualizable antecedents.

An *independent variable* is any presumed "causal factor," "prior condition," "determinant," "disposing feature," or other conceptualizable antecedent that is thought to account for, predict, explain, or contribute to the existence or specific form of an outcome or condition or phenomenon.

In experimental and quasi-experimental research designs, it is almost always the independent variable that is manipulated. If a research project has an experimental and a control group, the nature of those two groups constitutes, or embodies, the major independent variable. (Although many researchers have come to associate the notion of variables with statistical analysis, all empirical research can be usefully conceptualized in terms of variables, however implicit they may be in the actual research reports. Thus, data concerning particular variables may be "highly quantitative" or quite qualitative in presentation.

Hypotheses

A *hypothesis* is a more or less explicit statement of a hunch, expectation, or prediction of relationships or patterns that one seeks to test or examine in the course of a specific research project. Hypotheses, like operationalized definitions, are best seen as aspects of specific research projects.

Methodology

This concept refers to the logic-in-use in any research project whereby "raw" empirical observations are assembled and transformed into successively more abstract descriptive and analytic statements. Methodology may be thought of as a series of transformational rules and processes (including definitions of key concepts) that guide data gathering and relate the resulting data systematically to the hypotheses and other conceptual models in terms of which research results are expressed. Statistical procedures are one type of transformational system for arranging complex arrays of numerical data into patterns that can be expressed as theoretical models.

Models

A *model* is any representation of the interrelationships among a series of variables or constructs in a research domain. A model is thus an analogical, simplified, physical representation of the phenomenon in a particular instance of research. Commonly encountered models include maps, diagrams, scale models of physical things, as well as verbal descriptions that aptly portray essential elements of a complex domain. A famous model is the physical representation of the double helix used by the biologists Watson and Crick in arriving at the description of the DNA molecule (Watson 1968). In anthropology, particularly in earlier decades, the most commonly encountered models were representations of kinship terminologies. For our purposes, the term *model* is the meeting ground between the theoretical and methodological realms of discourse. A model embodies the elements derived from a particular theoretical perspective. Thus, the terms or features of a model are simplified portions of a general theory. At the same time, the model includes the elements or details about which specific data are to be gathered in a research project. Each element or concept in a model requires some sort of "operationalized" representation in the research activity.

Operational Definition

An operational definition (of a variable) is a statement of specific data-gathering procedures that produce indicators for a given independent or dependent variable. The procedures often include statements of cut-off points, such as, "High blood pressure will be defined as a measured systolic pressure above 140 and/or diastolic pressure above 90." Here is another example: "Socioeconomic status in this research was dichotomized into two groups, landowners (having more than 1 acre of arable lands) and the landless."

Some researchers appear to consider the idea of operational definitions as referring only to quantitative research. However, the logic of this concept is the same, whether quantified or not. All concepts reported by researchers arise from data of some sort. The reader of any research can always ask, "What data serve as evidence for this particular statement?" Much of the writing in anthropology, including medical anthropology, presents information without specifying details of research methodology. Often we are left to guess at the operational definitions. But they are still part of the research structure, even if they remain unreported.

Triangulation

In this strategy in ethnographic research, data concerning a particular topic are gathered from more than one source, or using more than one technique, so that systematic comparisons (and possible corrections) can be made. Examples of triangulation include the systematic comparisons of the statements made by different key informants and the comparison of key informant statements with the results of structured quantitative surveys. Another common form of triangulation that has come into vogue is to compare focus group discussions with key informant interviews and/or quantitative survey results (Helitzer-Allen, Makhambera, and Wangel 1994).

THE HOUSEHOLD AS A BASIC UNIT OF ANALYSIS

In most situations, the people of interest to medical anthropologists experience their health and illness and make decisions about health care in the context of the household or coresidential group. The specific operational definition of household may vary for different populations, but the general term refers to a group of people living together in a single domicile, sharing food and other resources, whether or not consanguineally related. Often researchers seek to delineate households as the people who eat from the same pot, even in cases in which more than one such cooking-eating group may be found within a compound or other complex domicile.

In most community-based studies, the common practice is to carry out some sort of census or enumeration of all the households, in order to define the universe (the population) from which samples may be selected. Even when research is mainly participant observation and unstructured interviewing, it is good practice to establish a baseline census. When large numbers of households are involved, the basic census is limited to a small list of key questions:

• Name, age, and sex of each person (and their relationship to household heads).
• Ethnic identifications of household heads.
• Occupations of adult members (including cash crops).
• Education of adult members.
• Religious affiliation of adult members.
• Physical indicators of house quality (usually number of rooms, floor material, roof and walls, number of windows).

The physical indicators of house quality are useful as an approximate measure of socioeconomic status.

In addition to these items, each household (and usually each individual) should be designated with a unique identification number, to relate all subsequently collected information, and the selection of research samples, to the correct units. Commonly the identification number is composed of community, household, individual, as follows: 01(community)/ 001(household)/ 01(individual) = 0100101 (the first person in the first household in the first community).

In many countries the health ministry or one of the government health research institutes may have a standard census form that it wants all researchers to use. Such "nationwide" formats have the advantage that they permit some comparisons of the specific research population with other areas of the country. On the other hand, the standard forms often include portions that are obsolete or inappropriate for given regions. If possible, researchers will use the official protocol, with additions and modifications to fit local conditions.

If resources are available for gathering more information in each household, the additional items will reflect the specific research concerns, as well as special

ecological and other local features important to specific health-illness issues—
for example:

• Sources of water supplies.
• Sources and types of fuel and cooking facilities.
• Latrine, toilet facilities.
• Immunization status of children and women.
• Physiological status of women (pregnant, etc.).
• Usual source(s) of health services.
• Labor migration status of family members.
• Recency of arrival to this area and community.
• Community of origin of adult members.
• Foods produced by household.
• Animals owned or maintained by household members.
• Ownership of selected consumer items (radio, television, vehicles, etc.).

Many other items can be added to the list of basic questions concerning the
universe of households. However, very few researchers can afford to collect
even this much information from all households in their study communities.
Quite often a researcher (or research team) will direct the extra questions to a
subsample—perhaps every tenth household of the overall census. In this way at
least approximate frequencies can be obtained for a variety of features that can
then be studied in greater depth as research progresses.

The census, or enumeration, of all households in a study population has other
functions besides the collection of specific data. Regardless of whether the process occurs at the outset of research or later, the census is an important opportunity to introduce the research group, and purposes of the research, to all
households in the area. In addition to the information about the project, each
household can also be given information about any expected health interventions
connected with the study. The census enumerators can distribute health education leaflets and information about clinic times and places, and can recruit volunteers for local health committees. Census contacts can often help in identifying
potential key informants, such as local healers.

THE ANTHROPOLOGICAL APPROACH

Compared to most other disciplines, the hallmark of anthropology, medical
anthropology included, is the so-called holistic approach. This takes many forms,
but in most research there is the assumption that for any particular outcome or
phenomenon to be explained, there are a great many interrelated factors at work.
In practice, this means that medical anthropologists are likely to collect a great
deal of data about economic features, social relationships, cultural belief sys-

tems, political processes, and other aspects of a community, even if the research intention is focused on a specific health question. This holistic perspective often leads anthropologists to be highly critical of other disciplines when they appear to adopt single-factor explanations or seemingly simple explanations for illness conditions, health care responses, and other issues.

The holistic perspective has important effects on research design. Whenever numerical analysis is involved, medical anthropologists are likely to be concerned with a large number of variables, requiring fairly complex statistical procedures. Also, attention to large numbers of factors, or variables, requires a considerable investment of time for each case, patient, illness episode, or other unit of analysis. The time limitations (and limitations of personnel) in turn constrain the anthropologist to limit sample sizes severely. The typical project in medical anthropology is likely to have much smaller samples than, for example, corresponding research projects by epidemiologists, sociologists, and demographers.

Another hallmark of medical anthropology is the central role played by the concept of culture. In recent years many other types of researchers have come to recognize the importance of cultural differences and cultural effects in relation to health issues, but for anthropologists, the concept has much greater importance in shaping the directions of research.

Earlier, before the subdiscipline of medical anthropology came into being, many anthropologists who studied matters of health and illness among non-Western peoples regarded the detailed description of traditional healers and cultural beliefs about illness to be the primary ethnographic objective. They often paid little or no attention to instances in which people used cosmopolitan medicines and practitioners. That is, the primary emphasis of earlier work was on the traditional belief system rather than on actual behavior. In such studies, then, "the culture" was seen as the sole topic of data gathering.

The concept of culture has now assumed a more modest place in the theoretical and methodological works of many medical anthropologists. "Culture," and cultural differences, have come to be seen as one major cluster of variables, along with complex networks of other factors that account for, or explain, actual behaviors. This shift in the use of the culture concept constitutes a major achievement in anthropological methodology and metatheory. The development of the idea of culture as distinct from behavior has made it methodologically possible to speak of (and carry out research on) the variable effects of culture on behaviors.

Not all anthropologists share this definition of culture, but there is a widespread tendency to consider culture as idea systems, systems of symbolic meaning, or other variations in language that all focus on people's mental processes. For example, a widely cited book by Arthur Kleinman states that "we can view medicine as a cultural system, a system of symbolic meanings anchored in particular arrangements of social institutions and patterns of interpersonal interactions" (Kleinman 1980:24). Similarly, Horacio Fabrega, in his book *Disease and Social Behavior,* commented that "illness, for example, offers an additional opportunity to study how behavior is structured and organized by underlying cultural rules" (Fabrega 1974:3) He then noted that "culture by definition represents a 'man-made,' socially relevant, experientially derived set of rules for living."

Regardless of researchers' specific definitions of culture, one of the central contributions of anthropology to applied studies of health issues is the delineation of the complex ways in which cultural belief systems interact with other factors in affecting rates of disease, definitions of illness, differential responses of illness, and other outcomes of interest. Although other disciplines pay some lip-service to the idea of culture in relation to health and illness, medical anthropologists are thought to be the methodological experts in the study of cultural factors. To a considerable extent, the continued increases in acceptance of medical anthropologists in the interdisciplinary community of health research are due to increased recognition of the cultural factor as crucial to understanding all aspects of illness and health care.

The concept of culture has led to a generally accepted distinction between disease and illness. Illness refers to the culturally defined feelings and perceptions of physical and mental ailments and disability in the minds of people in specific communities. Disease is the formally taught definition of physical and mental pathology from the point of view of the medical profession. Both terms are, of course, "culture." The terms refer methodologically to the contrasts between two distinct cultures that meet when patients interact with physicians, whether in modern urban settings or Third World health systems.

A large share of the research in medical anthropology of the 1980s and the 1990s has focused on situations of cultural pluralism, in which populations with various indigenous health cultures are in more or less extensive contact with the trappings of cosmopolitan health culture. Accordingly, their cultural systems (or "rules for living") include beliefs and rules about the introduced cosmopolitan medications and practitioners, intermingled with the cultural ideas concerning the indigenous healers and treatments. Studies of health care and health issues in urban communities in North America are set in a context of cultural pluralism—as most "mainline" and middle-class people are aware of various alternative health care choices.

EXPLANATORY MODELS: CULTURAL VIEWS OF ILLNESS

Arthur Kleinman's formulation of explanatory models (EM) of illness has taken a central place in research on specific sicknesses, as medical anthropologists and others have sought to present a coherent picture of the specific cultural features that affect peoples' health behaviors. The explanatory model for a particular illness consists of (1) signs and symptoms by which the illness is recognized; (2) presumed causes of the illness; (3) recommended therapies; (4) the pathophysiology of the illness; and (5) prognosis (Kleinman 1980:105–7).

As Kleinman points out, individuals are likely to have quite vague and indefinite models of explanation for their illnesses, depending on past experiences of the patient and her or his circle of kin and friends. On the other hand, some individuals in any given community have quite coherent explanations and expectations concerning a specific illness; and the "experts," the healers in the community, would probably on average have more coherent definitions than laypeople, with regard to illnesses and the relevant therapies. In any case, recent research by medical anthropologists has frequently made use of the EM construct as a focus around which a variety of questions can be raised concerning treatment behaviors and other features. Some of the examples of research designs described below focus on methods for systematic relating of explanatory models and treatment-seeking behaviors.

In the past two decades researchers have increasingly recognized the methodological importance of intracultural and intracommunity diversity in people's beliefs and practices. This tendency in research arose in part in relation to the growth of cultural pluralism, especially in matters of health and illness. Medical anthropologists have come to realize that even in seemingly "isolated" communities, individuals and families differ in their degree of adherence to traditional, indigenous health practices, as well as in their attitudes about medical-health ideas and materials newly introduced into their regions.

As a direct consequence, researchers have recognized the need for representative samples of individuals and households, from whom cultural data are collected. The older ethnographic methodology, based on a few selected key informants plus participant observation, is not entirely abandoned, however. In-depth interviewing of key informants, along with participant observation, are still essential aspects of anthropological research, particularly in early, exploratory phases of study. The qualitative, descriptive materials from this ethnographic work are essential for making sense of the more quantified materials gathered from samples of observations or structured interviews.

RESEARCH DESIGN: CLINICAL AND COMMUNITY APPROACHES

At the outset of research on health issues a major decision must be made: to focus the study on cases and events in clinical (health service) settings or to define the research population as community based. That decision has major implications for both qualitative and quantitative aspects of research design. Some researchers have found it useful to combine clinical and community-based samples. One very useful model is to start with a community in which cases of illness are identified. Differences between the users of health services and the nonusers can be explored in detail. In addition, the interactions in health care settings can be studied in the user subpopulation.

A *clinical population* can be defined as any group of patients, clients, or cases selected from the persons found at a particular health center, hospital, or individual healer's location. Clinical populations are selected for research whenever a portion of the research issues focus directly on the activities of the clinic or when it appears that a substantial part of the "cases" of a particular illness are to be found at the clinical setting.

Medical anthropologists have focused increasing attention on the cultural systems, technical workings, and other aspects of health care in hospitals and other health care settings. Direct observation of practitioner-patient interactions has become an especially important methodological focus, as researchers seek to define more precisely what really happens in therapeutic encounters. K. Finkler spent two years (1986–1988) observing physician-patient interactions in a large hospital in Mexico City (Finkler 1991). She was present at 800 consultations, and she collected detailed narratives from patients about their illness and systematic data concerning their family backgrounds. Follow-up visits were made to the homes of 205 of the patients to get fuller documentation of their illness experiences and perceptions of their interactions with the physicians. Her massive data collection also included in-depth interviews of seventeen physicians concerning their treatment philosophies and practices. Hospital records provided further depth of information.

Earlier (1977–1979), Finkler had carried out systematic observations among healers at a spiritualist temple in a rural region in Mexico. Her data in that study included 1,212 healer-patient interactions. Because of the similarities of data collection methods in the two studies, she was able to make systematic comparisons between the systems of treatment, identifying broad similarities and significant differences (Finkler 1994). She noted that "both Spiritualist healers and physicians impose a mind-body dualism on their patients." Also, "In both regimens, the patient takes the role of a passive recipient of the practitioner's ministrations, and in both regimens, the practitioners require their patients' compliance . . . reprimanding patients for not having followed prescribed treatments" (1994:182). On the other hand, Finkler found major differences between the two healing systems: the explanations of illness causation (and diagnoses) are very different; recruitment to the healing role differed greatly; treatment repertoires of spiritualist healers were usually more complex than those of the physicians, who relied mainly on medications. Contrary to widespread belief among anthropologists and the general public, the physicians she observed spent almost twice as much time with first-time patients than did the healers. On the other hand, "Perhaps the most crucial difference . . . is this: [spiritualist] healers resolve conflicts for patients that physicians cannot because the biomedical script requires physicians to focus on discrete physical pains" (p. 188).

Studies of provider-client interactions have been directed to the work of other practitioners besides doctors and healers. Rayna Rapp conducted an extensive study of genetic counselors, during which she "observed five genetic counselors working for New York City's Department of Health during their counseling sessions . . . sitting in on more than 200 intake interviews" (Rapp 1988a:145).

Where specific aspects of the client-provider interaction are studied, the sample unit is often the specific encounter rather than the population of individuals. Accordingly, in some cases the sampling frame is specified as "all client-provider interactions occurring during _____ period," and a system of randomizing can be applied to the time periods themselves.

A study by Trevathan of childbirth events in a bicultural community (El Paso, Texas) provides another illustration of research where the data can be gathered only in a clinic setting. In the case of childbirth, the significant questions often center on the expectations of mothers in relation to a particular clinic regimen. Accordingly, Trevathan selected a birth center with a large flow of clients. She enrolled in the one-year midwifery training program of the birth center, after which a study of mother-infant interaction was initiated. "Every woman who registered for prenatal care at the Birth Center and whose delivery was expected between October 1978 and May 1979 was informed of the 'bonding study.' . . . Volunteers were also recruited during childbirth education classes. . . . In the eight-month period, 152 women agreed to be in the study, approximately 50 percent of all those who delivered during that time period" (Trevathan 1988: 220). In this example, focus on cases in a particular clinical setting, where the researcher was a participant, permitted her to maintain close control of the research environment. On the other hand, the generalizations (e.g., concerning differences between Spanish-speaking and Anglo mother-infant pairs) cannot be extrapolated to the general population.

Studies based on clinical samples are often limited by the number of patients in a particular facility. For example, Cohen and colleagues compared and contrasted the explanatory models of diabetes patients with those of clinical staff in a diabetes clinic of a large midwestern university hospital. Their samples consisted of thirty-nine diabetes patients and fifteen professional staff. Despite the small sample sizes, the study shows interesting areas of discrepancy between the diabetes patients and the clinical staff, particularly in their interpretations of etiology, severity, and pathophysiology of the illness. Patients and clinical staff were in close agreement concerning the appropriate treatment for diabetes (Cohen et al. 1994). Studies focused on cultural patterns such as explanatory models of particular illnesses can often accomplish their objectives using rather small samples.

In the cases mentioned, the clinic populations were appropriately selected because of the nature of the research topic. However, clinic populations should never be considered as representative of the general (community-based) population. In almost every case, a particular hospital or other health setting receives only a selected, nonrandom portion of the population that exhibits a given illness or condition. Other cases may remain home, untreated; still others are found at the various alternative treatment facilities. Even an exhaustive tally of all cases in all facilities does not produce a representative picture of a given health problem, except perhaps with illnesses so severe, and so clearly identified, that nearly all of them can be found.

Clinic-based samples, if used as the sole data collection strategy, also have another potential weakness. Patients at health facilities appear as individuals, separated from the family networks in which they normally reside. Full, holistic understanding of people's expectations and reactions concerning illness and health care requires consideration of the household setting as it affects cultural responses. Thus, researchers such as Finkler have often carried out follow-up interviewing of patients in their homes, after observing their interactions in the clinic setting.

Generalizations about the frequencies of health care problems and choices of treatment require sampling from the relevant community population. Epidemiologists often refer to that community-based population as the "denominator," which is essential to study if one is interested in precise estimation of rates (or changes of rates) of particular illnesses or health care practices.

Clinical Samples with Matched Controls

Generalizations from clinic-based samples can often be greatly strengthened by selecting a control group from the same population that the clinic patients represent. K. Finkler, in the study of spiritualist healing mentioned above, introduced this method in her study of the patients. The data from the clinic (temple) sample were systematically compared with a control group ($N = 372$) "geographically matched with subjects interviewed in the temple corresponding to the villages . . . [from which the patients originated]" (Finkler 1986:201). Use of the control group permitted Finkler to state that the regular clientele of the temples did not differ significantly from the general population in perceived illness (Finkler 1985:130).

Strategies for Community-based Samples

Most research in medical anthropology has been structured in terms of communities or (sometimes) communities within communities. One or more communities in a particular region are chosen as primary sites for research, usually (not always) because of the prevalence of a particular health issue or problem in the selected region. Once the community or communities have been selected, sampling and other aspects of research design depend a great deal on two main factors: (1) the nature of the specific health problem addressed and (2) the geographic characteristics of the communities.

Community-based research is particularly congenial to medical anthropologists because the holistic methodological perspective requires a research context in which the field researcher enters into fairly long-term contacts with the people and is able to combine a great deal of firsthand participant observation with equally extensive interviews and conversations with people. Regardless of the specific topical focus, fieldworkers usually involve themselves in the daily lives of the people they study, even if only for short periods of time.

Often the researcher focuses on a single, well-chosen community of intermediate size. Where local villages and hamlets contain small numbers of house-holds, it becomes necessary to include several such communities. Research that is concerned with a particular illness of specific population segment (e.g., asthma among small children) requires that the population be large enough to contain an adequate sampling of households with small children experiencing the illness.

Sizes of study samples vary greatly, depending on overall community size, prevalence of specific illnesses studied, the types of data gathered, and the re-sources (including time) available. Nichter and Nichter described a survey car-ried out in South India, in which a small number of questions concerning food intake during pregnancy, preferred size of baby, and relations of food intake to baby size constituted the very simple interview protocol. The simplicity of the interview schedule made it feasible to manage a sample size of 282 participants (Nichter and Nichter 1983). Approximately 100 households appears to be a common ballpark figure in much medical anthropology research.

In many cases medical anthropologists find it necessary to collect data from multiple samples of informants or respondents, in part because of the difficulties in getting adequate representation of the various subgroups in a population. Also, different samples are sometimes selected in order to focus on particular topical areas. In a study of childbirth and obstetrics among the Bariba ethnic group in Benin, Sargent gathered data from several samples: (1) 26 postmenopausal women in a rural Bariba village; (2) 123 pregnant urban women of the same ethnic group (a clinic-based sample); (3) 35 pregnant Bariba women contacted in their homes; (4) 50 urban Bariba women currently employed in a cashew factory; and (5) 77 Bariba women who delivered at the Parakou hospital, whom she interviewed "concerning pregnancy and delivery expenses and hospital ex-periences" (Sargent 1989:13–15). Thus, Sargent found it important to combine community-based and clinic-based samples in order to get a holistic perspective on childbirth and maternity in the population.

When researchers have sufficient co-investigators and research assistants, samples can be larger. Browner and associates carried out research on repro-duction and health in a township of 1,800 inhabitants in highland Oaxaca, Mex-ico. "In addition to participant observation and intensive interviewing of selected key informants, single interviews were conducted with a 54 percent sample of the *municipio's* adult women and their husbands. One-hundred eighty women and 126 men were interviewed, with the sample constructed to represent the age, residential and linguistic backgrounds of . . . [the] adult population" (Browner and Pendue 1988:85–86).

Many anthropological studies utilize multiple community samples. In some cases several communities or hamlets must be included for representativeness in a complex population. Gittlesohn, in a study of intrahousehold food distri-bution patterns, defined his research population in rural Nepal in terms of a network of six villages, in order to include all relevant caste groups (Gittelsohn 1989).

Quite often the selection of multiple communities is used to operationalize a significant, usually independent, variable. Bentley chose three villages in north India as the population for study of household management of childhood diarrhea, in order to have an experimental and control group. One village was the site of an oral rehydration therapy (ORT) intervention program, and two villages nearby were selected as controls in order to test the efficacy of the ORT program (Bentley 1988).

In a study of "ethnicity, ecology and mortality in Northwestern Thailand," Kunstadter gathered data from a number of different communities, both highland and lowland. "Community type is the basic unit of comparison. Disaggregation of the population according to type of community shows that fertility and mortality patterns are systematically associated with ethnicity and ecology (location and basic economy). . . . Populations in the study area allow control of ecological and ethnic variablility by comparing, for example, the same ethnic group in different ecological settings (Northern Thai in Town, Suburb, and Lowland Rural communities), and different ethnic groups in the same ecological setting (e.g., Highland Skaw Karen, Po Karen and Lua' with similar swidden economies)" (Kunstadter 1986: 125). In a similar vein, Hackenberg and associates selected four communities in the Philippines—two sedentary and two migrant groups—for testing specific hypotheses about the effects of migration and modernization on hypertension levels (Hackenberg et al. 1983). Gebrian used a multicommunity design in a study of nutrition, rates of immunization, and other characteristics in a thirty four-community region in southwestern Haiti. She compared communities in terms of "distance from health center," "level of community participation," size of population," and other independent variables in testing hypotheses about the effectiveness of primary health care operations (Gebrian 1993).

Sampling in Urban Communities

Medical anthropology in urban sites, particularly in North American settings, very often focuses on one or more ethnic groups within the general population. The selection of such ethnic (or other) subcommunities poses special problems, particularly in identifying the total population of ethnic households from which sampling will occur. A typical strategy is to identify one or more urban "neighborhoods" thought to be concentrations of the particular ethnic group. In Hartford, Connecticut, Schensul and associates selected two neighborhoods; a public housing project and an area of privately owned houses. After arbitrarily delimiting the two neighborhoods, a system of random sampling was adopted by which 143 households were selected for interviews (Schensul and Borrero 1982).

Janes described the difficulties in selecting a sample of Samoan migrants in northern California for his study of hypertension. "The sample selection process involved the following steps: a list of the church membership of two large church congregations was obtained, numbering about 130 households. From this pool, 60 households were chosen at random. This resulted in 89 interviews with men and women in these households. . . . In addition, with the aid of a Samoan research assistant, who was also a well-known and respected member of the community, I selected a sample of 25 individuals from other religious denominations'' (Janes 1986:205)

The contrast in style between intensive, small-sample research and the collection of survey data in an urban setting is particularly striking in the work of Scrimshaw in the Ecuadorean city of Guayaquil. In the ethnographic phase of research, ''sixty-five families in one small area of the squatter settlement were studied for six months . . . using . . . participant observation, conversation, informal interviewing, and observation'' (Scrimshaw 1985:125). An interview schedule was then designed for gathering quantitative data on migration, fertility, and induced abortions and was administered to approximately 2,000 households in a squatter settlement and the ''central city slum'' area, using probability cluster sampling. Scrimshaw demonstrated that her ethnographic sample of fewer than 100 households was in many ways quite similar to the large-scale sample in terms of frequencies of fertility attitudes and behaviors.

BASIC DATA-GATHERING TOOLS

Key Informant Interviewing

Open-ended qualitative interviewing of key informants has long been the foundation stone of anthropological data gathering. Even in projects with a major focus on quantitative survey methods, there is almost always an initial phase of ethnographic exploration—in the form of informal interviewing.

Some unstructured conversations and interviews should always be carried out with a variety of informants before more structured quantitative data gathering is initiated. One major aim of the qualitative research is to develop a good sense of local vocabulary in relation to health problems. The forms of even the most routine questions and observations should be shaped by knowledge of the local language and ecological conditions.

Traditionally anthropologists have relied heavily on serendipity in locating key informants. Loitering about in public places usually leads to contacts with some local persons who happen to feel like talking with the outsider. A somewhat more structured approach is to go from household to household, to visit and to explain the intended research project to individual families.

In health care research, whether clinic based or community based, medical anthropologists often follow a sequence of contacts, beginning with local administrators, health authorities, and other leaders in the political and administrative hierarchy. Following that sequence of contacts with informants, it has become useful to distinguish three main types of key informants:

1. *Type 1 key informants: Administrators and officials.* The first key informants one contacts are likely to be personnel in government services, police, and administrators

in nongovernmental organizations, who are broadly familiar with local situations and activities because of their official duties. These first-line key informants can help data gatherers to get started in the target community, as they are often gatekeepers who can grant (or refuse to grant) access to clinics, hospitals, and community health workers.

2. *Type 2 key informants: Health workers and community outreach workers.* In most areas, both urban and rural, there are outreach workers of health services and other social programs, in government services as well as nongovernment organizations. These informants are particularly important because they can provide direct contacts with people in the target populations. Also, the community outreach workers are often in situations of mediating between service programs and the people's household-based health beliefs and practices.

3. *Type 3 key informants: Members of the target population.* Ethnographic research is rather incomplete until extensive informant interviews have been carried out with members of the target population. In the case of women's and children's illnesses it is commonly expected that the anthropologist visits a number of households, seeking out women who have had a lot of experience with illness management, and who are willing to spend considerable time in discussing "cases" and "episodes" of illness. Care should be taken that these key informants are drawn from several different parts of the community in order to ensure representativeness of the sample, even though key informants are never selected on a random sampling basis.

The numbers of conversations and other contacts with key informants will vary greatly, depending on their availability, their breadth of information, and willingness to spend many hours with the interviewer. Typically medical anthropologists, like other ethnographic fieldworkers, rely on a small number of key informants (usually fewer than ten) for a large part of their detailed information, with smaller amounts of contact with their secondary key informants, who are nonetheless very important for cross-checking and triangulation of data.

In some cases anthropologists select samples of informants from different sectors of the local population after carrying out a household census to identify types of households and other variations. Small numbers of representative families (e.g., families with children under five, households with pregnant women, nuclear versus extended households) can then be visited for in-depth ethnographic interviewing.

Ethnographic interviewing and unstructured observations in homes is the crucial stage in many projects, during which the complexities of health care decision making, types of home treatments, attitudes and relationships to health facilities, economic and political issues, and many other details of local life are studied extensively, in preparation for carefully designed, structured observations and interviews. The informal contacts with selected households can also include some pretesting of portions of data-gathering formats intended for the more structured portions of the study.

Structured Data Gathering in Samples of Households

Many health-related research projects include several different structured data-gathering operations, sometimes using somewhat different samples for the various observations. For example, Bentley, in her research on diarrhea management in north India, interviewed in a random sample of 199 households to collect data on beliefs and knowledge about the causes and prevention of diarrhea and other aspects of explanatory models. In a later phase of research, mothers of children with diarrhea episodes were interviewed as well as observed in 50 households, to get actual behavioral data (Bentley 1988:75–76). In his research on intrahousehold food distribution in Nepal, Gittelsohn selected six villages within a *panchayat,* from which he identified a random sample of 115 households. A number of different interviews and observations were carried out, including a socioeconomic interview, several twenty-four-hour dietary recalls, anthropometric measurements of both children and adults, repeated direct observations of meals (total of 354 meals recorded), collection of morbidity data, in addition to key informant interviews and informal chats with many of the people in the sample. The resulting data set contained twenty-one separate subfiles, totaling 70,000 lines (Gittelsohn, 1989).

Combining Qualitative and Quantitative Data: Some Examples

Case 1: Explanatory Models of Illness and Decision Making.

One of the more thorough and impressive studies of people's modes of choosing among health care alternatives is that of James Young, in the town of Pichataro in western Mexico (Young 1981). The study is important because it illustrates structured interviewing with small numbers of key informants, after which the methodology shifted to collection of actual illness episodes.

In the first phase of research Young and his wife, Linda Garro, carried out a census of the 509 households in the community and began key informant interviews concerning common illnesses and their characteristics. General ethnographic interviewing was necessary to identify specific types of health care resources utilized by the people, as well as to develop the basic list of locally recognized illnesses concerning which cultural models of explanation and choice making could be derived.

With a provisional set of forty-two physical and behavioral symptoms of illness (each written on a separate card), the researchers asked five literate informants to sort these into piles in terms of severity. The same informants were also asked to sort the illnesses (diagnostic labels) into piles in terms of severity.

The researchers carried out paired-comparison interviews, in which questions were posed in the basic form: "[In case of illness] . . . when—for what reasons—would you (consult) (use) [type of practitioner] instead of (consulting) (using) [another type of practitioner]?" The possible alternatives in the blanks were: "1. self-treatment; 2. a folk curer; 3. a pharmacy (with consultation only with the clerk or pharmacist); 4. a local *practicante;* 5. the Patzcuaro Health Center; and 6. a private-practice physician" (pp. 132–33). Each of the six alternatives was paired with every other, resulting in thirty choice questions. "The interview was completed with fifteen persons, eight men and seven women, of varying age, occupation, and economic status" (Young 1981:133).

In order to get in-depth information concerning the culturally defined characteristics of each of the illnesses, a set of forty-three different illness attributes (questions) were asked of each of the thirty-four illness terms identified in early stages of the research. This time-consuming interview required a number of sessions with each of the ten informants—six women and four men (Young 1981:81).

The most time-consuming process was the collection of a corpus of actual illnesses, for the testing of the decision model derived from analysis of the data on illness definitions and characteristics. From the original census data, a representative sample was drawn. "Over a six-month period, sixty-two households were visited on an approximate biweekly basis and records were made of each illness occurring among its members" (Young 1981:77). A total of 323 cases were collected.

This research project is very revealing, as it includes a thorough mixing of qualitative and quantified procedures, progressing from pattern identification of illnesses, to the testing of models concerning the ways in the patterns influenced actual behaviors (in the 323 episodes).

Case 2: Modernization and Arterial Blood Pressure

"Hypertension," or more accurately, differential blood pressures, is particularly interesting as a focus of research because the disease is relatively symptom free. As a result, in most indigenous communities there has been no traditional concept. Nonetheless, a great many cultural groups, including many Native American communities, now have cultural models of "hypertension," learned (and modified) from the doctors, nurses, and others in cosmopolitan medical services. Studies of factors affecting differences in blood pressure levels (and outright hypertension) involve use of an overt biomedical measurement (using a sphygmomanometer), plus the observation of cultural, psychological, social, and other factors thought to affect arterial blood pressure levels. The following case is important because it exemplifies an increasingly frequent type of study, in which medical anthropologists collaborate with epidemiologists and other biomedical researchers in projects sponsored by international agencies.

Dressler and associates chose an urban area in of Ribeirão Prêto, a city of 400,000 in Southeast Brazil, for the research. "A variant of cluster sampling was used to draw a sample of 139 individuals. Four broad clusters based on residential and economic sector ... were chosen, and then random samples of 20 households were chosen from each cluster" (Dressler et al. 1987:400). The clusters that the researchers selected represented agricultural day laborers, continuously employed plantation workers, factory workers, and a fourth cluster of bank employees.

For the dependent variable, the research group used the mean values derived from five separate measurements of blood pressure using a DINAMAP Vital Signs Monitor Model 845XT. The automated equipment for measuring blood pressure is much more reliable than ordinary sphymomanometers, as it "virtually eliminates inter-observer variability" (p. 401). This is an example of use of state-of-the-art equipment and methods to manage the biomedical variables in an interdisciplinary project. Other variables were "index of style of life," composed of ownership of items of material culture, and "economic resources," representing occupations of all adult members of the households. From these two measures, an index of "life-style stress" was computed, based on the discrepancies between the two indexes. Dietary data were collected using a series of four twenty-four-hour recalls. Other variables included individual perception of "relative deprivation," "life changes," and the usual age, sex, education, and race, as well as height and weight.

The lifestyle index in this study is particularly interesting because it includes ownership of consumer goods (color television, vehicle, food blender, camera, telephone, etc.) and also items such as yearly trips to São Paulo, vacation trips, magazines read per month, newspapers read per week, and number of books read per year (Dressler et al. 1987:402).

The statistical analysis (multiple regressions) replicated Dressler's previous study of hypertension in St. Lucia, again demonstrating the importance of lifestyle stresses as predictors of differences in blood pressures. In his earlier research, Dressler had carried out extensive qualitative ethnographic research in addition to the quantified data gathering. The Brazilian study, on the other hand, included very little qualitative data gathering.

Case 3: Diarrhea Research of the 1980s

This case departs from the focus on individual projects in order to examine some features of a concerted program of research on diarrhea that has played a central role in the child survival programs of the 1980s and 1990s, particularly involving Oral rehydration therapy (ORT). Infant and childhood diarrheas have been a leading cause of mortality in most parts of the developing world. Beginning in the 1980s, it became apparent that a major reduction in infant and small child mortality could take place if ORT were regularly used to offset the dehydrating effects of diarrheas, even though ORT is not itself a cure for the illness.

Practically every developing country now has a program for promotion and dissemination of ORT. In most cases the emphasis is on teaching people to use ORT packets disseminated throughout the primary health care systems; however, some programs have sought to train people to mix home-made oral rehydration solutions, following simple recipes. There has also been promotion of rice-based and other cereal-based ORT. Despite the apparent success in some of these campaigns, most national programs have encountered difficulties in convincing the majority of people to use ORT. And in many instances even the acceptors of the therapeutic regimen do not use ORT in an appropriate manner.

Problems with people's acceptance and proper use of ORT in most developing countries have led to widespread realization of the need for research, including anthropological data gathering, to identify the points of difficulty and to develop ways for improving programs. The study by Bentley in north India is one of a large number of studies by anthropologists during the 1980s. Several of these studies were published in a special edition of *Social Science and Medicine* (Coreil and Mull 1988).

Biomedical thinking and directions of research with regard to childhood diarrhea have progressed from a simple focus on ORT, to the examination of complex issues around breast feeding and other dietary behaviors, patterns of use (and misuse) of pharmaceutical remedies, and many other culturally mediated beliefs and behaviors. With the realization of complexity has come a greatly increased interest in the possibility that specifically anthropological methods may hold the keys to better management of the diarrhea issue.

A major first step to disentangling the "diarrhea problem" was the shift of focus from the biomedical construct, "diarrheal disease," to the variety of cultural constructions—the emically defined patterns related to diarrhea as illness. One of the more influential studies earlier in the decade was Nations's study of an economically impoverished area of northeast Brazil. She noted the points of incongruity between the prevailing allopathic approaches to diarrhea and the perspectives of the mothers and local healers among the people. She called for new approaches to diarrhea control:

In short, the foremost concern of this alternative approach to diarrheal disease control is to support rather than suppress popular village healing. Doctors must adapt medical terminology to popular usage. . . . They must learn the popular folk explanations for childhood illnesses and explore their relation to biomedical etiologies. Health professionals must also give villagers dietary advice in a way that does not violate harmless food beliefs and that assures the traditional healers power in village medicine. Still, peasant families must also have easy access to effective modern means to save children dying from severe dehydration. (Nations 1982:155)

Key informant interviewing to elicit varied terminology for diarrhea, emic types of diarrhea, and the exploration of the explanatory models (EM) for diarrhea in given cultures have become core elements of most community-based diarrhea research, even by nonanthropologists (Weiss 1988). In north India Bentley found that mothers identified five types of diarrhea: "bloody," "watery," "bits-and-pieces," "green," and "yellow" (Bentley 1988:76–77). Scrimshaw and Hurtado found that explanatory models of diarrhea in Guatemala included those caused by the mother (due to emotion, physiological condition, etc.), food-related diarrhea (hot, cold, "bad," excess), as well as those due to tooth eruption, "fallen fontanel," evil eye, worms, and "cold enters the stomach." This

complex array of different causes is associated with different choices of therapies.

In a rural area of central Mexico, Martinez asked mothers to sort into groups
the various foods that had previously been identified as "foods given to children
during diarrhea." The pile-sort task results were then submitted to multidimensional scaling. Martinez asked his community health workers to examine the
scaling results and to interpret the dimensions. The general result included the
finding that women were differentiating between foods that were appropriate
during acute phases of diarrhea and those that are usually fed during the recovery
phase (Martinez et al. 1988:39–40).

Most of these ethnographic researchers have used some sort of sampling procedures, but the exploration of folk taxonomies, explanatory models, and other
aspects of emic views of diarrhea do not generally depend on statistical analysis,
other than, at most, frequencies of recognition of taxonomic categories. While
some variations are always found in the numbers and types of categories identified by different informants, the range of variation is not usually extensive.

Quantitative survey techniques, on the other hand, are generally used to assess
the strength and prevalence of beliefs about causes of diarrhea, and especially
for assessing frequencies of crucial elements such as cessation of breast feeding,
curtailment of solid foods, and other potentially harmful behaviors arising from
cultural belief systems. Survey techniques have also been used to find out the
percentage of people who have heard of ORT, as well as the rates of recent use
of this therapy. Coreil and Genece report a survey concerning adoption of ORT
among Haitian mothers, carried out in the coastal town of Montrouis and the
surrounding villages. As is usual in this kind of study, several weeks of ethnographic investigation were carried out before the survey was initiated. "A
random sample of 300 mothers or caretakers of children 0–5 years were interviewed. . . . Census records allowed us to identify all the 1714 families in the
health program with preschool children" (Coreil and Genece 1988:88–89). The
researchers made use of two survey teams, "each consisting of 3 interviewers
and a supervisor. The project director (author) trained and closely monitored the
teams. . . . The 65-item questionnaire was pretested on 15 mothers from an ad-
jacent community" (p. 89). The statistical analysis consisted of a multiple regression to examine the relative strengths of several hypothesized predictors of
ORT knowledge and use.

The third major sector of anthropological research on diarrhea has been directed to prospective study of behaviors in the case of actual diarrheal episodes.
This methodology requires three main ingredients: (1) a representative sample
of households containing small children of the requisite age; (2) a method for
monitoring households so that episodes of diarrhea are quickly identified as they
occur; and (3) a well-designed protocol for direct observations and interviewing
concerning the identified cases. Monitoring and follow-up of diarrheal episodes
is time-consuming, as each visit should include direct observation if possible,
as well as interviews of caretakers concerning modes of treatment, visits to

health care facilities, feeding behaviors, condition of the child, and many other details. As studies of diarrhea have shifted toward possible prevention strategies, interest is developing concerning direct observation of hygiene and sanitation in households, including hand washing, modes of cleaning up after children's diarrhea, maintenance of drinking water, and other behaviors. All of the recent studies of actual behaviors have demonstrated that there are wide discrepancies between people's answers to surveys as opposed to actual behavior as observed directly by the researchers. At the same time, direct observation of complex health-related behaviors is a relatively underdeveloped aspect of anthropological research, and more experimentation is needed to refine the methodology.

Collaboration of medical anthropologists with epidemiologists, biomedical researchers, and others has been particularly fruitful in the sector of diarrhea control. This is partly because of the widespread realization that qualitative ethnographic work and other anthropological research tools play a vital role in furthering practical understanding of key issues, particularly about the ways in which complex health beliefs, or explanatory models, affect health care decision making.

Case 4: Focused Ethnographic Study of Acute Respiratory Infections in the 1990s

G. Pelto and associates at the World Health Organization (WHO) have recently developed a systematic ethnographic approach to the examination of people's cultural explanatory models of acute respiratory infections (ARI) in very young children. Serious respiratory infection (usually pneumonia) is a major killer of children under five years of age, currently accounting for more than 4 million deaths annually (Gove and Pelto 1994:409). In order to promote effective responses to serious ARI among mothers and other caretakers, the WHO planning team developed a set of interrelated data-gathering techniques that produce a relatively clear picture of the explanatory models, as well as behaviors and evaluations associated with the culturally defined ARI illness domain. Here are the main elements in their focused ethnographic study (FES) strategy:

1. Data gathering begins with key informant interviewing about respiratory illnesses and their treatments in the local area. The interviews also include a "free-listing exercise" (Weller and Romney 1988) to obtain the vocabulary of signs and symptoms, as well as local, culturally specific names for children's respiratory illnesses.

2. Illness episodes of ARI are collected from small samples of mothers in order to assemble more information about behaviors connected with the different categories of signs, symptoms, and illnesses.

3. Mothers are shown short video clips of sick children (including some with pneumonia) and are asked to identify symptoms and explain "what is wrong" with the child (what illness does the child have?). The mothers are also asked whether they have perceive the child to exhibit "rapid breathing" (an important symptom of pneumonia).

4. The sample of mothers is asked to respond to hypothetical vignettes of children with

ARI symptoms. The descriptions are varied systematically to highlight differences in response (recommended actions) for more severe and less severe symptoms.

5. The respondents are asked to do simple sorting tasks with sets of index cards, to indicate which specific symptoms are associated with local illness terms. The card sorting is also used to get systematic ratings of severity of the various signs, symptoms, and illnesses. Weller (1980) and others have used similar sorting tasks for cognitive mapping of various cultural domains.

6. Structured interviewing in the form of paired comparisons (Weller and Romney 1988: 45–46) is used to elicit the mothers' choices of health care providers. The list of alternatives (doctors, healers, clinics, etc.) is obtained from the key informant interviews.

7. Interviews with mothers (and other caretakers) bringing small children to clinics provide more direct information on actual health-seeking behaviors in relation to particular symptoms. A key question in that context is, "Which of the symptoms [that you saw in your child] were the ones that led to your decision to come for health care?"

8. Interviews with pharmacists and vendors concerning their prescribing patterns for ARI symptoms and interviews with various indigenous and cosmopolitan practitioners are included for rounding out the picture of the local people's management of ARI episodes. Also, home inventories of herbal remedies, pharmaceutical products, and other medicines are obtained from the sample households.

The FES strategy adopted in the WHO ARI program is a mixture of qualitative and small sample quantitative techniques, many of which are clearly described in *Systematic Data Collection,* by Weller and Romney (1988). The tools and techniques for cognitive mapping of cultural domains, as well as other basic ethnographic methods for this type of study, are also described in *Research Methods in Anthropology* (Bernard 1988).

This example of the use of explicitly ethnographic research methodology at the WHO is part of a rapidly developing trend in international health organizations. There is now widespread interest in adoption of the research approaches of medical anthropology, partly connected with a growing recognition among biomedical personnel and health care planners, of the importance of cultural and social factors in affecting the success of health care programs.

The FES battery of data-gathering techniques is a useful example of the strategy of triangulation in ethnographic research. Data concerning people's recognition and definitions of symptoms and illnesses are collected in illness episodes, free-listing exercises, viewing of the videos, and structured sorting tasks. Thus, the data provide systematic cross-checking of both illness definitions and the behaviors associated with them. Also, the authors noted that in their methodology, "Data on antibiotic use patterns are obtained from several FES procedures, including the narratives of past ARI episodes, scenarios, home inventories [of medicines], and interviews in clinics, with pharmacists and with practitioners" (Gove and Pelto 1994:419). Based on those multiple data sources across a number of different research sites, they found that there are widespread problems in misuse of antibiotics: "(1) antibiotics used for mild upper respiratory infections; (2) failure to continue with a full course of antibiotic treatment; and (3) saving medication from a partially completed course to use for another episode" (p. 420).

Discussion of the Cases

The four cases illustrate a few of the many trends in contemporary medical anthropology, particularly in fieldwork in primary health care in developing countries. To an increasing extent, medical anthropological research is directed to intensive study of specific sicknesses—either in emic, culturally delimited terms of illness or through study of a biomedically derived disease, for which the relevant cultural explanations, behaviors, and other features are explored. Research directed to specific pathological states has the large advantage of delimiting and controlling the range of relevant health behaviors to be studied. Also it permits the anthropologist to become at least moderately knowledgeable about the relevant biomedical aspects without having to spend months in studying medical textbooks.

Most field research in medical anthropology—in these cases and other studies like them—includes varying mixtures of the following ingredients:

1. Initial selection of field site where the sickness condition(s) of interest are prevalent enough to be studied. Quite often the field site is selected because of an ongoing health care program.

2. General, descriptive field research, particularly key informant interviewing, in the area, much like other anthropologists in the first phases of getting acquainted with the local environment and its people.

3. Census or enumeration of the local population in order to gather general descriptive information and to acquire the framework for later representative sampling.

4. Key informant interviewing and participant observation focused on the particular pathology, to explore "explanatory models," taxonomies, as well as a variety of other areas of cultural knowledge concerning the topical focus.

5. Use of pile sorts, triad sorts, sentence frames, or other structured methods with small numbers of informants, in order to refine various aspects of the explanatory models and other aspects of the cultural belief systems.

6. Structured direct observations of management of illness, hygienic-sanitation behavior and conditions, provider-patient interactions, and other behaviors central to the research.

7. Structured interviews for eliciting data on main independent and dependent variables from representative samples, in order to test specific hypotheses and to verify major patterns and processes tentatively identified in earlier steps of research.

8. Extraction of data from patient records in hospital, clinic, or other health care facility where available. In the usual case, extraction of such data requires permission not only from the administrative personnel who control the records but also from the

individual patients or their families. Such records may also include data from special bioclinical observations, including blood pressures, blood samples, urinalysis, x-rays, clinical assessments by doctors, and other procedures.

9. Analysis of both qualitative and quantitative data, using either micro- or mainframe computers, and often both.

10. Presentation of results of research and policy recommendations to persons in the research community and other groups involved in health program operations.

In addition, medical anthropologists generally collect large amounts of descriptive, contextual information about the community, environmental features, political and economic structures, and other relevant material. Most research projects do not, of course, include all of the qualitative and quantified procedures just mentioned. Depending on the time frames of research, the specific questions studied, and personnel and funding available, individual projects can range from small-scale studies using one or two of these basic tools, all the way to comprehensive, multiyear programs of data gathering that expand beyond this core list.

Rapid Ethnographic Assessment Procedures

Applied ethnographic research is frequently seen as a desirable first step before health care programs are put into operation. Also, increasing numbers of epidemiologists and other quantitative researchers are realizing the importance of ethnographic research for fine-tuning their approaches to planning of structured interviewing and other research operations. Three main reasons for initial ethnographic research are:

1. To provide locally relevant cultural information to be used to improve health care programs.

2. To provide a baseline of data from which to measure change and effectiveness in such programs.

3. To identify locally relevant cultural taxonomies and explanatory models, in order to frame meaningful questions in structured interviewing and observations.

Very often such initial ethnographic research must be completed in a few weeks, so as not to delay the introduction of the health care program itself. However, anthropologists have traditionally resisted what some people have referred to as "quick-and-dirty" applied research. Based on the general holistic principle common to most sociocultural anthropology, some ethnographers have argued that many months are required just to become familiar with all the relevant cultural features and to become known in a given community setting. Also, learning the local language(s), often thought essential to good ethnographic work, requires a great deal of time.

Despite some trepidations concerning rapid ethnographic research, there was a substantial increase in sophistication in systematizing this type of data gathering. In several instances the guidelines for specific data gathering have been set forth in field manuals, particularly when similar data were to be gathered in several sites by different research groups. One of the early examples of such a field manual was prepared by Marchione for the Infant Feeding Practices Study, undertaken by a consortium of researchers from the Population Council, Cornell University, and Columbia University School of Public Health (Marchione 1981). The plan of research called for approximately ten weeks of ethnographic reconnaissance, with a suggested sample of thirty to fifty informants. The informants were to be selected from the same communities in which a later, structured interview survey was to be carried out.

A more comprehensive manual for rapid anthropological assessment was designed by Scrimshaw and Hurtado for use in an ambitious program of research sponsored by the United Nations University, initiated in 1983–1984. Social science researchers in fifteen countries carried out projects that ranged from two or three months to six or eight months, using the draft set of guidelines. The researchers and their methodological consultants convened in Bellagio, Italy, in 1985 to review the resulting data and to modify aspects of the methodology. The revised set of research guidelines, the *RAP Manual* was then published for general use in health and nutrition programs. The manual includes an appendix with data collection guides including morbidity history of adult household members, inventory of household remedies, use of health resources, interview with health staff, provider-patient interaction, and others (Scrimshaw and Hurtado 1987:Appendix 1).

Scrimshaw and Hurtado commented, ''A great deal of practical, diagnostic, and applied work can be accomplished in a shorter time and by using a simpler approach'' (Scrimshaw and Hurtado 1987:1). The authors of the manual point out that a great many health care programs have been initiated without any sort of culture-specific map to guide health personnel in adjusting to local belief structures, ecological conditions, economic restraints, and other factors affecting peoples' health-seeking behaviors.

Among these several different examples of rapid research techniques, there are several common methodological themes:

1. It is commonly assumed that some descriptive materials on the local cultural system(s) are available, so that the researcher does not need to spend time finding out about the economic system, kinship and social organization, and other general features.

2. Familiarity with the local language on the part of the researchers, or else use of local research workers as interviewers, is generally assumed.

3. The extensive version of the holistic assumption is rejected in favor of a more limited style of multifactor research. For example, in research on diarrhea or acute respiratory infection, it is assumed that data gathering can focus very specifically on the illness itself, plus a clearly specified list of contextual factors. Very little general ethnography is needed.

4. The specific ethnographic data to be collected are thought to require small numbers of informants. Samples of thirty to forty respondents are usually sufficient to establish the local vocabulary, explanatory models, and other patterns.

5. When research is limited to small numbers of informants, contacted during a fairly short time period, considerable care is usually exerted to ensure representativeness of the sample, in terms of local subgroups, age and sex distribution, socioeconomic status, and other dimensions of variation.

6. The use of focus group interviews or group discussion sessions is commonly used in the exploratory phases of the research.

7. Inferential statistical analysis is seldom appropriate in the rapid ethnography methodology, but descriptions can include presentation of frequencies of responses in various categories.

8. The rapid methodologies sometimes include limited use of survey methods near the end of the data-gathering process.

The rapid methodologies have developed primarily in response to the requirements of applied primary health care programs. In many cases the rapid ethnographic assessment is needed to produce basic data for designing health care intervention programs. However, the *Rapid Assessment Procedures* manual by Scrimshaw and Hurtado (1989) was developed in relation to evaluation of ongoing nutrition and health care programs.

Use of Microcomputers

A second major methodological development of the 1980s and 1990s is the ongoing evolution of computer utilization in research. To an increasing extent, medical anthropologists (and many other types of researchers) are carrying microcomputers into fieldwork for both qualitative and quantitative data management. The most common use of microcomputers is for writing field notes. The legendary tediousness of writing field notes and analyzing them is somewhat lessened through use of versatile word processing software. Failures with microcomputers were numerous in mid-1980s fieldwork (Gittelsohn 1989), but laptop and notebook computers are now quite sturdy and reliable. Fieldworkers are nonetheless urged to print out hard-copy field notes frequently and to make backup copies onto floppy diskettes.

In larger, multidisciplinary projects involving collection of various epidemiological, social, and cultural data, the maintenance of computerized data systems becomes a major task. With proper team organization, data entry at the research site makes it possible to check computer printouts against the original raw data and to send researchers back to households to retrieve missing information. For community-based data capture, it is advisable that database programs be tailor-made so that the blanks for entering numbers and words mimic the basic interview forms. In Gebrian's primary health care project in Haiti, the field-based computer allows the program coordinator to send printouts of household data summaries back to individual communities, so that health committees receive feedback concerning local health status (e.g., percentage of malnourished children) for planning purposes (Gebrian 1993).

A major advantage of the microcomputer in fieldwork is the ability to carry out data analysis, both qualitative and quantitative, with at least some automated help. For extensive text data (field notes) most word processing programs include at least minimal search or find routines. Full-scale indexing of field notes, for more complex searches of key words, can be done with programs such as FOLIOVIEWS, GOFER, or ZYINDEX.

High-powered statistical analysis for microcomputers is available in SAS, SPSS, SYSTAT (Windows-based), and other statistical software. Practically all of the complex statistical analysis that required mainframe computers fifteen years ago can now be carried out in the field using easily portable computers. The use of microcomputers in field research is now quite common among many research groups in developing countries as well.

Until recently anthropologists have not had simple microcomputer programs available for construction and analysis of triad sorts and pile sorts and for developing and testing Guttman and Likert-type scales. However, a new program developed by Borgatti, called ANTHROPAC, is now available for these fieldwork operations. The program is menu driven and quite easy to use. Borgatti has also incorporated procedures for network analysis, another important tool for ongoing analysis in the field (Borgatti 1988).

Communications from field sites to home base often depend on slow-moving mails, but large amounts of data and voluminous reports can be conveniently shipped on floppy diskettes. Where telephone services are reliable, a great deal of communication, including transmission of data files, can be accomplished through e-mail, directly from computer to computer. E-mail simply requires that each end of the system have a modem for connecting computer to telephone, plus appropriate software to facilitate sending and receiving. Many researchers use a variety of different electronic communications systems for messages and data file transmissions, both domestic and international.

SUMMARY AND CONCLUSIONS

The 1980s and 1990s have seen impressive advances in research design and data-gathering techniques in medical anthropology. These developments are due in part to influences outside anthropology, through interdisciplinary communication. Widespread acceptance and recognition of medical anthropology as an essential ingredient in research on illness and health care has brought about increased sharing of methodological techniques among the biological, clinical, epidemiological, and social sciences. The mutual interactions of anthropology and epidemiology have been particularly important, as documented in *Anthropology and Epidemiology,* edited by Janes, Stall, and Gifford (1986). Cooperation between epidemiologists and anthropologists has led to methodological shifts on both sides. Medical anthropologists have come to pay more attention to matters of sampling and representativeness, along with new techniques of statistical analysis. The Applied Diarrheal Disease Research Program, PAHO, WHO, NIH, and other organizations have insisted that ethnographic fieldwork should be described in concrete, easily understood terms, and these influences have led anthropologists to be more specific about techniques, leading in turn to increased standardization of procedures.

In the area of structured direct observations, anthropologists, epidemiologists, nutritionists, and psychologists seem to have all learned from each other. Earlier anthropological observations tended to be unstructured and ad hoc, without much concern for representativeness. Some of the other disciplines, on the other hand, had developed methods that were highly structured but badly suited to specific field conditions. Medical anthropologists have played an important role in helping to develop culturally appropriate modes of observation that can be structured sufficiently to permit statistical analysis.

The advent of microcomputers has certainly had a direct technological impact on medical anthropology. The availability of easy-to-use statistical software has encouraged researchers to develop more systematic numerical as well as qualitative data gathering. Some of the impetus for improvements in computerized data gathering and analysis has come directly from anthropologists with long experience at mainframe operations. Researchers in other disciplines also contributed techniques and tools that anthropologists have found useful.

The continued spread of the HIV-AIDS epidemic and growth of needs for research to develop intervention programs have also contributed to developments in medical anthropology. The Global Programme on AIDS at WHO has included increasing numbers of anthropologists, particularly reflecting the need for systematic ethnographic fieldwork in relation to high-risk behaviors that contribute to spread of HIV infection. Everywhere in HIV-AIDS intervention programs one hears frequent reference to needs for qualitative, ethnographic research. The needs for careful, systematic ethnographic work are particularly evident in relation to hard-to-reach populations such as injection drug users, men who have sex with men, and commercial sex workers.

One of the major motivations for improved research methodologies, both qualitative and quantitative, arises from the requirements of applied community-based health programs. Health programs, particularly in developing countries, measure effectiveness in terms of reduced levels of infant mortality, morbidity, and other indicators. Whenever data gathering is intended to have direct programmatic consequences, within organizations whose personnel are largely non-anthropologists, there is a considerable pressure to improve the credibility of data gathering and data analysis. The conventions of report writing and oral presentations of research result in international health circles also foster consciousness of methodology.

Our impressions, based on many recent experiences and informal communications among medical anthropologists, are that the transmission of effective research methodology is not strongly developed in our graduate training programs. Most medical anthropologists have improved their methodological skills in the school of trial and error, in the course of work in interdisciplinary projects. As a result, colleagues who happen not to be involved in interdisciplinary team research can find themselves with fewer resources for keeping abreast of methodological developments.

Methodological skills are scarce resources and have direct economic value—in employment, promotion, and the like—in addition to their contribution to excellence of research output. To an increasing extent, researchers who are marginalized in relation to the main international communications networks may be falling behind in methodological terms, leading to relatively weaker, less useful research. The problem of effective dissemination of research methodologies is especially important for anthropologists in Third World countries. Fortunately, the research promotion efforts of international health organizations and foundations have been effective in promoting more sophistication in research methodology, including use of microcomputers, in the developing countries (Trostle et al. 1989).

During the past several decades, the research methods of anthropology have served as the primary source of development for research approaches in medical anthropology. At the same time, the field has also drawn on other social-behavioral sciences for both methods and theory. The expanding focus on application of research findings and the use of community-based information in intervention programs is leading medical anthropologists into closer collaboration with other types of professionals and introducing other approaches to the collection, analysis, and interpretation of data. These encounters are giving rise to new approaches that develop as the result of the interaction between well-established anthropological approaches with those of public health, health services, and social action. The materials we have reviewed provide examples of some of these new directions, and we can expect to see others as the field matures.

16

Epidemiology and Medical Anthropology

William R. True

Epidemiology has established a place for itself in the health sciences by providing both perspectives and methods for documenting and measuring the occurrence of health phenomena. The field of epidemiology appears to have considerable influence in current health care policy debates because it addresses outcomes, social and financial configurations for providing care, and various constructions of the model of risk, whether in terms of social attributes or biological susceptibility. Early victories over an array of infectious diseases such as cholera, smallpox, polio, tuberculosis, and syphilis emboldened epidemiology to move into the study of more complex, multifactorial, chronic disease processes, where the range of inquiry is more encompassing and progress has been more elusive. However, resurgence of sexually transmitted diseases, tuberculosis, and childhood diseases thought under control has reminded public health officials that victories, no matter how significant, cannot be taken for granted.

In its focus on populations rather than individuals, epidemiology contrasts sharply with clinical medical practice. This is a disciplinary tension analogous to that between anthropology and psychology. By attempting to define populations and to assess risk and outcome as characteristics of that population, epidemiologists may share more with anthropologists than either realizes.

Similarly, although epidemiology is primarily a quantitative discipline, its areas of interest have required that qualitative perspectives be employed as well. Because epidemiology utilizes comparative methodologies for studying the spectrum of health and disease and includes a holistic perspective encompassing environmental attributes, biological parameters, human physical endowments, and social resources, epidemiology compares in breadth and range, if not in focus and application, with medical anthropology.

The perspectives of epidemiology offer a bridge between medical anthropology's traditional focus on the social and environmental aspects of disease etiology and the focus on classification, definition, and etiology of specific disorders more typically the domain of interest of biomedical colleagues. This chapter focuses on the contribution epidemiology can make to medical anthropology in the definition and specification of research questions. Likewise, anthropologists can enrich and deepen traditional epidemiological methodologies for understanding the relationship of behaviors, social settings, and disease outcomes.

Although the lesson of this chapter is what epidemiology has to teach anthropology, it does not provide a précis of specific epidemiological methods, which are well covered in a number of excellent textbooks reviewing the fundamental assumptions and methods of the field (Lilienfeld and Stolley 1994; Brownson, Remington, and Davis 1993; Hennekens and Buring 1987; Rothman 1986, now a decade old, but ever cited) and also a practical introduction and workbook of basic quantitative methods (Morton, Hebel, and McCarter 1990).

What has not been well developed in the literature is the potential for cross-fertilization in perspectives between the fields of epidemiology and anthropology. The relationship between epidemiology and anthropology has been the subject of treatments (Janes, Stall, and Gifford 1986; Rubenstein 1984; Rubenstein and Perloff 1986). While these anthropological commentaries emphasize the different methods of epidemiology and the nature of epidemiological data, anthropologists have not recognized that the roots of epidemiology place the field squarely in the anthropological tradition of understanding how the well-being of human beings is directly affected by their physical, social, and cultural environments. By not availing ourselves of epidemiological training or perspectives and by engaging in the all-too-familiar occupational hazard of talking to ourselves about the problems of other disciplines, we lose a valuable opportunity to move our discipline in exciting new directions.

A HISTORICAL VIEW OF EPIDEMIOLOGY AND MEDICAL ANTHROPOLOGY

Historically, epidemiology is rooted in the fundamental observation that disease does not occur randomly but in patterned ways. Epidemiology portrays the occurrence of disease and ascertains susceptibility to risk, viewed in the context of cultural and social processes, environmental attributes, and historical sequence. From the earliest formulations of epidemiology it was clear that understanding these patterns demanded comparative investigations of social and cultural contexts of both the afflicted and the nonafflicted. Early writings are now seen as establishing this precedent for the field, even though the authors were not formally identified as epidemiologists.

For example, Villerme documented in 1840 (reprinted in Buck et al. 1988a) the patterns of morbidity and mortality among textile workers in Amiens, France, and in so doing described the living conditions of the afflicted. While the effects of noxious working conditions, the human costs of child labor, and the growing burden of industrial pollution were becoming serious concerns, Villerme noted direct connections between such variables and particular categories of illness or causes of death. His work provides precedent for both social epidemiologists and medical anthropologists.

A classic early example of the development of social epidemiological perspectives is found with tuberculosis, as reviewed by Susser (1988). Rudolph Virchow, who seeded so many of our notions of social medicine, described tuberculosis as a "social disease." Later, however, after Robert Koch isolated the tubercle bacillus and established a new paradigm with the germ theory, thinking of the day came to focus on relationships between specific agents and diseases. We now understand that single factorial reasoning was not adequate to explain tuberculosis. Today, science again is required to include such non-microbial factors as family characteristics, health status, housing, and genetic susceptibility to the etiological equation, because single-factorial models are not sufficient to account for occurrence of an increasing number of disorders.

Historically, epidemiologists were among the first to note the pernicious health consequences of industrialization, occupational exploitation, and urbanization. These perspectives emerged from the search to explain why certain diseases tended to occur at higher rates in these new social settings. In terms of how we would now look at these early efforts, we would say that these early investigators were defining disorders and their correlated risks.

For example, Merchant (1980) has traced the history of coal workers' pneumoconiosis in terms of detailing the parallel history of establishing the dangerous aspects of the workers' environment and the tragically difficult task of translating that knowledge into political and regulatory action. These kinds of issues are familiar to anthropologists. Where epidemiologists go further than anthropologists is in defining, measuring, and analyzing the pathologies that are implicated and arraying these data in terms of assessment of comparative health status.

Given research goals of describing and discovering the etiology of disorders, epidemiologists characteristically use methods and analyze data differently from anthropologists. These differences have precipitated some tension between epidemiologists and anthropologists because of conflicting values about types of data and have led to accusations by anthropologists that epidemiology is guilty of "scientism" (Rubenstein 1984) and "rigor mortis" (Nations 1986). Traditionally, anthropologists have been critical about kinds of data employed by epidemiologists, asserting, for example, that epidemiological data "run a serious risk of being inaccurate by excluding a vital human element: the way people really approach illness and cope with death" (Nations 1986). Nations's specific example is a moving description of an infant's death in her area of research in northeast Brazil. While it is true that epidemiologists portray such vital events as birth, death, and morbidity in statistical form, which indeed does not permit the rich ethnographic texture Nations captured in her work, to assert the relative merit of one kind of datum over the other is to ignore that data serve specific purposes and that purposes can vary. It is ironic that Nations criticizes the epidemiologist's conception of infant mortality as missing much of the meaning of the event when, in fact, epidemiologists have long recognized infant mortality as the most sensitive indicator of the health of a population (Windom 1987).

Anthropological and epidemiological data have the potential of complementing each other when the contrasting ideas and methods are framed in terms of an appropriate research question. In its adherence to a specific research question, epidemiology seems to anthropologists to be limiting itself to the most superficial of data, while to epidemiologists, depth of data without adherence to principles of generalizability and without specification in terms of a particular question seems excessive and of limited utility. Yet in spite of these difficulties, there is much common ground for collaboration, and both medical anthropology and epidemiology may profit from increased shared perspectives. Indeed, many medical anthropologists are now receiving postdoctoral training in epidemiology (Johnson 1984). The two fields share a holistic view of the processes of disease and health, and this provides the basis for further collaboration.

MEDICAL ANTHROPOLOGIST AS EPIDEMIOLOGIST

Working as an epidemiologist in a department of community health in a school of public health, my academic life is similar to other academically appointed anthropologists. I also am appointed at our Department of Veterans Affairs Medical Center, where I am a funded investigator and in the psychiatry department of the school of medicine, where I participate in research and train residents. Like many of the anthropologists writing in the Society for Medical Anthropology column of the *Anthropology Newsletter,* I am spread among various affiliations and institutions. My teaching assignments are more epidemiological and public health than anthropological.

It is in planning and carrying out a research agenda that the contrasts and complementarities of the different disciplines are evident. Epidemiological research typically is conducted by multidisciplinary teams, which often include the divergent viewpoints of physicians, social scientists, biostatisticians, research methodologists, and administrators. Medical anthropologists today work in such interdisciplinary research teams to a much greater degree than anticipated in traditional anthropological training, which too often presumes that anthropologists will work alone in the field. The professional and personal skills necessary for anthropologists to accommodate to a team approach to research unfortunately are usually learned by trial and error on the job. Training in team formation is available, however, and would be an asset in graduate anthropology training for those aiming to work in efforts requiring many perspectives and disciplinary approaches. Excellent projects are more often derailed, in my experience, by issues around developing the overall team and allocating its tasks than around deficiencies in scientific expertise.

Epidemiological contributions on research teams are arrayed along formal lines: deciding on research design and analytical strategies, defining the outcome or dependent variable (usually a disorder of some type), and speculating about the etiological dimensions or risk conditions represented in the independent variables. Teams work through a committee format and meet regularly to make decisions about all matters pertaining to the project. In lively and searching team meetings, I often have been struck by how holistic, in an anthropological sense, these deliberations are. Participants speculate and explore many hypotheses as they attempt to resolve the puzzles presented in choosing and estimating the independent variables or in specifying and verifying the dependent variable outcome conditions or disorders.

Each participant represents his or her own primary interests and concerns, knowing that, in the end, the team must choose from among the emphases of the individual participants. This is necessary, because if each member of the team could include all the questions he or she personally prefers on a questionnaire, or do all the analyses of interest, accomplishing the basic shared goals would be impossible. What is shared in epidemiological investigations is that all components must have clear, measurable dimensions and have to be integrated into a coherent statement or statements comprising hypotheses. The participants, whatever their disciplines, must argue for the importance of their views and contributions while sharing the common focus of the primary research question.

In my experience, where epidemiology sharply differs from anthropology is in the emphasis on the full implications of the statement of the research question. Research questions point directly to research designs because certain designs answer particular questions. Questions about the nature and extent of a condition in a population suggest certain cross-sectional approaches. Questions about potential etiological factors suggest case control design approaches and, subsequently, the development of powerful prospective designs. Further, each of these designs has different requirements: in methods, procedures, financial demands, personnel requirements, and institutional support. Formal training in epidemiology focuses on analyzing alternative designs and strategies and weighing the attendant strengths and limitations of each.

Anthropologists tend to see such activities as characteristic of other fields, but training in epidemiological perspectives affords anthropologists the opportunity to structure their own inquiries better. Some anthropologists may want to make major contributions to epidemiological research. Both approaches are appropriate because epidemiology provides a model for asserting the role of anthropology in research on health and illness and provides a model for assessing the role of social and cultural factors in health and disease.

THE RESEARCH QUESTION

All scientists are concerned with the issue, ''What is the research question?'' Epidemiologists understand that the specification of the research question implies which of the specific research designs is most appropriate.

When I was trained in anthropology, we understood that research questions may be thought of as exploratory, hypothesis generating, or quite specific, yet although training in anthropology is increasingly sophisticated on this issue, epidemiologists do have a particular slant. Having defined a research design, epidemiologists understand that categories of data pertinent for answering research questions for one design may not be appropriate for another. Statistical considerations about what is needed in order to answer the question raise issues of sample size and statistical power. Scope of the effort to answer the research question thus leads to data quality questions, including reliability and validity, and of course budget requirements.

Although anthropologists propose research projects, specify research questions, and delineate research designs, epidemiologists and anthropologists seem to me to have very different notions of this process. A particular point of contention is the issue of data gathering. In epidemiological research meetings, the purpose and utility of each piece of datum is usually clear, given the design chosen. Additional potentially interesting avenues for data gathering often are ruled out early in research planning. The participants return again and again to the declared research questions. Anthropologists, on the other hand, tend to be less willing to eliminate a priori certain avenues of data gathering simply because they do not seem initially to contribute directly to answering the research question. For an anthropologist, the test of whether data-gathering techniques should be considered to assist in answering the research question is tempered by the thought that it is always prudent to gather more data and subsequently to modify the research question. Anthropologists do not want to preclude unanticipated results that may emerge. I recall faculty stories from the field during my graduate school days that the important findings were serendipitous, enabled by a flexible research approach.

The first edition of this book presented the imaginary conversation that follows. I considered deleting it in this revision but reconsidered because the fundamental differences in worldview are subtle and pervasive.

Epidemiologist: You folks write the most interesting stuff. Who would have imagined that you could have learned so much about those health practices no one else has ever heard of. I would never have thought even to ask the questions you report upon. Take a look at my questionnaire. The Office of Management and Budget would never have approved the questions you asked.

Anthropologist: That's a difference between us. I didn't have a questionnaire.

Epidemiologist: How did you know what to ask everybody? How were you sure you got the same information from everyone you talked to? Did you pretest your interview?

Anthropologist: I was looking at healing rituals. I found some practitioners and got to talk to their clients. I let them lead much of the interview.

Epidemiologist: So your study was a survey of a kind of healers. We call that a cross-sectional study.

Anthropologist: No, it wasn't a survey. I have no idea how many healers like these there are. I just talked to some of them—enough to see what they had in their minds. I wanted to know what their patients were looking for.

Epidemiologist: You don't know how many there are? But aren't the ones you talked to at least typical?

Anthropologist: In the sense that there are a lot more like them.

Epidemiologist: No, no. I mean typical in the sense that at least the ones you talked to are like the others you didn't talk to.

Anthropologist: I have no way of knowing that. There aren't any lists to start with and choose informants from. I can try to cover the area geographically, but we don't sample the way you do.

Epidemiologist: It's not just sampling. I know that I'm looking at a particular disorder. I can get a dozen physicians to agree with me on how to define it. Then I want to know a lot about risk. You seem to me to ask everything. What is your outcome variable? What exactly is it that you are trying to predict?

Anthropologist: You see, we ask different questions. I'm looking at range of behaviors and beliefs on the part of both the healer and the patient. I don't even call him a patient. And I probably couldn't get two physicians to agree with any of my categories.

Epidemiologist: When I read your work, I'm never sure exactly who you're talking about. So I'm to generalize to whom?

Anthropologist: Don't you see I'm trying to portray the range of beliefs and behaviors that are out there? That they are believed and acted upon is what matters. I can't put a statistic on that.

Epidemiologist: So what's your research question? What is the research design that you picked to answer it?

Anthropologist: I have a problem that I was trying to answer, but when you ask that question, you have something really specific in mind, right?

Epidemiologist: Yes, there are only a few basic designs. It depends on whether we are looking prospectively or retrospectively. We also do descriptive studies and experimental studies.

Anthropologist: I don't think they are relevant to what I'm looking at. But I'm curious. You see, anthropologists are always curious about unusual worldviews. So what are the different designs, and what are they good for?

Epidemiologist: Ah, this is at the heart of my business. I love talking about designs and research questions. Do you have an overhead projector?

We leave the medical anthropologist about to embark on a crash course in epidemiology. The notion that, for epidemiological questions, there is a defined array of research design options is foreign to anthropology. I refer here to those types that may be further defined under categories of cross-sectional, retrospective, or prospective designs. One theme of the above conversation is that anthropologists and epidemiologists warm up to different aspects of research endeavors and that there are ample opportunities for profound misunderstandings. When an anthropologist examines epidemiological data and finds rates, odds ratios, etiologic fractions, and complex standardization procedures, he or she may be intimidated by either the apparent quantitative rigor or the superficiality. The anthropologist may at the same time take solace in the fact that the data are sparse compared to the rich ethnographic information available after a year of intensive fieldwork.

Epidemiologists see in anthropological data important information about the range and depth of phenomena but ask about generalizability and want to know the specific research question that the data purport to answer. Epidemiologists think in terms of the total population, the study population, and the sample to be studied. The concept of normality and abnormality serves to differentiate the members of these populations into those that are affected and those that are not. Descriptive and analytical procedures may then be conducted in order to place the disorder into a complete, population-based context. Therefore epidemiology constitutes, with the clinical profile, biological characteristics, and pathology markers, an essential aspect of the description of a disorder.

The question of etiology raises another key issue for anthropologist. I have been asked by an anthropologist who had just heard a presentation about epidemiological views of response to trauma that was rich in quantitative graphics and terminology: "But is this kind of data better than a richly detailed case series such as a fieldworker in a clinic might gather?" The answer can be found in the theme of this chapter: it depends on the research question. The anthropologist in the clinic, documenting with thick description a problem seen in patients, is performing a role similar to that of clinicians' presenting case reports of their treatment experiences. This kind of information establishes the importance of a question by documenting that certain clinical patterns exist but cannot answer a question. No progress toward establishing etiology, or causal factors, can be made, however, until the case material is arrayed in terms of a research question, an appropriate research design is selected, and it is followed by an orderly execution of the design.

BASIC EPIDEMIOLOGICAL PERSPECTIVES

Normality-Abnormality

There are major underlying differences between anthropological and epidemiological perspectives. Perhaps first among these are conceptions of normality and abnormality. Typically, in epidemiological thinking, those being studied are sorted into two groups: those with and those without the condition under question. Something has to be amiss. The epidemiological questions have as a touchstone a "something" that needs to be defined and understood. Therefore, in epidemiological thinking, "normal" is thought of as "unaffected" or "noncase," and "abnormal" is thought of as "affected" or "case."

I would like to relate one of my own moments of enlightenment during my training as an epidemiologist as my "Aha!" experience, even though my naiveté at the time now makes me uncomfortable. I was fresh from anthropological training, steeped in ethnomedicine and sick roles, and indoctrinated into the blindnesses of Western medicine when I was taking a required year-long seminar in a major disease process—in my case, the epidemiology of coronary heart disease. The second class session appropriately dealt with anatomy and physiology, and the speaker, an anatomy professor, came to class carrying a dissecting tray, covered in a green cloth. After a dense but interesting lecture on the anatomy and physiology of the heart and its arteries, he turned to the tray. Upon uncovering it, I saw that it contained a human heart. He dissected it, and we studied its arterial structures.

My own heart was beating rapidly, as I was facing many issues well known to medical students who have to confront the human body in all sorts of permutations. But finally, the lesson of the class struck me. Those coronary arteries were really blocked, I believe the professor said approximately 80 percent. That very blockage was the dependent variable, the case definition, the abnormality that was in question. The rest of the course was to look at the medical, social, psychological, dietary, and familial factors that shed light on the development of those blockages, either by increasing the likelihood that those blockages would occur, and thereby become risk factors, or would diminish that likelihood, and become protective factors. Thereby, as we have learned, oat bran, negative family history, and exercise are "good," and excessive job stress, obesity, and cigarettes are "bad."

My thinking on outcomes changed that moment as I realized that my future research interests would be with colleagues with whom we would dissect different areas of interest to measure and analyze, trying always to retain a sense of the whole—whether that whole is the individual, the study sample, or the population from which both the individual and the sample were drawn.

Therefore, in epidemiological designs, the abnormality is called the outcome—the unhealthy condition. The outcome condition does not necessarily have to be a diagnosis, such as type of depression or diabetes. It does not have to be a structure as dramatic or obvious as those atherosclerotic plaques we observed. It may be a diagnostic sign (such as a blood chemistry value like cholesterol or high-density lipoprotein levels), a syndrome, or a symptom cluster (such as might be found in the example of coronary artery disease risk factors). The role of hypothesized etiologic factors in the disease process may be unclear or even of uncertain importance, and the purpose of the research may be to illuminate whether there is an etiological role for the outcome.

This epidemiological conceptualization of affected and unaffected was born out of the discipline's roots in infectious disease analysis and is now incorporated into some of the most useful and powerful of the epidemiologist's analytical tools such as case control studies and the concept of relative risk. The binary logic of normality and abnormality is also a traditional product of a clinician's approach to a patient as therapeutic decisions are made.

Now, we know that disease processes are not all-or-none phenomena and that case definition is a highly complex business. This has come about because the increasingly sophisticated detection of precursor states, subclinical manifestations of disease, presence of risk factors, and even positive family histories may justify defining a case or an abnormality even in the absence of frank clinical pathology. To epidemiologists, the notion of abnormality or case therefore does not necessarily imply a practitioner-defined case that would justify specific treatment. It is a concept that alludes to a replicable (reliable) definition of a state of health that can be the focus of a defined research question, to be operationalized and tested. A current example is the case of an HIV-positive individual, with no clinical symptoms, with a probability of progressing to AIDS over a highly variable period of time.

It is important to detail several common ways to define abnormality and the attendant difficulties with each. The issue is complex because the definition of abnormality suggests different kinds of reality. Following an effective and succinct review of conventional approaches (Rose and Barker 1978), I will characterize these as statistical, clinical, prognostic, and operational. An excellent recent review of chronic disease epidemiology includes reviews of case definitions for a number of chronic diseases of current epidemiological interest (Brownson et al. 1993). The point of presenting these different perceptions of the problems of defining normality and abnormality is to show that each may be appropriate for different purposes. The researcher must make these definitions in terms of the research question motivating the inquiry.

Using statistical criteria, standardized laboratory practice often defines normal as within two standard deviations of the mean value, thereby fixing abnormal scores as comprising approximately 5 percent of each stratum. Such an approach does not establish the content for such a definition but specifies the tails of the distribution as defining a case. Another application of the statistical approach is to define an arbitrary score as a case—for example, all individuals in the top quartile of a symptom scale. This reasoning describes the definition of standard normal, which is used in a range of diagnostic procedures.

The definition of cases, as contrasted with statistical findings, often provides research teams with much to talk about. The biostatisticians on a team may find that there is a statistically significant difference between groups of cases and controls. Following the example of the last paragraph, this difference may be one of 5 millimeters of mercury on systolic blood pressure. The biostatisticians say, "This is significant," meaning that there is less than a 5 percent (or 1 percent) chance of the findings' occurring by chance. "But," the clinicians on the team reply, "that isn't a clinically important difference," meaning that the magnitude observed would not be enough to begin a treatment course or change one already in place. "However," the dieticians, who have defined a pressure-lowering dietary intervention, may interject, "that may translate into a much lower incidence of strokes in the study group." What is "significant," "clinical," or "important" is what research team members spend much time defining and interpreting.

The conception of prognostic cases and noncases is based on probabilistic assumptions about the likelihood of developing a disorder based on an aspect of current health status. Consequently this approach is quite sensitive to ongoing research, which constantly redefines these thresholds. For example, clinicians used to consider a normal systolic blood pressure as one's age plus 100. Thus, a fifty-year-old man with a systolic blood pressure of 150 would have been considered both asymptomatic and normal. Following the well-known Veterans Administration clinical trial on borderline hypertension (Veterans Administration 1970), the risks of even slightly elevated blood pressures became known, and now the conception of normal blood pressure is one that is clinically normal and does not increase with age.

The final perspective is the operational one. The referent is to the clinician as one who makes decisions about when to treat and how to treat. Thus, regardless of the research criteria for defining a particular disorder, the thresholds for treatment may be different. For example, in a research project, borderline hypertension may be defined as 140 millimeters of mercury, but the threshold for treatment—the clinicians' operational definition—may be 150.

These ideas are summarized by physicians writing about clinical epidemiology (Fletcher, Fletcher, and Wagner 1982) to define abnormality in three ways: as unusual, as associated with disease, and as treatable. These authors discuss the utility and limitations of the clinician's available quantitative data for arriving at case definitions. Using data for defining criteria raises issues of validity (accuracy) and reliability (repeatability), and sources of variation in observation. The message from these sophisticated treatments of the conceptions of normality and abnormality is that the distinction can be made but must be done with thought and care, and in terms of the research question at hand. Clearly, decisions using any of the approaches would not likely agree with the others.

I have pointed out that there are factors implicated in the etiology of outcomes or abnormal conditions. I have called these *risk factors;* in the language of research designs, they are labeled *independent variables,* and to epidemiologists they are captured in the term *exposure.* Thus, smoking cigarettes is the risk factor, or exposure, associated with the development of lung cancer. A measured level of smoking, operationalized, for example, as lifetime "pack-years," therefore can be entered into analysis as an independent exposure variable.

These notions about normality and abnormality contrast sharply with the anthropological doctrine of cultural relativity, which was the lodestar for my own training in anthropology. This is surely the minimal message from anthropology that most faculty would agree must emerge from the introductory course. Therefore most anthropologists are uncomfortable with the discussion about abnormality. Yet there is nothing comparable in anthropology to the occluded artery, which I discovered in my epidemiology seminar. We as anthropologists are trained to see what is before us as a natural sample, explicable in its own terms. Once we would have said the system was functional. We as anthropologists are not to judge, not to categorize into such notions, so foreign to the emic point of view, as normal or abnormal, and especially for our own purposes as inquiring scientists.

Causation

Epidemiologists, in focusing on risk and exposure, are using terminology and concepts that focus on etiology or cause. Thus in addressing the scientific and philosophical issue of causation, epidemiologists also are in territory that is typically not comfortable ground for anthropologists. Epidemiologists are asking about the contribution to developing a health outcome of certain risks or exposures.

The issue of how epidemiologists view cause is well summarized in a recent textbook of epidemiology (Lilienfeld and Stolley 1994:255–268) and in Rothman (1988). Mausner and Kramer (1985:185–91) discussed the criteria for causation with reference to the evidence for the relationship between cigarette smoking and lung cancer, a presentation I will summarize here.

The first criterion for ascertaining causation is evaluating the *strength of the association* between the hypothesized causal factor and the disease. Technically, this is calculated as the ratio of the disease rates for two groups: those with and those without the causal factor. This ratio is called the relative risk, and high ratios indicate strong strength of association. The relative risk can be directly calculated from a prospective or cohort study. With reference to smoking and cancer, Mausner and Kramer cite two studies that report relative risks for cancer in heavy smokers of twenty to one and one study that reports forty to one relative risks.

The second criterion, *dose-response relationship,* is related to the first, referring specifically to whether the increasing gradient of exposure is related to an increase in disease outcome. For example, the increase in risk for lung cancer increases from a 4.4-fold greater risk of mortality at fewer than ten cigarettes per day to a 43.7-fold increased risk at forty cigarettes or more per day (Mausner and Kramer 1985:188).

Consistency of the association refers to the fact that if a causal relationship is present, it will be replicated in different settings, with different populations, and with different study methods. With tobacco, replications have been conducted, with consistent findings in different countries, with study populations of contrasting demographic characteristics, and with both retrospective and prospective designs.

A claim of causation requires evidence of *temporal association* between exposure and outcome. While obvious, this observation cannot be made in cross-sectional studies or even in retrospective case control studies, when an interview is administered to a sample at a single point in time. Individual reconstruction of history may not be accurate, and cross-sectional studies cannot claim findings about temporality. In a case control study, the subject is recalling earlier exposures, but establishing the timing of specific exposures in terms of the etiological history is not possible. Evidence for tobacco is indicated by studies that have demonstrated the onset of disease after long exposure and decreased mortality following longer periods of time of abstinence for those who have stopped smoking. These determinations can only be made in prospective or cohort studies.

The next criterion, *specificity of the association,* has caused important scientific debate. Ideally, this criterion would hold that there is always a relationship between an exposure and the outcome. Rarely, in industrial chemical exposures, such as chloracne following exposure to dioxin, can this association can be asserted. Usually, however, an exposure or exposures can lead to more than one outcome, and further, disease causality has traditionally postulated that the argument that a single cause is both necessary and sufficient to precipitate a particular disease outcome may be applicable to only a very few disease processes. In the case of smoking and lung cancer, this criterion has been the basis for much of the ongoing controversy between the Tobacco Institute and the epidemiological community. The tobacco interests point out that the claims for disease causation are negated by the fact that a multitude of diseases are attributed to tobacco. The epidemiologists respond that a case for each can be made with epidemiological logic. Another argument of the Tobacco Institute is that most smokers do not develop lung cancer and that some cases of disease occur in nonsmokers. Both statements are true. Epidemiologists have responded that disease processes are embedded in a multifactorial web of causation where the single factor of tobacco exposure is neither necessary nor sufficient to explain all cases of lung cancer. Still, they argue, the evidence is overwhelming for a causal relationship. Anthropologists should be aware of an important critique of the epidemiologists' traditional approach to multifactorial sources of disease causation. Nancy Krieger (1994) has asked of the "web of causation" the important question: "Has anyone seen the spider?" Krieger has observed that "the web" has caused modern epidemiology to become mainly focused on methodological issues, to the exclusion of thinking about fundamental theories of disease causation, which would encompass models including consideration of social determinants of disease.

The final criterion specifies that the postulated association be *biologically plausible,* or coherent with existing understanding information. This point does not require that the biological link be proved or specified, only that it be plausible. Thus, chronic smoking can be understood as a continual irritant to the lung, the organ receiving the smoke, and the link to pulmonary pathology is plausible.

Figure 16.1
The Fundamental Epidemiological 2 × 2 Table

Outcome/disorder

	Case	Noncase	
Exposed	a	b	a + b
Not exposed	c	d	c + d
	a + c	b + d	

EPIDEMIOLOGISTS' TOOL KIT

Observational Research Designs

Observational designs are discussed here, as distinguished from experimental designs, including clinical trials, which are of less relevance to anthropologists and are described elsewhere (Lilienfeld and Stolley 1994). An excellent narrative text reviews the important issues in observational studies, without the computational intensity so characteristic of modern epidemiology (Kelsey, Thompson, and Evans 1986). Several issues concerning observational designs already discussed are embodied in Figure 16.1, a traditional epidemiological 2 × 2 table. First, the idea of normality-abnormality is portrayed in the column heads of "case" and "noncase." Like it or not, the disorder-disease is either present or absent. The definition is crucial, much debated, and imperfectly operationalized at times, thereby creating errors of misclassification. Similarly, definitions of "exposure" and "nonexposure" are specifically defined according to criteria explicated by the investigator. Recall that exposures may be obvious toxins or dangerous substances, risk factors, comorbid conditions, or the like. Thus, the basic epidemiological question is what kinds of noxious things (conditions or exposures) are associated with causing sick outcomes (diseases or precursor states). Upon establishing correlation, may the relationship further be postulated to be causal?

The second idea found in the figure concerns the crucial criterion of temporality for arguing for a causative influence. A research design provides more conclusive proof of causation when an exposure, or "cause," is shown to be demonstrably both correlated with the outcome and shown to precede it in timing. Prospective studies therefore are the most convincing because they ascertain exposure in disease-free individuals and provide for the passage of time to observe the development of disease outcomes, thereby demonstrating temporality. Retrospective studies ascertain the presence or absence of disease in cases and noncases and assess the presence or absence of risk factors. Thus, correlation with risk factors can be established, but the absence of temporal information

Table 16.1
Cell Definitions

Cell	Prospective	Retrospective
A	Exposed/develops disease	Diseased (case) with exposure
B	Exposed and does not develop disease	Not diseased (control)
C	Nonexposed and develops disease	Diseased (case) without exposure
D	Not exposed and does not develop disease	Not diseased (control) without exposure

limits conclusions about causality. This is because in a retrospective study, one cannot know whether the outcome followed the exposure.

The time perspective is conveyed in Figure 16.1 by alternating one's perspective from viewing the figure either from the left to the right or the top to the bottom. First, viewing it from the top, we are conditioning on disorder or disease, which will be defined as either present or absent. Therefore a sample of affected persons will be matched with a group of unaffected controls, and a retrospective examination will be conducted among these cases and controls to determine what exposures might be associated with the presence of the disease state. This retrospective study, also called a case control study, provides suggestive leads for causative influences, may lead to more expensive and conclusive prospective studies, and is a model of investigation that is quite frequently reported in medical and epidemiological scientific literature.

Second, viewing the figure from the left, we are conditioning on exposure, whether present or absent. This means that we have done the preliminary investigation to determine who among our study subjects can be counted on during the study to be either exposed or not exposed to a putative causal agent. An example will be persons defined as smokers or nonsmokers or factory workers who either are or are not in a place where they will be exposed to vinyl chloride. The key then is to follow an identified cohort in a prospective manner in order to determine who develops the outcome or health state of interest. This is the fundamental idea of a cohort, or prospective study. The study conceptually begins at a point in time and continues into the future. Thereby, beginning on the left side of the figure, we know the exposure status of the study subjects and that all subjects are free of the disease or disorder at the beginning of the period of observation. The definitions, portrayed in Table 16.1 define who is in each cell according to whether the design is retrospective or prospective.

Note that cells A and D conform to the logic that the epidemiological approach is in fact testing. Thus, in a perfect world, which ran according to immutable epidemiological logic, the diseased would all be exposed (cell A) and the healthy would be not exposed (cell D). Here, all smokers would become ill, and those with good, healthy habits are forever protected from infirmity. Alas, such a gratifying distribution is rarely seen. Rather, as epidemiologists note, the key data are located in the off-diagonals, that is, cells B and C, which provide the data to establish the appropriate measurement of risk that can be attributed to the factor or exposure. The intricacies of such calculations are best studied in the epidemiological texts cited at the beginning of the chapter. I will now discuss some further details about these basic epidemiological research designs. First I will address retrospective, or case control studies.

Case Control Designs

Case control designs are found so frequently in the literature because of their inherent strengths. They require identified cases, appropriate controls, and a method for ascertaining a history of pertinent information, including exposure history. Therefore they can be relatively small scale, low cost, easily managed in many clinical settings, and quite informative in terms of informing future research. Typically a series of case control studies provides a rationale for tackling a more expensive and logistically difficult prospective study. Case control designs address the particular issue of trying to ascertain the etiology of rare conditions where normal sampling procedures would be too inefficient to conduct a study. Also, the latency of disease onset often makes a prospective study an interminable and excessively expensive venture (Greenberg and Ibrahim 1985; Schlesselman 1982). In this design, a group of people who has the outcome or condition of interest (cases) is defined and might be recruited from a clinic or hospital population on the basis of a screening technique applied to a given at-risk group or an entire community, or from listing on a register of one kind or another. These cases are compared with controls: individuals who are similar but assuredly free of the pathological condition being investigated. Case control designs may be matched or unmatched with controls. Who would be appropriate controls? Often these decisions are based on categorical criteria: age within a bracket, sex, some rough economic status indicator, or other similar marker. Sometimes controls are defined as those in the same patient lists as the cases, or neighbors. Fallacies through incorrect identification of controls are the most difficult issue of designing case control studies.

The key component of the design is a systematic elicitation of past history, exposures, experiences, or treatments from both cases and controls. The sensitivity and care required for these elicitations will be familiar to anthropologists, whose techniques might add much to common methods used, which are questionnaires or highly structured interviews. These different histories are then systematically compared to detect differences in any of a multitude of exposures that might distinguish cases from controls. In the references cited above, the multiple subtleties and complications of the design are discussed.

The most critical problem with case control studies is selective recall. The design requires that comparable histories be elicited from cases and controls. Imagine the complication in a case control study of birth defects, however. When the mother of an affected child (a case) is interviewed and asked to search her memory for some drink, drug, or experience that might account for a birth defect in her child, she will likely be especially vigilant in trying to remember. This woman's control, who might be down the hall of the hospital enjoying her new, healthy baby, would not feel the same urgency to remember every glass of wine, use of prescriptions or over-the-counter medication, or every unusual event or circumstance.

Cohort Designs

The second broad category of epidemiological study begins with healthy people who are differentially exposed to a suspected etiological factor. Whether or not exposures are noxious in one way or another is the specific question for study. Cohort studies are a logical follow-up to case control studies. A case control study may discover that the cases showing a disorder share a common factor, as Doll and Hill (1950) found with smoking and lung cancer. Although the link may be biologically plausible, as discussed above in the context of causation, the case control method shows only the correlation of the outcome and the supposed exposure. The sequence of exposure to outcome can be shown only in a cohort study, which follows exposed and nonexposed cohorts over time, in a type of natural experiment to see if the exposed group, in fact, develops higher levels of disorder. Doll and Hill (1964) followed up their case control study with a cohort study, confirming their original observation.

Epidemiologists see these designs in terms of the differences in the logistical requirements they demand. The case control study can be fast and inexpensive, requiring relatively few subjects and the gathering of limited data, and utilizing relatively straightforward analytical techniques. In contrast, a cohort study is a long-term project, usually of high cost, and characterized by problems in minimizing attrition (dropouts) from the study, usually accomplished only by great expenditure of effort to keep in touch with study subjects.

What do these observations about the two basic kinds of epidemiological research designs say to medical anthropologists? The basic message from discussing research questions and research design is that hypotheses about antecedents and sequelae can be addressed. For example, anthropologists who track a community or group over many years are conforming to one of the attributes of a cohort study. Whether the full attributes of a cohort may be of use to an anthropologist would depend on the nature of the question and whether definition issues around exposure and outcome would contribute to answering that question. Topics of interest to follow-up must, of course, be assessed at baseline, and methods for collecting and analyzing later data must be organized at the beginning.

What is essential in either of the two basic research designs is a defined condition, disorder or disease, and a defined, specified exposure. Epidemiological research designs focus on studying disorders and exposures in systematic and replicable ways. A priori conceptions of what may be abnormal as case definitions are made do not flow easily from the tongues of medical anthropologists, who may be more comfortable conducting a study with the goal of discovering the natural categories of abnormality as the subjects themselves portray them. Medical anthropologists have continuously pointed out that illness as it is experienced by those afflicted may not conform to the categories of those doing the treating. In an epidemiological design, there must be agreement about what is the condition of interest. In whatever design is employed, epidemiologists are concerned that the case definition is repeatable or replicable when in the hands of different investigators, even in different research settings. It is crucial that the definitions be consistently applied by both participants and researchers. Analyses of such reliability may seem tedious, but these efforts should seem familiar to anthropologists who constantly ask if their categories have utility in other, usually cross-cultural, settings.

The next question asked by epidemiologists is: Are the categories accurate or valid? Do they reflect field or clinical reality? The issue of validity is a crucial one for all scientists, but for epidemiologists the definitions are the basis for specifying the outcome or dependent variable and therefore are the keys to understanding the different research designs. The concept of validity has become even more complex as the nosological coding schemes, such as the *Diagnostic and Statistical Manual* (American Psychiatric Association 1980, 1987, 1994), have become increasingly concrete in terms of the kinds and numbers of specific criteria determined to be necessary for the diagnosing of certain mental and emotional disorders.

Measures of Association

The essential task of epidemiology is comparison, exemplified by comparing the risks for lung cancer for smokers versus nonsmokers. Therefore a crucial item of the epidemiologist's took kit is the measure of association: a quantitative description of the relationship between the risk factor and the disease outcome. The two most frequently reported measures of association are simple relative risks and odds ratios. Relative risks are reported for a cohort study, and odds ratios are reported for a case control study. Although the interpretation of each is quite similar, the two measures of association are calculated differently.

Recall that in a prospective study, cohorts are identified by whether they are exposed to a risk of interest. The task of the cohort study is to observe the development of new cases, or incident cases, in each of the cohorts. The calculation of the incidence rate characterizes the association between exposure and outcome for each cohort. The incidence rate is calculated by dividing the number of cases over the number of persons at risk during the period of observation times a constant for a given period of time.

In a retrospective, or case control, study, there is no opportunity to observe incident cases, because the design compares cases with noncases for exposure history. Nevertheless, if certain assumptions are met, the case control design may yield an estimate of the relative risk, called an odds ratio. The necessary assumptions are, first, that the disease in question have a low prevalence in the population, and, second, that controls in the study are representative of controls in the population and that cases in the study are representative of cases in the population. Technical details of case control studies are addressed in Schlesselman's definitive volume (1982). The calculation of the odds ratio as an estimate of the relative risk is accomplished by the cross-product of the cells in Figure 16.1 of ad/bc, based on a theoretical insight (Cornfield 1951), explicated thoroughly in a sophisticated text (Kahn and Sempos 1989).

The Rate

The fundamental measurement for relating and describing occurrence of disease is the ratio of affected cases to the total population at risk or the rate. The concept of the rate is a deceptively simple one. A rate consists of three parts. With no more complexity than that encountered in high school algebra, the basic rate consists of a numerator, a denominator, a standard constant (such as per 1,000) to yield comparability, and a designation of time. For example, the infant mortality rate for the United States for 1989 is 10.0 per 1000 per year (Children's Defense Fund 1991). Therefore, the form of a rate is:

$$\frac{\text{Event or condition of interest}}{\text{Population at risk}} \times \text{standard factor} \times \text{time.}$$

The numerator represents the case and refers back to the discussion of abnormality. Thus, as we saw, there are a number of bases for defining a case—statistical, clinical, prognostic, or operational. These criteria are embedded in the concept of the "natural history of disease," which describes how disease processes move through stages (see Mausner and Kramer 1985:6–9).

First among these is the stage of susceptibility, where disease is not present, but fertile soil for the development of disorder is present. These factors may include malnutrition, high cholesterol levels, or maladaptive living circumstances. Next is the stage of presymptomatic disease, where atherosclerotic plaques may mark the onset of coronary artery disease but without any symptoms of the disorder. The onset of clinical disease may mark various functional levels of health, from no limitations to complete bed rest. Finally, for some there is the stage of disability that marks a change to life under altered conditions. The point is that caseness may be defined at any point in the natural history of disease, depending on the nature of the research question. This definition will reflect issues of definition in the concept of abnormality.

Corresponding to issues in defining the numerator are those pertaining to the denominator. The denominator is so important to epidemiologists, and controversies about it occur so often, that there is a term shared among practitioners: the *denominator problem*. The issue is one of definition. If the numerator consists of cases, then the denominator must consist of all those at risk of being cases. Thus the denominator consists of the population at risk. Mistakenly defining the population at risk can modify rates and change the description being presented.

I will present an example from literature about adolescent pregnancy addressing the controversy about the effectiveness of the increased availability of contraceptives for lowering teen pregnancy rates. A fundamental issue is what has been the trend over time in the adolescent pregnancy rates. Alan Guttmacher Institute (1994) presents data showing two trends in rates: an increasing rate (that calculated for all women ages fifteen through nineteen), which ranges from 95 per 1,000 in 1972 to 117 per 1,000 in 1990, and a decreasing rate (that calculated for all sexually active women), which ranges from 254 per 1,000 in 1972 to 207 per 1,000 in 1990.

Those uncomfortable with providing contraceptives to adolescents have been able to cite the increasing pregnancy rates as evidence that contraceptive programs are not working. But there is a denominator problem because the rate for all adolescent women obscures the fact that the proportion of sexually active adolescents has increased substantially over the same period of time. That is, out of 1,000 adolescent women in 1972 and 1,000 in 1990, there are more exposed to the risk of pregnancy in 1990. When recalculated with sexually active adolescent women as the denominator, the trend reverses. The denominator problem stems from the fact that not all women age fifteen through nineteen were at risk of being in the numerator (being pregnant). When the denominator is changed to those actually at risk of pregnancy, those who are sexually active, the rate is dropping, and a policy issue would then turn to defining how the declining rate could be reduced further (Flick n.d.) Thus, a technical epidemiological principle can be seen to have considerable policy impact.

There are a number of important rates, which are routinely defined in epidemiology texts (Hennekens and Buring 1987:54–98). Most epidemiologists would agree that the most sensitive and most important rate for indicating the overall health of population is the infant mortality rate, which I will use to illustrate the terminology given above. The infant mortality rate is calculated as follows:

$$\frac{\text{Number of deaths of children less than 1 year of age in that year}}{\text{Number of live births in that year}} \times 1{,}000 \text{ per year,}$$

Obviously, such a rate is more accurate for a society that has complete reporting of vital events than a developing country without complete data. Still, in spite of the problems of complete and accurate reporting, there is little ambiguity about a mortal event, or age. I am claiming that there is little difficulty in defining the outcome, or establishing the age, even if these data do not end up properly recorded for retrieval. Similarly, the problem for the denominator is tallying the number of births, not identifying whether a birth has occurred. With the increasing utilization of home deliveries and other nonstandard delivery of obstetrical services, the recording of births has moved beyond hospital delivery rooms. Controversy about legal status of aliens and the existence of support groups for those at risk may cause delay in reporting vital events, or perhaps missed events altogether. Therefore, there may be a basis for research focused on basic principles of descriptive epidemiology.

These examples are intended to illustrate the kind of reasoning that epidemiologists use when examining data. I have emphasized rates in the seminar I teach about epidemiology. The students come to see that the apparent obvious simplicity of the rate conceals much subtlety and sophistication in presenting data and describing reality.

The Centers for Disease Control (CDC)

It may seem odd to include a governmental agency as an item in the anthropologist's tool kit. However, the CDC has made some important innovations to field public health workers and epidemiologists that are pertinent to anthropologists interested in the field. First, the CDC has developed a computer program, Epi Info, now in Version 6. This versatile package includes modules for epidemiological analysis and calculation, data entry and management, word processing, and questionnaire development. Screens may be brought up that perform all standard epidemiological calculations. Online questionnaire administration automatically creates a database for analysis. This package is in wide use in public health departments and is readily available.[1] A second tool developed by the CDC is the WONDER/PC (Friede, Reid, and O'Carroll 1993; Friede, Reid, and Ory 1993) electronic link, which enables public health professionals to communicate with each other and with CDC. Interested users may obtain an account number and establish modem connection with CDC via an 800 line, access and download CDC data bases, transmit data, maintain e-mail, and join user groups.

CONCLUSIONS: HOLISM AND EPIDEMIOLOGY

I have argued that there are shared grounds for collaboration between epidemiologists and anthropologists. As a field of science epidemiology bridges between what are usually biologically and clinically oriented outcomes and a range of etiological factors associated with the development of those outcomes. As etiological factors may encompass many candidate variables, social scientists are often involved in the research endeavor. Epidemiology embodies a set of methods and approaches for answering questions concerning the distribution of disease. The field systematically approaches causation while drawing widely from a range of disciplines through the integrative mechanism of focused research questions. Therefore, the field operationalizes the concept of holism in an instructive and powerful way.

My own anthropological training emphasized anthropology as a holistic science, and therefore we studied the traditional four fields. Epidemiology has seemed a way to carry out some of the holistic research goals of anthropology. In thinking about outcomes, and physical illness and health states, epidemiology clearly has shared ground with physical anthropology, including considerations of genetics, biological processes, and measurement. Epidemiology shares interests with social and cultural anthropology when considering risk factors, exposures that encompass environmental dimensions, and variables concerning work and family: the whole constellation of concerns that define human settings.

Epidemiologists seem little concerned with matters that would draw from linguistics and archaeology. However, diagnostic schemes, such as the *Diagnostic and Statistical Manual,* embody nuances of nosology and discrimination among similar disorders that invites linguistic analysis. Inquiries in epidemiology would be enriched by a historical, archaeological view, particularly in the area of environmental issues. I see areas where there is now much cross-fertilization and areas where there are potential mutual contributions.

Epidemiology, while defined as a discipline only quite recently, provides explanations for health phenomena that have presented a range of presumed etiology from moral turpitude (tuberculosis) to contagion associated with poverty (pellagra). Now, in a time when the ills of humanity are increasingly chronic and the etiologies are understood to be of extreme multifactorial complexity, any cross-fertilization of these two fields may contribute new perspectives and approaches.

Anthropologists need to judge work by the questions that are asked, not by the methods used. I have heard the criticism, "But that is not anthropology," when the research question at hand in fact posed a coordinated inquiry about social and biological factors involved in an outcome of considerable impact. I suspect what was meant by the statement was, "But the methods employed are not those traditionally used by anthropologists." By shifting emphasis to the questions, not the methods, we will be able to define unique anthropological contributions to a wide range of human concerns where we will interact with colleagues who will teach us new perspectives and involve ourselves with other disciplines that will enrich our science and widen the scope of our endeavors.

NOTE

1. Information about Epi Info is available from USD, Inc., 2075-A West Park Place, Stone Mountain, GA 30087.

Part V

Policy and Advocacy

17

Bioethics in Anthropology: Perspectives on Culture, Medicine, and Morality

Patricia A. Marshall and Barbara A. Koenig

Scientific advances throughout the twentieth century have been driven by the promise of technology to ameliorate sickness, cure disease, and lengthen and improve the quality of life. The dramatic impact of medical innovation stimulates and reinforces an ethos of scientific progress. Although there continues to be enthusiasm for new developments in health care, there is growing recognition of the moral conundrums that accompany most medical achievements. Paradoxically, consumers of health care in the industrialized First World, particularly in the United States, have expressed concern about two issues that appear contradictory. On the one hand, individuals want and expect to have access to sophisticated medical therapies, and they are troubled about potential limits on the availability of services because of the need for fiscal restraint. On the other hand, many patients and their families are seriously concerned about being kept alive indefinitely by life-support machines. Thus, the media celebrate the latest miracles in medical science—breakthroughs in cancer research, genetic testing, or reproductive technology—and simultaneously report on state referendums to legalize physician-assisted suicide. It is within this historical climate of medical promise and human suffering that the field of bioethics has evolved.

This review essay explores the relationship between anthropology and bioethics.[1] We give special attention to the theoretical foundations and methodological practices of each field in order to demonstrate the great potential for full collaboration, while also documenting barriers to shared work. In reviewing the intellectual connections between anthropology and the evolving discipline of bioethics it is important to make our position clear. First and foremost, we are medical anthropologists. Neither of us comfortably adopts the title ''bioethicist,'' although we hold positions in bioethics programs in American medical centers and thus gain part of our identity through involvement with the bioethics community. Furthermore, we are both committed to a full engagement between anthropology and clinical medical practice. Ethics consultations and service on ethics committees form part of our daily work. We are not content simply to sit back and offer a cultural and historical critique of practice, leaving the work of better care to others.

As medical anthropologists working in bioethics, we toil in environments where we are constantly uncomfortable, spending a good part of every day translating ourselves and our anthropological worldview, which always appears upside-down to our colleagues in biomedical disciplines and in philosophy and the law, the dominant discourses within professional bioethics. The bottom-up approach of cultural interpretation, situating the moral dimensions of care in local ethical practices, is antithetical to the universalizing discourses of both basic science—which assumes that scientific rules and principles can be applied successfully to human bodies in all times and places—and to the universalizing discourse of the most dominant traditions in philosophy (although currently less hegemonic)—which define a good ethical theory as one that can produce "objective" results, an "ideal observer" approach that yields rational standards by which to judge cultures, irrespective of their history or locality.

In a detailed review of the assumptions and theoretical foundations of bioethics, Arthur Kleinman (1995) recently offered a critical analysis of the new field. His critique—which focuses on the thinness of bioethics accounts, the failure to account for the lived experience of illness, suffering, and death—reveals medical anthropology's potential to transform bioethics. We are in full agreement with Kleinman's vision of how an anthropological approach can expand the limitations of conventional bioethics perspectives through cultural analysis of moral conflicts located within unique local worlds. A primary goal of this chapter is to explore the full range of anthropological contributions, both theoretical and methodological.

THE EVOLVING FIELD OF BIOETHICS

The terms *medical ethics* and *bioethics* are often used interchangeably; however, following Fabrega's lead (1990b) we prefer to distinguish between them in a way that accords medical ethics a broader applicability cross-culturally. Our use of the terms suggests a frame of inquiry that runs parallel to the concerns of medical anthropology. Thus, we believe that the subject of medical ethics, in its broadest articulation, is the cultural construction of morality, particularly as manifested in beliefs and behavior about health, illness, and healing practices. This expansive definition—and specifically the focus on the cultural construction of medical morality—has not been the conventional understanding of medical ethics by professionals in the field of bioethics. Nevertheless, as anthropologists, we maintain that the purview of medical ethics across cultures includes the lived experience of human suffering in the context of disease, the moral discourse of healers and patients, the development and use of healing modalities, the professional organization of practitioners, and the social and economic regulation of medical environments.

The term *bioethics* refers more specifically to moral problems associated with the development and application of Western biomedical technology.[2] Fox and Swazey underscore the decidedly American orientation of bioethics: "Bioethics is the neologism coined in this country in the 1960s to refer to the rise of professional and public interest in moral, social, and religious issues connected with the 'new biology' and medicine and to the emergence of an interdisciplinary field of inquiry and action concerned with these issues" (1984:336). Indeed, Fox emphasizes the "Americanness" of bioethics, suggesting that the prevailing ethos of bioethics exemplifies the importance given to the "value-complex of individualism" in the United States (1990:206).

Since its inception, the interests of bioethicists (who came primarily from the fields of jurisprudence, moral and political philosophy, and theological ethics) have paralleled advances in basic biomedical science and clinical research.[3] Innovative technologies in organ transplantation and concerns about abuses in human subject experimentation were important issues as bioethics emerged as a unique field. Although many medically significant events occurred during the 1960s and early 1970s, two incidents proved to be particularly influential in determining the direction of bioethics. First, the transplantation of a human heart into a person with terminal cardiac disease in 1967 focused concerns on definitions of death, the meaning of personhood, and the allocation of scarce medical resources in heroic efforts to prolong life. Second, human subject abuses were reported. In a seminal paper published in 1966 in the *New England Journal of Medicine,* Henry Beecher critiqued a series of scientific studies that involved deceit, coercion, or excessive risk to research subjects. In 1972, the Tuskegee, Alabama, research scandal was revealed to the public: experiments conducted by the U.S. Public Health Service over several decades to examine the natural course of syphilis had used low-income African-American subjects who were unaware of the purposes of the research and were not offered treatment when it was developed (Jones 1981). Response to reports of these abuses prompted the establishment of the National Commission for the Protection of Human Subjects of Biomedical and Behavior Research. An important objective of the commission was to develop policies and guidelines for ethical research. In 1978, the commission authored the *Belmont Report,* articulating philosophical principles that undergird investigations involving human subjects. This document has had significant influence on the conceptualization of problems in medical research. The regulation of clinical research is an important thread in the development of bioethics as a specialized discipline (see Rothman 1991).

In addition to human experimentation and organ transplantation, problematic questions about withholding or withdrawing life-sustaining treatment were important early concerns in bioethics and have continued to challenge ethicists. For example, in 1978, Ramsey published his classic work examining ethical quandaries at the "edges of life"; in 1981 and 1983, the President's Commission for the Study of Ethical Problems in Medicine and Biomedical and Behavioral Research devoted two volumes to end-of-life issues. Today there is an extensive literature available on medical interventions and end-of-life decision making, particularly the use of advance directives for medical care (Teno, Hill, and O'Conner 1994; Emanuel et al. 1995), the definition of medically futile treatment (Schneiderman and Jecker 1995; Miles 1992), and euthanasia (Battin 1994; Thomasma and Graber 1990).

Reproductive technologies such as in vitro fertilization and surrogate motherhood have also been the focus of ongoing debates in bioethics (Lauritzen 1993). Bioethicists are concerned about the implications of developments in genetic research and their applications in patient care (Robertson 1994; Frankel and Teich 1994). Additionally, there is considerable discussion of the rising cost of health care, the just allocation of scarce resources, and the movement toward health care reform through managed care and managed competition (Morreim 1995; S. Wolf 1994). Other topics being addressed include the growth of hospital ethics committees and clinical ethics consultation for health practitioners, patients, and families faced with difficult medical decisions (Fletcher, Quist, and Jonson 1989; Siegler, Pellegrino, and Singer 1990; La Puma and Schiedermayer 1994). The range of problems represented in the bioethics literature is expansive and will most certainly evolve with developments in science and the changing organization and financing of medical practice in the United States.

Conceptual Orientations in Bioethics

The intellectual contours of bioethics are defined not only by scientific advances and their implications for medical care but also by the disciplinary perspectives of individuals who have articulated the concerns and methodologies of the field. The ideological orientations of philosophers and moral theologians were significant in shaping the early development of the field (Fletcher 1954; Ramsey 1970); physicians and lawyers have also been prominent in the field's maturation. But the discipline of moral philosophy, more than any other field, has been home territory for the developing school of bioethics. Many of the founding parents (mostly fathers) of the field were schooled in the ways of twentieth-century analytic philosophy, and that tradition, more than any other, is relevant for understanding the difficulties inherent in incorporating an anthropological perspective—or any other empirically based social science—into the heart of bioethics.

Analytic philosophy maintains an Enlightenment concern with rational man and the individual. Concern with individual rights often undermines an examination of the social as a dimension (Callahan 1984, 1994). Culture is often viewed as something extraneous to the rational core human, something that can be stripped away to reveal a universal being. This view is, of course, anathema to most anthropologists, who often err on the other side, reifying culture.

Identifying and defining a common area of inquiry—that is, the nature of morality—has proved to be difficult. According to one introductory text, "Ethics is a branch of philosophy: it is moral philosophy or philosophical thinking about morality, moral problems and moral judgment" (Frankena 1973:4). One anthropologist has warned, "Philosophers are not agreed on the definition of morality and no sensible anthropologist will want to intrude into a debate in which the best brains of the past fifty to sixty generations have been engaged without reaching a definite conclusion" (Furer-Haimendorf 1967:9). Like the concept of culture in anthropology, morality is the central focus of thought and study and at the same time a fundamentally problematic concept, defying easy definition.

Although there is general agreement among the disciplines that morality is inherently social, the consensus ends there. Barry Hoffmaster notes, "According to the prevailing positivist approach in Anglo-American philosophy, morality consists of rules and principles, which because they are *normative,* can be articulated and defended only on the basis of rational arguments directed at what *ought* to be the case" (1990:242). The normative and metaethical focus of moral philosophy effectively precludes a meaningful dialogue with empirical social scientists, who, according to the tenets of moral philosophy, are preordained to work only at the level of descriptive ethics. This debate has centered on the presumed dichotomy of fact and value. Or as philosophers have asked: How can an empirical description of what is influence the formulation of statements about what ought to be? The answer given is usually, "Not at all," or, at the most, "Very little." Anthropologists, working from a firm basis of empiricism, are oriented toward cultural description. Edel and Edel (1968) point out that this approach to the study of morality is a "startling" idea to most philosophers. And perhaps many social scientists, grounded in their "data," fail to understand just how large a gap this creates between the two approaches; if the gap is left unrecognized, it cannot be bridged.

Another important issue to anthropologists is how the species "morality" is to be treated within the all-encompassing category of culture. Philosophers take the independence of morality for granted; anthropologists generally treat morality as enmeshed with other factors in the description of society and culture. The sacredness and primacy of the moral sphere is threatened by empirical work, from the philosopher's vantage point.

Because of the strong philosophical grounding of bioethics, the field has relied heavily on the language of principles and rights. Although the principles approach is currently being scrutinized for its theoretical and practical relevance, it remains strong in bioethics practices (Beauchamp and Childress 1993; Engelhardt 1986; Pellegrino and Thomasma 1981, 1989; Veatch 1981).[4] In this framework, medical ethical dilemmas are analyzed in terms of the Western philosophical principles of respect for individual autonomy, beneficence, nonmaleficence, and distributive justice.

The application of philosophical abstract principles to the resolution of ethical dilemmas complements the Cartesian duality associated with the biomedical model of disease. The principles paradigm and the reductionist model of disease causation share an analytical, mechanistic, and rationalistic foundation. Moreover, both perspectives provide a constrained and diminished assessment of contextual—social, emotional, political—issues that give life and meaning to the embodied and lived experience of a moral problem.

Alternative Paradigms in Bioethics

In the past decade, bioethicists (see e.g., Callahan 1984; Pellegrino and Thomasma 1989; Fox and Swazey 1984; Fox 1990; Jennings 1990; Hoffmaster 1990; Clouser and Gert 1990; Dubose, Hamel, and O'Connell 1994) have expressed dissatisfaction with the limitations of the reductionist and positivist approach of "Anglo-American" philosophy. Alternative frameworks for ethical analysis are currently represented in the conceptual models and methodologies of casuistry (Jonsen and Toulmin 1988; Tomlinson 1994; Kopelman 1994), virtue ethics (MacIntyre 1984; Drane 1988; Pellegrino and Thomasma 1993), narrative ethics (K. Hunter 1989, 1991; Brody 1988b; Reich 1987), relational and communitarian ethics (Benner 1991; Gould 1983; Loewey 1991), and feminist ethics (Sherwin 1992; Benhabib 1992; Gilligan, Ward, and Taylor 1988; Holmes and Purdy 1992; Kittay and Meyers 1987).[5]

Each of these approaches provides a somewhat different account of moral problems in clinical care. However, all of them recognize the fundamental importance of human relationships and contextual features in defining the parameters of moral dilemmas and bioethical practices. Casuistry emphasizes an analytical method in which the details of a case are explored and then compared to other paradigmatic cases in order to ascertain how customary moral norms might apply. Virtue ethics calls attention to the unique qualities that embody the patient-provider relationship; this approach highlights the valued dispositions of, for example, the "good physician." Narrative ethics situates moral dilemmas in the biographical and developmental framework of a story; situational context, personal character, and the social and political determinants that influence behavior and meaning are all relevant to an ethical analysis. Similarly, feminist and relational ethics take into account the interactional and broader social and political dimensions of moral dilemmas in medical care.

Interpretive and Empirical Trends

There is a strong relationship between new perspectives in bioethics and traditional concerns of the social sciences and humanities. As P. Marshall (1992: 53) observes, bioethicists have "begun to acknowledge the hermeneutical nature of clinical medicine, something that anthropologists and other social scientists have recognized for some time" (Good 1977, 1994; Good and Good 1981; Kleinman 1980, 1988, 1995).

Indicative of the move toward a contextualized and meaning-centered approach to medical morality, Carson, a bioethicist, (1990:51) argues that bioethics is essentially an interpretive enterprise. In his proposal for a framework of "practiced discernment" as a multifaceted approach to moral questions, Carson combines elements of hermeneutics, casuistry, practical reasoning, and thick description (Geertz 1973a). Leder (1990), Churchill (1990) and, more recently, Ten Have (1994) and Cooper (1994) have explored the hermeneutical dimensions of medical morality. Taken together, these perspectives provide a rich and expansive view of moral dilemmas within the context of U.S. health care. Thomasma (1994:97) makes his interpretive objective explicit in developing his model of clinical ethics as hermeneutics: "My focus is on how the good emerges from medical and clinical judgement, and how the interaction of persons in context leads to that emergence." Toombs (1992) illustrates the dialogical nature of Thomasma's "emergent values" in the patient-physician relationship in her sensitive phenomenological account of the meaning of illness.

Contextual models attempt to account for the uncertain, ambiguous, and situational features that are intrinsic to clinical dilemmas. Because medical morality—how it is understood, articulated, and experienced—is embedded in cultural contexts, more and more bioethics scholars (Hoffmaster 1990, 1992; Jennings 1990; Thomasma 1984, 1994) call attention to the need for a model of ethical reasoning that emphasizes social practices rather than abstract moral propositions. The development of new frameworks for exploring moral dimensions of medical practice will continue to evolve. We believe that the emphasis on context and interpretation in bioethics will be sustained because of the greater sensitivity these approaches offer to the perplexing reality of moral conflicts.

ANTHROPOLOGICAL PERSPECTIVES ON MEDICAL ETHICS

There are fundamental tensions to joining empirical and philosophical approaches to bioethics. But there are indications that a more cooperative alliance is emerging.[6] Bruce Jennings (1990:261) observes:

It is becoming increasingly difficult to find diehards who will flatly assert that bioethics and social science have nothing to contribute to (and learn from) one another. The rigid separation of facts and values once enshrined in academic discourse by the influence of logical positivism and Kantian formalism is now untenable. Fluid boundaries and blurred genres are now the order of the day throughout the humanities and social sciences.

Anthropologists have begun to participate actively in the field of bioethics and to formulate substantive critiques of its foundational schema (for current reviews, see Kleinman 1995; Muller 1994; Marshall 1992). Many important investigations within medical anthropology have explored moral problems associated with health care beliefs and treatment modalities (Lock 1993b; Scheper-

Hughes 1992; Farmer 1992; Estroff 1981), but they have not necessarily been defined as being explicitly within the domain of medical ethics.

Foster and Anderson (1978) first joined the concerns of bioethics—then in its opening decade—with those of medical anthropology by including a chapter on biomedical conflicts in birth, death, and aging in their textbook, *Medical Anthropology*. Kundstadter (1980), Lieban (1990), and Fabrega (1990b) focused specifically on outlining a framework for studying questions of medical ethics across cultures. Kundstadter (1980) argued for a medical ethics with relevance for complicated international public health concerns; at that time, issues of cultural difference were not being addressed by mainstream bioethicists. Fabrega (1990b) echoed Kundstater's interest in an examination of ethical problems in a cross-cultural context. Fabrega (1990b) described an ''ethnomedical'' approach to medical ethics, which would encompass a broad range of areas, including the complex relationships that exist between healers and patients, among groups of healers, and between healers and the larger society. Moreover, Fabrega calls attention to the strong link between medical morality and ritual and theological beliefs in small-scale, preliterate societies.

Lieban (1990) uses the term *ethnoethics* to refer to the exploration of moral issues related to healing practices in non-Western societies. According to Lieban (1990:223), ethnoethics ''should be informative not only about cross-cultural variation in ethical principles of medicine, but also about variations in the issues which in different societies come to be defined as morally relevant or problematic.''

Lieban (1990:221–22) suggests two primary reasons that the voice of anthropology has been absent from bioethics research and policy debates. First, he cites the strong history of cultural relativism in traditional approaches to anthropology. Most studies of health and illness take each local medical system as a whole, consciously avoiding ''ethnocentric'' value judgments about other systems. Thus, there has been little concern with the moral rightness or wrongness of actions, the domain of ethics. Second, the non-Western locations of most medical anthropological work have not been the site of rapid technological advance. Hence the questions of concern to American bioethicists—organ transplantation, respirators—seem less salient on first consideration.

Marshall (1992) proposes a third reason that anthropologists have not focused attention on the concerns of bioethics. Until recently, bioethicists have concentrated their attention on the individual as the primary unit of analysis; for social scientists, the individual is viewed as one element within a larger social and cultural context. The notion of autonomy, for example, presumes an individuated self, set apart from the collective experience of family or community. Nevertheless, these explanations provide only superficial justifications for the lack of anthropological participation or interest in bioethics; in fact, the reluctance to engage with bioethicists reflects deep-seated value differences and conflicting epistemologies.

Marshall (1992) considers the potential for bridging the methodological and theoretical concerns of each discipline in order to achieve a robust articulation of the moral underpinnings of biomedical practices. Marshall calls attention to the unique vulnerability of patients and their families as they struggle to make sense of "moral" worlds gone awry. She notes also the problem of power: how it is defined and exercised in the context of medical ethical dilemmas and how it is expressed in the positioned and privileged voice of those who speak with "moral" authority.

Kleinman (1995) levels a harsh critique of the fundamental assumptions of bioethics while at the same time arguing for the advantages of an anthropological turn in evolving bioethics perspectives. This seemingly contradictory stance— reproaching bioethics and urging that the new field adopt a critical cultural approach based on ethnographic assessments of clinical conflicts—is justified, Kleinman would argue, because bioethics has opened a discursive space within biomedicine where topics generally forbidden, like the meaning of suffering or death, can be explored.

Kleinman suggests that bioethics shares with biomedicine the profound limitations associated with an orientation that is fundamentally ethnocentric, psychocentric, and medicocentric. Ethnocentrism and psychocentrism are demonstrated by a failure to engage with the major non-Western moral traditions and to question the "orthodox sources of the self within the western philosophical tradition" (Kleinman 1995:1669). Although the bioethicist is charged with listening to the patient and taking account of his or her perspective, Kleinman argues that the medicocentrism inherent in bioethics constrains the illness narrative: "The experience of illness is made over, through the application of ethical abstractions . . . into a contextless philosophical construct that is every bit as professionally centered and divorced from patients suffering as is the biomedical construction of disease pathology" (Kleinman 1995:1669).

An alternative approach is distinctly cultural, characterized by an essential focus on problems that emerge out of the experiences and interactions of patients, families, and healers in everyday life. Kleinman and Kleinman (in press) distinguish between the moral and the ethical: "Whereas ethical discourse is a codified body of abstract knowledge held by experts about 'the good' and ways to realize it, moral accounts are the commitments of social participants in a local world about what is at stake in everyday experience" (Kleinman in press).

The moral dimensions of medical care are viewed by anthropologists as inextricably bound to culture. Ethical components of medical beliefs and practices are culturally constituted, embedded in religious and political ideologies that influence individuals and communities at particular biographical and historical moments. We argue that the cultural construction of medical morality is precisely the area in which anthropologists have the potential to make significant contributions to the field of medical ethics.

ANTHROPOLOGICAL STUDIES OF MEDICAL MORALITY AND ETHICS

A small number of scholars (Jennings 1990; Hoffmaster 1992; Conrad 1994) working in the field of bioethics have begun to challenge ethicists to incorporate ethnographic approaches in their philosophical research. Hoffmaster (1992: 1425), for example, states, "What is needed is a different brand of moral theory, one that is more closely allied with and faithful to real-life moral phenomena. Ethnography has a vital role to play in developing a more empirically grounded theory of morality."

There are several examples of early medical ethnographies that focused on moral aspects of clinical care and biomedical practice. In 1959, Renee Fox (1959) employed the methods of participant observation with patients and staff on a hospital ward, focusing particularly on the work of physicians involved in refining treatments for metabolic diseases. Like Fox, Bosk (1979) used ethnographic methods in his classic description of surgeons in training; Bosk provides a sensitive account of the social construction of medical mistakes in the process of professionalization.

More recently, anthropologists have used ethnographic approaches and other empirical methods for examining moral dimensions of biomedicine. Investigations have focused on a broad range of issues, including end-of-life decision making, definitions of death, organ transplantation, disclosure of medical information, informed consent for medical treatment, and research ethics. Studies by anthropologists on these topics and other aspects of bioethics are outlined below. Because the field of bioethics developed predominantly within the United States, the majority of anthropological studies have been conducted there; we include the few cross-cultural studies as well, especially those that suggest the influence of Western bioethics abroad. Our review cites studies by anthropologists or others who have used anthropological methods.

Critical Care

Ethnographies of neonatal intensive care units (NICUs) have shown how moral dilemmas evolve within the cultural framework of biomedicine when families and health providers negotiate the meaning of medical interventions for critically ill newborns (Anspach 1987, 1993; Guillemin and Holmstrom 1986; Levin 1986; Levin, Driscoll, and Fleischman 1991). These investigations illustrate that the opinion of physicians regarding therapeutic interventions often overrides the views of parents, despite the current emphasis on an equitable partnership between parents and the health care team. Moreover, the ethnographies reveal how the infant's personhood is signified by assessments of viability on the part of parents and the NICU staff. The studies also show that evaluations of an infant's diagnosis and prognosis are culturally and professionally situated. Anspach (1993), for example, notes that physicians relied primarily on diagnostic information from biomedical test results to determine a baby's prognosis; nurses' judgments of a baby's condition included their observations based on sustained interaction with the infant.

In her research involving adult intensive care units (ICUs), Slomka (1992) identified issues regarding medical decision making comparable to those that arose in the NICU setting. Slomka found that disagreements between family members and physicians about the use of life-sustaining treatment resulted in the "negotiated death" of the patient. Similarly, in his extensive field obser-vations in an adult ICU, Zussman (1992) calls attention to the continual rene-gotiation of medical decisions as new information is considered by family members and the health care team. Zussman's astute observations of decision-making processes reveal strong differences in opinions about what constitutes ethical problems and the "appropriate" way to solve them. Despite the influence of the courts and administrative policy, Zussman illustrates that some physicians resist the new clinical ethical practices that emphasize "respect for patient choice." He reports instances when physicians claimed to act in a patient's "best interest," regardless of the patient's expressed wishes. Additionally, Zussman (p. 89) reveals how the physician's relationship with the family not only be-comes a substitute for the relationship with the patient but also comes to mirror it. In this way, the family becomes the "carrier" for the patient's desires and "rights."

Death, Dying, and Care at the End of Life

The cultural configuration of death and the practices associated with it, in-cluding medical decisions at the end of life, both express and determine the nature of ethical dilemmas in these areas. Anthropologists have much to con-tribute to ongoing bioethical discussions of death and dying. K. Brown's (1991) analysis, for example, demonstrates the relevance of cross-cultural practices sur-rounding death for policy debates over the allocation of medical resources. Ap-proaching the topic of death from a very different perspective, Muller and Koenig (1988) explore the cultural construction of dying. Their analysis reveals how physicians in training learn to identify patients as "terminally ill." Two factors are important to residents as they construct a terminal illness: the poten-tial for therapeutic interventions and the patient's ability to interact. Muller's (1992) investigation of the use of "slow" or "limited" resuscitation codes reveals the culturally situated meanings attached to cardiopulmonary arrest. As Muller (1994:455) suggests, she approached the problem of slow codes within the interactional and informal context of physicians' work in hospitals rather than from the perspective of abstract moral principles.

Medical decision making has been an important focus for bioethics; it is in this context precisely that professional authority and patient autonomy are ex-pressed and contested. Koenig and her associates (Orona, Koenig, and Davis 1994; Koenig 1993) have conducted ethnographic research about end-of-life decision making among cancer patients in a multiethnic population, including African Americans, European Americans, Chinese Americans, and Latinos (Mexican and Central Americans). Their research highlights the cultural negotiation of decisions to limit care, emphasizing that end-of-life decisions about interventions are influenced strongly by family concerns and cultural beliefs about death and dying. The case analyses illustrate the tension between a physician's power to influence medical decisions and a patient's ability *and* desire to exercise choice in decision making.

In his analysis of the narrative accounts of middle-aged daughters' perceptions of the death of their mothers, R. L. Rubinstein (1995) found that moral dilemmas arose in virtually all of the stories, particularly in relation to decision making about medical treatment. Rubinstein (p. 269) reports that most mothers and daughters were unprepared for the suddenness of the need to make decisions; the majority of the dying mothers did not have advance directives, and the medical facts presented often appeared confusing to the patient and her daughter.

Advance directives for medical treatments—individuals' stated preferences for medical treatments when they cannot decide for themselves—have significant implications for clinical decision making. The biomedical practice of advance care planning derives directly from the Western ethical principle of respect for autonomy and individual choice. There are two forms of advance directives: a living will specifies medical interventions to be applied or withheld in the case of incompetence; the durable power of attorney for health care is a legal document that designates someone who can make decisions for the patient.

There are few anthropological investigations of the influence of cultural traditions on patients' response to advance directives for medical care. In a unique multiethnic study combining qualitative and quantitative methods, Frank, Blackhall, and Murphy (1994) found differences in attitudes toward advance directives. The study explored advance care planning among European Americans, African Americans, Mexican Americans, and Korean Americans. The investigators report that an autonomy approach to decision making, consistent with mainstream U.S. norms and bioethical practices, was adopted by the European Americans and African Americans. In sharp contrast, a family-based decision-making model was adopted by the Korean Americans and Mexican Americans. Additionally, Frank, Blackhall, and Murphy found that African Americans were less likely to complete advance directives than were European Americans. This finding is consistent with the results of surveys that have shown that Anglos are more inclined to complete a living will or a durable power of attorney for health care than are other ethnic groups (Caralis et al. 1993; Rubin et al. 1994; Klessig 1992; Garrett et al. 1993).

Aging and the Care of the Elderly

Cultural aspects of aging, like reproduction, represents an area of broad interest to anthropologists historically. Bioethical issues related to the developmental, emotional, and institutional aspects of aging are now beginning to be addressed by anthropologists. Iris (1990) has examined ethical problems related to elder abuse, assessing the cultural basis of guardianship as a protective intervention. More recently, Iris (1995) has addressed decision making for the critically ill elderly, calling attention to the vitality and importance of social context when treatment decisions are made. Similarly, Kayser-Jones's (1995) study of decision making in a nursing home demonstrates how judgments about treatment interventions are informed by the personal values of the patient, the family, and the physician, in addition to specific institutional constraints. S. Kaufman (1994) explores cultural discourse on questions surrounding perceptions of responsibility and risk for the frail elderly.

In her examination of the transformation of medical practice throughout this century, Kaufman (1993) records the life histories of seven leading U.S. physicians. Each physician was in his or her eighties; their narrative accounts provide a rich and telling history of the way in which moral concerns in biomedicine have shifted in line with scientific advances, technological developments, and epidemiological changes in the incidence and prevalence of specific diseases.

Truth Telling, Disclosure, and Hope

In the bioethics tradition, the term *truth telling* has been used to refer to the process of disclosing information to patients about medical diagnosis and prognosis. The myriad problems surrounding communication and the way it is situated within cultural, biomedical, and bioethical context have much to gain from anthropological inquiry. M. DelVecchio Good (1991), for example, has explored what she calls the "discourse of hope" associated with the treatment of cancer patients in the United States. Good shows how discussions about prognosis are imbued with cultural beliefs about the relationship between mind and body; her research reveals that these fundamental beliefs influence perceptions of control over the therapeutic and personal response to a diagnosis of cancer.

D. Gordon (1990, 1991, 1994) has examined cross-cultural aspects of disclosure in her research on concealment of medical information from cancer patients in Italy. Good's (1991) observation that U.S. oncologists believe a frank and honest discussion about cancer helps forge a partnership between physicians and patients stands in sharp contrast to the more ambiguous, restricted, and protective form of disclosure that continues to be the dominant pattern in Italian clinics, despite pressure from the U.S. "ideal" of open conversation. These studies suggest different cultural orientations to sharing or withholding medical information (Taylor 1988; Feldman 1992; Hunt 1992). Underlying specific disclosure practices are divergent beliefs about the exercise of power and control in a therapeutic relationship.

Mental Health

Narratives and discourse analysis have been used by anthropologists to examine the way in which illness experiences are embedded in biographical context; stories about sickness reveal the social construction of illness through time (Kleinman 1988b; Mattingly 1991). To date, applications of narrative analysis to moral issues in medical care have been limited. However, in his research on combat-related posttraumatic stress syndrome, Young (1990) illustrates the usefulness of narrative for anthropological investigations of moral issues in a psychiatric setting. Young shows how the narrative accounts of war experiences provide a contextual grounding for the production of moral meaning. Young demonstrates that moral dilemmas are adjusted and regulated through the etiological narratives of the men suffering from posttraumatic stress syndrome.

Informed Consent

The notion of informed consent for medical treatment is a fundamental concept in traditional bioethics. The philosophical bioethics literature on informed consent is extensive, but few anthropologists have explored the notion from a cultural perspective (Hahn 1983b; Beyene 1992). An important exception is Kaufert and O'Neil's (1990) study of the consent agreements between Native Canadians and health professionals using a Native speaker as an interpreter. Kaufert and O'Neil's landmark study examines the negotiation of informed consent in the political context of the biomedical setting. They found that the clinician's approach to the consent process emphasized a biomedical understanding of disease and therapy, a view anchored in the legal and ethical tradition of patient "rights." In contrast, the Native patients approached consent agreements as a reflection of trust relationships that could emerge only through a process of communication that extends over time. Thus, the formal and contractual framework of the biomedical and bioethical model is distinguished from the informal and interactional framework of the Native model that emphasizes relationship within a broader community. Kaufert and O'Neil also demonstrate how the interpreter, acting as a cultural intermediary, emerges as an agent of empowerment for the patient. Finally, they suggest that cross-cultural agreements serve as "integrative rituals through which participants reconcile power imbalance" and mediate clinical respect and confidence.

Research Ethics

The application of informed consent in non-Western cultures challenges the philosophical foundations of this practice. Informed consent presupposes a cultural orientation that embraces personal autonomy and self-determination (Levine 1991; Christakis 1992). These values often conflict with local traditions that allocate decision-making authority to community or religious leaders. In their essays Angell (1988), a physician, and Newton (1990), a philosopher, suggest that applying Western ethical standards of informed consent may represent a form of ethical imperialism.

Recognizing the potential for exploitation of indigenous populations because of an "imperialistic" morality, Christakis (1988) outlines ethical problems associated with obtaining informed consent for AIDS vaccine trials in Africa. More recently, Coreil et al. (1994) has addressed ethical issues in the implementation of a study that examines the willingness of individuals to participate in an AIDS vaccine trial in Haiti. Ethical issues associated with AIDS prevention research in Africa have been discussed by Schoef (1991a).

In a different context, Lane (1994) reports on her involvement in the development of an ethics committee for biomedical research in Cairo, Egypt. Lane argues that biomedical investigations in Egypt, as elsewhere, are necessarily constrained by the social, cultural, and political context within which they are developed and applied. Lane suggests that, in order to be effective, ethical codes of research must be culturally sensitive in their guidelines and implementation.

In her examination of research ethics in applied medical anthropology, Marshall (1991) calls attention to some of the unique problems anthropologists face using qualitative methods, particularly in cross-cultural settings. Similarly, Kayser-Jones and Koenig (1994) have addressed ethical issues associated with qualitative anthropological research methods. Anthropological investigations of issues such as informed consent and confidentiality in health-related studies, in both Western and non-Western research environments, would provide for a culturally grounded discussion of problems associated with human subjects research.

Clinical Ethics Consultation

In the past decade, hospital ethics committees and ethics consultation have become more common in clinical settings. Crigger (1995) argues that close examination of the practice of ethics consultation reveals that it risks subverting the goal of empowering patients by interpolating a third (expert) party into the doctor-patient encounter. Moreover, ethics consultation does the broader cultural work of furthering a shared moral order in the context of a multicultural society. In doing so, as Crigger points out, ethics consultation reinforces medicine as a privileged domain of moral discourse. Flynn (1992) makes a similar case in her analysis of interaction and authority on hospital ethics committees. In their report of an ethnographic study of hospital ethics committees at five sites, Sanders and associates (1994) call attention to the negotiated and contingent nature of ethics consults and the dominance of the clinical perspective at committee meetings. From a different perspective, Orr, Marshall and Osborne (1995) analyze four clinical ethics consultations involving cross-cultural cases. The area of ethics in clinical consultation provides a rich avenue for anthropological exploration.

Genetic Testing and Prenatal Screening

New developments in genetic research have made it possible to test individuals for a wide range of genetic diseases. Proponents of testing and screening argue that knowledge of a genetic predisposition for certain diseases can be empowering. Opponents, however, say that it simply opens a Pandora's box of problems. If someone learns, for example, that she has tested positive for breast cancer (Press, Burke, and Durfy in press), this knowledge may profoundly influence her self-identity and relationships with others. Moreover, there may be serious political and economic consequences.

In the area of prenatal testing, individuals may use the results of testing to decide whether to continue a pregnancy. As Bosk (1992) observes in his ethnography of genetic counseling in a pediatric hospital, the use of prenatal tests for selecting a child's physical and mental characteristics has significant implications for the cultural construction of individual worth and the boundaries of social acceptability. Press and Browner (1995) have examined genetic screening for maternal serum alpha-feto protein for Down's syndrome and neural tube defects. Their study explored perceptions of risk and the articulation of autonomy in the informed consent process. Rapp's (1989, 1993) extensive work in the area of genetic counseling examines the cultural underpinnings of screening from the perspectives of patients, counselors, and geneticists.

Reproductive Technologies

Like genetic screening, innovative reproductive technologies such as in vitro fertilization (IVF) and surrogacy call into question traditional social configurations of personhood and community. Historically, anthropologists have had a strong interest in women's reproductive health; there is now an extensive literature available (Davis-Floyd and Sargent 1996). More recently, however, anthropologists have begun to explore ethical aspects of new technologies, identifying their application in the context of particular cultures. L. Handwerker (1995), for example, describes the painful experience of infertility in China, where couples are generally permitted to have only one child. Handwerker notes that women who bear a child are rewarded socially and personally—for example, they are given governmental supplements and one vacation day a year. Ironically, in a country that has actively promoted population control, childless women are socially stigmatized because of infertility, and they receive no governmental rewards. In her ethnographic research, Handwerker shows how IVF is being used in China to sustain traditional beliefs about the importance of child rearing. Her work also reveals that IVF babies are thought to be "better products"—smarter and healthier than children conceived under normal conditions.

Modell's (1989) ethnographic research in a clinic offering IVF examines the culturally based interpretations of parenthood and calls attention to ideas about kinship in the United States. Additionally, Modell makes the point that although the practice of IVF represents an innovative technology, it sustains a conservative ideology about sex, marriage, and parenthood. There is a growing literature addressing the complicated social, cultural, ethical, and policy issues related to IVF and other reproductive technologies (e.g., Shore 1992; Rothman 1989; Overall 1993).

Organ Transplantation

Developments in organ transplantation raise serious ethical questions, not only about the allocation of scarce resources but also about the very nature of what it means to be human. What does the exchange of human body parts suggest about embodiment and personhood? How do cultural beliefs facilitate or diminish the possibility of organ transplantation? When is someone ''dead'' enough to remove his or her organs? These questions are of interest to anthropologists because they address the cultural foundations underlying the impact of medical technology on human lives and definitions of the ''self'' (Fox and Swazey 1974, 1992; Clark 1992).

Lock and Honde's (1990) investigation of heart transplantation in Japan illustrates how definitions of death are culturally embedded; their work examines critically the powerful way in which social values constrain the politics of implementing transplantation technology. Solid organ transplantation is not possible in Japan because ''whole-brain death'' is not recognized. In her recent analysis of the Japanese reluctance to accept a definition of whole-brain death, Lock suggests that the debate reveals ambivalence about the problematic relationship between concepts of self and other, tradition and modernity, and Eastern and Western values. Ohnuki-Tierney (1994) explores more generally the cultural articulation of organ transplantation in Japan, noting distinctively Japanese aspects of the ''gift'' relationship expressed in organ donation. Sharp (1995) examines the transformative potential of organ transplantation for self-definition. Hogle (1995) and Joralemon (1995) address the cultural dimensions of organ procurement nationally and internationally.

Science and Technology Studies

Recent critical studies of Western science and biomedical technology offer another important anthropological contribution to bioethics. More and more anthropologists are working in the interdisciplinary field of ''cultural [or social] studies of science and technology'' (Traweek 1993; Hess 1995; Hess and Layne 1992; Woolgar 1991).[7] Anthropologists in science and technology studies explicitly support Kleinman's (1995) complaint about contemporary bioethics discourse that it is ''medicocentric.'' Kleinman argues that bioethics, like biomedicine more generally, begins with professional biomedical definitions of pathology, appropriate treatment for disease, and institutional structures of care.

By contrast, good ethnography and a sophisticated anthropological stance require that the researcher make the object of study problematic.

Bioethics has not taken a critical perspective toward medical knowledge; indeed, this theoretical shift is relatively recent within anthropology. As Lock (1988a:3) has written, "For many years social scientists left unquestioned the dominant ideology of their time; scientific 'facts' were reified, assumed to be pristine and beyond the realm of social analysis." The idea that medical knowledge (and scientific facts) can be analyzed and discussed as social and cultural constructions is invaluable in understanding the nature of bioethics theory and practice. Philosophical ethics approaches have too often involved an application of universal "principles" to a body of unquestioned medical "facts." Bioethics generally has failed to appreciate that many categories of medical facts—including predictions about prognosis, as well as basic notions of disease—are not biological realities but socially created and negotiated knowledge.

Many of the medical ethnographies we have reviewed discuss these issues and provide useful insights into bioethics debates. In her study of therapeutic plasma exchange technologies, Koenig (1988) describes how a "moral imperative" for providing a new treatment develops as the technical procedure becomes routine for clinicians. The idea of a standard medical therapy is highly contingent, dependent on social context. Physicians do not simply assess the safety and efficacy of a new treatment; rather they respond to subtle social queues. Anthropologist Diana Forsythe (1992), who studies the field of medical informatics, has demonstrated how the assumptions of physicians—often the most powerful social actors in medical settings—may be embedded in supposedly "neutral" computer programs. For example, the range of choices offered to a patient may be constrained by cultural assumptions built into a computer system, effectively obstructing the bioethics ideal of informed consent following full disclosure of information (Forsythe 1992).

Other writers, such as Cambrosio and Keating (1992) take as their subject the actual content of biomedical knowledge and practices. Their ethnographic analysis of how new "facts" develop in the field of immunology challenges the simplistic positivistic view that scientific truths are discovered rather than created within a complex social environment. The field of genetics, particularly the effort to map the full human genome, demonstrates how the "interior spaces of the body have become the locus of new forms of knowledge and power" (Heath and Rabinow 1993:1). Although bioethics debates about the new genetics have focused on relatively narrow concerns like procedures for protecting the privacy of genetic information, anthropologists are more concerned with how existing relations of power will be reproduced through medical interventions based on genetic difference (Flowers and Heath 1993).

Anthropologists are not the only scholars who have taken up the challenge of empirical studies in bioethics; however, a complete review of studies by Western clinicians and other social scientists is beyond the scope of this essay.[8]

THE CHALLENGE OF MULTICULTURALISM FOR
BIOETHICS

Since we are anthropologists working in bioethics, those in other fields expect us to be culture experts. Not surprisingly, we have become involved in research examining the relevance of cultural difference, focusing on differences of race or ethnicity within the United States.[9] We have found the questions involved in studying ethnicity and bioethics to be enormously salient to our clinical work and yet to be fraught with conceptual difficulty.

The salience of cultural diversity to bioethics is not simply a response to changing demographics. The issues are complex and deeply political, and they have relevance beyond the realm of health care.[10] Debates in bioethics about topics such as decisions at the end of life, health care reform, or reproductive choice will inevitably become entangled with political struggles about how to recognize "minority" voices in society.

Giving Form to the Transparency of Culture in Bioethics

Until recently, ethical issues arising from ethnic or cultural diversity in medical practice were for the most part ignored. Indeed, we believe that cultural difference has been virtually transparent in bioethics, despite the fact that cross-cultural encounters between patients and providers are routine experiences. This is primarily due to a philosophical legacy that has emphasized universalism and reductionism. With the strong reliance on Anglo-American philosophical traditions, little attention has been paid to questions of cultural difference (for exceptions see Cross and Churchill 1982; Hahn 1983b). The result is a fundamental and problematic assumption concerning the universal applicability of bioethics. As Renee Fox (1990:207) has written, "There is a sense in which bioethics has taken its American [Western] societal and cultural attributes for granted, ignoring them in ways that imply that its conception of ethics, its value systems, and its mode of reasoning transcend social and cultural particularities." Indeed, clinical practices of American bioethics are often exported internationally along with biomedical innovations developed in the United States.

Embedded within many current health care practices that have emerged under the influence of American bioethics are unexamined assumptions that stem from specific Western cultural traditions. Advance directives, for example, which emphasize a patient's "right" to limit or withdraw unwanted therapy, appear to presuppose a particular patient. As Koenig (1993) suggests, this ideal patient has a number of archetypical characteristics: (1) a clear understanding of the illness, prognosis, and treatment options, which is shared with the members of the health care team; (2) a temporal orientation to the future and a desire to maintain control over that future; (3) the perception of freedom of choice; and (4) a willingness to discuss the prospect of death and dying openly.

This idealized view of the patient reinforces a perspective common within bioethics that individuals actually have the capacity for self-determination in settings where medical authority, not patient control, has governed interactions. Practitioners who rely on a caricature of the ideal patient often fail to recognize how biomedical knowledge is socially constructed (Gordon 1988a, 1988b). The primacy of autonomy and individualism is especially problematic because it represents largely the narrow concerns of white, middle- and upper-middle-class North Americans (Dula 1991, 1994; Fox 1990; Fox and Swazey 1984).

Although attention to cultural diversity is made possible by current theoretical shifts in bioethics, philosophical studies of the relevance of cultural difference to bioethics and medical decision making are in their infancy. Pellegrino, Mazzarella, and Corsi (1992) and Veatch (1989) have edited volumes that catalog the array of religious and cultural perspectives relevant to clinical bioethics. However, these works do not address the issue of potential conflicts in the United States or other plural societies when myriad traditions collide (Orr, Marshall, and Osborn 1995). More fundamental is the question of whether an "ethnic perspective" on bioethics is philosophically justifiable or desirable (Cortese 1990; Tully 1995). African-American philosophers express opposing views in a recent volume (Flack and Pellegrino 1992). Nevertheless, a growing body of literature addresses explicitly the African-American perspective (Dula 1991; 1994; Sanders 1994; Garcia 1992; and the edited volumes by Dula and Goering 1994; Flack and Pellegrino 1992).

Rethinking the Cultural Relevance of Bioethics

While considerable variation in cultural expressions of medical morality may be observed, some philosophers, physicians, and social scientists are attempting to find ways to bridge ethnic differences. In his essay on the possibility of a transnational bioethics, Pellegrino (1992:191) suggests that the science, technology, and morality of biomedical ethics are deeply ingrained with distinctly Western values that are "often alien, and even antipathetic, to many non-Western world views." According to Engelhardt (1991), the very existence of cultural pluralism and diversity in social values suggests that secular bioethics may be the harbinger of the "peaceable community." However, as Moreno (1995:55) points out in his exploration of the possibility of attaining moral agreement in bioethics, "in a liberal and pluralistic society, assessing the authority of moral consensus in a field such as bioethics involves going beyond political philosophy to the study of actual social processes."

Anthropologists and philosophers have approached morality and cultural pluralism from two very different perspectives. The cultural relativism of anthropology emphasizes the unique morality of individual cultures. Anthropologists view morality as an entity—like other dimensions of culture—that can be empirically described (Geertz 1984b; Hatch 1983). Ethical relativism, as defined by philosophers, means that it is impossible to evaluate cultural morality because it is always relative to specific social traditions and historical points in time.

The notion of incommensurability—that competing paradigms may not be rationally compared—has relevance for bioethics in a world of cultural pluralism (Veatch and Stempsy 1995; Bayley 1995). In his discussion of problems associated with the international application of informed consent, for example, Levine (1991) acknowledges the incommensurability between particular Western and non-Western cultural beliefs. Levine (1991) and Christakis (1992) back off from a universal definition of informed consent because of different perspectives on the nature of the person. Instead, these physicians recognize the necessity of accommodation when applying Western beliefs about informed consent and other ethical issues in non-Western cultural environments.

Emphasizing the importance of respect for cultural differences, Jecker, Carrese, and Pearlman (1995) offer recommendations for resolving ethical dilemmas in patient care in two clinical cases involving Navajo patients. The choice of cases reflects intracultural variability. Thus, not only do the investigators point out cultural differences between Navajo and Anglo worlds, they also recognize the inherent variability that exists among people who share the same worldview. The Navajos are no more unidimensional in their values and beliefs than are people of any other ethnic or cultural heritage.

In their discussion of intercultural moral reasoning, Marshall, Thomasma, and Bergsma (1994) examine a selection of cases that illustrate problems surrounding conceptual issues and specific technologies in cross-cultural context; their examples include the ethics of abortion for sexual preference in India, the Remmelink Report on the status of euthanasia in the Netherlands, and misunderstandings about the definitions of pluralism and relativism among participants at an international bioethics conference. They argue that bioethical cacophony can occur on many different levels: intercultural, intracultural, linguistic, and contextual. Marshall and her colleagues suggest that consensus on issues may not be feasible but that communication may be improved if there is minimal agreement concerning the language, meaning, and value of ethical concepts and a genuine commitment to discerning cultural context. This view is probably idealistic given the nature of cultural conflict nationally and internationally. Ultimately, cultural beliefs about any issue are expressed through a discourse of power, articulating a dialectical tension between the domination and subjugation of individual and community opinion.

Philosophers have begun to examine frameworks for addressing the moral problems of pluralistic societies (Kekes 1993; Tully 1994). Culture—and cultural beliefs about medical morality—cannot be represented by a single worldview or a categorical illustration of a particular mind-set. In acknowledging that cultural beliefs are fluid, dynamic, and negotiable, Gutmann (1992) argues that societies and individuals are multicultural. By this she means that several cultures may contribute to the profile and substance of identity, whether that identity is constituted in the form of an individual, a local community, or a nation.

In his critical examination of the ''politics of recognition,'' Charles Taylor struggles with the problem of identity in a multicultural world. Taylor (1992:

37) argues that tension ensues because the notion of respect and dignity for individuals and communities simultaneously demands recognition of particular differences and recognition of universal equality. The latter presupposes one homogeneous, assimilated, and difference-blind society—usually reflecting the values of the dominant culture. The former presupposes just the opposite: that individuals and groups are distinctive and uniquely culture bearing.

Taylor (1992:62) believes that a liberal and multicultural society cannot and should not claim cultural neutrality. Rather, he contends that the personal and public need for recognition requires both protection of basic ("universal") human rights and regard for the needs of individuals as representatives of particular social groups. Taylor, however, does not articulate a framework for how this might actually occur. Kleinman (in press) argues for a process of ethical deliberation that he calls "deliberative relativism," central to which is his notion of "cultural engagement." As Kleinman (in press) suggests, a "cultureless deliberative universalism" denies the fact that the deliberative process is itself both cultural and contextualized. A broader rendering of the complexities surrounding our response to cultural practices that are repugnant or abhorrent in the light of our own standards of morality is needed.

We agree with Taylor (1992) and Kleinman (in press) that claims of value neutrality misrepresent the fundamental essence of what it means to be a culturally informed—culturally *formed*—human being. Value neutrality is an untenable position in bioethics because it is impossible to achieve in the real world. Although current efforts to develop models for understanding moral difference may appear inadequate, there is too much at stake—the potential for human suffering and conflict is too great—not to sustain the effort to develop a framework that satisfies requirements for cultural diversity.

CONCLUSION: FUTURE DIRECTIONS IN ANTHROPOLOGY AND BIOETHICS

Future work on the boundaries of anthropology and bioethics must concentrate on four areas. First, if there is going to be a more explicit integration of anthropological and bioethical concerns, it is essential to generate models of bioethics teaching that incorporate the perspectives of anthropology and other social sciences. In bioethics training programs for health professionals, students should be introduced to concepts that represent the cross-disciplinary nature of the field of bioethics through readings and discussion. Moreover, students should be given opportunities to experience the practice of morality in local cultural context through fieldwork placements. In hospice settings, for example, students could explore decisions at the end of life. In an ideal situation, students in the social sciences, bioethics, medicine, and law would have the opportunity to collaborate in a learning experience.

Second, individuals working at the intersection of anthropology and bioethics could improve the quality and character of new bioethics practices in clinical

settings—advance directives, hospital ethics committees, and ethics consultations—by encouraging the incorporation of ethnographic techniques. Kleinman,
for example, suggests conducting a "mini-ethnography" when attempting to
resolve an ethical dilemma in clinical care in order to situate the problem in its
local biomedical, familial, and interpersonal context. In the area of research,
investigations by anthropologists on end-of-life decision making among culturally diverse populations illustrate the importance of ethnicity and cultural heritage for advance care planning.

Third, it is vitally important to develop models of qualitative and quantitative
research that are interdisciplinary, combining the perspectives and interests of
all participants in the multidisciplinary field of bioethics. As our review of anthropological studies of bioethics practices has shown, ethnographic methodologies in particular have the advantage of situating moral practices in their
political and economic context. Investigations of the cultural dimensions of genetic testing, for example, will expand our understanding of how medical practice serves a social regulatory function in this new era of surveillance of the
human body. Similarly, studies of reproductive technologies will offer new perspectives on our conceptualizations of kinship and parenthood. Moreover, research examining the cultural construction of autonomy and self-determination
and its expression in matters of health and illness would contribute significantly
to a fuller recognition of culturally diverse beliefs about personal choice. Further
exploration of topics such as personhood and the self will also strengthen and
reinforce the development of anthropological theories about the relationships
between the individual and the larger social community.

Additionally, there is a great need for cross-cultural studies of bioethics practices, in both the United States and abroad. The implications of cultural pluralism
for the application of Western bioethics is an area of inquiry that has been
virtually neglected in traditional bioethics literature. An important question concerns the transformation of "American" bioethics as it is exported, along with
biomedical practices and technology, to other Western and non-Western nations.

Finally, and perhaps most important, theoretical perspectives on the relationship between the normative concerns of traditional bioethicists and the empirical
and descriptive concerns of anthropology should be advanced. The universalizing discourse of analytic philosophy, with its emphasis on objective standards
of morality, requires cultural grounding. It is precisely in this domain that anthropologists can make a substantive contribution to the development of a robust
and expansive approach to moral analysis. The new interpretive and empirical
trends in bioethics, combined with increasing interest in bioethics on the part of
medical anthropologists, suggests that now is a fertile time for collaboration
between the two fields.

Scientific advances in medical technology, fundamental changes in systems
of health care delivery in the United States and internationally, the ongoing
transformation of relationships between patients and healers, and the increasing
recognition of cultural diversity: these realities of the practice of biomedicine

will continue to challenge the field of bioethics. As anthropologists, we believe that it is vitally important for bioethics not to lose sight of the cultural and experiential dimension of human suffering in the course of medical and moral crises.

ACKNOWLEDGMENTS

Our work on multiculturalism and bioethics has been supported by the Greenwall Foundation. We thank William Stubing for his confidence in us and his belief that investing in an anthropological perspective on bioethics would bear fruit. Arthur Kleinman generously took time away from a fellowship at the Center for Advanced Study in the Behavioral Sciences to participate in Koenig's project meetings on joining empirical and philosophical perspectives in bioethics research. (This research, focusing on cultural diversity in medical care at the end of life, is supported by the National Institutes of Health, RO1NR02906 and the American Foundation for AIDS Research 1772.) And finally, we wish to thank Barry Hoffmaster and all members of the Humanizing Bioethics project group for lively discussions and critical reviews of our previous work.

NOTES

1. For earlier reviews see Kleinman (1995); Muller (1994); P. Marshall (1992); Lieban (1990); Fabrega (1989); Koenig and Clark (1989); Kunstadter (1980).

2. For extended discussions of the historical development of bioethics, see D. Rothman (1991), Fox (1990:203–12), and Fox and Swazey (1984).

3. The primary journals for the field of bioethics are the *Hastings Center Report, Journal of Medicine and Philosophy, Theoretical Medicine, Journal of Clinical Ethics,* the *Cambridge Quarterly for Healthcare Ethics, Kennedy Institute of Ethics Journal,* and, to a lesser extent, *Perspectives on Biology and Medicine* and the *Milbank Quarterly.*

4. The pervasive and ongoing strength of the principles approach in bioethics is evidenced by the fact that Beauchamp and Childress's treatise, *Principles of Biomedical Ethics* (1993), is now in its fourth edition; it was originally published in 1979. The current edition represents an updated version of the principles approach, recognizing some of the limitations of this perspective; the authors include a discussion of alternative perspectives in bioethics.

5. A full discussion of the range of approaches in contemporary bioethics is beyond the scope of this chapter.

6. Two collaborative efforts between social scientists and bioethicists illustrate the promise of joint inquiry. In 1988, historian George Weisz assembled a small group of scholars to discuss how the methods and conceptual frameworks of social science were relevant to bioethics. The conference volume, *Social Science Perspectives on Medical Ethics* (Weisz 1990), illustrates the depth of disciplinary divides as well as the potential contribution of cross-fertilization between social science and bioethics.

Philosopher Barry Hoffmaster initiated a three-year project, Humanizing Bioethics, in 1993. Hoffmaster has included scholars in philosophy, anthropology, sociology, history, and cultural studies; the interdisciplinary format is challenging participants to question seriously the assumptions that underlie professional practices and ideologies.

Since 1989, the Anthropology and Bioethics group within the Society for Medical Anthropology has sponsored yearly sessions at the annual meeting of the American Anthropological Association. A strong interest group, the Forum on Bioethics, has also formed within the American Public Health Association.

7. Coauthor Koenig is editing a special issue of the *Medical Anthropology Quarterly,* "Biomedical Technologies: Reconfiguring Nature and Culture," that will examine the anthropology of biomedical technology.

8. In addition to the ethnographic work by medical anthropologists and sociologists described in this chapter, there are parallel approaches within medicine. Another approach to "empirical" as opposed to "philosophic" bioethics research is the use of traditional survey research techniques, generally employing quantitative methods. Although anthropologists and other social scientists are often involved in this work, the field has been dominated by physicians with training in the methods of clinical epidemiology. An example of this type of work is found in the increasing number of studies attempting to quantify the use of advance directives for medical care (e.g., living wills or durable power of attorney for health care). A summary of past work, including an agenda for future research, was recently published in the *Hastings Center Report* (Teno, Hill, O'Conner 1994). An excellent review of empirical work in bioethics, particularly work on the use of "do not resuscitate" orders, was done by Pearlman and his associates (1993).

Another area of investigation that we have not reviewed here concerns the political economy of bioethics practices. Lurie (1994), an anthropologist, has analyzed ethical problems in occupational medicine. Her research addresses conflicts of interest between patients and their employers when work-related injuries or sickness occurs.

9. Recently we were asked to recommend a research agenda on cultural diversity and bioethics to the Greenwall Foundation, one of the few U.S. foundations that funds bioethics research. Our focus is on cultural pluralism in the United States.

10. Issues such as immigration, political refugees, and ethnic violence and its relationship to nationalism are of global and transnational importance. The politics of ethnic difference is one of the central political issues of our time, and is crucial in the North-South realignment of world politics.

18

The Professionalization of Indigenous Healers

Murray Last

In an anthropological context, "profession" takes on a set of meanings wider than those used in sociology. Even within sociology, after nearly a century, the range of definitions remains large and the debate continues. Our concern here, however, is not with professions per se but with medicine—the way it is organized, the way its systems of knowledge are structured—and comparison is sought not with other occupations but with medicine as it is practiced in different cultures. Nonetheless, it needs to be noted that, among professions, medicine is an extreme case, more regulated and more exposed to public scrutiny, with stricter social closure (through stiff requirements for qualifications that take long to acquire in higher education) and with particular privileges in courts of law. While the church, perhaps the oldest of professional institutions, has lost its monopoly and while lawyers have multiplied and diversified, medicine has become increasingly specialized, with numerous health-related services seeking similar forms of organization and regulation in order to become "professional." It has also retained an unusually high social status (Becker 1970; Larson 1977; Freidson 1986; Johnson 1972; Dingwall and Lewis 1983; Abbott 1988, Jacob 1988; Hefferty and McKinley 1993).

The detailed history of the professionalization of medicine and related occupations in Britain and the United States (the paradigmatic examples of professionalism) is the subject of a large literature (for example, Mapother 1968; Carr-Saunders and Wilson 1933; Shryock 1967; Parry and Parry 1976; Burrow 1977; Gelfand 1980; Starr 1982; Ramsey 1988; Spree 1988; Burrage and Torstendahl and Burrage 1990; Perkin 1990; Kimball 1992). (On the current range, and absurdities, of licencing practice generally in Britain, see Mason 1988.) The way professions have been elaborated in Britain and the United States, as nowhere else in the world, has led sociologists to treat "profession" as a culture-bound folk concept (Becker 1970:92). Yet that Anglo-American folk concept has gone into circulation worldwide, as indeed has so-called Western (or cosmopolitan) medicine. As a consequence, in a wider anthropology of medical professions, we need to retain the broader senses of the English term *profession* (as a full-time occupation locally recognized for its specialized skills), if we are to compare contemporary processes and structures in the practice of medicine beyond America and Europe.

The criteria employed here for inclusion as a profession are that it be an extended self-conscious grouping of healers with defined criteria for membership (whether through licensing, certification, or registration) and an expertise over which it seeks primary control; it is also an expertise that claims to be more than a craft and has in addition an esoteric, theoretical basis. These criteria, used here in lieu of a formal definition of a profession, reflect the attributes of the conventional professions of Europe and America, since de facto the agenda under which all these therapeutic organizations have to operate has already been set by the existing agreements between government and the conventional professions after nearly a century of political debate and lawmaking. This is as true of India or Nigeria as it is of Europe or America; the detailed history of these debates, though, is particularly well documented only for Europe and America, with some valuable literature on India and China (Leslie 1972, 1975, 1976; Leslie and Young 1992; Jeffery 1988; Hillier and Jewell 1983; Unschuld 1975).

The spread of professionalism in medicine has been especially notable in Anglophone countries—both in nations that had once been part of the British Empire and in states more recently affected by American influence. In such countries, professional associations modeled on British or American associations have been set up, initially as branches and subsequently as autonomous but mutually recognized institutions (Johnson 1973; Grey-Turner and Sutherland 1982). Furthermore, since 1948 the World Health Organization (WHO) has played an increasingly significant part in attempts to foster a worldwide medical profession, though because of its size and internal diversity, it has not always spoken with a single voice. For example, its attitude toward "traditional medicine" and its policy of encouraging member-states to organize their traditional practitioners was finally adopted in 1978 despite internal debate and controversy; today, that policy is still in question and subject to review. Yet overall the consequences are clear: the potential professionalization of indigenous practitioners is firmly on the agenda (Bannenman, Burton, and Wen-Chief 1983; WHO 1976, 1978b).

The issues are not academic. With the much-proclaimed target of health for all by the year 2000, the shortage of medical practitioners in the period of economic crisis in the Third World is so acute that medical practitioners of all kinds are potentially acceptable recruits to national health services. Add to this the extra demand on resources posed by the AIDS epidemic, and issues such as the training and licensing of auxiliary practitioners come to the fore as matters of urgency. In such a context, there is a particular relevance in an anthropology of professionalism in medicine that extends beyond the limited experience of Europe and North America.

Three arguments are presented here. First, professions of medicine function primarily within a national medical culture, with certain professions claiming for themselves a universal validity. These claims are significant in the struggles over professional recognition and dominance within the national culture. But despite the claims, all systems of medicine are in varying measure culture specific.

Second, these national medical cultures are partly the product of a nation's ruling political philosophy and partly the product of the ways people express their health needs and find solutions to them. Worldwide there are broadly three types of political philosophies that affect medical practice and seek to determine the role of healers in society and how (if at all) they will be organized: government, for example, can behave either as a bureaucrat for which medicine is primarily a matter for the state, or as a market overseer for which medicine is primarily a staple item of consumption for sale in the marketplace; otherwise it can behave as a new landlord who willingly puts up with the two or three types of medicine that some of his older "tenants" regularly turn to. But we need to recognize that popular support, from patients and their kin, is also a crucial factor in formulating the diverse medical subculture labeled indigenous or "traditional medicine" (the term conventionally used to replace the earlier "native medicine" and "folk medicine"; it includes practices that may in fact not be traditional). The two perspectives—the one from above, the other from below—are often at odds.

Third, professionalization is one solution to the dilemma of practitioners of traditional medicine in the face of unequal competition from other systems of medicine. It requires being organized in a form, recognized and respected within the national culture, that can best represent the interests of practitioners and their clientele, both now and in the future. The problem is by no means limited to Third World countries, though it is there that the issues are being most clearly articulated and the possibilities for developing "traditional medicine" most practicable (Velimirovic 1984; Chambers 1986; cf. Vaskilampi and Mac-Cormack 1982; Chavunduka 1994).

MEDICAL CULTURES: NATIONAL AND INTERNATIONAL

I use the concept of a national medical culture here to denote the national arena in which competition between medical systems takes place, with professionalism as one factor in that competition. The nation-state is an appropriate unit of analysis, for although the term *cosmopolitan medicine* (as modern hospital-based medicine is often called, e.g., in Leslie 1976) suggests it has become today's universal medical system much as humoral medicine was before it, in practice even such an apparently rigorous scientific system is subject to national cultural variations.

Attempts to foster a worldwide medical profession are nonetheless significant for the support a wider profession can give to the local status of national medical groupings. Not only do agencies like WHO and UNICEF act as forces for unification, but international congresses and working parties are set up to seek agreement on such issues as the proper definition (and treatment) of schizophrenia or updated nomenclatures for diseases and anatomical structures (WHO 1973, 1974; Warwick 1977). Indeed for AIDS, WHO has resorted to publishing "consensus statements" in an attempt to avoid controversies among national experts (Panos 1988:105). These attempts, however, betray how nationally oriented the medical professions are. For example, other countries' medical qualifications are rarely recognized as adequate in themselves; thus the United States requires a further comprehensive examination for foreigners, and Indian medical degrees after May 1975 are refused direct recognition in Britain (Stevens, Goodman, and Mick 1978; Jeffery 1988:207). A limited step toward a common international profession is being taken by the European Union, but early doubts about whether this will actually work and what changes to national regulations will be involved have not so far proved justified. Whether the result is more regulation or less (for example, of practitioners of alternative medicine) remains to be seen.

Hospital medicine is not the only system of medicine that has sought to organize itself worldwide. The most successful is homeopathy, though it lacks the sort of funding that gives WHO its authority (Salmon 1984:75). Patients' self-help groups, most notably Alcoholics Anonymous, have also succeeded in crossing national and cultural boundaries to provide common techniques of treatment (Janzen 1982b:158; Kurtz 1979:226–27). The international status of these groupings and others like them gives them an added weight within the politics of national health services.

Indigenous practitioners of traditional medicine, by contrast, have few if any such links and tend to emphasize instead not the universality of their therapies but their cultural or regional specificity. Pan-African associations of healers have been of only limited scope and short duration, while international congresses (to which less culture-specific herbalists are often invited) have tended to be dominated by professionals from pharmacology and pharmacognosy intent on incorporating into their own universal systems any traditional expertise that is available (Sofowora 1979, 1982). Indeed even WHO's patronage has served mainly to encourage national ministries of health to try to incorporate healers into the hospital-based profession, offering them retraining and a minor role in state health services (Sargent 1986; Twumasi and Warren 1986). In short, any tendency to "universalize" or even internationalize traditional medicine seems to call into question practitioners' autonomy. Within a national medical culture, this issue is not so apparent.

One reason that there does not yet exist any worldwide profession of medicine, with uniform credentials that permit holders to practice clinically anywhere they wish, is that clinical practice varies in detail from state to state, with the variation due as much to historical and cultural differences as to any scientific rationale (O'Brien 1984; Payer 1988). Indeed, in all clinical practice, traditional or scientific, there is a significant element that is culture specific.

Some national differences in medical practice are notorious. Disputes over the definition of schizophrenia, let alone its proper treatment, have already been mentioned (Leff 1981). The different ways in which countries collect medical statistics are reflected in the various national nomenclatures of disease; the terminology of medicine, and with it the etiological and anatomical categories, reveals how basic assumptions in medical thought vary (Royal College of Physicians 1948). So too in research; the academic dispute between French and American research teams over the AIDS virus proved to be more a national political (and economic) issue than a serious question of medical science, despite the common discourse (Connor and Kingman 1988).

Finally, practice also is subject to national custom. Well known is the French preference for pessaries over pills (a preference that extends to francophone Africa) or the particular German interest in hydrotherapy (Payer 1988). Soviet bloc medicine was noted for preferring terminations to contraceptive devices; and, uniquely, sanatoriums for treating asthma and emphysema there have long been sited in disused deep-mine workings, with great success. In Third World countries where nationals have been trained in a range of institutions abroad and foreigners are regularly employed, the diversity is readily apparent, and though doctors seldom know it, the different national styles are the subject of critical evaluation by patients locally.

Again ''cosmopolitan'' medicine is not the only medical system with a worldwide distribution that is subject to national variation. In homeopathy some of the national variations reflect which edition of Hahnemann's *Organon* was used when homeopathy was introduced, while, for example, in its Indian or Brazilian forms, homeopathy has been identified by nationalists as an indigenous modern medicine and has been absorbed and modified accordingly (Santos 1981). Similarly the practice of acupuncture and Ayurvedic medicine in Europe and America varies considerably from that practiced in China or India; both have been adapted to local conditions, whether climatic or scientific, and the subtle theoretical basis of each system is usually ignored by patients and practitioners alike (Kao and Kao 1979).

For these reasons, a comparative analysis of national medical cultures is a necessary starting point. No one should take for granted that what is normative according to the textbook (which textbook?) is in fact the practice in any one locality; it may be so. There can thus be no adequate discussion of the comparative efficacy of the different systems. In theory, no doubt, all systems may ''work''; in practice, all have successes and failures, with some systems scoring much higher in particular areas of medicine. Yet all too frequently, when comparisons are made between the different systems of medicine practiced in any one state, a normative model is used for one system while observed practice is used for the other. We lack enough detailed ethnographies of the various systems at work.

Within a national medical culture, then, are included all the various medical systems and practices available to patients. These often quite distinct systems of medicine are competing for custom, for privileged access to government finance, for bureaucratic recognition of their certificates as competent to certify sickness or health; they are competing too for the "truth" of their particular understanding of the nature of life and how best to sustain it. By using the nation as the analytical unit, emphasis is being put on the political aspect of professionalism in medicine, for it is through the political process that the most significant variations in professionalism have come into being—and through it too will come (if ever) the professional recognition of indigenous practitioners.

PROFESSIONS OF MEDICINE AND THE MARKET

In this wider anthropology of medical professions I will include three distinct groupings:

1. The conventional medical professions privileged by almost every state and by WHO as the scientifically efficacious system for a nation's health services. Included in this category are professionals such as nurses and midwives, as well as those in occupations formally labeled in Britain as "professions supplementary to medicine," alias physiotherapy, occupational therapy, radiotherapy, ophthalmic opticians, and others (Larkin 1983; MacNab 1970).

2. Professions of alternative medicine, such as homeopathy, Ayurveda, acupuncture, or osteopathy, which may be recognized by government and public alike as a formal system of therapy, with a set curriculum taught in special colleges or as a special subject.

3. Professions of traditional medicine, where there is an attempt to create a new professional group in amalgamating ordinary, individual healers of varying kinds and specialties into a single body as the basis for obtaining government recognition and for improving public acceptance of its members.

It is important to recognize that a great deal of healing takes place outside the purview of governmental or professional regulations. The largest segment, self-medication (including home remedies), accounts for the great majority of ailments, injuries, and malaise. Where a range of drugs is readily available over the counter (for example, as antibiotics are in France), the scale of self-medication is vast; the tendency today is to enlarge rather than limit the number and type of drugs so available. In addition, in countries like Nigeria where such drugs are not restricted to registered pharmacists but form part of a trader's ordinary merchandise, injection sets are also available; and with razor blades for scalpels, rudimentary surgery is undertaken at home. Given that people's commonsense knowledge normally includes herbal medicines and tonics available in the habitat; given too that people have always coped with wounds from fights and hunting, lancing boils and reducing fractures, contemporary self-medication is simply an expansion of ordinary practice. (The other important area of healing outside medical or bureaucratic regulation, church healing, will be discussed below.)

The professions in medicine, then, are dealing with a relatively restricted field. Indeed, until recently (especially, for example, in the old Soviet Union; Ryan 1978:44–45) the majority of licensed doctors have not always found it easy to make a living from medicine full time. The development of new drugs and equipment has given doctors a considerable technical (if not always therapeutic) edge in most fields of medicine. But it is only with the provision by the state of free medicine, and the establishment of government hospitals and dispensaries, that the demand for medicine (and the expectations of good health) expanded the market for medicine. Thus in India, people's present widespread use of ''Western'' medicine is attributed to its ready availability at low cost in rural areas, whereas before Ayurveda and homeopathy had a greater share of a smaller ''market'' (Jeffery 1988:57–58).

The limited market in which the various medical professions operate is not, however, a free one. Regulatory systems of one sort or another are found governing the provision of health care in every modern state.

THE MATRIX FOR PROFESSIONALISM: REGULATIONS AND THE STATE

The range of subcultures permitted within a national medical culture varies greatly, from the monolithic system of state-controlled health that was characteristic of the old Soviet Union to the systems of, say, Nigeria, India, or Britain, where pluralism is at its most extreme. In practice there are three broad types of regulatory systems that help to determine politically the nature of a state's medical culture, and with it the organizational possibilities for indigenous practitioners (Stepan 1985; Ramsey 1984; Moran and Wood 1992).

Exclusive Systems: Medical Monopolies

Marxist Model

Developed out of the autocratic tradition of Eastern European government and greatly expanded under a Soviet administration, Marxist medicine is typically a monopoly of the state (Konrad and Szelenyi 1979; Ryan 1978; Field 1976b, 1991). In the former Soviet Union, the Ministry of Health, both at the center and in the republics, employed medical practitioners as civil servants and attached them to public clinics or to specific ministries and industries, where they formed part of a management team concerned with productivity. All other forms of healer had been formally banned since 1923. The only ''professional'' association was the Medical Workers Union, in which paramedicals outnumbered doctors; any other professional groupings dating from before the revolution had disappeared by the 1930s, under strong pressure from other medical workers. In an otherwise apparently uniform medical system it was the patient's political merit, rather than just wealth or clinical need, that thus determined the way different medical facilities (such as a bed in the special hospitals run by the "Fourth Department") were allocated (Matthews 1978:47).

The bureaucratically rational, total monopoly model was adopted, with variations, in Third World countries influenced by the Soviet Union and by Marxist modes of planning. Typically the status of doctors in such countries is usually higher (they form part of the intelligentsia "class") and their numbers lower than was the case in the old Soviet Union, and the ban on traditional healers is usually ineffective. Nonetheless, opposition to healers remains linked ideologically to the role they played in supporting the "feudal" social systems of the past, while the endorsement healers receive elsewhere is put down to the bourgeoisie's predictable preference for the cheapest possible health care for the masses (Barker and Turshen 1986). Furthermore traditional medicine is seen as reinforcing the class divide, by helping to prevent people having a proper scientific understanding of their condition and pandering instead to superstition.

French Model

This model starts from the premise of centralized state control with all unlicensed healers illegal; the state employs doctors in official position as civil servants, to practice medicine, to teach, and to conduct research. In addition, registered doctors can practice privately; pharmacists routinely advise customers and sell a wide range of drugs. The result is a mixed state and professional system in which some doctors attain high social and political status by playing both sides of the system (Bourdieu 1988; Jamous and Peloille 1970). Licenses are granted only to those qualified in state-run schools of medicine, and prosecutions are brought against the unlicensed if they are practicing regularly (Stepan 1985:288).

The Third World countries that follow the French model have tended to emphasize that aspect of the model that favors a state monopoly. Colonial regimes were by nature autocratic, and the Napoleonic legal code that sanctioned centralized control has been carried over into the new independent states. In Cameroon, in particular, control reaches down to district levels, and until recently any attempt in certain areas to set up an alternative healing practice, even under church auspices, was likely to be closed rapidly by the police; but even there policy has been under pressure to change (cf. de Rosny 1991). Elsewhere in francophone Africa, no such tight control exists. Indeed in Cote d'Ivoire, government made use of the healing cult run by Albert Atcho (Piault 1975:45–72). Representatives of healers may sit, as in Benin, on the village health committees and traditional birth attendants may be employed as health workers, but the healers' professional associations get little or no encouragement and collaboration is minimal (Sargent 1986; Heywood 1991). The degree of actual harassment of healers by local police (and healers' fears of such harassment) is variable, but ultimately the legality of traditional practice remains in question until the relevant laws are changed.

The basic French model is not confined to former French colonies. Variations of the model are found in Spanish- and Portuguese-speaking areas, particularly in Latin America, though in practice restrictions on indigenous practitioners have proved unenforceable. Indeed in Mexico, for example, the government has judiciously made it possible now for villages to have the services of a local practitioner available at the state clinic. Further modification has come through American influence, whether in the form of missionary medicine, through local doctors receiving their training in the United States, or through the establishment of private American-funded medical institutions.

American Model

While the French model assumes government could be bureaucratically rational (and not just seeking to monopolize power), the American model seeks to modify, through strict and detailed regulation at the state (not national) level, a free medical market (Freidson 1986; Starr 1982; Navarro 1986). Both models in the process, however, greatly enhanced the privileges of the dominant medical subculture, hospital medicine, at the expense of alternative systems and practices. Osteopathy, for example, allied itself with hospital medicine so as to gain recognition, and a version of it has been integrated into the educational system. Other systems have fared somewhat better under a religious umbrella (because of federal provisions for freedom of religion) so long as they do not use drugs. But refusal on religious grounds to seek adequate treatment is a matter of contention; people have fewer rights over their bodies than over their minds or souls.

The rationale for the state's policing role in medicine is the maintenance of public health. In practice, however, curanderos and similar practitioners serving specific minorities have been left to function as normal (many, however, prefer to keep their practice secret: Fontenot 1994; Snow 1993), though it seems regulation of them too will eventually become an issue despite the political climate against regulation and monopolies. Debate is likely to focus on the legal problems surrounding malpractice suits, just as it did in the nineteenth century before states introduced their various regulations (Burns 1977; Shrylock 1967; Department of Health, Education and Welfare 1973; Forbes 1948; Rosenthal 1987).

An important difference between the American and other state-centered models is the lack of standardization due to privately run institutions in all aspects of medicine. In theory the hallmark of the bureaucratically run system is that its standards should be uniform throughout the nation. Despite an important public health sector, it is privately funded medicine—schools, research institutes, hospitals, health insurance systems—that dominates the American system and marks it as distinctive. In other countries the state runs more or less directly the institutions that award the credentials of individual doctors; in the United States the state accredits independent institutions, which in turn form regional groupings in order to raise their status collectively. The result is a competitive market within the medical profession rather than a market between the medical and other therapeutic professions. It is to this latter market that we now turn.

Tolerant Systems: Medical Markets

British Model

In the British model, instead of outlawing all other forms of healing, regulations merely define who can legally be described by a specific professional label, "doctor" (Ramsey 1984; Parry and Parry 1976; cf. Stacey 1992; Saks 1994). The formal rationale of the legislation is to prevent fraudulent descriptions so that the customer-patient can make an informed choice; a patient who wants the services of a nondoctor is free to do so, and healers of any persuasion (except in the fields of surgery and dentistry) are free to offer their services. Until very recently the centrally financed National Health Service, for which the majority of doctors worked on contract, did not pay for alternative or traditional treatments, though doctors may practice such treatments themselves or formally supervise others doing so. Now with both family doctors and hospitals treated as budget-holding units, in principle doctors (or their managers) can fund any kind of treatment. A crucial degree of regulation is maintained through controls over the sale of drugs, making access to most significant medicines possible only through a doctor's prescription (the list of over-the-counter drugs is, however, lengthening). Yet another regulatory mechanism is a restriction on the right to incise the skin to any depth. Similarly certain diseases have to be referred, as a matter of public health if nothing else, to doctors. Thus self-medication or treatment by unqualified healers is in fact more restricted than it might at first seem.

Professional autonomy in this model is maintained through a series of institutions that distance the government (which provides effectively all the funds for both medical practice and for medical education) from detailed policymaking, structuring, and disciplining of the profession. The compromise works only insofar as there is a consensus between government and profession; when resources are scarce and the consensus breaks down, professional autonomy proves hollow. On an individual basis, autonomy does, however, allow the doctor, once qualified, to practice as he or she thinks fit; licensing does not in itself prohibit unorthodox practice. In this system, then, professional knowledge does not rule out quite alien medical beliefs or even practices beyond the point of entry into the system. An unorthodox doctor (who may have to work in private practice if no one is willing to appoint him or her to a post) is thus free to compete for patients on an open medical market, though he or she is still bound by profession restrictions on advertising services.

It follows from this that other systems of medicine are free to form professional associations, set up special colleges, and issue qualifications (but not to describe themselves as doctors) without reference to any other profession. Thus osteopathy in Britain (but not in the United States) remains independent of orthopedic medicine, and in principle it retains its distinct theoretical basis, though there is no evidence that its clientele is particularly interested in those theories or in their development (Inglis 1964:94–122). Indeed people's therapeutic pragmatism—their willingness to divorce therapeutic practice from therapeutic theory—is essential in understanding how the medical market works, for efficacy is not seen to depend on "truth"; a mode of treatment can be right for the wrong reason.

Anomalies reveal a similar pragmatism in the model itself. For example, homeopathy has won for itself the privileged position of being officially included, if only marginally, within the state's health service, despite numerous professional commissions of inquiries rejecting its scientific status. Political patronage is an important factor since in this instance the Royal National Homeopathic Hospital has long received royal support (Inglis 1964:85; Nichols 1988). But the anomaly extends even to veterinary medicine, which is otherwise much more strictly regulated in Britain (as elsewhere in formerly British-run territories) than human medicine in that homeopathic vets have a growing, and legal, share of the market for treating both domestic and farm animals.

In the numerous Third World and other countries that follow the British model (the majority of them former colonies), the conventional medical profession has proved politically to be relatively weak (Johnson 1973; Macleod and Lewis 1988 Last and Chavunduka 1986:9–12; Schram 1971). Private practice cannot be a substitute for government employment for the majority of doctors until there is a large enough middle class to provide the demand. Demand is further weakened by people's ability to buy without prescription the drugs that in Britain are on the restricted list; in this doctors have lost a crucial monopoly. Furthermore it is in these countries that there has come the strongest pressure from traditional practitioners for government recognition. Nonetheless, the social status of doctors is very high—constitutionally, since colonial times, the medical officer has been the second-ranking official in the community should a crisis arise—and the informal influence of the profession remains in spite of its lack of monopoly. The success of alternative medical systems in establishing themselves in developing countries has been patchy. Apart from India where homeopathy has thrived, the main areas have been where Anglophone immigrants have settled— for example, in southern and eastern Africa, where they have been subject to special legislation, distinct from that covering either indigenous practitioners or doctors.

German Model

The importance here of the German model lies in the unique way German indigenous practitioners of any kind are licensed (Unschuld 1980; Stepan 1985.

On German professions generally, see McClelland 1991; Cocks and Jarausch 1990). They merely have to pass an examination to show that they know the state law regulating medical practice; the actual content of the expertise they claim to exercise is not otherwise restricted or examined. Not surprisingly no overall profession of *Heilpraktiker* (as lay practitioners are called) exists, and given their diversity it is unlikely that one would be practicable. Schools, however, exist to teach would-be lay practitioners the relevant, legal information to pass the examination.

The model has left no legacy in the Third World. (Indeed, when Germany established colonies in Africa, the colonial authorities never apparently applied this model. Local practitioners were considered instead to be resistance leaders and were closely controlled, to the extent of prices' being fixed [Feierman 1986: 208].) Nonetheless, it is surely one possible model—should a model be needed—if licensing of indigenous practitioners is to be introduced elsewhere.

Integrated Systems: Asian Pluralism

Indian and Chinese Models

Under British imperial legislation, Indian practitioners of Ayurvedic, Siddha, and Unani medicine were at liberty not only to practice but to develop associations and schools of medicine. For nearly a century these alternative medical institutions have developed to rival those set up for "cosmopolitan" (or "Western") medicine by the imperial regime (Jeffery 1988). All the formal trappings of professionalism—theoretical texts for teaching in university courses, research institutes, an autonomous governing council with statutory powers, hospitals, state funding, a specialized drug industry—have long been in place. Nonetheless, since independence the government of India has built up the cosmopolitan, hospital-based services, not only supporting a strong medical profession with qualifications that met international standards but also developing a network of rural dispensaries and related services to such an extent that use of "Western" medicine is reported to be as widespread as Ayurveda. Not merely is it now as widely available, but it is offered at lower cost. In this situation Ayurvedic colleges are said to be having difficulties recruiting applicants of comparable caliber. Homeopathy, with an origin that links it theoretically with Islamic medicine, has been adopted and adapted, particularly in Bengal, as an Indian system of medicine and similarly given rise to formal professional structures.

Other, less systematic therapeutic systems survive without professionalization on the margins of the national medical culture and meeting specific needs that the various formal systems cannot adequately provide for. Many are religious in essence, using temples or festivals as focal points for healing and relying on charity rather than on government or local state funds (Kakar 1982).

Legal models like India's are widespread in south and East Asia, with professional recognition given to more than one system of medicine (cf. Lock 1980 on Japan). In recent years the more restrictive legislation carried over from the colonial period has been replaced, in part as a response to nationalist feeling, in part to make the law match social reality. The degree to which all formally recognized medical professions are run as bureaucracies by the state depends on the local political matrix. India, with its open, democratic system, reflects that political tradition in its attitudes to medical politics and so leaves practitioners largely to regulate themselves. China, by contrast, although Marxist in ideology, has always recognized Chinese traditional medicine in all its variety but integrates it into the state-run services (Hillier and Jewell 1983). "Barefoot doctors" were one solution to the problem of integration; trained partly in traditional but mainly in "Western" medicine, they served as medical auxiliaries. Another solution was to maintain state-financed hospitals in which acupuncture, moxibustion, and herbal therapy were available as required. During the Cultural Revolution, the independence of practitioners of traditional systems was sharply curtailed and their associations closed down—only temporarily, as it has happened. More recently priorities have once again changed; for example, now that the one-child policy is in force, parents in the countryside are reportedly seeking out the best-qualified urban obstetricians and pediatricians; traditional midwives and barefoot doctors—once the models for Third World medicine—are being spurned. The current liberalization of the economy has further encouraged the open market in medicines.

These two systems—Indian and Chinese—have provided models for incorporating indigenous practitioners elsewhere, but there are questions as to their appropriateness, particularly in Africa, where, historically, centralized states have tended not to create elaborate medical bureaucracies, with ancient written texts and systematic theorization. Furthermore, in both India and China there was considerable unity to the medical traditions, which had largely ceased to be as culture or region specific as are many such traditions in Africa.

Third World Model

A final model that de facto (if not de jure) is integrative is to be found in Third World countries whose economic resources and colonial history have left them with the legacy of small, secondary professions not powerful enough to effect a monopoly. Although their legal traditions and the current political matrix may differ, these differences may count for less than the characteristics they have in common. The characteristics of the Third World model are (1) a relatively weak and underfinanced system of hospital medicine, largely urban centered, staffed by doctors (nationals and foreigners) trained to different standards and routines in a number of different countries; (2) a legal system that privileges that hospital system yet is unable, in practical terms, to outlaw any alternative; (3) a very large number of local practitioners of traditional medicine, bonesetters, midwives, barber-surgeons, and so forth who have always tried to meet the health needs of the community; (4) a wide spectrum of modern alternative therapies alongside a market in medical drugs imported, sometimes unmarked and instructionless, from all over the world; and (5) a population that is dispersed and often difficult of access yet has high rates of morbidity and mortality (Sanders 1985; Twumasi 1975; Good 1987).

It should be noted, too, that case law on medical, or indeed any other form of, negligence is virtually nonexistent in most Third World countries, and consumer rights remain to be defined either by new legislation after independence or by judicial decision (*Newswatch* September 26, 1988:37). At present, in a country like Nigeria, death due to a healer's bold attempt at surgery can lead to his or her arrest by the police for manslaughter, but otherwise malpractice results at most in loss of reputation and earnings. Conventional doctors have been equally safe, though attitudes are apparently beginning to change (*African Guardian,* November 7, 1988). In Cameroon, witches have recently begun to be recognized as expert witnesses and required to testify in court against fellow witches (Geschiere 1988:60, 1995; Chukkol 1981; *Dar es Salaam Sunday News,* October 30, 1988:8). In time, then, as healers and other purveyors of medicines or medical services gain formal recognition, litigation is likely to be added to social pressure as a curb on fraudulent or negligent practice.

In this context, the practitioners of traditional medicine have been encouraged by their national ministries of health and by WHO either to organize themselves into professional associations or be organized into a role ancillary to hospital-based medicine. Their dilemma is the central theme of the remainder of this chapter.

THE SOCIAL MATRIX: PROFESSIONALIZATION FROM BELOW

The legal matrix is not the sole determinant; medicine is more than merely a matter of political culture. Strictly local realities are a factor in determining what is available to the sick. Seen from the perspective of the sick and their kin, the national medical culture takes on a much less orderly, systematic appearance, with matters like price, availability, efficacy, local experience, and sympathy all counting toward how a particular therapy for a particular case comes to be chosen. The issues are complex and likely to change as people alter their priorities and their perceptions of risk.

Seen from below, then, the legitimacy of a healing system is quite distinct from the kind of political legality so far discussed. This grass-roots legitimacy may arise, as Weber suggests, either from the community's own traditions or from the healer's personal charisma. Whatever the source, at this level it is clinical practice, not political philosophy, that is determinant. At the core of clinical practice is the therapeutic triangle of relationships of patient, healer, and a local public that includes both kin and others in the community. The structure of these relationships and the medical concepts that inform them vary widely within any country today, indeed even within communities. But taken together, the distinct patterns of relationships and concepts rendered visible in this therapeutic triangle constitute the various separate medical subcultures that, for convenience we can label as Ayurveda, for example, or homeopathy. Constituting more diffuse a subculture are those individual practitioners whose therapies we generally categorize together under the heading "traditional medicine."

Professionalization of this traditionally diffuse subculture seeks to give it not only a certain political unity but also at the community level a coherent image, akin to a successful trademark with its associated goodwill, that would guarantee a uniformly high quality of service. Contemporary sociological analyses are obsessed with the power of professions as interest groups within society at large, whereas earlier analysts were intrigued by the way ethical rather than commercial norms were (in theory at least) established and enforced, by the way too that unethical or incompetent practitioners were controlled. Unfashionable though these concerns may be (or simply taken for granted), nonetheless for patients at the clinical level, these concerns are central. The legality of a practice is less important than the practitioner's moral standing or trustworthiness. Where a community and its practitioners have worked together for years, this local legitimation is rarely problematic. Elsewhere, and particularly in towns, where practitioners or patients may be newcomers, initial legitimation of this kind might potentially come from professional membership.

In short a professionalization from below has always existed in some form or other in long-established communities. The question is how to expand it to meet modern circumstances. Is politically orientated professionalization from above compatible with socially sanctioned professionalization from below? A major difference between the two perspectives on professionalization lies in the way professional knowledge is perceived (whether bureaucratically from above or clinically from below) and what the relationship is between the two. It is to professional knowledge, then, that we now briefly turn.

PROFESSIONAL KNOWLEDGE

Conventionally, professions are characterized by their use of higher education for their specialist qualifications—by their control over the curriculum and staffing of the specialized institutions responsible for both teaching and developing the area of expertise on behalf of the nation (Freidson 1986). In the process an orthodoxy comes into being, consisting of a standardized body of knowledge that has been developed, disseminated, and accepted. It does not necessarily include the latest in therapeutic fashion or even the latest research ideas; indeed orthodoxy can be not only obsolete but wrong in terms of current sophisticated thinking (which is orthodoxy in the making). In short, while knowledge, both abstract and factual, constitutes a crucial element in professionalism, the professional medical knowledge that underwrites daily clinical practice is a bundle of "facts" and working hypotheses of uncertain truth value, if usually of proved efficacy. Furthermore, most of the knowledge is factual, not theoretical; scientific debates about the nature of life, matter, and time are not intrinsic to this professional knowledge.

From one angle, then, professional knowledge may look formidably systematic and complete, the bureaucratic requirements of licensing elaborate and foolproof. From below, as practitioners perform their daily work, the coherence is not so obvious or the logic so compelling. The differences at this low level between medical systems are not so marked. Indeed for many patients, the theoretical basis for a particular therapy is not only irrelevant but better left unknown; their confidence in the therapy is more important than an acceptance of its logic. Thus the dilemma facing practitioners of traditional medicine is whether they really need to match the systematization achieved by other professions in medicine—for example, by Ayurveda—so long as their own practice remains rooted in people's common sense knowledge of illness, its causes and its cures. For example, an attempt by Zimbabwe's healers' association, ZINATHA, at running a school for trainee healers was halted not only for financial reasons (which are surmountable) but also over the issue of an appropriate structure and content of the curriculum. Nor was it clear that the traditional methods of training recruits through apprenticeships and of licensing through an initiatory experience were not more effective and publicly more acceptable than a school diploma (Chavunduka 1984, 1986, 1994).

Furthermore traditional medical knowledge is rarely uniform. Broadly speaking, traditional practitioners are considered specialists in one of the two main aspects of healing: divining or diagnosing the ultimate causes of an illness, and identifying the nature of the illness and treating it, usually with an herbal or other empirical medicine. As a diviner, a healer practices usually in a specific locality where his or her social knowledge of the community is crucial; in contrast, a herbalist can ply the trade anywhere. Many practitioners (especially diviners) are skilled in both aspects of healing, but the theoretical premises are distinct. While herbal expertise can be acquired by anyone so inclined and is often an extension of people's ordinary knowledge of their habitat, diviners' skills are much more personal, even charismatic in origin and scarcely amenable to being taught or examined in schools. As a consequence, attempts to formalize the qualifications of practitioners through school education are likely to lose the support of many diviners, yet it is they who often have the widest public recognition.

Nonetheless, the elaboration of traditional knowledge into a formal system is proceeding among some groups—most notably, among Yoruba religious experts and practitioners in Nigeria. Here Yoruba traditional religion has already been elevated into an academically led philosophy (Abimbola 1976; Pearce 1986; Oyebola 1981). The literature on the subject is sufficient for university degree courses; initially oral, the central texts are now published along with a large exegetical literature and studies of healers in practice. Given the strong emphasis on schooling and certification generally in other aspects of Yoruba life, given too the plethora of privately owned schools and personally run churches, the problem will lie not so much in creating a suitable curriculum as in agreeing upon a common one. Finally, the Yoruba tradition has been maintained, and recently revived for political purposes, in both Brazil and many Caribbean states, thus giving the Yoruba system a potential international status. At present, it is seen primarily as a religious, not a medical, system. Yet it is among Yoruba healers that the strongest pressure for formal government recognition comes; and such recognition has already been won in Lagos state (Oyebola 1986). In a national context, however, nurturing so culture specific a system of therapy provokes both opposition on the grounds that it is tribalistic and derision on religious grounds, and thus effectively strangles attempts to form a nationwide profession.

In short, the formal elaboration of traditional medical knowledge has so far proved difficult and divisive, and without obvious benefits. More success has been had in creating practitioners' organizations that can bridge the differences in styles of expertise. But not all countries recognize people's rights to form associations (or indeed churches), and those that do often require them to be registered under one category or another. There is not space here to go into the relevant national variables, but it can be a significant feature of the political climate in which popular but marginalized groups have to operate.

PROFESSIONAL ORGANIZATIONS IN THE THIRD WORLD

In recent years the number of practitioners' organizations has grown rapidly, with at least one attaining professional powers. Most, however, operate as networks or as pressure groups. The difficulty has been to expand beyond this and find leaders widely acceptable and able to unite the majority of healers; in older organizations the problem has been in ensuring continuity once the local founder has died. Furthermore, as one such leader complained, the "bureaucratic habit" necessary to run committees proved uncongenial to most healers. It is arguable that the organizations will develop stage by stage—from regional to national society, from society to licensing authority, from licensing to full professional institutions—and given time and continuing government support that may be possible. More detailed analysis, country by country, is necessary. The present range of organizational types is as follows, starting with those with the least professional powers:

1. Cultural societies for like-minded practitioners whose aim is the advancement of their particular therapy. Membership is voluntary and does not depend on any qualification; it carries no weight publicly except to demonstrate commitment to a common cause. Yet the society's officers may be influential in advising government and thereby profitably enhance their reputations. Such societies are common; often they are regionally organized and create a network through which practitioners can exchange remedies and experiences, place suitable apprentices, and even refer cases for specialist attention. Some of the earliest associations of traditional practitioners were of this kind

but were not formally constituted. An example of such an informal, early association is described by Harriet Sibisi (1981); Gilles Bibeau (1980, 1982) has discussed a modern network of associations in Zaire.

2. Promotional groupings, membership of which is seen as a seal of approval, seeking to guarantee certain standards of competence. Membership is voluntary, but members submit themselves to some form of testing or at least undertake to comply with the grouping's code of conduct. Such codes of conduct may be displayed along with membership certificates. But the grouping has no statutory control over a particular therapy or its practitioners. Many of Nigeria's different associations of traditional medicine are of this kind, with some formally registered as commercial companies (Last and Chavunduka 1986:22,93).

3. Unions to which persons employed in medical practice (for example, by the state) have to belong in order to practice legally, though the union does not itself do any testing of its members. The union defends its members' interests in relation to their employers and acts as a vehicle for government to mobilize or instruct practitioners. Unions of this kind exist particularly in states with government-run health services employing practitioners such as traditional birth attendants and others in primary care as part-time auxiliaries (usually after some introductory retraining). The system effectively acts as a register of state-recognized healers and can take the form of an association run centrally by the ministry of health, as in Zambia (Twumasi and Warren 1986).

4. Professional associations, in which committees of the practitioners' organization have exclusive rights to license a practitioner. The organization undertakes to test the practitioner's ability to practice adequately and safely and to review (and, if necessary, revoke) any practitioner's license for malpractice or other misconduct. The business of the profession may be divided between a general council (a statutory body for traditional medicine established by government) and an association run by officers elected by practitioners and answerable to them. The profession's certificates are recognized by employers and insurers for certain benefits on a par with those issued by doctors. Zimbabwe has established professional institutions of this last kind after much debate and delay. Though they do not have powers to prevent nonmembers from practicing, many in the rural areas believe that they have. At present, testing procedures are carried out (orally) within each community by a committee of the leading local healers, and their recommendations are accepted centrally. Recognition by employers of certificates for sick leave and other matters has been won only recently through strike action (Chavunduka 1984, 1986).

Formal identification as a branch of medicine is not, of course, the only route practitioners can take to avoid the legal sanctions associated with medical practice. An alternative route is for healers to capitalize on their religious strengths and form a church instead of a medical profession. Where the political climate has been opposed to traditional medicine yet tolerant of church diversity, large numbers of Zionist or prophetic churches have sprung up to divine the causes of illness and to offer healing through prayer, exorcism, laying on of hands, or using incense or holy waters and oils. Historically, Christian churches have always been centers of medical care, pioneering some of the earliest hospital and ambulance services. Theologians' emphasis on Christ's role as a healer has ensured that the tradition of healing has continued into the present among both Catholics and Protestants, as shown most recently by the former archbishop of Lusaka Emmanuel Milingo or by the Filipino evangelists who perform "psychic surgery" (Milingo 1984; Hagey 1980).

Other healers, basing their practice not on church rituals but on the concepts of traditional religions, have the option of turning their practice formally into a cult, focusing on a shrine or a regular ritual like spirit possession. The success of candomble in Brazil, vodoo in Haiti, and Lemba in Zaire is well known (Janzen 1982b, 1992). But they are dependent nonetheless on the vitality of traditional belief in the face of increasingly widespread secular education and the explicit hostility of churches, Muslim organizations, and Marxist parties. Where church and cult groupings have to be registered in order to be allowed to operate, such hostility has potentially severe consequences, such as an outright ban or the destruction by the police of the shrine (as can happen, for example, in Cameroon). Though the demand for their services may be strong—for example, at a time when accusations of witchcraft grow particularly common and there is an epidemic of anxiety—yet the political clout of their clientele, especially if it is composed mainly of women, has in the past proved inadequate to protect them from closure. In this situation, better protection can come from redefining a religious cult as primarily therapeutic and joining a healers' association, run perhaps with links to the university and its hospitals. Thus the *zar* cult has continued to thrive in the Sudan despite an otherwise pervasive Islamic fundamentalism.

The final alternative is for practitioners not to organize themselves but to practice as individuals, train apprentices individually as before, and serve, as required, on government-run local health committees by virtue of their own public reputation. Thus the personal, almost idiosyncratic nature of their healing skill is recognized. Healers only in their spare time, many escape notice as they treat local patients privately. In this manner they survived through the colonial period unorganized. The danger now is that their skills will disappear with them—but not just their skills: the intellectual insight into how their society functions, its inner meanings and rituals, and, from that insight, how society's casualties can be repaired. Given the weakness in many Third World countries of university departments teaching "Western" psychiatry—a weakness that is both conceptual and practical—and given the scant psychiatric facilities made available by governments (Cohen 1988; Jong 1987), surely no country can afford to lose the insight and creative abilities of its indigenous practitioners, in this field at least. It is not that professional organization is thought to be the solution (though it is politically achievable now as never before) but that it offers a framework within which new developments in traditional medical thought can be tried out and passed on. In the process, new forms of professionalism will no doubt emerge, reflecting the priorities of indigenous practitioners and the public that patronizes them.

IN CONCLUSION

The systems of professionalized medicine described here have been developing over the last hundred years, in parallel with a similar professionalization in other fields of social activity ranging from government to sports (Perkin 1990; Burrage and Torstendahl 1990; Torstendahl and Burrage 1990). This age of professionalism, some say, is now drawing to a close; its place is being taken, once again, by a more entrepreneurial age, in which we are to see a return to some of the values and disciplines that preceded the rise of the professions and their bureaucratic rationality. Even large firms are downsizing and ceasing to look like quasi-governments. In short, the century of the professions, it is argued, will appear to future analysts to have been an organizational experiment that failed, a set of systems bankrupted finally by their inability to control costs.

There is indeed evidence for substantial shifts, if not for a new world order, in the patterns of health provision. The breakup of the Soviet Union and the Eastern bloc has given rise, at least initially, to a huge expansion of private medicine and a coming-out of fringe practitioners, offering the public all kinds of therapies including even witchcraft (Eberstadt 1994; Field 1994; Powell 1994). China, too, has seen health become an arena in which individual entrepreneurs can make money out of both ordinary and unorthodox treatments. Though much of the evidence is still anecdotal, the transformation of countries turning from the Marxist model to a post-Marxist free-for-all has been dramatic, but so too has been the persistent demand in those countries for the old securities of basic health care: ex-communists are reelected in the hope that they will provide some of the former services. In a country like Cuba, where the application of the Marxist model brought about great gains in health, the model still survives, though the system is close to bankruptcy.

The Soviet-Marxist health care model is not alone in being abandoned by the countries that developed it. Costs have also led to the transformation of the British system by changes that reflect a much wider trend of privatization and decentralization. After forty years of the National Health Service, hospitals in Britain have now been turned into individual enterprises in which costs and management priorities can override the patient's needs and best medical practice. In the same spirit, hospital managements now bring into the system a range of alternative therapies to offer patients, thus incorporating very different theories alongside those of biomedicine. Similarly, in South Africa, where health care is extremely uneven in distribution, there are pressures to recognize the services of some two thousand *sangomas* as part of the nation's new medical culture.

Elsewhere in Africa the effects of structural adjustment and, in particular, intrastate conflict have weakened or even destroyed the infrastructure required to deliver health services in rural areas. Add to this the fact that these economic and political trends, even in a rich country like Nigeria, have also crippled the middle classes (and the universities) where the ideology of professionalism was most firmly established, and the tide of professionalism, so marked in the 1970s and 1980s, seems to have turned. So what is happening now to the professional associations?

That centralized bureaucracies (and the professional ethos they run by) are in crisis does not in itself mean that professionalization in medicine is also in jeopardy. It means, rather, that the professions and would-be professionals have to adapt. In Britain it was members of the medical profession who were co-opted into reshaping the system, realizing too late (or so they said) the damage they were inflicting at the government's behest; the habitual (and usually profitable) closeness of professionals to government can also be their undoing. In the ex-Marxist countries, the new professional associations have yet to emerge, but a professionalization from below, on the model of Third World communities, has, it seems, already started.

Trends at the local level are beginning to show, as the social matrix within which medicine operates adjusts to the new relaxation of controls. For example, in a context where licensing has become meaningless, it is possible for new healers to develop new cures and to market them as never before. Most notably the AIDS epidemic has offered healers the chance to outdo biomedicine and offer their own cures to the public. The cures are popularly plausible in that they rely on fluctuations in the early symptoms of HIV, and encourage those who are HIV positive believing themselves cured, to go out and infect others. In both Zimbabwe and Kenya, healers' claims to have a cure for AIDS have therefore been stifled by an anxious government; healers are only allowed to claim that their remedies alleviate the symptoms, with the ZINATHA setting up a department for AIDS prevention and control (Chavunduka 1994:22). AIDS cures apart, the fact that governments are no longer so hostile to unorthodox therapies has meant that a would-be healing cult no longer needs to take on the coloring of a church; they can openly market their practices as medicine, not religion. It remains to be seen whether this will result in the development of new indigenous medicines as modernist and experimental in their way as the healing churches were under colonial rule (cf. Comaroff 1985); if it does, then the vehicle for these new systems of medicine is likely to be the professional association.

Similarly, patients facing a greater entrepreneurship in medicine are developing the consumerism that already exists for other products in the marketplace. Litigation is only one response; there are other, more direct ways of taking revenge. Where effective policing is absent, social violence is already a deterrent against medical incompetence or malpractice. Where the healer is lucky enough to escape, he can hope to shed his reputation by moving on, perhaps to one of the great cities, where the social mechanisms that normally control healers from below have little chance to develop, while control from above, by governments seen as hostile to the people of the shanty towns, is out of the question. In that case, the new associations springing up in response will be urban centered, possibly with protection from local mafias.

The breakdown of control over medical knowledge has already given rise to entrepreneurs who blend different medical technologies, modifying or blending regimens and procedures (including surgical ones) according to novel theories that tally with old ideas. (In not-so-different circumstances arose the now-established systems of osteopathy, chiropractic and homeopathy.) Conversely, new solutions have arisen to cope with the failure of controls. For example, in Nigeria, where fake or faulty drugs are a common hazard, the role of professional drug taster has developed: the would-be customer gets him to sample the pills to be purchased, to check that they conform to the known taste of authentic drugs of that brand.

In these conditions, then, the anthropology of professionalization in the field of medicine is particularly interesting as patients and practitioners alike have to find new ways of assessing skills and controlling knowledge, marking out jurisdictions, and developing means of redress. Medicine is paradoxical in the way that people are willing to pay highly for treatment, often believing that the costlier it is, the better. Professions in the health field therefore have had little problem keeping their fees high; the main threat is from interlopers. At the same time, the fact that patients—unlike the clients of most other professions—may not recover adds an element of serious risk missing from other professional arenas. The quest for some kind of professionalization, then, is particularly keen—however, we need always to remember that this has been so since long before the rise of professional society.

19

International Health: Problems and Programs in Anthropological Perspective

Sandra D. Lane and Robert A. Rubinstein

International health development work is among the most personally challenging, intellectually engaging, and potentially frustrating areas of medical anthropological practice. On a personal level, it can demand compassion and understanding in the midst of seemingly incredible amounts of disease, poverty, and suffering. Yet because an adequate understanding of the dynamics that lead to these conditions requires the integration of information from many spheres—biological, ecological, social, and cultural, for instance—using a variety of qualitative and quantitative methods, it engages the holistic commitment of anthropology as do few other anthropological activities. Notwithstanding this, it can be a frustrating area of work because the interaction of the broader political and economic contexts in which international health and development work is situated and the culture of the community of international health workers often leads to perverse outcomes.

These challenges, problems, and paradoxes are partly reflected in the following three examples:

1. In developing countries, 14 million children under the age of five died during 1987. More than 70 percent of these deaths were due to four main causes, all of which "are now susceptible to effective low-cost actions by well-informed and well-supported parents" (Grant 1988:3): diarrheal diseases, malaria, measles, and acute respiratory infection. In fact, children die of multiple causes, and malnutrition contributes to many of these.

2. U.S. foreign aid to Egypt since 1974 has totaled $13 billion. The principal bureaucratic means for distributing these funds is the U.S. Agency for International Development (USAID). In part because of AID policies and practices, this massive investment has not yielded equally impressive results. One problem is that AID assistance requires

that projects use costly U.S. materials and equipment: "One Egyptian government source has estimated that AID financed purchases are from 30 to 40 percent more expensive than substitutes readily available even in U.S. markets. Goods must also be shipped on U.S. vessels, at a cost that is sometimes three times the going international rate" (Rodenbeck 1988:17; see also Sullivan 1984). And the annual cost of maintaining the Cairo USAID office is approximately $150 million.

3. After investing huge amounts of money in the basic laboratory work needed to develop effective low-cost oral rehydration therapy (ORT) for stemming the devastating effects of diarrheal diseases, these techniques are frequently unused or misused. In part this failure derives from the frustrating circumstance that research supporting health planning is constrained by bureaucratic commitments so that it necessarily fails to discover culturally appropriate ways of integrating low-cost technologies, like ORT, into people's daily lives. As Foster (1987a:715) observes, "The assumption that asking people about their health beliefs and behavior, and observing their health behavior, is not science unless the data are used to test hypotheses, often severely constricts research designs and research results." (See also Pacey 1982; Rubinstein 1984.)

International health is the term that is most frequently used when health policy planners speak about health in the developing world. Although the United States and other industrialized nations are normally included in the concept international, in the case of health development work they are most commonly the planners, and less developed nations such as Egypt, Liberia, and Bangladesh are the recipients. Thus, in practice, international health refers to the flow of advice, health professionals, and health technology from the wealthier nations to the poorer.

International health development began with the eighteenth- and nineteenth-century missionaries, who set up clinics and offered medicine to the people they were trying to convert. Following the missionaries, colonial governments established health services in their colonies. Leng (1982:411) argues that the development of medical care by the British colonialists in Malaya occurred mainly because the indigenous labor force was decimated by infectious diseases, and communicable diseases were threatening the lives of the colonizers. El-Mehairy (1984:11) also stresses that "Western governments undertook international health work to protect their people from exotic diseases . . . [and in] the hope of political and economic benefit from foreign aid."

In 1914 Charles Eliot set out these assumptions in a remarkably unself-conscious way in his report to the Carnegie Endowment for International Peace:

The fundamental object of Western colonization, or other form of occupation in the East, is, as it always has been, the extension of European trade and the increase of European wealth; but the opinion is beginning to prevail extensively in Europe and among Europeans who live in the East, that these objects can best be accomplished by increasing the intelligence, skill, and well-being of the Eastern populations controlled, by raising their standards of living, relieving them from superstitious terrors, social bondages and industrial handicaps, and by creating among them new wants and ambitions. . . . The principal means to these worthy ends are . . . preventive medicine and an effective public health organization directed to the relief of current suffering, the prevention of sweeping pestilences, and the increase of industrial efficiency. (Eliot 1914:4)

Thus although international health work has always drawn on the talents and energies of compassionate and caring health professionals, the social organization of international health work developed in the context of, and continues to be shaped by, the political and economic self-interests of powerful groups. In a real sense, international health development was not based on altruism but served the political and medical needs of the donor countries.

An unequal distribution of power is implicit in the relationship between the donors of medical assistance and its recipients. Arturo Escobar (1985), following Michel Foucault's analysis of the discourse of power, examines the jargon of international health. He argues that health development work was preceded by the "creation of abnormalities" such as the term *underdeveloped,* which held the West to be the "developed" goal to which other countries must aspire, and in doing so devalued more than half of the world (p. 387). The standard on which development is based is largely arbitrary, culture bound, and one-dimensional. The basis of this evaluation, industrialization and wealth, assumes that the "underdeveloped" countries would benefit from becoming more like the developed countries and that they therefore must attempt to change in that direction. A rarely stated but increasingly clear point is that a scale based on development devalues, or discounts, some aspects of culture that promote quality of life, including "non-Western" traditions of art, religion, intellectual accomplishment, and social support (Rahnema 1986).[1]

Once these kinds of assumptions coalesced to form the "problem of under-development," its professionalization soon followed. As Escobar (1985) notes, major universities formed departments focused on development studies, which led to an institutionalized approach to the analysis and treatment of development projects (Sen 1979; Silverberg 1986) that restricts the range of information considered legitimate. A particularly extreme view of this process is expressed by Allan Hoben, who argues that development studies are a "positivistic and eth-nocentric interpretation of a particular historical process, the emergence of capitalism, and the industrial revolution in Western Europe" (Hoben 1982:352; see also Hill 1986). This situation has resulted in calls for expanding the kinds of information considered appropriate for use in health planning (Rubinstein 1984; Foster 1987a, 1987b; Justice 1987), and it has spawned more passionate responses as well.[2]

Nearly all of the terms used in international health work reflect the unequal relationship between the haves and the have-nots. Thus, it is problematic to choose non-value-laden terms. In an effort to modify the term *underdeveloped,* scholars have used *developing* and *less developed countries* (LDCs), in the World Health Organization jargon. Marxists and others with a political-economic perspective began referring to the "Third World" to distinguish, prior to the breakup of the Soviet Union, the First World (the United States and its allies) and the Second World (the Soviet Union and its allies) from the remaining polities in the world. The term *Third World* implies an understanding of the sociopolitical divisions between rich and poor nations, but it nonetheless lumps together quite diverse countries that often have little in common except poverty (Worsley 1984). Since there are no nonpejorative terms to describe the major recipient countries of international health aid, in this chapter we use *developing countries* and *Third World* interchangeably.

ASSUMPTIONS AND ORGANIZATION OF INTERNATIONAL HEALTH WORK

The assumptions of international health work have, according to George Foster (1987a, 1987b), historically included the assumptions that (1) wealthier countries have the capital, the talent, and the know-how to solve the health problems of the poorer countries; (2) the wealthier countries should therefore plan and direct such efforts; and (3) Western health care institutions and approaches will work in solving health problems in LDCs. These general assumptions are elements of a professional worldview that persists despite repeated demonstrations that it is inadequate. There is no reason to assume that development projects designed and implemented by Western experts will be appropriate or useful in the Third World. Judithanne Justice (1983, 1984, 1987) demonstrates that in Nepal, the primary health care model developed by WHO, the United Nations Children's Fund (UNICEF), and USAID was applied without considering local cultural or political factors. It failed as a result.

A further, perhaps more basic, assumption in international health development has been that the provision of health care will improve the health of the recipients. Although there have been successes in international health work—the most frequently cited being the eradication of smallpox during the 1970s—many projects have failed to improve health, and some have worsened the health of the people they were trying to help. Furthermore, in Europe, the major improvements in infectious diseases (especially tuberculosis) occurred before the development of sophisticated health care technologies like antibiotics, vaccines, or modern medicine (Dubos 1959; Ratcliffe 1985).

T. McKeown (1976b) describes how the social movements of the nineteenth century in England led to the provision of clean water and improvements in nutrition and housing, which were responsible for the reduction in infectious disease. The resulting decrease in mortality rates, especially among infants and children, happened before the advent of antibiotics. Thus, health care alone may not be the best method of improving the health of people internationally, particularly when their health problems stem directly from poverty.

International health bureaucracies encompass four distinct types of organizations (Foster 1987a, 1987b):

1. *International (multilateral) organizations,* such as WHO, UNICEF, the Food and Agriculture Organization (FAO), the United Nations Fund for Population Assistance (UNFPA), the United Nations Educational, Scientific and Cultural Organization (UNESCO), the World Bank, and many others. It is at conferences funded and organized by these agencies that major policy directions are charted. One of the most famous such meetings was the 1978 Alma Ata Conference, which officially inaugurated primary health care (WHO 1978a). Following ratification of each new policy direction, the multilateral organizations, often in cooperation with bilateral and private organizations, fund projects in individual countries.

2. *Governmental (bilateral) organizations,* in which one country directly extends aid to a second country, usually through the ministry of health in the recipient country. The United States channels this assistance through the USAID. Although this aid is officially for health projects, it also serves the needs of U.S. foreign policy and is used as an incentive to encourage others to act in accord with U.S. interests. Furthermore, USAID assistance often reflects U.S. concerns more than those of the recipient countries. For example, during the Reagan administration, USAID withdrew its support from UNFPA because of right-wing pressure against funding abortion services. The conservative trend toward privatization has influenced USAID funding as well. Although the bulk of USAID's support still goes to ministries of health, an increasing portion supports the health projects of private organizations and for-profit health services (Montague and Lamstein 1988).

3. *Private and voluntary organizations (PVOs) or nongovernmental organizations* (NGOs), which may be secular (for example, Save the Children Foundation and CARE) or religious (for example, Catholic Relief Services and the American Friends Service Committee). They may also be international, where the headquarters are located in the United States or Europe with local offices in recipient countries, or they may be indigenous. In India, for example, indigenous voluntary organizations are particularly strong. In many other countries, however, government control of indigenous organizations precludes their development of effective programs. In general, NGOs provide direct assistance to particular groups, such as refugees, children, or disaster victims. Since they often serve fairly small groups, NGOs may quite successfully improve the health of their target populations. When the same programs are attempted with a larger population with no increase in funding (for example, when a ministry of health attempts to replicate a successful pilot project on a country-wide scale), the projects often fail. This effect, called *upscaling* in the development literature, is one of the main reasons that pilot projects are so difficult to translate into large-scale strategies (Sohoni 1988:25–28).

4. *Philanthropic foundations,* which were among the first bureaucracies to become involved in international health. These include the Rockefeller Foundation, the Ford Foundation, Hewlett, Mellon, the Packard Foundation, and many others. Although U.S.–based philanthropic foundations are private and not associated with the government, they have, especially in the past, been accused of serving the needs of American business and foreign policy. Indeed, an entire body of literature examines the Rockefeller Foundation's heavy-handed approach to international development (E. Brown 1976, 1980; Donaldson 1976; Franco-Agudelo 1983). More recently, however, many philanthropic agencies have revised their funding strategies. The Ford Foundation,

for example, works primarily through indigenous institutions. It supports research, education, and action programs conceived of and conducted by local scholars to meet the needs of their own countries.

HEALTH PROBLEMS IN THE THIRD WORLD

Before discussing specific international health projects or the role of anthropologists in them, it is important to review the major health problems in the Third World that these projects are designed to address. Obviously the countries that make up the Third World are heterogeneous, as are the populations within those countries, so any overview that lumps them together does not do justice to their diversity. Nevertheless, sociopolitical and ecological similarities exist among Third World countries that affect the health of their people.

Third World populations are usually characterized by pyramidal age structures, with the bulk of the people under age fifteen. High infant death is reflected in the infant morality rates (Table 19.1)—for 1992, for example, 165 per 1,000 in Afghanistan and 122 per 1,000 in Mali, with 6 per 1,000 for Sweden and Finland and 9 per 1,000 for the United States (Grant 1988:64–65; International Bank for Reconstruction and Development 1988; Golladay and Liese 1980; Rohde 1983). The leading infectious causes of infant and childhood death are diarrhea, respiratory illnesses, malaria, measles, and neonatal tetanus. Childhood vaccines against polio, diphtheria, pertussis (whooping cough), tetanus (including tetanus immunization for pregnant women), measles, and tuberculosis are potential lifesaving interventions (World Bank 1993). Although immunizations are officially available in most countries, many children are unvaccinated, for reasons that span the cultural and political spectrum. There are, however, some encouraging accomplishments. Polio, targeted by the WHO and UNICEF for eradication by the year 2000, has been virtually eliminated in the Western Hemisphere (Grant 1994; Jamison et al. 1991).

Since the late 1970s the spread of HIV-AIDS has reached global pandemic proportions. The WHO estimates that by mid-1993 HIV had infected more than 14 million individuals worldwide, with approximately 1 million of these infections occurring in children, through vertical, or mother-to-child transmission (WHO 1993). Babies infected with the human immunodeficiency virus rarely survive to their fifth year. Hepatitis B infection, transmitted like HIV from mother to child as well as via contaminated blood and semen, may induce chronic hepatitis and, years later, liver cancer (Horn 1986a). Childhood immunization programs in a number of countries, where the infection is endemic, have begun to include vaccination against hepatitis B (Prince 1990).

The major parasitic diseases (malaria, schistosomiasis, onchocerciasis, trypanasomiasis, leischmaniasis, filiriasis, dracunculiasis, and the intestinal parasites) plague both children and adults with chronic infections that cause debility, loss of productivity, and shortened life spans (Katz, Despommier, and Gwadz 1982). Although much international health work has attempted to control these parasitic

Table 19.1
Child and Infant Mortality Rates and Adult Literacy Rates

Country	1992 under 5 Mortality	1992 IMR	% Adults Literate--1990 male/female
Afghanistan	257	165	44/14
Mali	220	122	41/24
Sierra Leone	249	144	31/11
Malawi	226	143	52/31*
Ethiopia	208	123	
Guinea	230	135	33/16
Somalia	211	125	36/14
Burkina Faso	150	101	28/9
Niger	320	191	40/17
Chad	209	123	42/18
Guinea-Bissau	239	141	50/24
Central African Republic	179	105	52/25
Senegal	145	90	52/25
Mauritania	206	118	47/21
Liberia	217	146	50/29
Rwanda	222	131	64/37
Yemen	177	107	53/26
Bhutan	201	131	51/25
Nepal	128	90	38/13
Burundi	179	108	61/40
Bangladesh	127	97	47/22
Benin	147	88	32/16
Sudan	166	100	43/12
Tanzania, U. Rep. of	176	111	93/88
Bolivia	118	80	87/71
Nigeria	191	114	62/40
Haiti	133	87	59/47
Gabon	158	95	74/49
Uganda	185	111	62/35
Pakistan	137	95	47/21
Zaire	188	121	84/61
Lao Dem. Rep.	145	98	92/76*
Oman	31	24	47/12*
Cameroon	117	74	67/43
Togo	137	86	56/31
India	124	83	62/34
Cote d'Ivoire	124	91	67/40
Ghana	170	103	70/51
Zambia	202	113	81/65
Eritrea	208	123	
Cambodia	184	117	48/22
Namibia	79	62	
Azerbaijan	53	37	
Kazakhstan	50	43	

*Indicates that the data are from prior to 1990.
Source: From Grant (1994:62).

Table 19.1 (Continued)

Country	1992 under 5 Mortality	1992 IMR	% Adults Literate--1990 male/female
Egypt	55	43	63/34
Peru	65	46	91/79
Libyan Arab Jamahiriya	104	70	75/50
Morocco	61	50	61/38
Indonesia	111	71	88/75
Congo	110	82	70/44
Kenya	74	51	80/59
Zimbabwe	86	60	74/60
Honduras	58	45	75/71
Algeria	72	60	70/46
Tunisia	38	32	74/56
Guatemala	76	55	63/47
Saudi Arabia	40	35	73/48
South Africa	70	53	78/75*
Nicaragua	76	54	
Turkey	87	70	90/71
Iraq	80	64	70/49
Botswana	58	45	84/65
Viet Nam	49	37	92/84
Madagascar	168	110	88/73
Ecuador	59	47	88/84
Papua New Guinea	77	54	65/38
Brazil	65	54	83/80
El Salvador	63	47	76/70
Dominican Republic	50	42	85/82
Philippines	60	46	90/89
Mexico	33	27	90/85
Colombia	20	17	87/86
Syrian Arab Republic	40	34	78/51
Paraguay	34	28	92/88
Mongolia	80	61	93/86*
Jordan	30	25	89/70
Lebanon	44	35	88/73
Thailand	33	27	96/90
Albania	34	28	
China	43	35	84/62
Sri Lanka	19	15	93/84
Venezuela	24	20	87/90
United Arab Emirates	22	18	58/38*
Argentina	24	22	95/95
Malaysia	19	14	86/70
Panama	20	18	88/88
Moldova	36	31	
Armenia	34	29	
Latvia	26	22	
Estonia	24	20	100/100*
Korea Dem. Rep.	33	25	

Table 19.1 (Continued)

Country	1992 under 5 Mortality	1992 IMR	% Adults Literate—1990 male/female
Korea, Republic of	9	8	99/94
Uruguay	22	20	97/96
Mauritius	24	20	89/77*
Romania	28	23	
Yugoslavia (former)	22	19	97/88
Russian Federation	32	28	
Chile	18	15	93/93
Trinidad and Tobago	22	19	97/93*
Jamaica	14	12	98/99
Kuwait	16	14	77/67
Costa Rica	17	14	93/93
Portugal	13	11	89/81
Bulgaria	20	16	
Hungary	16	15	99/99*
Poland	16	14	
Cuba	11	10	95/93
Greece	9	8	98/89
Czech Republic	12	11	
Israel	11	9	95/89*
New Zealand	10	8	
USA	10	9	
Austria	9	7	
Belgium	11	9	
Germany	8	7	
Italy	10	8	98/96
Singapore	7	6	92/74*
Ireland	6	5	
Spain	9	8	97/93
United Kingdom	9	7	
Australia	9	7	
Hong Kong	7	6	95/81*
France	9	7	
Canada	8	7	
Denmark	8	7	
Japan	6	4	
Netherlands	7	6	
Switzerland	9	7	
Norway	8	6	
Finland	7	6	
Sweden	7	6	

diseases, especially malaria, schistosomiasis, and trypanasomiasis, the failure of vector control measures and a number of other problems have contributed to the failure of these programs (Golladay and Liese 1980:18).

Emerging new and reemerging old diseases have proved that the once-assumed victory over infectious diseases was nothing but a temporary reprieve (Sommerfeld 1994). Overuse and inappropriate use of antimicrobial drugs have bred resistant strains of tuberculosis, *Streptococcus pneumoniae,* and *Staphylococcus aureus.* Decreased attention to public health prevention, including food safety and rodent and vector control, has led to epidemics of cholera, plague, and dengue (Bryan et al. 1994; Burns 1994). New and potentially fatal viruses—including HIV, hantavirus, Legionnaire's disease, and Ebola virus—have been identified since 1980 (Bryan et al. 1994).

Accidents, particularly motor vehicle accidents, are common in cities where the traffic congestion rivals that in the industrialized world (Fenner 1980). Burns are frequent in makeshift housing, where open fires or small kerosene stoves are used for cooking and heating. Inadequate or completely lacking emergency and fire vehicles, equipment, and personnel mean that people die who might otherwise be saved. Occupational exposures to such toxins as lead, pesticides, and other chemicals cause unknown amounts of disease, especially where safety equipment is inadequate or not even considered. For example, textile workers in Egypt frequently suffer from pneumoconiosis after years of inhaling fiber dust without any respiratory protective equipment (Lane 1985).

Illiteracy is often high, and in some countries a majority of women are illiterate (Grant 1988:76–77). Female literacy has a profound indirect effect on health. Illiterate mothers are unable to read directions on medicine containers and consequently may give the wrong medicine or wrong dose of medicine to a child (Lane 1987). Furthermore, increasing female literacy is associated with a decrease in the birthrate and decreased infant mortality rates (Herz and Measham 1987:35–37). In a remarkable study that examined data from thirty-three countries, a linear relationship was found between maternal education and child survival (Cochrane, O'Hara, and Leslie 1980). For every one-year increment in mothers' education there was a 7 to 9 percent decline in child mortality.

Unemployment and underemployment are large problems in the developing world, where the labor force may be unable to absorb those who receive an education (Kepel 1985:85). Frequently the brightest and the best young graduates emigrate to seek their fortunes in other countries, often in the West (Saleh 1979). This brain drain disproportionately affects the ranks of physicians and nurses, the loss of whom directly affects a country's health care. According to Mahler (1981:10) more than 75 percent of the world's migrant physicians now practice in five of the wealthiest Western countries: Australia, Canada, the Federal Republic of Germany, the United Kingdom, and the United States.

Poverty grew in many parts of the world during the 1980s. In 1990 the World Bank estimated that 1.1 billion people were living in poverty. In a worsening spiral, external debt and structural adjustment policies have severely limited the

amount that developing countries can afford to spend on essential health services, such as immunization and tuberculosis treatment (Grant 1994). According
to James Grant, late director of UNICEF, the debt service alone for sub-Saharan
African countries per month in 1993 came to $1 billion (Grant 1993). Due to
poverty, the toll of AIDS infection in families, and civil conflict, the WHO
estimates that by the year 2000 there will be 10 million abandoned or orphaned
children living on their own in Africa (Grant 1994).

Sociopolitical conditions both cause some health problems and make a number of existing problems worse, including inadequate food, clean water, stress
associated with migration, war, multinational business interests, and large-scale
development projects.

Poor Access to Food

It is widely acknowledged that nutritional status is the most important determinant of health (Scrimshaw 1974). Nevertheless, due to lack of food, millions
of children and adults in the developing world are malnourished. Dietary inadequacy often results from unequal distribution of food within a country and
between countries, which occurs even when adequate food stores exist (Feder
1981). Susan George (1977) describes how price controls meant to increase
profits result in planned scarcity, where millions starve while farmers in the
United States are paid not to produce. Noting the unequal distribution of food
internationally, the *Food and Nutrition Bulletin* commented:

No doubt everyone realizes how preposterous it is that the two most protein-needy con-
tinents, Africa and South America, are the main suppliers of animal protein food moving
in the world trade—and they supply those who already have plenty. (cited by *Xeroph-
thalmia Club Bulletin* 1983)

In Egypt, for example, the rural delta has the highest density of animals per
unit of land in the world (Horn 1986b); however, in many rural hamlets, the
peasants can afford very little meat, which they eat mainly on religious holy
days and when someone dies (Lane 1987). Nevertheless, a significant amount
of acreage is devoted to fodder to fatten the livestock, which are then sold for
cash (Adams 1986; Lane 1987).

In rural farming areas, the shift from subsistence agriculture to growing cash
crops has worsened the diets of the farmers and their families (George 1977:
15–19). The change in crops, often from food to nonfood items such as cotton
or coffee, began as an influence of European colonialism. For example, in 1832
Egypt began growing cotton, which is still its major cash crop (Owen 1969).
The Sudan began cotton production in 1910, when it was then under British
colonial rule. With the completion of the Sennar Dam in 1925, more than 2
million acres in the Gezira scheme were irrigated for the production of cotton
and other crops (Gezira Board 1987). Since cash crops are grown to be exported

and are usually cultivated on the best land, farmers must then grow their families' food on smaller and poorer plots of land and purchase the remainder of the food they need. Further, farmers must purchase seeds, fertilizer, pesticides, and the like to grow the next year's cash crop. The families' diet, which may have been relatively abundant and varied during subsistence farming, suffers, and the most vulnerable members of each family, the children and childbearing women, suffer the most.

The "green revolution" was a development strategy based on the assumption that producing more food per unit of land would be the answer to the world's food shortages (George 1977). In an attempt to increase crop yield, new hybrid plants were developed that produced twice their former yields. However, the green revolution replaced the varied traditional agriculture with monocrops of cereals (Taussig 1978; Schertz 1972). This switch decreased the peasants' dietary diversity and replaced much of the leguminous proteins that were the peasants' main protein source. Furthermore, the genetic diversity of the crops was decreased, since the hybrids were developed in a few laboratories, such as the International Rice Research Institute in the Philippines (George 1977:88). The new hybrids needed enormous amounts of fertilizer and pesticides, which the developing countries were often forced to purchase from the West. The expense of these purchases forced many small farmers off their land, which was then bought by agribusinesses that used the green revolution technology to produce cash crops (World Agricultural Research Project 1980). In Colombia, for example, "the expansion of intensive large-scale farming has driven the bulk of the peasantry off the land in recent years; 50 percent of the children six years and under are said to be suffering from malnutrition" (Taussig 1978:101).

In many parts of the world, land tenure remains nearly feudal, with a small percentage of landlords owning the fields on which tenant farmers grow crops. P. J. Brown (1987) examined such a situation in Sardinia and found that the energy taken from the peasants in the form of payment to the landlords was a much greater burden on them than the chronic malaria from which they suffered. He had originally gone to Sardinia to study the effect of malaria on impeding development and concluded that the land tenure system that so favored the few owners presented a much larger obstacle. A similar situation exists in many parts of India. Sandra Lane interviewed landless farmworkers in Gujarat state and found that they were paid only half of the official minimum wage (6 rupees per day rather than 12 rupees). When large expenses, such as providing a dowry for a daughter, forced them to borrow from the landlord, they and their entire families entered into a form of indentured servitude.

In Third World cities, rural-to-urban migrants have swelled the squatter settlements. Many of these residents were farmers who lost their land due to poverty and must now purchase all of their food. With high unemployment and lack of literacy and job skills to survive in a city, they and their children may starve due to lack money. Charles Hughes and John Hunter (1970) describe this phenomenon as "urban malnutrition."

Even fuel for cooking of food is often scarce and expensive. In areas where women depend on wood for cooking, deforestation has complicated their lives enormously. In a village in Gujarat state, India, the women claimed to spend between two to four hours per day gathering sufficient firewood to cook the daily meal.

Lack of Clean Water

In many countries, piped water and sanitation are luxuries of the urban middle and upper classes. In rural areas and urban slums, residents may have to travel some distance to a crowded public tap or may have to drink from a stream polluted with human and animal waste. Between 1988 and 1991, for example, only 51 percent of people in Indonesia, 25 percent of people in Paraguay, and 22 percent of people in Mozambique had access to safe water (Grant 1994).

David Sanders (1985) describes three types of disease associated with inadequate water supplies: water-borne diseases, which occur when drinking water is contaminated with fecal organisms, such as cholera, typhoid, amoebiasis, hepatitis A, polio, and diarrhea; water-washed diseases, which increase when wash water is inadequate, such as skin and eye infections; and water-based diseases, in which the infectious agent is present in the water and penetrates the skin during washing, such as schistosomiasis. The most ubiquitous water-borne disease, diarrhea, is the leading cause of death in children under five in developing countries and results in between 5 and 18 million childhood deaths per year (Rohde and Northrup 1976:341). In addition to fatal dehydration, diarrhea contributes to malnutrition and weakened immunity in children who survive (Chen and Scrimshaw 1983). So detrimental is diarrhea to the child's nutritional status that it can cause malnutrition even when there is sufficient food available to the child (Chen and Scrimshaw 1983).

Increase in Disease Due to Refugee Flight, Forced Relocation, and Rural to Urban Migration

Migration, especially refugee flight from war and natural disasters, has been increasing every year. Since 1945, 60 million to 70 million people have fled from their homes because of political repression and war (Beyer 1981:26); more than 14 million of these refugees fled in 1974 alone (1974 World Refugee Report, cited by Jacobson 1977:516), and in 1995 alone, there were 23 million official refugees (Peterson 1995:9). In 1993, an increasing number of individuals fled their homes without crossing international borders; these internally displaced persons are harder to reach with emergency services and are frequently more vulnerable than officially recognized refugees (Frelick 1994). Forced relocation of entire communities is a consequence of the construction of such dams as the Kariba Dam (Zimbabwe), the Aswan High Dam (Egypt and the Sudan), and the Keban Dam (Turkey) (Scudder 1975). In most Third World countries, a large proportion of the population is rural, with farming as its main occupation. However, rural-to-urban migration is increasing; the World Bank estimates that by the year 2000 the worldwide urban population will be 45 percent of the total (Golladay and Liese 1980:21). Due to this migration, the large cities in the Third World have swelled and are surrounded by squatter settlements of poor people who live without basic sanitation in crowded, makeshift housing (Peattie 1968). In many Third World cities, estimates of the proportion of the population that lives in squatter settlements range from 20 percent to 50 percent (Abrams 1970).

Scudder and Colson (1982) attribute the health effects of migration to three types of stress: physiological, psychological, and sociocultural. Such physiological stresses as crowding, inadequate food, inadequate water, and inadequate sewage disposal can both lower the migrants' resistance to disease and expose them to such infectious diseases as tuberculosis, parasitism, diarrhea, and respiratory illnesses (Hull 1979:32; McNeill 1980). Such psychological stresses as grief, anxiety, and emotional trauma contribute to both physical and mental illness (Murphy 1961). Such sociocultural stresses as language barriers, resettlement in an area where the habits, attitudes, and beliefs are unfamiliar, and where xenophobia makes the host population negatively prejudiced toward the migrants, may lead to such economic, family, and social problems as alcoholism (Scudder and Colson 1982; Ablon 1965).

Political Repression, Violence, and War

Directly and indirectly political-economic struggles affect health. War and violence, as parts of contemporary political realities, are now much different from the conventional wars of other eras of human history. Now combat between opposing armies is infrequent. In its place, "war is focused on the Third World, and pits guerrilla insurgences against state governments and states against indigenous nations" (Nietschmann 1987:1). The direct killing and maiming of combatants is the unfortunate goal of war. A less obvious effect is the loss of this human power for the society—the loss of teachers, engineers, and manual workers to carry on the daily tasks of the society. After the war, the society must support and care for the disabled veterans and suffers the effects of angry men in its midst who have been trained to kill (Siegel, Baron, and Epstein 1985). It is not hyperbole to say, for example, that the young Israeli soldiers who are learning that it is acceptable to break the hands and skulls of West Bank Palestinians have become dehumanized. One soldier stated, "The more I break other people's bones, the more I am broken myself" (Greenberg 1988:1). Nor is it difficult to imagine the future problems this brutality will create for Israeli society (Physicians for Human Rights 1988).

War profoundly affects civilian health as well. The civilians need not be members of the enemy; war may provide an excuse for genocide of a national minority population. The examples of such genocide are numerous, from the

German Holocaust of European Jews to the Guatemalan extermination of the indigenous Indian peasants (Carmack 1988).[3] Before Rwanda's Hutu ethnic majority began its genocidal slaughter of the Tutsi minority in April 1994, the country's total population numbered 8 million. As a result of the tragedy, 500,000 people were killed, and nearly 5 million became refugees or internally displaced (Atwood 1994).

Direct health effects on civilian enemies are also numerous but are often ignored since the people killed are typically women, children, and elders. The My Lai massacre of an entire village by U.S. soldiers is one example (Nagel 1972). During the war of 1948, 250 Palestinians were killed in the village of Dier Yassin, to "liberate" the territory for the newly created state of Israel (Said 1979:44). And more recently, the use of poison gas by Iraq during its war with Iran is reported to have wiped out the entire population of a Kurdish village (Browne 1988; Physicians for Human Rights 1989).

A less obvious effect of war on civilian health is the disruption of food distribution and health care. In Sudan, the largest country in Africa, the effects of the brutal civil war between the Muslim north and non-Muslim south have resulted in significant losses in progress from past development efforts and in diminished prospects for development in the future (Ahmed et al. 1988). For example, for the south the war meant the near cessation of the drilling of boreholes for fresh water after 1985 (Dodge and Ibrahim 1988:48–49), an exceptionally high infant mortality rate of 180 per 1,000, prevalent malnutrition among children twelve and younger (Duku 1988:44), and the decimation of the infrastructure for primary and secondary health care in the region (Duku 1988: 37–41).

In Zimbabwe from 1978 to 1980 the military carried out Operation Turkey, destroying crops, livestock, and food supplies in order to starve the guerrillas (Sanders 1982). The unfortunate consequence of this strategy was widespread malnutrition of rural children and increased infant and childhood mortality.

In Nicaragua the contra forces explicitly targeted health workers and health institutions (Siegel, Baron, and Epstein 1985; Siegel, Baron, and Eitel 1985; Kreier and Baron 1987). From 1981 to 1985, thirty-eight health workers were killed and twenty-eight kidnapped while they were performing medical services; sixty-one health units were destroyed and thirty-seven others forced to close due to contra activity. Due to the decreased availability of health services, immunization, sanitation, nutrition and other health programs were curtailed and health, especially of the rural peasants, suffered.

In the Guatemalan village of San Pedro, for instance, the effect of the burden of military operations on the economy is conspicuous. Between 1977 and 1987 the cost of one pound of rice increased fivefold, from .15 quetzal to .75 quetzal. Although there was a rise in wages during the decade, it was nowhere as great as the rise in prices. This means that one pound of rice rose from representing .25 percent to .71 percent of a laborer's average monthly wage. Similar increases

Table 19.2
Prices in San Pedro, Guatemala, as a Percentage of Monthly Wages,
1977 and 1987

| | | 1977 | | | | 1987 | | |
		Teacher	Laborer	Maid		Teacher	Laborer	Maid
Wage*		240.00	60.00	12.00		372.00	105.00	40.00
	Price	%	%	%	Price	%	%	%
Black beans/lb	.08	.03	.13	.67	.70	.19	.67	1.75
Corn/lb	.05	.02	.08	.42	.22	.06	.21	.55
Rice/lb	.15	.06	.25	1.25	.75	.20	.71	1.88
Soap/ea	.04	.02	.07	.33	.22	.06	.21	.55
Meat/lb	.75	.31	1.25	6.25	3.75	1.01	3.57	9.38
Chicken feed/100lbs	8.40	3.50	14.00	70.00	33.80	9.09	32.19	84.50
Milk/liter	.08	.03	.13	.67	.50	.13	.48	1.25
Salt	.03	.01	.05	.25	.20	.05	.19	.50
Chicken/lb	.29	.12	.48	2.42	1.80	.48	1.71	4.50
Sugar/lb	.08	.03	.13	.67	.30	.08	.29	.75
Bread/six	.05	.02	.08	.42	.24	.06	.23	.60
Carrots/doz.	.40	.17	.67	3.33	1.00	.27	.95	2.50
Shrimp/lb	1.20	.50	2.00	10.00	8.00	2.15	7.62	20.00
Tomato paste/each	.15	.06	.25	1.25	.75	.20	.71	1.88
Hot sauce/each	.10	.04	.17	.83	.50	.13	.48	1.25
Gasoline/gallon	.95	.40	1.58	7.92	2.95	.79	2.81	7.38
Electricity/kwh	.07	.03	.12	.58	.21	.06	.20	.53
Antacids/each	.05	.02	.08	.42	.15	.04	.14	.38
Private school/month	4.00	1.67	6.67	33.33	15.00	4.03	14.29	37.50
Bus to Quezaltenango	.50	.21	.83	4.17	1.50	.40	1.43	3.75

*Quetzals, laborer's wage based on daily wage estimate.
Source: From Ehlers (1987:27).

occurred in the cost of other staple commodities (Table 19.2). The nutritional consequences of this situation are remarkable:

One impact of all this is that protein consumption dropped by at least 15 percent, caloric intake by 16 percent, and the per capita intake of eggs, meat and fat was reduced in 90 percent of the population. (Ehlers 1987:27)

That devoting a disproportionate share of a nation's economy to maintaining a military effort has a negative effect on human services and on social supports in that nation has been well documented (Melman 1965, 1988; Pinxten 1986). Further, devoting resources to the procurement of military resources has world-wide effects, especially in the case of the development of nuclear arsenals.

The threat of nuclear war and the scientific study of long-term effects of dropping the atomic bomb on Hiroshima and Nagasaki have focused attention on the medical aspects of nuclear war (Ishikawa and Swain 1981). This has inspired a number of speculative reports on the potential health effects of nuclear war. Owen Greene and associates (1982) describe the effects of several different kinds of nuclear attacks on London, England. In their analysis, they calculate that "a single one-megaton bomb can destroy by blast and fire an area 10 miles across'' (Greene et al. 1982:25), and they note that it would disrupt electrical and other utilities over a much wider area. As for casualties, they say that even in an attack,

in which no bomb falls on Inner London, over one million die in seconds from blast injuries and more than 4 million from radiation over a period of up to two months after the attack. At least half a million people are injured by blast. (Greene et al. 1982:55)

More generally, in addition to deaths immediately attributable to the blast, Elizabeth Schueler and George Armelagos (1989:108; Armelagos and Schueler 1986) point out that the "short term health effects on the population will be further exacerbated by the destruction of an estimated 80 percent of the medical resources." Further, aside from radiation-induced illness, there will be an increase in morbidity due to vitamin, mineral, and food deficiencies. On the social and cultural levels, the possibility of nuclear war suggests the likely disruption of social life on a dramatic scale (Rubinstein 1988).

Multinational Business Interests

Businesses often place profits above other considerations, including the health of unsuspecting consumers. The infant formula scandal is perhaps the most well-known example of this phenomenon. Following World War II infant formula companies, such as Nestlé and Unigate, began increasingly intensive promotion of artificial milk as the healthiest choice for infant diets (George 1977:152–153; Jelliffe and Jelliffe 1977). This marketing involved not only print, radio, and television advertisements but also saleswomen dressed as nurses who demonstrated the products to new mothers in hospitals, frequently giving away the first tin for free (George 1977:153). For poor families, however, the formula was so expensive that one-quarter to one-third of the family's income might be required to purchase adequate amounts, forcing mothers to dilute the strength of the mixture (George 1977:153; Elling 1981). Furthermore, lack of refrigeration and contamination of the water used to mix the formula is the surest route to diarrhea. Finally, without the nipple stimulation of frequent suckling, the mother's breast milk dries up. Thus, the child is deprived of the immunoprotective factors intrinsic to human milk—factors that would protect it from infection—and if the parents lack money to purchase sufficient formula, the infant starves. The irony is how completely unnecessary artificial formula is for babies; breast milk is healthier than formula, and it is free and sterile.

A second example of multinational business interests' directly impairing health is the dumping of drugs in the Third World. M. Silverman, P. Lee, and M. Lydecker (1982) have conducted extensive investigations of the marketing of drugs in the developing world. Specifically they called attention to the inconsistencies in drug indications and descriptions of side effects in the promotional literature. Powerful antibiotics such as chloramphenocol are used extensively in Latin America and the Middle East for childhood diarrhea, according to package directions. The package directions do not mention the potentially fatal side effect—aplastic anemia—which is the reason that chloramphenocol is reserved for only life-threatening infections in the United States. This inappropriate use of powerful antibiotics, moreover, encourages the development of resistant organisms, so that the drugs may then be ineffective when they are truly needed. Since in many parts of the developing world it is possible to purchase drugs directly from the pharmacy without a doctor's prescription or advice, there is great danger that such inappropriate drugs are given to children and adults every day.

The companies that make these drugs are well aware of their side effects. For example Ciba-Geigy produces an antidiarrhea medication marketed as Entero-Vioform. The active ingredient, clioquinol, was found to cause a nerve disease, subacute myeloopticoneuropathy (SMON), characterized by numbness in the extremities and in some cases blindness and paralysis. SMON litigation throughout the 1970s resulted in the Ciba-Geigy company's being forced to pay the Japanese victims of the drug 109,346,000,000 yen (approximately $490 million) in legal compensation (Silverman, Lee, and Lydecker 1982:51). In 1985, Ciba-Geigy was still marketing Entero-Vioform in Egypt, without any warning on the package insert (Lane 1985).

Large-Scale Development Projects

Development projects are meant to improve the standard of living in developing countries, so it is at first surprising that they are responsible for much disease themselves. However, as D. Heyneman (1983), Thayer Scudder (1973), and Charles Hughes and John Hunter (1970) point out, projects are often developed in the donor countries without considering the ecological cost of the endeavor. Indeed there has developed a culture of the development community that is heavily invested in providing technological solutions to the "problems of developing countries" (Pacey 1983:5–15). One result is that even when local planners are involved in projects, local information is not incorporated into project designs, as Justice's (1986) analysis of health development planning in Nepal shows.

We have already described the effects of forced relocation on migrants who must resettle to accommodate big dam projects. Heyneman (1983) also describes how the construction of each major dam in Africa was accompanied by an upsurge of parasitic diseases. For example, more than half of the 85,000 new residents in fishing villages around the newly created Lake Volta have become infected with *Schistosoma haematobium*. This chronic parasite spends part of its life cycle in snails that live in slow-moving water. Whenever the water flow is impeded, such as with a dam, the snails flourish and provide the perfect ecosphere for the *Schistosoma* parasite. In humans, chronic schistosomiasis or bilharziasis causes cirrhosis, enlarged spleen, and portal hypertension; infected adults frequently bleed to death when the overdistended veins in their esophagi burst (Plorde 1980:907–911). In 1937, just twelve years after the completion of the Sennar Dam on the Blue Nile in the Sudan, these health problems were already apparent, and perceptively, if paternalistically, noted by Emil Ludwig (1937:37):

For disease, in an uncanny way, followed the dam, the cotton and the gold to which it gave birth. Bilharziasis, a severe parasitic affliction, which had broken out before the completion of the dam in Dongola Province, and been carried to Sennar by western pilgrims, then ague, malaria, and smallpox—all spread, to the horror of the people, who saw their suspicions of machines confirmed by Allah's wrath. In 1930, many thousands of sick passed through the Sudanese hospitals. Science and medical practice advanced vigorously from Khartoum against the pests; the locusts, which lay their eggs in light sand, were attacked by an army of chemists, policemen, and Arabs, who by means of poison and rapidly dug trenches, endeavored to keep the insects away from the crops. But when an aeroplane circled overhead, bringing fresh medicines from England, the natives looked up angrily and said that all the evil came from aeroplanes.

Here lies the terrible warning that will again thunder towards us in Egypt. It is true that the world crisis, rain, and sickness have upset a reckoning that at first seemed good and brought big profits. But what good is a new raw material to a country which, to export it, has to go without the bread which was its natural portion for thousands of years, and for the increase of which the dams and canals, the tractors and engineers' brains, would have been admirably employed.

Widespread clearing of the rain forests is another example of the destruction wrought by development. F. B. Livingstone (1958) first connected the cutting down of the rain forest with the increase in malaria because it gave the malaria vector—the mosquito—more open pools of stagnant water in which to breed. Commenting on how frequently the increase in malaria and other diseases are associated with changes in the ecosystem, J. R. Audy (1958) coined the term *man-made maladies*. R. H. Adams (1986) described the World Bank–supported Polonoreste project in northeastern Brazil that cleared the rain forest for agriculture. Unfortunately, the exposed soil is not rich enough to support agriculture, causing the project to fail. And the aboriginal populations who resided in these rain forests have witnessed the destruction of their homelands and suffered from exposure to many diseases brought in by the project laborers.

TRENDS AND ANTHROPOLOGICAL PROSPECTS IN INTERNATIONAL HEALTH

Many of the health problems of the developing world result from inequality. It follows that the greatest improvement in health would be accomplished by education, the provision of adequate food, clean water, sanitation, housing, employment, and freedom from bombs, guns, and torture. The major improvements in health in Europe did not result from medicines or other technological advances, or from the elaboration of health care per se, but from improved water supplies, sanitation, nutrition, and housing. Nonetheless, the major themes of health development work involve the exporting by the West to the developing world its concepts of medicine and health care.

There have been historic trends in international health work, and anthropologists have played roles in two opposing camps: those who worked on the projects and those who became the critics.

Control of Tropical Diseases

In the early years of the twentieth century, the Rockefeller Foundation and other agencies began national and international economic development projects. A major program rationale for these projects, which placed health development at their center, was that tropical diseases (especially hookworm, malaria and yellow fever) were obstacles to development (Brown 1976). According to E. Brown (1976:898), the Rockefeller hookworm eradication campaign began when Charles Stiles, a zoologist, convinced the foundation that the parasite was the cause of "some of the proverbial laziness of the poorer classes," following which the *New York Sun* proclaimed that they had found the "germ of laziness."

Significantly, health was defined as the capacity to work, and the program's successes were measured in increased productivity of workers. From Molina-Guzman's (1979) description of the projects, it appears that they employed many altruistic health professionals, unknowingly to serve economic and political ends with which they may not have agreed.

Medical Education and Population Programs

Following World War II two trends emerged in international health work: development of medical schools, hospitals, and clinics based on Western systems (Molina-Guzman 1979) and population programs. F. M. Mburu (1981) shows that the introduction of curative, hospital-centered care was particularly ill suited to African countries. Such health care is urban based, while the bulk of the population is rural; it is expensive, while the majority are poor; it is highly specialized and focused on esoteric diseases, while most of these people suffer from communicable diseases, deficiencies in sanitation, and malnutrition.

Toward the end of the 1950s, international awareness focused on two factors: the world's population was rapidly increasing, and developments in fertility control had reached the point where it was becoming possible to control population growth (Greep, Koblinsky, and Jaffe 1976:372–79). A 1962 United Nations resolution, "Population Growth and Economic Development," recognized that the poorest people in the least developed nations had the highest fertility. In recognition of the demographic transition that European populations experienced during industrialization, policymakers of this era thought that widespread adoption of population control measures could "jump-start" economic and social progress. In other words, poverty could be overcome if only the poor would control their fertility.

The correlation of high fertility with poverty may not indicate direct causation, however. John Ratcliffe (1978, 1985) suggested that rather than being poor because they have many children, people may have many children because they are poor. He cites the example of Kerala state, India, where social justice reforms including land reform, increased education, and availability of health services were followed by decreases in infant and child mortality and only then by declining fertility. While not necessarily advocating social justice, others have claimed that economic development could be a better contraceptive than programs aimed specifically at population control.

Nevertheless, improvements in education and health services are exceedingly difficult if the population is increasing at a rapid pace. Such is the case with Egypt, where the population was 51 million in 1988 and is projected to reach 126 million before declines in fertility reach zero population growth (International Bank for Reconstruction and Development 1988:76). Egypt's schools are overcrowded, the health care system can barely cope with the demand, and housing in Cairo is in such demand that there is a waiting list of people seeking to live in mausoleums in the cemetery known as the City of the Dead (Schiffer 1988).

Underlying the altruistic concerns expressed by the West about the alleviation of poverty, however, was another more self-interested worry of Western governments derived from Malthusian notions of the tragic consequences of unchecked population growth (Malthus 1972). In 1965, for example, President Lyndon Johnson's State of the Union message called for funding to "seek new ways to use our knowledge to help deal with the explosion in world population and the growing scarcity in world resources" (Johnson 1965:16). The United States began funding population control activities through USAID in 1965, and in 1967 UNFPA was established to coordinate the growing international funding and transfer of contraceptive technology to developing country population programs (Conly, Speidel, and Camp 1991; UN Advisory Committee for the Coordination of Information Systems 1992).

Cold war fears about rapid birthrates' furthering the potential spread of communism also inspired the funding of overseas population activities by the United States. A 1974 memorandum drafted by Henry Kissinger, then secretary of state and director of the National Security Council, called for support for population control in countries of political interest to the United States: Bangladesh, Brazil, Colombia, Egypt, Ethiopia, India, Indonesia, Mexico, Nigeria, Pakistan, the Philippines, Thailand, and Turkey (Collins 1992; Sobo 1991). The United States' experience in Vietnam further aroused fears of communism's emerging in societies with large dissatisfied peasant populations.

Ecological factors continue to be the explicit concerns in current population debates. During the 1991 Earth Summit in Rio de Janeiro the United States stressed overpopulation as a cause of environmental degradation (Collins 1992), and a recent issue of *Population Reports* calls for a "Decade for Action" on the environmental problems caused by population growth (Population Reports 1992). Without minimizing the environmental crisis facing our planet, it is critical to point out that as Malini Karkal, consultant to the World Health Organization, has said, "One birth in the United States is the 'ecological equivalent' of twenty-five [births] in India" in terms of consumption of valuable resources (Collins 1992:15).

Despite the self-interested motives of the industrialized donor nations, their support has contributed to slowing the world's population growth, which most observers agree is an important goal. Family planning programs have been established in most countries worldwide, and in many countries even poor rural women have access to modern contraceptives (Potts and Resenfield 1990). Although the world's population has now reached 5.5 billion and increases at 90 million per year, recent studies indicate that independent of social and economic factors, family planning programs have significantly reduced fertility in developing countries (Bongaarts, Mauldin, and Phillips 1990; Robey, Rutstein, and Morris 1993). Since the mid-1960s social, political, and economic changes and access to modern contraception have caused a decline in the average number of children per woman in the developing world from six to four (Robey, Rutstein, and Morris 1993).

Unfortunately, many of the population programs of the 1960s through the 1980s concentrated on population control at the expense of human dignity and rights. Policies aimed at trying to control numbers of poor people convinced many in the Third World that such policies were a form of genocide. They found confirmation of these convictions too often in the use of medical technology in the service of project objectives. By the mid-1970s, one-third of Puerto Rican women of reproductive age had been sterilized, the highest recorded incidence in the world (Henderson 1975). Although Puerto Rican health officials claim that these sterilizations have been voluntary, critics argue that this represents a "form of cultural genocide or class warfare" (Henderson 1975: 252). Drugs and devices, such as Depo-Provera and the Dalkon Shield, have been used in the Third World even after their safety was seriously questioned in the United States (Elling 1981). And Norplant, the five-year subdermal contraceptive implant, has been used coercively in some programs. A recent volume addresses the safety, acceptability, and ethics of Norplant in several countries (Mintzes, Hardon, and Hanhart 1993). Two of the contributors to the Norplant book, writing about Indonesia and Egypt, describe numerous instances in which women have had great difficulty in getting Norplant removed before the five years had ended (Hanhart 1993; Morsy 1993b). Of course many women, and men, want permanent sterilization, and many women like the contraceptive benefits of Norplant. The problem is not with the methods themselves but with formal and informal policies that give the decision-making power to someone other than the individual in whom they are used. Clearly women and men need safe, reliable methods to control their fertility, and countries need to limit their populations so that they may better serve their existing citizens. However, to succeed, such programs must respect the humanity and choice of the consumers of family planning technologies.

Primary Health Care

Primary health care emerged in the 1970s with a growing realization that the supposed benefits of all the money spent on sophisticated curative medicine was not reaching the poor, mostly rural, populations who had the most disease (Golladay and Liese 1980). Its ambitious goal, proclaimed by the Alma Ata declaration of 1978, was, "Health for All by the Year 2000" (Mahler 1981). The basic components of primary health care are community involvement, appropriate health technology, and reorientation of health services away from urban, hospital-based care toward country-wide health programs. It includes an emphasis on preventive medicine and employs community health workers to serve the needs of their communities. This model of primary health care has now been adopted worldwide but implemented with varying degrees of success. In highly motivated socialist societies, such as China (Mosley 1983) and Nicaragua (Donahue 1986b), great improvements in health indicators have been reported.

Elsewhere primary health care has been less impressive. Justice (1984) describes how the introduction of nurse-midwives failed because young women were stationed at health posts away from their home areas, without taking into account the social constraints that make it socially unacceptable for young Nepali women to travel or live alone.

David Werner (1983) argues that while Cuba has made great strides in health care, its system remains highly centralized and dependent on physicians. He also points out (1977) that in Mexico, primary health care was less successful when community health workers were appointed by the government rather than chosen by the village, and he argues that many programs fail because they only give lip-service to community involvement while remaining paternalistic and authoritarian.

In Bolivia, Libbett Crandon (1983) saw a USAID-sponsored primary health program disbanded by the government. It failed for the frequently cited reason that the imported model of health care was imposed on the local system without taking into account cultural or political realities (see, for example, Paul 1955). Moreover, many primary health care programs may never have had much chance to succeed, especially where governments lacked the political will for their support (Heggenhougen 1984b). In areas where physicians dominate the governments and ministries of health, their suspicion of nontraditional alternatives may have truncated the system before it began (Mosley 1983). In addition, the community involvement and thus the level of organization demanded by primary health care may have alarmed governments that feared losing control to a newly militant peasantry (Davis 1988:6–20).

Child Survival

By the early 1980s it had become clear that unless existing strategies were revised, health for all, especially for the world's children, would not be achieved by the year 2000 (International Conference on Population 1984). Political economists like Vicente Navarro (1984) claimed that major health improvements are not possible without changes in economic, social, and political structures. Nevertheless, many international health specialists felt that the introduction of specific, inexpensive technologies could have a major impact on child mortality (Walsh and Warren 1979).

With this in mind UNICEF outlined its child survival strategy *State of the World's Children* (Mandl 1983). Originally the program included strategies that became popularly known as GOBI-FFF: growth monitoring, oral rehydration therapy, breast feeding, immunization, food supplements, family planning, and female education (Wisner 1988). By the mid-1980s the program was formalized as the Child Survival Development Revolution (CSDR), focusing on Control of Diarrheal Disease (CDD), the Expanded Program on Immunization (EPI), Growth Monitoring (GM), and, later, Acute Respiratory Infection (ARI). Rather than targeting the community as did the Primary Health Care program, Child Survival emphasizes the mother and her children. It has influenced a great deal of research on the determinants of child health (see Mosley and Chen 1984). Anthropologists are increasingly being included in research teams investigating the question, "How can we change mothers' behavior?"

This initiative focused mainly on exporting simple, low-cost medical technologies—so-called appropriate technologies—to the developing countries. Massive investments, for example, were made in developing oral rehydration therapy—a simple solution (McQuestion 1983:ix) of 1 liter of water mixed with sodium chloride (3.5 grams), sodium bicarbonate (2.5 grams), potassium chloride (1.5 grams), and glucose (20 grams). So large was the investment that between 1980 and 1982 alone, at least 150 articles about ORT appeared in the scientific literature. Most of these focused on the technical aspects of ORT, like the proper composition of the rehydration solution, clinical trials, or the measurement of the impact on nutritional status of treatment with ORT under controlled circumstances (McQuestion 1983).

As an easy-to-use, inexpensive, and life-saving technology that could prevent death from dehydration and could replace costly hospital-based intravenous rehydration, the value of ORT was unquestionable in principle. But because its development had emphasized scientific questions to the exclusion of sociocultural information, attempts at implementing its widespread use were often unsuccessful and frustrating. For instance, WHO recommendations for the implementation of ORT, based on technical research, were often out of touch with the realities of people's lives. Richard Cash (1983:211) asserts that "the overall recommendation by WHO is that ORT be made with ordinary drinking water, and that prepared oral therapy should not be kept more than 24 hours.

There is no apparent reason to alter this recommendation.'' Yet in many cases ORT is inaccurately mixed, infrequently used, and not often recommended by physicians.

The National Control of Diarrheal Diseases Project (NCDDP) in Egypt, which did have substantial input from social scientists, is widely acknowledged to be one of the most successful Child Survival projects worldwide (Fox 1988; Robson 1991). Televised health messages employed local indigenous terms for diarrhea that were identified by social scientists doing informal and focus group interviews. A term that had formerly described the yearly drought Egypt experienced before the construction of the High Dam—*gafaf*—was chosen to describe diarrhea-caused dehydration. This new meaning of *gafaf* became so widely adopted that in 1986, Anis Monsour, editor-in-chief of Egypt's leading newspaper, *Al Ahram,* reported that some high school students who, when asked to write about the yearly drought on a final exam, misunderstood and wrote instead about child dehydration (Elkamel, personal communication 1991).

NCDDP's impact on childhood diarrheal deaths has been considerable. Several studies report that from 1983 to 1988, childhood diarrheal disease deaths had decreased by nearly half and that NCDDP is responsible for much of this improvement (Rashad 1989; El Rafie et al 1990). The NCDDP was the Cadillac of all health interventions. It had the backing of the Egyptian government, support from UNICEF, the WHO, and allocation from USAID of $36 million over ten years (USAID 1989). It was conducted by some of the most talented Egyptian social scientists and public health specialists, with technical support from the John Snow Public Health Group, U.S.-based consulting firm. A good part of the NCDDP's success was due to the careful assessment, pretesting, and ongoing evaluation that its team conducted. Largely because of time and financial constraints and the fact that policymakers often consider research to be a nonessential extra that can be cut, most other health education campaigns fall short of this type of careful planning. Unfortunately, with the decrease of external support in the 1990s, many of NCDDP's gains have been eroded (Grant 1994:6). The program was a brilliant demonstration of how diarrheal disease deaths could be dramatically decreased. Sustainability, however, was not well planned for and has proved to be a major stumbling block.

A preliminary examination of the problems with the Child Survival Development Revolution also includes wasteful redundancy in some countries, where it has produced a series of vertical programs, each with its own staff, budget and agenda. For example, in the Sudan during the late 1980s, there were separate programs for the Expanded Program of Immunization (EPI), the Control of Diarrheal Diseases (CDD), Growth Monitoring, and the like. Each program had its own bureaucracy, vehicles, and personnel. When the CDD people went to a village, they did not take vaccines along, and when the growth monitors weighed and measured children, they did not give out oral rehydration solution packets. Clearly this is inefficient at best.

Furthermore, John Briscoe (1987:103) argues that the ''Child Survival Revolution gives low priority to improvements in water supply and sanitation because it has concluded that these interventions are not cost-effective.'' Such shortsighted planning results from programs that count success only in numbers of children vaccinated or numbers of oral rehydration solution packets distributed. Health improvements resulting from clean water, adequate housing, or fair wages are much more difficult to measure and are thus discounted in international development priorities.

Safe Motherhood

Safe motherhood, which focuses on the preventable death of women during pregnancy, was initiated by a World Bank–supported conference in February 1987 in Nairobi, Kenya. Between 1987 and 1988, in fact, twelve conferences on safe motherhood in Africa, Asia, Latin America, and the Middle East were funded by international health agencies. Among the sponsors for these conferences have been the WHO, UNDP, UNICEF, the World Bank, and the Ford Foundation. The slogan for this program—''putting the M back in MCH'' (putting the mother back into maternal/child health)—indicates a recognition that women have been largely ignored in favor of children. Moreover, the health of women before and during pregnancy profoundly affects the health of their infants.

A maternal death is a death of a woman who is pregnant or within forty-two days after pregnancy (AbouZahr and Royston 1991:17). One-half million women die of pregnancy-related causes worldwide each year, and the majority of these deaths are preventable (AbouZahr and Royston 1991:1). Maternal mortality ratios in developing countries range from 100 to 700 per 100,000 live births compared with 8 deaths per 100,000 live births in the United States (Herz and Measham 1987; Grant 1994). In parts of the Sudan, maternal deaths reach 2,276 per 100,000 live births (Sudan Ministry of Health personal communication). Safe motherhood strategies include stronger community-based care (primarily nonphysician care), stronger referral facilities, better transport systems for high-risk pregnancies, and better emergency services for treating obstetrical complications (Hertz and Measham 1987; AbouZahr and Royston 1991).

The implementation of safe motherhood programs is just beginning in many countries. UNICEF is sponsoring training of traditional birth attendants in the hope of improving the community-based care of pregnant women, and research is beginning in many areas into how to improve women's reproductive health.

Anthropological Prospects

Just as the general area of development studies has evolved in a way that is consistent with the concerns of development professionals, so the development of international health programs takes place in an arena in which the concerns of the First World provide the major imperatives for action. Shifts in the focus of international health work have taken place primarily not because the problems were solved but rather because of political and economic considerations. Indeed, there is evidence that program shifts occur even at times when such changes frustrate the chances of success of the earlier programs.

Trends in international health development can be traced in large part to the constraints within which programs are developed: organizational cultures that reward innovation rather than constancy, planning tied to short-term (fiscal year) cycles rather than to time periods that reflect realistic program spans, and a basic ethnocentrism involved in exporting technology and development based on "rational," "scientific" principles. Medical anthropologists working in international health must recognize these constraints, identify their effect on people's health, and work to ensure that bureaucratic and ethnocentric program rationales do not blind health professionals to the critical and dynamic role culture and political processes play in enabling people to achieve satisfactory levels of health and well-being.

ACKNOWLEDGMENTS

We thank Sol Tax, George Foster, Judith Justice, and Robert Pickering for critical discussions of earlier drafts of this chapter, and Rupa Goswami and Stephanie Maurer for bibliographical assistance.

NOTES

1. Reflecting on his twenty years of experience working with USAID, Harrison (1985) states straightforwardly these premises. Introducing his retrospective analysis, *Underdevelopment is a State of Mind,* he says: "I hope the book will demonstrate how one culture may make progress easier for its people than another. According to my values, which are, I believe, generally shared by most people in both the developed and underdeveloped worlds, progress-prone cultures are better places for human beings to live than traditional, static cultures. And the most progressive cultures that humankind has thus far evolved follow the democratic model of the West" (Harrison 1985:xvii).

2. Majid Rahnema, a former United Nations civil servant, summed up this aspect of development work when he wrote: "Ever since that restless little macho man, called *homo economicus,* was born to our planet, some 300 years ago, the economized societies of his creation have, in turn, given birth to a host of new varieties of humanoids, most of them frightfully dangerous: bureaucrats, strategists, entrepreneurs, developers and planners of all kinds; modern shamans and marabouts with professional degrees in every discipline, from animal psychiatry and bereavement counseling to genetic engineering; technowizards producing nuclear toys and statesmen and generals specialized in playing with them; heads of state who believe that nuclear war is the ultimate answer to peacekeeping, and those who would not speak the language of their peoples, yet master the language of anyone who provides them with arms and weapons in order to keep their people quiet and docile. All these figures and figureheads have pledged allegiance to a three-headed monster, the heads representing the new world empires of economics, pol-

itics, and technology. They are all pledged to save the 'underdeveloped' world, through aid and assistance'' (Rahnema 1988:117).

3. We do not consider here the effects of the participation of health professionals in political repression and violence through state-sanctioned torture and abuse of citizens. Nonetheless, the organization and consequences of such activities affect international health and are important for medical anthropologists practicing in such circumstances (see Claude, Stover, and Lopez 1987; Bloche 1987; Stover 1987; Rayner 1987).

References

Aamodt, A. M. 1972. The Child View of Health and Healing. In *Communicating Nurse Research: The Many Sources of Nursing Knowledge,* ed. M. Batey. Boulder, Colo.: Western Interstate Commission on Higher Education, 5:38–54.

———. 1978. *The Care Component in a Health and Healing System: The Anthropology of Health.* St. Louis: Mosby.

———. 1981. Neighboring: Discovering Support Systems among Norwegian-American Women. In *Anthropologists at Home in America: Methods and Issues in the Study of One's Own Culture,* ed. D. Messerschmidt. Cambridge: Cambridge University Press, 133–49.

———. 1982. Examining Ethnography for Nurse Researchers. *Western Journal of Nursing Research* 4:209–21.

———. 1984. Themes and Issues in Conceptualizing Care. In *Care: The Essence of Nursing and Health.* Thorofare, N.J.: Slack, 75–79.

Abaza, Mona, and Georg Stauth. 1988. Occidental Reason, Orientalism, Islamic Fundamentalism: A Critique. *International Sociology* 3(4):343–64.

Abbot, A. 1988. *The Systems of Professions: An Essay on the Division of Expert Labor.* Chicago: University of Chicago Press.

Abdel, Malek. 1963. Orientalism in Crisis. *Diogenes* 44:107–8.

Abdel-Salam, E., P. A. S. Peters, A. E. Abdel Meguid, A. A. E. Abdel Meguid, and A. A. F. Mahmoud. 1986. Discrepancies in Outcome of a Control Program for Schistosomiasis haematobia in Fayoum Governorate, Egypt. *American Journal of Tropical Medicine and Hygiene* 35:786–90.

Abel, Theodora M., Rhoda Metraux, and Samuel Roll. 1987. *Psychotherapy and Culture.* Rev. ed. Albuquerque, N.M.: University of New Mexico Press.

Aberle, David. 1952. Artic Hysteria and Latah in Mongolia. *Transactions of the New York Academy of Science* 14:294–97.

Aberle, D. F., A. K. Cohen, A. K. Davis, M. J. Levy, and F. X. Sutton. 1960. The Functional Prerequisites of a Society. *Ethics* 60:100–11.

Abimola, W. 1976. *Ifa: An Exposition of Ifa Literary Corpus.* Nigeria: Ibadan University Press.

Ablon, Joan. 1965. American Indian Relocation: Problems of Dependency and Management in the City. *Phylon* 26:362–71.

———. 1976. Family Behavior and Alcoholism. In *Cross-Cultural Approaches to the Study of Alcohol,* ed. M. Everett et al. The Hague: Mouton.

———. 1980. Thoughts on a "Clinical Anthropology." *Medical Anthropology Newsletter* 12(1): 22–23.

———. 1984. Family Research and Alcoholism. In *Recent Developments in Alcoholism,* vol. 2, ed. Marc Galanter. New York: Plenum.

———. 1985. Irish-American Catholics in a West Coast Metropolitan Area. In *The American Experience with Alcohol,* ed. Linda Bennett and Genevieve Ames. New York: Plenum.

AbouZahr, Carla, and Erica Royston. 1991. *Maternal Mortality. A Global Factbook.* Geneva: World Health Organization.

Abrams, Charles. 1970. *Man's Struggle for Shelter in an Urbanizing World.* Cambridge: MIT Press.

Abu-Lughod, Lila. 1986. *Veiled Sentiments: Honor and Poetry in a Bedouin Society.* Berkeley and Los Angeles: University of California Press.

———. 1990. Shifting Politics in Bedouin Love Poetry. In *Language and the Politics of Emotion,* ed. Catherine A. and Lila Abu-Lughod. Cambridge: Cambridge University Press.

———. 1991. Writing against Culture. In *Recapturing Anthropology: Working in the Present,* ed. Richard G. Fox. Santa Fe: School of American Research Press, 137–62.

———. 1993. *Writing Women's Worlds: Bedouin Stories.* Berkeley and Los Angeles: University of California Press.

Abu-Lughod, Lila, and Catherine Lutz. 1990. Introduction: Emotion, Discourse, and the Politics of Everyday Life. In *Language and the Politics of Emotion,* ed. Catherine A. Lutz and Lila Abu-Lughod. Cambridge University Press.

Ackerknecht, Erwin H. 1943. Psychopathology, Primitive Medicine and Primitive Culture. *Bulletin of the History of Medicine* 14:30–67.

———. 1944. Primitive Surgery. *American Anthropologist* 49:25–45.

———. 1945. Malaria in the Upper Mississippi Valley, 1760–1900. *Bulletin of the History of Medicine* (suppl. 4).

———. 1946. Natural Diseases and Rational Treatment in Primitive Medicine. *Bulletin of the History of Medicine* 19(5):467–97.

———. 1958. Primitive Medicine's Social Function. In *Miscelanea,* ed. Paul Rivet. Mexico City: Universidad Nacional Autonoma de Mexico, 3–7.

———. 1971. *Medicine and Ethnology: Selected Essays.* Baltimore: Johns Hopkins University Press.

Adams, F., trans. 1939. *Hippocrates: The Genuine Works of Hippocrates.* 2 vols. Baltimore: Williams & Wilkins.

Adams, R. H. 1986. *Development and Social Change in Rural Egypt.* Syracuse, N.Y.: Syracuse University Press.

Adams, Richard N., and Arthur J. Rubel. 1967. Sickness and Social Relations. In *Handbook of Middle American Indians,* ed. Robert Wauchope. Austin: University of Texas Press, 333–56.

Adams, Vincanne. 1988. Modes of Production and Medicine: An Examination of the Theory in Light of Sherpa Medical Traditionalism. *Social Science and Medicine* 27(5):505–13.

Adler, Nancy E., et al. 1993. Socioeconomic Inequalities in Health: No Easy Solution. *Journal of the American Medical Association* 269:3140–45.

Agar, Michael H. 1973. *Ripping and Running: A Formal Ethnography of Urban Heroin Addicts.* New York: Seminar Press.

———. 1977. Into That Whole Ritual Thing: Ritualistic Drug Use among Urban American Heroin Addicts. In *Drugs, Rituals, and Altered States of Consciousness,* ed. Brian M. du Toit. Rotterdam: A. A. Balkema.

———. 1980. *The Professional Stranger: An Informal Introduction to Ethnography.* New York: Academic Press.

———. 1981. The Commonality Quest: The Search for Parallels between Drug Use and Other

Behaviors. *Newsletter of the Alcohol and Drug Study Group, American Anthropological Association,* no. 3.

———. 1986. *Speaking of Ethnography.* Sage University Series on Qualitative Research Methods, vol. 2. Beverly Hills, Calif.: Sage.

Agar, Michael H., Charles Underwood, and Kathryn Woolard. 1981. The Commonalities Quest: Toward a Theory of "Problem Behavior." *Journal of Psychoactive Drugs* 13(4):333–43.

Ahmed, Abdul Rahman Abu Zayd, et al. 1988. *War Wounds: Development Costs of Conflict in Southern Sudan.* London: Panos Institute.

Ailinger, R. L. 1980. *Nursing—A Social Policy Statement.* Kansas City: American Nurses' Association.

———. 1982. Hypertension Knowledge in a Hispanic Community. *Nursing Research* 31:207–10.

———. 1983. *Facts about Nursing.* Kansas City: American Nurses' Association.

Ajabnoor, M. A., and A. K. Tilmisany. 1988. Effect of Trigonella foenum graceum on Blood Glucose Levels in Normal and Alloxan-Diabetic Mice. *Journal of Ethnopharmacology* 23: 45–49.

Akerele, O. 1987. The Best of Both Worlds: Bringing Traditional Medicine Up to Date. *Social Science and Medicine* 24:177–81.

Alan Guttmacher Institute. 1994. *Sex and America's Teenagers.* Washington, D.C.: Alan Guttmacher Institute.

Alarcon, Renato D. 1983. A Latin American Perspective on DSM-III. *American Journal of Psychiatry* 140(1):102–5.

Alcorn, Janis B. 1981. Some Factors Influencing Botanical Resource Perception among the Huastec. *Journal of Ethnobiology* 1:221–30.

Alexander, Franz, Samuel Eisenstein, and Martin Grotjahn, eds. 1966. *Psychoanalytic Pioneers.* New York: Basic Books.

Alexander, Jaqui. 1988. The Ideological Construction of Risk: An Analysis of Corporate Health Promotion Programs in the 1980's. *Social Science and Medicine* 26(5):559–67.

Alexander, Linda. 1979. Clinical Anthropology: Morals and Methods. *Medical Anthropology* 3(1): 61–109.

———. 1982. Illness Maintenance and the New American Sick Role. In *Clinically Applied Anthropology: Anthropologists in Health Science Settings,* ed. Noel Chrisman and Thomas Maretzki. Dordrecht: D. Reidel.

Ali, Kamran. 1994. Dissertation in Progress. Department of Anthropology, Johns Hopkins University.

Alland, A. 1966. Medical Anthropology and the Study of Biological and Cultural Adaptation. *American Anthropologist* 68:40.

———. 1970. *Adaptation in Cultural Evolution: An Approach to Medical Anthropology.* New York: Columbia University Press.

———. 1987. Looking Backward: An Autocritique. *Medical Anthropology Quarterly* 1(4):424–31.

Alland, A., and B. McCay. 1973. The Concept of Adaptation in Biological and Cultural Evolution. In *Handbook of Social and Cultural Anthropology,* ed. J. Honigmann. Chicago: Rand McNally.

Allen, L., et al. 1987. *The Collaborative Research and Support Program on Food Intake and Human Function: Mexico Project.* Final Report. University of Connecticut and Instituto Nacional de Nutricion (Mexico).

Allison, A. C. 1954. Protection Afforded by Sickle-Cell Trait against Subtertian Malarial Infection. *British Medical Journal* 1:290–94.

Altorki, Soraya, and Camilia Fawz El-Solh. 1988. *Arab Women in the Field: Studying Your Own Society.* Syracuse, N.Y.: Syracuse University Press.

Alubo, S. Ogoh. 1987. Drugging the Nigerian People: The Public Hazards of Private Profits. The Impact of Development and Modern Technologies in Third World Health. *Studies in Third World Societies* 34:89–114.

American Nurses' Association. 1980. *Nursing—A Social Policy Statement.* Kansas City: American Nurses' Association.

———. 1983. *Facts about Nursing.* Kansas City: American Nurses' Association.

American Psychiatric Association. 1978. *Diagnostic and Statistical Manual of Mental Disorders.* 2nd ed. Washington, D.C.: APA.

———. 1980. *Diagnostic and Statistical Manual of Mental Disorders.* 3d ed. Washington, D.C.: APA.

———. 1987. *Diagnostic and Statistical Manual of Mental Disorders.* 3d ed. rev. Washington, D.C.: APA.

———. 1994. *Diagnostic and Statistical Manual of Mental Disorders.* 4th ed. rev. Washington, D.C.: APA.

Amering, M., and H. Katsching. 1990. Panic Attacks and Panic Disorder in Cross-Cultural Perspective. *Psychiatric Annals* 20:511–16.

Ames, Genevieve M. 1982. Maternal Alcoholism and Family Life: A Cultural Model for Research and Intervention. Doctoral dissertation, University of California Medical Center.

———. 1985a. American Beliefs about Alcoholism: Historical Perspectives on the Moral-Medical Controversy. In *The American Experience with Alcohol,* ed. Linda Bennett and Genevieve Ames. New York: Plenum.

———. 1985b. Middle-class Protestants: Alcohol and the Family. In *The American Experience with Alcohol,* ed. Linda Bennett and Genevieve Ames. New York: Plenum.

———. 1993. Research and Strategies for the Primary Prevention of Workplace Alcohol Problems. *Alcohol Health and Research World* 17(1):19–27.

Ames, Genevieve M., and Craig R. Janes. 1987. Heavy and Problem Drinking in an American Blue-collar Population: Implications for Prevention. *Social Science and Medicine* 25(8):949–60.

———. 1992. A Cultural Approach to Conceptualizing Alcohol and the Workplace. *Alcohol Health and Research World* 16(2):112–19.

Amin, Galal. 1981. Some Economic and Cultural Aspects of Economic Liberalization in Egypt. *Social Problems* 28(4):430–41.

Amin, Samir. 1972. Under-Populated Africa. *Manpower and Unemployment Research in Africa* 5: 5–17.

Anderson, E. N. 1988. A Native-based Strategy for Alcohol Abuse Control. Paper presented at IUAES Congress, Zagreb, Yugoslavia.

Anderson, E. R., M. L. Anderson, and J. H. C. Ho. 1978. Environmental Backgrounds of Young Chinese NPC Patients. In G. de-The and Y. Ito, eds., *NPC: Etiology and Control.* Lyon: IARC, 231–39.

Anderson, J. R. 1985. *Muir's Textbook of Pathology.* Baltimore: Edward Arnold.

Anderson, R. M., and R. M. May. 1978. Regulation and Stability in Host-Parasite Interactions, I. Regulatory Processes. *Journal of Animal Ecology* 47:219–47.

Anderson, Robert. 1991. The Efficacy of Ethomedicine: Research Methods in Trouble. *Medical Anthropology* 13:1–17.

Andorka, R. 1978. *Determinants of Fertility in Advanced Societies.* New York: Free Press.

Aneshensel, Carol S., and Jeffrey D. Stone. 1982. Stress and Depression: A Test of the Buffering Model of Social Support. *Archives of General Psychiatry* 39:1392–96.

Angell, Marcia. 1988. Ethical Imperialism: Ethics in International Collaborative Clinical Research. *New England Journal of Medicine* 319(16):1081–83.

Anisimov, A. F. 1963. The Shaman's Tent of the Evenks and the Origin of the Shamanistic Rite. In *Studies in Siberian Shamanism,* ed. H. N. Michael. Toronto: University of Toronto Press, 84–123.

Annis, Linda Ferrill. 1978. *The Child before Birth.* Ithaca: Cornell University Press.

Anspach, Renee. 1987. Prognostic Conflict in Life-and-Death Decisions: The Organization as an Ecology of Knowledge. *Journal of Health and Social Behavior* 28:215–31.

———. 1993. *Deciding Who Lives: Fateful Choices in the Intensive-Care Nursery.* Berkeley: University of California Press.

Antonovsky, Aaron. 1979. *Health, Stress, and Coping.* San Francisco: Jossey-Bass.

Apprey, Maurice. 1986. Discussion: A Prefatory Note on Motives and Projective Identification. *International Journal of Psychoanalytic Psychotherapy* 11:111–16.

Arbain, D., et al. 1989. Survey of Some West Sumatran Plants for Alkaloids. *Economic Botany* 43: 73–78.

Arditti, Rita, Renate Duelli Klein, and Shelley Minden, eds. 1984. *Test-Tube Women: What Future for Motherhood?* London: Pandora Press.

Armelagos, G. J., and J. R. Dewey. 1970. Evolutionary Response to Human Infectious Diseases. *BioScience* 157:638–44.

Armelagos, G. J., A. Goodman, and K. H. Jacobs. 1978. The Ecological Perspective in Disease. In *Health and the Human Condition,* ed. M. Logan and E. Hunt. North Scituate, Mass.: Duxbury, 71–84.

Armelagos, George, and Elizabeth Schueler. 1986. Biological Consequences of Nuclear Winter. In *Nuclear Winter: The Anthropology of Human Survival,* ed. M. Pamela Bumsted. Los Alamos, N.M.: Los Alamos National Laboratory, 23–29.

Armelagos, G., M. Ryan, and T. Leatherman. 1990. The Evolution of Infectious Disease: A Biocultural Analysis of AIDS. *American Journal of Human Biology* 2:353–63.

Armstrong, R. W., M. J. Armstrong, M. C. Yu, and B. C. Henderson. 1983. Salted Fish and Inhalants as Risk Factors for NPC in Malaysian Chinese. *Cancer Research* 43:2967–70.

Arney, William Ray. 1982. *Power and the Profession of Obstetrics.* Chicago: University of Chicago Press.

Arney, William Ray, and Bernard J. Bergen. 1984. *Medicine and the Management of Living: Taming the Last Great Beast.* Chicago: University of Chicago Press.

Asad, Talal. 1973. *Anthropology and the Colonial Encounter.* London: Ithaca Press.

———. 1979. Anthropology and the Analysis of Ideology. *Man* n.s. 14(4):607–27.

———. 1987. Are There Histories of Peoples without Europe? A Review Article. *Comparative Studies in Society and History* 29(3):597–607.

Atal, C. K., U. Zutshi, and P. G. Rao. 1981. Scientific Evidence on the Role of Ayurvedic Herbals on Bioavailability of Drugs. *Journal of Ethnopharmacology* 4:229–32.

Atwood, Donald. 1994. Prepared statement of Mr. Atwood. In Hearing before the Subcommittee on African Affairs of the Committee on Foreign Relations. U.S. Senate, 103d Cong., July 26.

Aubo, Ogoh. 1987. Power and Privileges in Medical Care: An Analysis of Medical Services in Post Colonial Nigeria. *Social Science and Medicine* 24(5):453–62.

Audy, J. R. 1958. Medical Ecology in Relation to Geography. *British Journal of Clinical Practice* 12:102–10.

August, Lynn R., and Barbara A. Gianola. 1987. Symptoms of War Trauma Induced Psychiatric Disorders: Southeast Asian Refugees and Vietnam Veterans. *International Migration Review* 21:820–31.

Ayala, F. J. 1983. Microevolution and Macroevolution. In *Evolution from Molecules to Men,* ed. D. Bendall. Cambridge: Cambridge University Press, 387–402.

Badcock, C. R. 1980. *The Psychoanalysis of Culture.* Oxford: Basil Blackwell.

———. 1986. *The Problem of Altruism: Freudian-Darwinian Solutions.* New York: Basil Blackwell.

Backstrand, Jeffrey R. 1994. Hiring Not Influenced by Gender, Ethnicity. *Hartford Courant,* August.

Baer, Hans A. 1982. On the Political Economy of Health. *Medical Anthropology Newsletter* 14(1): 1–2, 13–17.

———. 1984. A Comparative View of a Heterodox Health System: Chiropractics in America and Britain. *Medical Anthropology* 8:151–68.

————. 1986a. The Replication of the Medical Division of Labor in Medical Anthropology. *Medical Anthropology Quarterly* 17(3):63–65.

————. 1986b. Sociological Contributions to the Political Economy of Health: Lessons for Medical Anthropologists. *Medical Anthropology Quarterly* 17(5):129–31.

————. 1989. The American Dominative Medical System as a Reflection of Social Relations in the Larger Society. *Social Science and Medicine* 28(11):1103–12.

————. 1990. The Possibilities and Dilemmas of Building Bridges between Critical Medical Anthropology and Clinical Anthropology: A Discussion. *Social Science and Medicine* 30(9): 1011–13.

————. 1993a. How Critical Can Clinical Anthropology Be? *Medical Anthropology* 15:299–317.

————. 1993b. The Misconstruction of Critical Medical Anthropology: A Response to a Cultural Constructivist Critique. Paper prepared for the Annual Meeting of the American Anthropological Association, Washington, D.C., November 12–21.

————. 1993c. Biocultural Approaches in Medical Anthropology: A Critical Medical Anthropology Commentary. *Medical Anthropology Quarterly* 4(3):344–47.

Baer, Hans A., Merrill Singer, and John H. Johnsen. 1986. Introduction toward a Critical Medical Anthropology. *Social Science and Medicine* 23(2):95–98.

Bahr, Donald M., Juan Gregorio, David I. Lopez, and Albert Alvarez. 1974. *Piman Shamanism and Staying Sickness.* Tucson: University of Arizona Press.

Baker, P. T. 1984. The Adaptive Limits of Human Populations. *Man* n.s. 19:1–14.

————. 1986. Rationale and Research Design. In *The Changing Samoans: Behavior and Health in Transition,* ed. Paul T. Baker, Joel M. Hanna, and Thelma S. Baker. New York: Oxford University Press.

Balint, Michael. 1964. *The Doctor, the Patient and His Illness.* London: Pitman Medical Publications.

Banaji, J. 1970. Crisis in British Anthropology. *New Left Review* 64:71–85.

Banerji, Debabar. 1984. The Political Economy of Western Medicine in Third World Countries. In *Issues in the Political Economy of Health Care,* ed. J. McKinlay. New York: Tavistock, 257–82.

————. 1986. Comments on New Patterns in Health Sector Aid to India. *International Journal of Health Services* 16(2):309–11.

Bannerman, R. H., J. Burton, and C. Wen-Chief, eds. 1983. *Traditional Medicine and Health Coverage.* Geneva: World Health Organization.

Bannoune, Mahfoud. 1984. What Does it Mean to Be a Third World Anthropologist? *Dialectical Anthropology* 9(1–4):357–64.

Barclay, George W. 1958. *Techniques of Population Analysis.* New York: Wiley.

Barker, C., and Meredith Turshen. 1986. Primary Health Care or Selective Health Strategies. *Review of African Political Economy* 36 (September):78–85.

Barker, Judith C., and M. Margaret Clark. 1992. Cross-Cultural Medicine a Decade Later. Special issue of *Western Journal of Medicine* 157(3):215–390.

Barnes, J. A. 1973. Genitrix: Genitor: Nature: Culture? In *The Character of Kinship,* ed. Jack Goody. Cambridge: Cambridge University Press.

Barnes, S. T., and C. D. Jenkins. 1972. Changing Personal and Social Behavior: Experiences of Health Workers in a Tribal Society. *Social Science and Medicine* 6:1–15.

Barnett, Clifford R. 1980. Commentary (On Clinical Anthropology). *Medical Anthropology Newsletter* 12(1):23–25.

————. 1985. Anthropological Research in Clinical Settings: Role Requirements and Adaptations. *Medical Anthropology Quarterly* 16(3):59–61.

Barnett, Clifford, M. L. Poland, H. H. Weidman, H. F. Stein, I. Press, A. Kleinman, and O. von Mering. 1985. Symposium: Anthropologists in Clinical Settings—A Matter of Style. *Medical Anthropology Quarterly* 16(3):59–73.

Barnett, Elyse Ann. 1988. La Edad Critica: The Positive Experience of Menopause in a Small

Peruvian Town. In *Women and Health,* ed. Patricia Whelehan. Granby, Mass.: Bergin and Garvey, 40–55.

Barnouw, Victor. 1973. *Culture and Personality.* Homewood, Ill.: Dorsey Press.

Barrabee, Paul, and Otto von Mering. 1953. Ethnic Variations in Mental Stress in Families with Psychotic Children. *Social Problems* 1(2):48–53.

Barrett, James E., ed. 1979. *Stress and Mental Disorder.* New York: Raven Press.

Barry, Herbert, III. 1982. Cultural Variations in Alcohol Use. In *Culture and Psychopathology,* ed. I. Al-Issa. Baltimore: University Park Press.

Barry, Michele. 1988. Ethical Considerations of Human Investigation in Developing Countries: The AIDS Dilemma. *New England Journal of Medicine* 319(16):1083–86.

Basch, Paul F. 1990. *Textbook of International Health.* New York: Oxford University Press.

Basker, D., and M. Negbi. 1983. Uses of Saffron. *Economic Botany* 37(2):228–36.

Bassaglia, Franco. 1964. Silence in the Dialogue with the Psychotic. *Journal of Existentialism* 6(21): 99–102.

Bassett, Ken. 1988. The Fetal Patient. Paper prepared for the Society of Medical Anthropology Invited Session, "Reproductive Technology, Medical Practice, Public Expectations and New Representations of the Human Body," Annual Meeting of the American Anthropological Association, Phoenix, Arizona, November 16–20.

Basso, Keith H. 1969. *Western Apache Witchcraft.* Tucson: University of Arizona Press.

Bastien, Joseph. 1985. Qollahuaya-Andean Body Concepts: A Topographical-Hydraulic Model of Physiology. *American Anthropologist* 87:595–611.

Bateson, Gregory. 1958. *Naven.* Stanford: Stanford University Press.

———. 1972. *Steps to an Ecology of Mind.* St. Albans, England: Palladin Books.

Bateson, Mary Catherine. 1980. Continuities in Insight and Innovation: Toward a Biography of Margaret Mead. *American Anthropologist* 82:270–77.

Battah, Abdallah M. 1988. Ibn Khnaldun's Principles of Political Economy: Rudiments of a New Science. Ph.D. dissertation, American University.

Battin, Margaret P. 1994. *The Least Worst Death: Essays in Bioethics on the End of Life.* New York: Oxford University Press.

Bauwens, E. E. 1977. Medical Beliefs and Practices among Lower-Income Anglos. In *Ethnic Medicine in the Southwest.* Tucson: University of Arizona Press.

———. 1978. *The Anthropology of Health.* St. Louis: Mosby.

Bayley, Carol. 1995. Our World Views (May Be) Incommensurable: Now What? *Journal of Medicine and Philosophy* 20(3):271–84.

Beachamp, Tom L., and John Childress. 1993. *Principles of Biomedical Ethics.* 4th ed. New York: Oxford University Press.

Beachamp, Tom L., and Seymour Perlin, eds. 1978. *Ethical Issues in Death and Dying.* Englewood Cliffs, N.J.: Prentice-Hall.

Beals, Ralph L. 1980. Intracultural Variation: Reflections Stimulated by George Foster. *Human Organization* 39:289–91.

Beardsley, Edward. 1987. *A History of Neglect: Health Care for Blacks and Mill Workers in the Twentieth-Century South.* Knoxville: University of Tennessee Press.

Beaton, George H. 1983. Supplementary Feeding Programs in Pregnancy and Lactation: Consideration for Nutrition Intervention Programs. In *Nutrition Intervention Strategies in National Development,* ed. Barbara A. Underwood. New York: Academic Press.

Beaton, G. H., J. Milner, V. McGuire, T. E. Feather, and J. A. Litte. 1983. Source of Variance in 24-Hour Dietary Recall Data: Implications for Nutrition Study Design and Interpretation. *American Journal of Clinical Nutrition* 37:986–95.

Beaujard, Philippe. 1988. Plantes et médécine traditionnelle dans le sud-est de Madagascar. *Journal of Ethnopharmacology* 23:165–265.

Becker, Gay. 1990. *Healing the Infertile Family.* New York: Bantam Press.

Becker, H. S., ed. 1970. *Sociological Work.* Chicago: Aldine.

Bee, R. L., and B. F. Cra. 1989. Using Ethnography in Fieldnote Management. In *Computer Applications for Anthropologists*, ed. M. S. Boone and J. J. Wood. Belmont, Calif.: Wadsworth.

Beecher, Henry J. 1966. Ethics and Clinical Research. *New England Journal of Medicine* 74:1354–60.

Beeman, William O. 1985. Dimensions of Dysphoria: The View from Linguistic Anthropology. In *Culture and Depression: Studies in the Anthropology and Cross-Cultural Psychiatry of Affect and Disorder*, ed. Arthur Kleinman and Byron Good. Berkeley: University of California Press.

Beiser, Morton. 1985. A Study of Depression among Traditional Africans, Urban North Americans and Southeast Asian Refugees. In *Culture and Depression: Studies in the Anthropology and Cross-Cultural Psychiatry of Affect and Disorder*, ed. Arthur Kleinman and Byron Good. Berkeley: University of California Press.

Beiser, M., H. Collomb, J. Ravel, and C. J. Nafziger. 1976. Systemic Blood Pressure Studies among the Serer of Senegal. *Journal of Chronic Diseases* 29:371–80.

Bello, Walden, Shea Cunningham, and Bill Rau. 1994. *Dark Victory: The United States, Structural Adjustment and Global Poverty*. London: Pluto Press/Oakland: Food First.

Belmonte, Thomas. 1979. *The Broken Fountain*. New York: Columbia University Press.

Belsey, Mark A. 1976. The Epidemiology of Infertility: A Review with Particular Reference to Sub-Saharan Africa. *Bulletin of the World Health Organization* 54:319–41.

Benedict, Ruth. 1934. *Patterns of Culture*. Boston: Houghton Mifflin.

Beneria, Lourdes. 1979. Reproduction, Production and the Sexual Division of Labor. *Cambridge Journal of Economics* 3:203–23.

Beneria, Lourdes, and Martha Roldan. 1987. *The Crossroads of Class and Gender*. Chicago: University of Chicago Press.

Benhabib, Seyla. 1992. *Situating the Self: Gender, Community and Postmodernism in Contemporary Ethics*. New York: Routledge.

Benner, P. 1984. *From Novice to Expert: Excellence and Power in Clinical Nursing Practice*. Reading, Mass.: Addison-Wesley.

Benner, Patricia. 1991. The Role of Experience, Narrative, and Community in Skilled Ethical Comportment. *Advances in Nursing Science* 14(2):1–21.

Bennett, John W. 1985. The Micro-Macro Nexus: Typology, Process, and System. In Billie R. DeWalt and Pertti Pelto, eds., 23–54. *Micro and Macro Levels of Analysis in Anthropology: Issues in Theory and Research*. Boulder: Westview.

Bennett, Linda A. 1984. Contributions from Anthropology to the Study of Alcoholism. In *Recent Developments in Alcoholism*, vol. 2, ed. Marc Galanter. New York: Plenum.

———. 1988. Alcohol in Context: Anthropological Perspectives. *Drugs and Society* 2(3/4):89–131.

———. 1989. Family, Alcohol, and Culture. In *Recent Developments in Alcholism*, vol. 7, ed. Marc Galanter. New York: Plenum.

———. 1994. Accountability for Alcoholism in American Families. *Social Science and Medicine* 40(1):15–25.

Bennett, Linda A., ed. 1984. Ethnography, Alcohol, and South-Central European Societies. *East European Quarterly* 18(4): entire issue.

Bennett, Linda A., and Genevieve M. Ames, eds. 1985. *The American Experience with Alcohol: Contrasting Cultural Perspectives*. New York: Plenum.

Bennett, Linda A., Aleksandar Janca, Bridget F. Grant, and Norman Sartorius. 1993. Boundaries between Normal and Pathological Drinking. A Cross-Cultural Comparison. *Alcohol Health and Research World* 17(3):190–95.

Bennett, Linda A., Steven J. Wolin, David Reiss, and Martha A. Teitelbaum. 1987. Couples at Risk for Alcoholism Transmission: Protective Influences. *Family Process* 26:111–29.

Benoist, Jean. 1978. *The Structural Revolution*. London: Weidenfeld Nicols.

Benthall, J, and T. Polhemus, eds. 1975. *The Body as a Medium of Expression*. New York: Dutton.

Bentley, M. E. 1988. The Household Management of Childhood Diarrhea in Rural North India. Special issue of *Social Science and Medicine* 27(1):75–86.

Bentley, M. E., and G. H. Pelto. 1991. The Household Production of Nutrition. *Social Science and Medicine* 33(10):1101–2.

Bentley, M. E., et al. 1988. Rapid Ethnographic Assessment: Applications in a Diarrhea Management Program. Special issue of *Social Science and Medicine* 27(1):107–16.

Berelson, Bernard. 1966. KAP Studies on Fertility. In *Family Planning and Population Programs,* ed. Bernard Berelson et al. Chicago: University of Chicago Press, 655–68.

Berg, Elliott J. 1965. The Economics of the Migrant Labor System. In *Urbanization and Migration in West Africa,* ed. Hilda Kuper. Berkeley: University of California Press, 160–81.

Berkman, Lisa F. 1981. Physical Health and the Social Environment: A Social Epidemiological Perspective. In *The Relevance of Social Science for Medicine,* ed. Leon Eisenberg and Arthur Kleinman. Dordrecht, Holland: D. Reidel, 51–75.

———. 1985. Measures of Social Networks and Social Support: Evidence and Measurement. In *Measuring Psychosocial Variables in Epidemiologic Studies of Cardiovascular Disease,* ed. Adrian M. Ostfeld and Elaine D. Eaker. NIH Publication No. 85-2270. Bethesda, Md.: National Institutes of Health.

Berkman, L. F., and S. L. Syme. 1979. Social Networks, Host Resistance and Mortality: A Nine-Year Follow-up Study of Alameda County Residents. *American Journal of Epidemiology* 109(2):186–204.

Berliner, Howard. 1977. Emerging Ideologies in Medicine. *Review of Radical Political Economics* 9(1):116–24.

Bernard, H. R. 1988. *Research Methods in Cultural Anthropology.* Beverly Hills: Sage.

Bernard, H. R., et al. 1986. The Construction of Primary Data in Cultural Anthropology. *Current Anthropology* 27(4):382–96.

Bernstein, Gale L., and Yasue Aoki Kidd. 1982. Childbearing in Japan. In *Anthropology of Human Birth,* ed. Margarita Artschwager Kay. Philadelphia: F. A. Davis Co., 101–18.

Berry, J. W., Uichol Kim, Thomas Minde, and Doris Mok. 1987. Comparative Studies of Acculturative Stress. *International Migration Review* 21:491–511.

Beuscher, N., C. Bodinet, D. Neumann-Haefelin, A. Marston, and K. Hostettmann. 1994. Antiviral Activity of African Medicinal Plants. *Journal of Ethnopharmacology* 42:101–9.

Beyene, Yewoubdar.

———. 1989. *From Menarche to Menopause: Reproductive Lives of Peasant Women in Two Cultures.* Albany: State University of New York Press.

———. 1992. Medical Disclosure and Refugees–Telling Bad News to Ethiopian Patients. *Western Journal of Medicine* 157:328–32.

Beyer, Gunther. 1981. The Political Refugee: 35 Years Later. *International Migration Review* 15:26–34.

Bhanumathi, P. P. 1977. Nurses' Conceptions of "Sick-Role" and "Good Patient" Behavior: A Cross-Cultural Comparison. *International Nursing Review* 24:20–24.

Bibeau, Gilles. 1980. *Traditional Medicine in Zaire.* Ottawa: IRDC.

———. 1981. The Circular Semantic Network in Ngbandi Disease Nosology. *Social Science and Medicine* 15B:295–307.

———. 1982. New Legal Values for an Old Art of Healing. *Social Science and Medicine* 16(21):1843–49.

Binn, M. 1980. Using the Explanatory Model to Understand Ethnomedical Perceptions of Hypertension and the Resultant Behaviors. In *Transcultural Nursing Care: Teaching, Practice and Research,* ed. M. Leininger. Salt Lake City: University of Utah, College of Nursing, 60–76.

Binswanger, Ludwig. 1958. Insanity as Life-History Phenomenon. In *Existence: A New Dimension in Psychiatry and Psychology,* ed. Rollo May, Ernest Angle, and Henri Ellenberger. New York: Simon & Schuster.

Bion, W. R. 1959. *Experiences in Groups*. London: Tavistock.

Bisset, Norman G. 1991. One Man's Poison, Another Man's Medicine? *Journal of Ethnopharmacology* 32:71–81.

Black, Judith, and Kingsley Davis. 1964. Norms, Values, and Sanctions. In *Handbook of Modern Sociology,* ed. Robert E. L. Faris. Chicago: Rand McNally, 465–84.

Black, Peter Weston. 1984. The Anthropology of Tobacco Use: Tobian Data and Theoretical Issues. *Journal of Anthropological Research* 40(4):475–503.

Blacking, John. 1977. Towards an Anthropology of the Body. In *The Anthropology of the Body,* ed. John Blacking. New York: Academic Press, 1–17.

Blacking, John, ed. 1977. *Outline of a Theory of Practice.* Cambridge Studies in Social Anthropology, vol. 16. Cambridge: Cambridge University Press.

Blake, Judith. 1974. Coercive Pronatalism and American Population Policy. In *Pronatalism: The Myth of Mom and Apple Pie,* ed. Ellen Peck and Judith Senderowitz. New York: Thomas Y. Crowell Co., 29–68.

Blake, Judith, and Kingsley Davis. 1964. Norms, Values, and Sanctions. In *Handbook of Modern Sociology,* ed. Robert E. L. Faris. Chicago: Rand McNally, 465–84.

Blank, Robert H. 1984. *Redefining Human Life: Reproductive Technologies and Social Policy.* Boulder, Colo.: Westview Press.

Bledsoe, C. 1990. The Politics of AIDS, Condoms and Heterosexual Relations in Africa: Recent Evidence from the Local Print Media. In *Births and Power: Social Change and the Politics of Reproduction,* ed. W. P. Handwerker. Boulder, Colo.: Westview Press, 197–222.

Bloche, Gregg. 1987. *Uruguay's Military Physicians: Cogs in a System of State Terror.* Washington, D.C.: American Association for the Advancement of Science.

Block, G., L. M. Coyle, A. M. Hartman, and S. M. Scoppa. 1994. Revision of Dietary Analysis Software for the Health Habits and History Questionnaire. *American Journal of Epidemiology* 139:1190–96.

Bloom, Lawrence. 1991. Moral Perception and Particularity. *Ethics* 101:701–25.

Bock, Philip K. 1980. *Continuities in Psychological Anthropology.* San Fransisco: W. H. Freeman and Company.

———. 1988. *Rethinking Psychological Anthropology: Continuity and Change in the Study of Human Action.* San Francisco: W. H. Freeman and Co.

———. 1994. *Handbook of Psychological Anthropology.* Westport, Conn.: Greenwood Press.

Boddy, Janice. 1988. Spirits and Selves in Northern Sudan: The Cultural Therapeutics of Possession and Trance. *American Ethnologist* 15:4–27.

———. 1989. *Wombs and Alien Spirits: Women, Men, and the Zar Cult in Northern Sudan.* Madison: University of Wisconsin Press.

Bolton, J. L. 1980. *The Medieval English Economy, 1150–1500.* London: J. M. Dent & Sons.

Bolton, R., and G. Orozco. 1994. *The AIDS Bibliography: Studies in Anthropology and Related Fields.* Arlington, Va.: American Anthropological Association.

Bonaparte, B. 1979. Ego Defensiveness, Open-closed Mindedness, and Nurses' Attitudes toward Culturally Different Patients. *Nursing Research* 28:166–72.

Bonfil-Batalla, G. 1966. Conservative Thought in Applied Anthropology: A Critique. *Human Organization* 25(2):89–92.

———. 1970. Conservative Thought in Applied Anthropology. In *Applied Anthropology,* ed. J. A. Clifton, 246–53. Boston: Houghton Mifflin.

Bongaarts, John. 1980. Does Malnutrition Affect Fertility? *Science* 208:564–69.

———. 1982. The Fertility Inhibiting Effects of the Intermediate Fertility Variables. *Studies in Family Planning* 13:179–89.

———. 1983. The Proximate Determinants of Natural Marital Fertility. In *Determinants of Fertility in Developing Countries,* ed. R. A. Bulatao and R. D. Lee. Vol. 1. San Francisco: Academic Press, 103–38.

Bongaarts, John, W. P. Mauldin, and J. Phillips. 1990. The Demographic Impact of Family Planning Programs. *Studies in Family Planning* 21(6):299–310.

Bongaarts, John, and R. G. Potter. 1983. *Fertility, Biology and Behavior.* New York: Academic Press.

Boone, M. S., and J. J. Woods, eds. 1989. *Computer Applications for Anthropologists.* Belmont, Calif.: Wadsworth.

Borgatti, S. 1988. ANTHROPAC. Microcomputer software.

Borgerhoff Mulder, Monique. 1987. Resources and Reproductive Success in Women with an Example from the Kipsigis of Kenya. *Journal of Zoology* (London) 213:489–505.

Borjas, George J., and Marta Tienda. 1987. The Economic Consequences of Immigration. *Science* 235:645–51.

Borofsky, Robert. 1994. Cultural Anthropology's Future Agenda. *Anthropology Newsletter* (September): 76.

Borrini, Grazia. 1987. Health and Development: A Marriage of Heaven and Hell? In *The Impact of Development and Modern Technologies in Third World Health,* ed. Barbara Jackson and Antonio Ugalde. Studies in Third World Societies 34. Williamsburg, Va.: College of William and Mary, Department of Anthropology.

Boserup, Ester. 1965. *The Conditions of Agricultural Growth.* Chicago: Aldine.

———. 1981. *Population and Technological Change.* Chicago: University of Chicago Press.

Bosk, Charles L. 1979. *Forgive and Remember: Managing Medical Failure.* Chicago: University of Chicago Press.

———. 1992. *All God's Mistakes: Genetic Counseling in a Pediatric Hospital.* Chicago: University of Chicago Press.

Bourdieu, P. 1977. *Outline of a Theory of Practice.* Cambridge Studies in Social Anthropology, vol. 16. Cambridge: Cambridge University Press.

———. 1988. *Homo Academicus.* Cambridge: Polity Press. (French ed., 1984.)

Bourguignon, Erika. 1976. The Effectiveness of Religious Healing Movements: A Review of the Literature. *Transcultural Psychiatric Research Review* 13:5–21.

———. 1983. Sex Bias Ethnocentrism, and Myth Building in Anthropology: The Case of Universal Male Dominance. *Central Issues of Anthropology* 5(1):59–79.

Boyer, L. Bryce. 1979. *Childhood and Folklore: A Psychoanalytic Study of Apache Personality.* New York: Library of Psychological Anthropology.

Boyer, L. Bryce, George De Vos, Orin Borders, and Alice Tani-Borders. 1978. The "Burnt Child Reaction" among the Yukon Eskimos. *Journal of Psychological Anthropology* 1(1):7–56.

Brachman, P. S. 1985a. Principles and Methods. In *Principles and Practice of Infectious Diseases,* ed. G. L. Mandell, R. G. Douglas, and J. E. Bennett. 2d ed. New York: John Wiley, 96–103.

———. 1985b. Transmission and Principles of Control. In *Principles and Practice of Infectious Diseases,* ed. G. L. Mandell, R. G. Douglas, and J. E. Bennett, 2d ed. New York: John Wiley, 103–6.

Brady, Maggie. 1988. Indigenous and Government Attempts to Control Alcohol Use among Australian Aborigines. Paper presented at International Union of Anthropological and Ethnological Sciences Congress, Zagreb, Yugoslavia.

Bratton, Michael. 1982. Types of Development and Underdevelopment: Towards Comparison. Unpublished manuscript.

Brecher, Jeremy, and Tim Costello. 1994. *Global Village or Global Pillage.* Boston: South End Press.

Brenner, Charles. 1974. *An Elementary Textbook of Psychoanalysis.* Rev. and exp. ed. New York: International Universities Press.

Brenner, Robert. 1976. Agrarian Class Structure and Economic Development in Pre-industrial Europe. *Past and Present* 70:30–75.

Briesemeister, Linda H., and Beth A. Haines. 1988. The Interactions of Fathers and Newborns. In *Childbirth in America,* ed. Karen Michaelson. South Hadley, Mass.: Bergin and Garvey, 228–39.

Briggs, Jean. 1970. *Never in Anger: Portrait of an Eskimo Family.* Cambridge, Mass.: Harvard University Press.

Brill, L. 1981. The Clinical Treatment of Substance Abusers. New York: Free Press.

Brink, P. J., ed. 1976. *Transcultural Nursing: A Book of Readings.* Englewood Cliffs, N.J.: Prentice-Hall.

Briscoe, John. 1987. A Role for Water Supply and Sanitation in the Child Survival Revolution. *PAHO Bulletin* 21(2):93–105.

Brody, Eugene. 1993. *Biomedical Technology and Human Rights.* Paris: United Nations Educational, Scientific and Cultural Organization.

Brody, Howard. 1980. *Placebos and the Philosophy of Medicine.* Chicago: University of Chicago Press.

———. 1988a. The Symbolic Power of the Modern Personal Physician: The Placebo Response under Challenge. *Journal of Drug Issues* 18(2):149–61.

———. 1988b. *Stories of Sickness.* New Haven, Conn.: Yale University Press.

———. 1992. *The Healer's Power.* New Haven, Conn.: Yale University Press.

———. 1994. The Four Principles and Narrative Ethics. In *Principles of Health Care Ethics,* ed. Raana Gilon. New York: John Wiley and Sons, 207–16.

Brooker, Stanley G., Richard C. Cambie, and Robert C. Cooper. 1989. Economic Native Plants of New Zealand. *Economic Botany* 43:79–106.

Brothwell, D. R., and A. T. Sandison. 1967. *Diseases in Antiquity: A Survey of Diseases, Injuries, and Surgery in Ancient Populations.* Springfield, Ill.: Charles C. Thomas.

Brown, Diane R., and Lawrence E. Gary. 1987. Stressful Life Events, Social Support Networks, and the Physical and Mental Health of Urban Black Adults. *Journal of Human Stress* 13: 165–74.

Brown, E. L. 1982. Cross-cultural Perspectives on Middle-aged Women. *Current Anthropology* 23(2):143–56.

Brown, E. Richard. 1976. Public Health in Imperialism: Early Rockefeller Programs at Home and Abroad. *American Journal of Public Health* 66:897.

———. 1979. *Rockefeller Medicine Men: Medicine and Capitalism in America.* Berkeley: University of California Press.

———. 1980. Rockefeller Medicine in China: Professionalism and Imperialism. In *Philanthropy and Cultural Imperialism,* ed. Robert F. Armour. Boston: G. K. Hall, 123–46.

Brown, George W. 1974. Meaning, Measurement, and Stress of Life Events. In *Stressful Life Events: Their Nature and Effects,* ed. B. S. Dohrenwend, and B. P. Dohrenwend. New York: Wiley.

Brown, G., J. L. T. Birley, and J. Wing. 1972. Influence of Family Life on the Course of Schizophrenic Disorders: A Replication. *British Journal of Psychiatry* 121:241–58.

Brown, G. W., and T. Harris. 1978. *Social Origins of Depression: A Study of Psychiatric Disorder in Women.* New York: Free Press.

Brown, Howard P., Jr., John H. Peterson, Jr., and Orville Cunningham. 1988. An Individualized Behavior Approach to Spiritual Development for the Recovering Alcoholic/Addict. *Alcoholism Treatment Quarterly* 5(1/2):177–91.

Brown, Judith K. 1970. Note on the Division of Labor by Sex. *American Anthropologist* 72(5): 1073–78.

Brown, Judith K., and Virginia Kerns, eds. 1985. *In Her Prime: A New View of Middle-Aged Women.* South Hadley, Mass.: Bergin and Garvey.

Brown, Kate. 1991. Death and Access: Ethics in Cross-Cultural Health Care. In *Making Choices,* ed. Emily Friedman. Chicago: American Hospital Association Publishing Co.

———. 1994. Outside the Garden of Eden: Rural Values and Healthcare Reform. *Cambridge Quarterly of Healthcare Ethics* 3(3):329–37.

Brown, Michael F. 1988. Shamanism and Its Discontents. *Medical Anthropology Quarterly* 2:102–20.

Brown, P. J. 1981. Cultural Adaptations to Endemic Malaria in Sardinia. *Medical Anthropology* 5:311.

———. 1986. Cultural and Genetic Adaptations to Malaria: Problems of Comparison. *Human Ecology* 14:311–32.

———. 1987. Microparasites and Macroparasites. *Cultural Anthropology* 2:155–71.

Brown, Paul, and D. Carleton Gajdusek. 1978. Acute and Chronic Pulmonary Airway Disease in Pacific Island Micronesians. *American Journal of Epidemiology* 108:266–73.

Brown, P. J., and M. Konner. 1987. An Anthropological Perspective on Obesity. *Annals of the New York Academy of Sciences* 499:29–46.

Browne, M. W. 1988. Poor Man's Atomic Bomb Is Once Again Used in Battle. *New York Times,* April 17.

Browner, Carole H. 1976. Poor Women's Fertility Decisions: Illegal Abortion in Cali, Colombia. Ph.D. dissertation, University of California.

———. 1979. Abortion Decision Making: Some Findings from Colombia. *Studies in Family Planning* 10(3):96–106.

———. 1980. The Management of Early Pregnancy: Folk Concepts of Fertility Control. *Social Science and Medicine* 14B(1):25–32.

———. 1983. Male Pregnancy Symptoms in Urban Colombia. *American Ethnologist* 10(3):494–511.

———. 1985a. Criteria for Selecting Herbal Remedies. *Ethnology* 24(1):13–32.

———. 1985b. Plants Used for Reproductive Health in Oaxaca, Mexico. *Economic Botany* 39:482–504.

———. 1985c. Women, Household, and Health in Latin America. Social Science Research Council Conference on the Political Economy of Health and Disease in Africa and Latin America, Toluca, Mexico, January 8–12.

———. 1986. The Politics of Reproduction in a Mexican Village. *Signs* 11(4):710–24.

———. 1988. Women's Secrets: Bases for Reproductive and Social Autonomy in a Mexican Community. *American Ethnologist* 15:84–97.

———. 1989a. The Management of Reproduction in an Egalitarian Community. In *Women Healers,* ed. Carol McClain. New Brunswick, N.J.: Rutgers University Press.

———. 1989b. Women, Household, and Health in Latin America. *Social Science and Medicine* 28:461–73.

Browner, Carole, and Ellen Lewin. 1982. Female Altruism Reconsidered: The Virgin Mary as Economic Woman. *American Ethnologist* 9(1):61–75.

Browner, C. H., and Bernard R. Ortiz de Montellano. 1986. Herbal Emmenagogues Used by Women in Colombia and Mexico. In *Plants in Indigenous Medicine and Diet,* ed. N. L. Etkin. Bedford Hills, N.Y.: Redgrave, 32–47.

Browner, Carole, Bernard R. Ortiz de Montellano, and Arthur J. Rubel. 1988. A Methodology for Cross-Cultural Ethnomedical Research. *Current Anthropology* 29(5):681–702.

Browner, C. H., and S. T. Perdue. 1988 Womens' Secrets: Bases for Reproductive and Social Autonomy in a Mexican Community. *American Ethnologist* 15(1):84–97.

Browner, C. H., and Nancy Press. 1995. The Normalization of Prenatal Diagnostic Testing. In *Conceiving the New World Order,* ed. Faye Ginsberg and Rayna Rapp. Berkeley: University of California Press, 307–22.

Brownson, R. C., R. L. Remington, and J. R. Davis. 1993. *Chronic Disease Epidemiology and Control.* Washington, D.C.: American Public Health Association.

Bruce-Chwatt, L. J. 1980. *Essential Malariology.* London: William Heinemann Medical Books.

Bruhn, John G., and Billy U. Phillips. 1984. Measuring Social Support: A Synthesis of Current Approaches. *Journal of Behavioral Medicine* 7:151–69.

Bruhn, J. G., and S. Wolf. 1979. *The Roseto Story: An Anatomy of Health.* Norman: University of Oklahoma Press.

Brunton, Ron. 1989. *The Abandoned Narcotic: Kava and Cultural Instability in Melanesia.* Cambridge: Cambridge University Press.

Bryan, Ralph, Robert W. Pinner, Robert P. Gaynes, C. J. Peters, Judith R. Aguilar, and Ruth L. Berkelman. 1994. Addressing Emerging Infectious Disease Threats: A Prevention Strategy for the United States. Executive Summary. *Morbidity and Mortality Weekly Report* 43(RR-5):1–18.

Bryant, Carol A. 1982. The Impact of Kin, Friend and Neighbor Networks on Infant Feeding Practices. *Social Science and Medicine* 16:1757–65.

Buchbinder, G. 1977. Endemic Cretinism among the Maring: The By-product of Culture Contact. In *Nutrition and Anthropology in Action,* ed. T. K. Fitzgerald. Assem, the Netherlands: Van Gorcum, 106–16.

Buck, C., Alvaro Llopis, Enrique Najera, and Milton Terris. 1988a. *The Challenge of Epidemiology: Issues and Selected Readings.* Pan American Health Organization, Scientific Publication 505. Washington, D.C.: Children's Defense Fund.

———. 1988b. *Teen Age Pregnancy: The Advocate's Guide to the Numbers.* Washington, D.C.: Adolescent Pregnancy Prevention Clearing House.

Buckley, Thomas. 1982. Menstruation and the Power of Yurok Women: Methods in Cultural Reconstruction. *American Ethnologist* 9(1):47–61.

Buckley, T., and A. Gottlieb, eds. 1988. *Blood Magic: The Anthropology of Menstruation.* Berkeley: University of California Press.

Bulatao, R. A., and R. D. Lee, eds. 1983. *Determinants of Fertility in Developing Countries.* 2 vols. San Francisco: Academic Press.

Bunzel, Ruth. 1940. The Role of Alcoholism in Two Central American Cultures. *Psychiatry* 3:361–87.

———. 1976. Chamula and Chichicastenango: A Reexamination. In *Cross-Cultural Approaches to the Study of Alcohol,* ed. M. Everett et al. The Hague: Mouton.

Burke, B. 1947. The Dietary History as a Tool in Research. *Journal of the American Dietetic Association* 23:1041–46.

Burnam, M. Audrey, Richard L. Hough, Marvin Karno, Javier I. Escobar, and Cynthia A. Telles. 1987. Acculturation and Lifetime Prevalence of Psychiatric Disorders among Mexican Americans in Los Angeles. *Journal of Health and Social Behavior* 28:89–102.

Burnet, M., and D. O. White. 1978. *Natural History of Infectious Disease.* 4th ed. Cambridge: Cambridge University Press.

Burns, Chester, ed. 1977. *Legacies in Law and Medicine.* New York: Science History Publications.

Burns J. F. 1994. Thousands Flee Indian City in Deadly Plague Outbreak. *New York Times,* September 24, 1, 5.

Burr, Angela. 1984. The Ideologies of Despair: A Symbolic Interpretation of Punks and Skinheads' Usage of Barbiturates. *Social Science and Medicine* 19(9):929–38.

Burrage, Michael, and Rolf Torstendahl, eds. 1990. *Professions in Theory and History: Rethinking the Study of Professions.* London: Sage.

Burrow, James. 1977. *Organized Medicine in the Progressive Era: The Move toward Monopoly.* Baltimore: Johns Hopkins University Press.

Bush, M. T., J. A. Ullom, and O. H. Osborne. 1975. The Meaning of Mental Health: A Report of Two Ethnoscientific Studies. *Nursing Research* 24:130–38.

Butzer, K. W. 1975. Geological and Ecological Perspectives on the Middle Pleistocene. In *After the Australopithecines,* ed. K. W. Butzer and G. L. Isaac. The Hague: Mouton, 857–73.

Bye, S. N., and M. F. Dutton. 1991. The Inappropriate Use of Traditional Medicines in South Africa. *Journal of Ethnopharmacology* 34:253–59.

Byerly, E. L. 1969. The Nurse-Researcher as Participant-Observer in a Nursing Setting. *Nursing Research* 18:230–36.

Byerly, E. L., and C. A. Molgaard. 1982. Social Institutions and Disease Transmission. In *Clinically Applied Anthropology: Anthropologists in Health Science Settings,* ed. N. Chrisman and T. Maretzki. Dordrecht: D. Reidel, 395–409.

Byerly, E. L., C. A. Molgaard, and C. T. Snow. 1979. Dissonance in the Desert: What to Do with the Golden Seal? In *Transcultural Nursing Care: Culture Change, Ethics and Nursing Care Implications. Proceeding of the Fourth National Transcultural Nursing Conference,* ed. M. Leininger. Salt Lake City: University of Utah, College of Nursing, 114–33.

Cain, Mead. 1988. The Material Consequences of Reproductive Failures in Rural South Asia. In *A Home Divided: Women and Income in the Third World,* ed. Daisy Dwyer and Judith Bruce. Stanford: Stanford University Press, 20–38.

Caldwell, John C. 1981. The Mechanisms of Demographic Change in Historical Perspective. *Population Studies* 35(1):5–27.

———. 1982. *Theory of Fertility Decline.* San Francisco: Academic Press.

Caldwell, J., P. Caldwell, and P. Quiggin. 1989. The Social Context of AIDS in Sub-Saharan Africa. *Population and Development Review* 15(2):185–234.

Caldwell, J., I. Orubuloye, and P. Caldwell. 1992. Underreaction to AIDS in Sub-Saharan Africa. *Social Science and Medicine* 34(11):1169–82.

Caldwell, Robert A., and Bernard L. Bloom. 1982. Social Support: Its Structure and Impact on Marital Disruption. *American Journal of Community Psychology* 10:647–67.

Calestro, Kenneth. 1972. Psychotherapy, Faith Healing, and Suggestion. *International Journal of Psychiatry* 10:83–113.

Callahan, Daniel. 1973. Bioethics as a Discipline. *Hastings Center Studies* 1:66–73.

———. 1980. Contemporary Biomedical Ethics (Shattuck Lecture). *New England Journal of Medicine* 320:1228–33.

———. 1984. Autonomy: A Moral Good, Not a Moral Obsession. *Hastings Center Report* 14(5): 40–42.

———. 1986. How Technology Is Shaping the Abortion Debate. *Hastings Center Report* 16:33–42.

———. 1993. *The Troubled Dream of Life: Living with Mortality.* New York: Simon & Schuster.

———. 1994. Bioethics: Private Choice and Common Good. *Hastings Center Report* 24(3):28–31.

Cambrosio, Alberto, and Peter Keating. 1992. A Matter of FACS: Constituting Novel Entities in Immunology. *Medical Anthropology Quarterly* 6:262–384.

Camenish, Paul F., ed. 1994. *Religious Methods and Resources in Bioethics.* Boston: Kluwer Academic Publishers.

Cameron, A. 1960. Folk-lore as a Medical Problem Among Arab Refugees. *Practitioner* 185:347–53.

Camp, Charles. 1979. Federal Foodways Research, 1935–1943. *Digest* 2:4–17.

Campbell, Gregory. 1988. Historic Health Patterns on the Northern Cheyenne Reservation. Paper presented at the Annual Meeting of the American Anthropological Association, Phoenix, Arizona, November 16–20.

Campbell, Kenneth L., and James W. Wood. 1987. Fertility in Traditional Societies. In *Natural Human Fertility: Social and Biological Mechanisms,* ed. P. Diggory and S. Teper. London: Macmillan.

Canguilhem, George. 1989. *The Normal and the Pathological.* New York: Zone Books.

Cannon, J. R., A. Capasso, F. N. Mascolo, G. Autore, F. de Simone, and F. Senatore. 1983. Anti-inflammatory and Analgesic Activity in Alcoholic Extract of Tamus communis L. *Journal of Ethnopharmacology* 8(3):321–25.

Cannon, W. B. 1942. Voodoo Death. *American Anthropologist* 44:169–81.

Capers, Cynthia Flynn. 1985. Cultural Diversity and Nursing Practice. *Topics in Clinical Nursing* 7:3.

Caplan, Robert D., R. K. Naidu, and Rama C. Tripathi. 1984. Coping and Defense: Constellations vs. Components. *Journal of Health and Social Behavior* 25:303–20.

Caralis, P. V., et al. 1993. The Influence of Ethnicity and Race on Attitudes toward Advance Directives, Life-Prolonging Treatments and Euthanasia. *Journal of Clinical Ethics* 4:155–65.

Carbajal, D., A. Casaco, L. Arruzazabala, R. Gonzalez, and Z. Tolon. 1989. Pharmacological Study of *Cymbopogon citratus* Leaves. *Journal of Ethnopharmacology* 25:103–7.

Carey, James W. 1988. Folk Illness: Incidence Patterns and Household Health in the Southern Peruvian Andes. Paper presented at Annual Meetings, American Anthropological Association, Phoenix, Arizona.

Carlson, Katherine A. 1977. Identifying the Stranger: An Analysis of Behavioral Rules of Sales of Heroin. In *Drugs, Rituals and Altered States of Consciousness,* ed. Brian du Toit. Rotterdam: A. A. Balkema.

Carlson, Robert G., Jichuan Wang, Harvey A. Siegal, Russel S. Falck, and Jie Guo. 1994. An Ethnographic Approach to Targeted Sampling: Problems and Solutions in AIDS Prevention Research among Injection Drug and Crack-Cocaine Users. *Human Organization* 53:79–86.

Carmack, Robert M., ed. 1988. *Harvest of Violence: The Maya Indians and the Guatemalan Crisis.* Norman: University of Oklahoma Press.

Carovano, K. 1991. More Than Mothers and Whores: Redefining the AIDS Prevention Needs of Women. *International Journal of Health Services* 21(1):131–42.

Carr-Saunders, E. M., and P. A. Wilson. 1933. *The Professions.* Oxford: Clarendon Press.

Carr, John E., and Peter P. Vitaliano. 1985. The Theoretical Implications of Converging Research on Depression and the Culture-Bound Syndromes. In *Culture and Depression: Studies in the Anthropology and Cross-Cultural Psychiatry of Affect and Disorder,* ed. Arthur Kleinman and Byron Good. Berkeley: University of California Press.

Carson, Ronald A. 1990. Interpretive Bioethics: The Way of Discernment. *Theoretical Medicine* 11(1):51–60.

Carter, William E., ed. 1980. *Cannabis in Costa Rica.* Philadelphia: Institute for the Study of Human Issues.

Cash, Richard A. 1983. Oral Rehydration in the Treatment of Diarrhea: Issues in the Implementation of Diarrhea Treatment Programs. In *Diarrhea and Malnutrition: Interactions, Mechanisms, and Interventions,* ed. Lincoln Chen and Nevin Scrimshaw. New York: Plenum Press, 203–21.

Cassel, John C. 1955. A Comprehensive Health Program among South African Zulus. In *Health, Culture, and Community,* ed. Benjamin D. Paul. New York: Russell Sage Foundation, 15–41.

———. 1976. The Contribution of the Social Environment to Host Resistance. *American Journal of Epidemiology* 104:107–23.

Cassel, John C., Ralph Patrick, and David Jenkins. 1960. Epidemiological Analysis of the Health Implications of Culture Change. *Annals of the New York Academy of Sciences* 84:938–49.

Cassel, John C., and H. A. Tyroler. 1961. Epidemiological Studies of Cultural Change. *Archives of Environmental Health* 3(1):25–33.

Cassel, Eric J. 1991. *The Nature of Suffering and the Goals of Medicine.* Oxford: Oxford University Press.

Cassell, Joan. 1987. On Control, Certitude and the "Paranoia" of Surgeons. *Culture, Medicine and Psychiatry* 11:229–49.

Cassidy, C. M. 1980a. Benign Neglect and Toddler Malnutrition. In *Social and Biological Predictors of Nutritional Status, Physical Growth, and Neurological Development,* ed. L. S. Greene and F. E. Johnston. New York: Academic Press, 109–39.

———. 1980b. Nutrition and Health in Agriculturists and Hunter-Gatherers: A Case Study of Two Prehistoric Populations. In *Nutritional Anthropology: Contemporary Approaches to Diet and Culture,* ed. N. Jerome, R. Kandel, and G. H. Pelto. New York: Regrave Publishing Co.

———. 1982. Protein-Energy Malnutrition as a Culture-Bound Syndrome. *Culture, Medicine and Psychiatry* 6:325–45.

———. 1987. World-View Conflict and Toddler Malnutrition: Change Agent Dilemmas. In *Child Survival,* ed. Nancy Scheper-Hughes. Dordrecht, Holland: D. Reidel, 293–324.

Caudill, William. 1953. Applied Anthropology in Medicine. In *Anthropology Today,* ed. A. L. Kroeber. Chicago: University of Chicago Press.

———. 1958a. *Effects of Social and Cultural Systems in Reactions to Stress.* New York: Social Science Research Council.

———. 1958b. *The Psychiatric Hospital as a Small Society.* Cambridge: Harvard University Press.

———. 1962. Anthropology and Psychoanalysis: Some Theoretical Issues. In *Anthropology and Human Behavior,* ed. T. Gladwin and W. C. Sturtevant. Washington, D.C.: Anthropological Society of Washington, 174–214.

Centers for Disease Control. 1993. Use of Race and Ethnicity in Public Health Surveillance. *Morbidity and Mortality Weekly Report* 42.

Chafetz, L. 1981. Aggressive Behaviors in Walk-in Settings: Nursing Responses. *In Developing, Teaching and Practicing Transcultural Nursing: Proceedings of the 6th Transcultural Nursing Conference,* ed. P. Morley. Salt Lake City: University of Utah, College of Nursing and the Transcultural Nursing Society, 96–114.

Chagnon, Napoleon A. 1968. Yanomamo Social Organization and Warfare. In *War: The Anthropology of Armed Conflict and Aggression,* ed. Morton Fried, Marvin Harris, and Robert Murphy. New York: Natural History Press, 109–59.

———. 1977. *The Fierce People.* 2d ed. New York: Holt, Rinehart & Winston.

Chambers, Erve J., and Philip D. Young. 1979. Mesoamerican Community Studies: The Past Decade. *Annual Reviews of Anthropology* 8:45–69.

Chambers, Robert. 1986. *Normal Professionalism, New Paradigms, and Development.* Discussion Paper 227. Brighton: Institute of Development Studies.

Chance, Norman A. 1965. Acculturation, Self-identification, and Personality Adjustment. *American Anthropologist* 67:372–93.

Chasin, Barbara, and Richard W. Franke. 1979. The West African Sahel: Social Roots of Ecological Disaster. *ARC Newsletter* 3(2):3.

Chavez, Leo R. 1986. Mexican Immigration and Health Care: A Political Economy Perspective. *Human Organization* 45(4):344–52.

Chavez, Leo R., Estevan T. Flores, and Marta Lopez-Garza. 1992. Undocumented Latin American Immigrants and U.S. Health Services: An Approach to a Political Economy of Utilization. *Medical Anthropology Quarterly* 6(1):6–26.

Chavunduka, G. L. 1984. *The Zimbabwe National Traditional Healers Association* (ZINATHA). Harare. 1986. The Organisation of Traditional Medicine in Zimbabwe. In M. Last and G. L. Chavunduka, eds., *The Professionalisation of African Medicine.* Manchester: Manchester University Press for the International African Institute, 29–50.

———. 1994. *Traditional Medicine in Modern Zimbabwe.* Harare: University of Zimbabwe Publications.

Cheesmond, A. K., and A. Fenwick. 1981. Human Excretion Behavior in a Schistosomiasis Endemic Area of the Geizira, Sudan. *Journal of Tropical Medicine and Hygiene* 84:101–7.

Chen, Lincoln, and Nevin Scrimshaw, eds. 1983. *Diarrhea and Malnutrition: Interactions, Mechanisms, and Interventions.* New York: Plenum Press.

Cheng, L. Y., F. Cheung and C. N. Chen. 1993. *Psychotherapy for the Chinese.* Hong Kong: Department of Psychiatry, Chinese University of Hong Kong.

Children's Defense Fund. 1988. *Teen Age Pregnancy: The Advocates' Guide to the Numbers.* Washington, D.C.: Adolescent Pregnancy Prevention Clearing House.

———. 1991. *The State of America's Children 1991.* Washington, D.C.: Children's Defense Fund.

Childress, James F. 1990. The Place of Autonomy in Bioethics. *Hastings Center Reports* 20(1):12–17.

Chinn, P. L. 1983. Nursing Theory Development: Where We Have Been and Where We Are Going. In *The Nursing Profession: A Time to Speak,* ed. N. L. Chaska. New York: McGraw-Hill, 394–405.

Chinn, P. L., ed. 1982. From the Editor. Nursing and Culture. *Advance Nursing Science* 4(3):xii–xiii.

Choukri, Ghari. 1985. Conceptual Problems on the Arab Road towards a Sociology of Knowledge. *Al-Mustaqbal Al-Arabi* 77(7):126–36. (in Arabic)

Chrisman, Noel J. 1977. The Health Seeking Process: An Approach to the Natural History of Illness. *Culture, Medicine, and Psychiatry* 1(4):351–77.

———. 1982. Anthropology in Nursing: An Exploration of Adaptation. In *Clinically Applied Anthropology: Anthropologists in Health Science Settings*, ed. N. Chrisman and T. Maretzki. Dordrecht: D. Reidel, 117–40.

———. 1986. Transcultural Care. In *Mosby's Comprehensive Review of Critical Care*, ed. Donna Zschoche. St. Louis: Mosby, chap. 2.

———. 1988. The Role of Anthropology in Nursing Education. *Practicing Anthropology* 10:21.

———. 1991a. Cultural Systems. In *Cancer Nursing*, ed. S. Baird, R. McCorkle, and M. Grant. Philadelphia: W. B. Saunders, 45–54.

———. 1991b. Culture Sensitive Nursing Care. In *Medical-Surgical Nursing: Pathophysiologic Concepts*, ed. M. Patrick, S. Woods, R. Craven, J. Rokosky, and P. Bruno. 2d ed. Philadelphia: Lippincott.

Chrisman, Noel J., and Arthur Kleinman. 1983. Popular Health Care, Social Networks, and Cultural Meanings: The Orientation of Medical Anthropology. In *Handbook of Health, Health Care, and the Health Professions*, ed. David Mechanic. New York: Free Press, 569–91.

Chrisman, Noel J., and Thomas W. Maretzki, eds. 1982. *Clinically Applied Anthropology: Anthropologists in Health Science Settings*. Dordrecht: D. Reidel.

Christakis, Nicholas. 1988. The Ethical Design of an AIDS Vaccine Trial in Africa. *Hastings Center Report* 18(3):31–37.

———. 1992. Ethics Are Local: Engaging Cross-Cultural Variation in the Ethics of Clinical Research. *Social Science and Medicine* 35(9):1079–91.

Chukkol, Kharisu Sufiyanu. 1981. *Supernatural Belief and the Criminal Law in Nigeria: A Critical Appraisal*. Zaria: Ahmadu Bello University Press.

Chung, Rita Chi-ying, and Marjorie Kagawa-Singer. 1993. Predictors of Psychological Distress among Southeast Asian Refugees. *Social Science and Medicine* 36:631–39.

Churchill, Larry R. 1990. Hermeneutics in Science and Medicine: A Thesis Understated. *Theoretical Medicine* 11(2):141–44.

Clancy, Patricia. 1986. The Acquisition of Communicative Style in Japanese. In *Language Socialization across Cultures*, ed. E. Ochs and B. Schieffelin. Cambridge: Cambridge University Press.

Clark, A. L., ed. 1978. *Culture, Child-bearing, Health Professionals*. Philadelphia: Davis.

Clark, Margaret. 1992. Medical Anthropology and the Redefining of Human Nature. Paper presented to the Society for Applied Anthropology, Memphis, Tennessee.

Clark, M. Margaret, ed. 1983. Cross-Cultural Medicine. Special issue of *Western Journal of Medicine* 139:805–938.

Clark, Margaret, and Barbara G. Anderson. 1967. *Culture and Aging*. Springfield, Ill.: Charles Thomas.

Clark, Edith. 1957. *My Mother Who Fathered Me*. London: George Allen and Unwin.

Clark, M. 1978. Getting Through the Work. In *Readings in the Sociology of Nursing*, ed. R. Dingwall and J. McIntosh. London: Churchill Livingstone, 67–86.

Classen, Constance. 1993. *Worlds of Sense: Exploring the Senses in History and across Cultures*. London and New York: Routledge.

Claude, Richard, Eric Stover, and June Lopez. 1987. *Health Professionals and Human Rights in the Philippines*. Washington, D.C.: American Association for the Advancement of Science.

Clawson, Patrick. 1978. Egypt's Industrialization: A Critique of Dependency Theory. *MERIP Reports* 72:17–23.

Clements, Forrest E. 1932. Primitive Concepts of Disease. *University of California Publications in American Archaeology and Ethnology* 32(2):185–252.

Cleveland, David. 1986. The Political Economy of Fertility Regulation: The Kusasi of Savanna West Africa (Ghana). In *Culture and Reproduction*, ed. W. Penn Handwerker. Boulder, Colo.: Westview, 263–93.

Clifford, James, and George E. Marcus, eds. 1986. *Writing Culture: The Poetics and Politics of Ethnography.* Berkeley: University of California Press.

Clouser, Danner, and Bernard Gert. 1990. A Critique of Principlism. *Journal of Medicine and Philosophy* 15:219–236.

Coale, Ansley J. 1969. The Decline of Fertility in Europe from the French Revolution to World War II. In *Fertility and Family Planning,* ed. S. J. Behrman, Leslie Corsa, and Ronald Fredman. Ann Arbor, Mich.: University of Michigan Press.

———. 1974. The History of the Human Population. *Scientific American* 231:41–51.

Coale, Ansley J., and Paul Demeny. 1983. *Regional Model Life Tables and Stable Populations.* 2d ed. New York: Academic Press.

Coale, Ansley J., and T. James Trussel. 1974. Model Fertility Schedules. *Population Index* 40:185–258.

———. 1975. Erratum. *Population Index* 41:572–73.

Cobb, Sidney. 1976. Social Support as a Moderator of Life Stress. *Psychosomatic Medicine* 38:300–14.

Cochrane, S. H., D. J. O'Hara, and J. Leslie. 1980. *The Effects of Education on Health.* World Bank Staff Working Paper 405. Washington, D.C.: World Bank.

Cocks, G., and K. Jarausch, eds. 1990. *German Professions 1800–1950.* New York: Oxford University Press.

Cohen, Alex. 1992. Prognosis for Schizophrenia in the Third World: A Re-evaluation of Cross-Cultural Research. *Culture, Medicine and Psychiatry* 16(1):53–75.

Cohen, David. 1988. *Forgotten Millions.* London: Paladin Grafton Books.

Cohen, Mark N. 1989. *Health and the Rise of Civilization.* New Haven: Yale University Press.

Cohen, M. N., and G. J. Armelagos, eds. 1984. *Paleopathology at the Origins of Agriculture.* New York: Academic Press.

Cohen, M. Z., T. Tripp-Reimer, C. Smith, B. Sorofman, and S. Lively. 1994. Explanatory Models of Diabetes: Patient, Practitioner Variation. *Social Science and Medicine* 38(1):59–66.

Cohen, Sheldon, and S. Leonard Syme, eds. 1985. *Social Support and Health.* Orlando, Fla., Academic Press.

Cohen, Sheldon, and Thomas Ashby Wills. 1985. Stress, Social Support, and the Buffering Hypothesis. *Psychological Bulletin* 98:310–57.

Colby, Benjamin N. 1987. Well-being: A Theoretical Program. *American Anthropologist* 89:879–95.

Colby, Benjamin N., et al. 1985. Adaptive Potential, Stress, and Illness in the Elderly. *Medical Anthropology* 9:283–95.

Coleman, Samuel. 1983. *Family Planning in Japanese Society: Traditional Birth Control in a Modern Urban Culture.* Princeton, N.J.: Princeton University Press.

Collier, Jane F., and Michelle Z. Rosaldo. 1981. Politics and Gender in Simple Societies. In *Sexual Meanings. The Cultural Construction of Gender and Sexuality,* ed. Sherry B. Ortner and Harriet Whitehead. Cambridge: Cambridge University Press, 275–329.

Collier, Jane Fishburne, and Sylvia Junko Yanagisako, eds. 1987. *Gender and Kinship. Essays toward a Unified Analysis.* Stanford: Stanford University Press.

Collins, C. 1992. Women as Hidden Casualties of the Cold War. *MS* 3(November–December):14–15.

Colson, Audrey B., and Cesario de Armellado. 1983. An American Derivation for Latin American Creole Illnesses and Their Treatment. *Social Science and Medicine* 17:1229–48.

Comaroff, Jean. 1982. Medicine: Symbol and Ideology. In *The Problem of Medical Knowledge: Examining the Social Construction of Medicine,* ed. Peter Wright and Andrew Treacher. Edinburgh: Edinburgh University Press, 49–68.

———. 1985. *Body of Power, Spirit of Resistance: The Culture and History of a South African People.* Chicago: University of Chicago Press.

———. 1988. The Diseased Heart of Africa: Medicine, Colonialism and the Black Body. In *Analysis in Medical Anthropology,* ed. S. Lindenbaum and M. Lock. Dordrecht: Kluwer Academic Publishers.

Comaroff, Jean, and Peter Maguire. 1981. Ambiguity and the Search for Meaning: Childhood Leukaemia in the Modern Clinical Context. *Social Science and Medicine* 15B:115–23.

Comaroff, John, and Jean Comaroff. 1992. *Ethnography and the Historical Imagination.* Boulder, Colo.: Westview Press.

Conly, S. R., J. Speidel, and S. Camp. 1991. *U.S. Population Assistance: Issues for the 1990s.* Washington, D.C.: Population Crisis Committee.

Connor, S., and S. Kingman. 1973. *Medical Malpractice: Secretary's Commission on Medical Malpractice.* Washington, D.C.: Department of Health, Education and Welfare.

———. 1988. *The Search for the Virus.* London: Penguin Group.

Conrad, Peter. 1994. How Ethnography Can Help Bioethics. *Bulletin of Medical Ethics* (May): 13–18.

Conway, M. E. 1983. Socialization and Roles in Nursing. In *Annual Review of Nursing Research,* ed. H. H. Werley and J. J. Fitzpatrick. New York: Springer, 1:183–208.

Cooper, John M. 1933. The Cree Witiko Psychosis. *Primitive Man* 6:20–24.

———. 1934. Mental Disease Situations in Certain Cultures: A New Field for Research. *Journal of Abnormal and Social Psychology* 29:10–17.

Cooper, M. Wayne. 1994. Is Medicine Hermeneutics All the Way Down? *Theoretical Medicine* 15(2):149–80.

Corbett, Kitty King. 1986. Adding Insult to Injury: Cultural Dimensions of Frustration in the Management of Chronic Back Pain. Ph.D. dissertation, University of California.

Corea, Gina, Renate Duelli Klein, Jalna Hanmer, Helen B. Holmes, Betty Hoskins, Madhu Kishwar, Janice Raymond, Robyn Rowland, and Roberta Steinbacher. 1987. *Man-Made Women: How Reproductive Technologies Affect Women.* Bloomington: Indiana University Press.

Coreil, J., and E. Genece. 1988. Adoption of Oral Rehydration Therapy among Haitian Mothers. Special issue of *Social Science and Medicine,* 27(1):87–96.

Coreil, J., and J. D. Mull, eds. 1988. Anthropological Studies of Diarrheal Illness. Special issue of *Social Science and Medicine* 27(1):87–96.

Coreil, Jeannine, et al. 1994. *Perceptions of HIV Vaccine Trials in Cite Soleil, Haiti.* Report submitted to Johns Hopkins University, Department of International Health.

Corin, Ellen. 1990. Facts and Meaning in Psychiatry: An Anthropological Approach to the Lifeworld of Schizophrenics. *Culture, Medicine, and Psychiatry* 14:153–88.

Cornfield, J. 1951. A Method of Estimating Comparative Rates from Clinical Data. Applications to Cancer of the Lung, Breast, and Cervix. *Journal of the National Cancer Institute* 11:1269–75.

Cornoni-Huntley, Joan C., Tamara B. Harris, Donald F. Everett. Demetrius Albanes, Marc S. Micozzi, Toni P. Miles, and Jacob J. Feldman. 1991. An Overview of Body Weight of Older Persons Including the Impact of Mortality. *Journal of Clinical Epidemiology* 44:743–53.

Cortese, Anthony. 1990. *Ethnic Ethics: The Restructuring of Moral Theory.* Albany, N.Y.: State University of New York Press.

Coser, R. 1962. *Life in the Ward.* East Lansing: Michigan State University Press.

Cosminsky, Sheila. 1976. Cross-Cultural Perspectives on Midwifery. In *Medical Anthropology,* ed. F. X. Grollig and Harold Haley. The Hague: Mouton Publishers, 229–49.

———. 1977. Childbirth and Midwifery on a Guatemalan Finca. *Medical Anthropology* 1(3):69–104.

Crabtree, Benjamin F., and P. J. Pelto. 1988. Anthropologists Learn Systat Computer Program for Applied and Research Purposes. *Practicing Anthropology* 18–21.

Crandon, Libbet. 1983. Grass Roots, Herbs, Promoters and Preventions: A Re-evaluation of Contemporary International Health Care Planning: The Bolivian Case. *Social Science and Medicine* 17:1281–89.

Crandon-Malamud, Libbet. 1991. *From the Fat of Our Souls: Social Change, Political Process, and Medical Pluralism in Boliva.* Berkeley: University of California Press.

Crapanzano, Victor. 1973. *The Hamadsha: A Study in Moroccan Ethnopsychiatry.* Berkeley: University of California Press.

Crapanzano, Vincent, and Vivian Garrison, eds. 1977. *Case Studies in Spirit Possession.* New York: John Wiley and Sons.

Crawford, Robert. 1980. Healthism and the Medicalization of Everyday Life. *International Journal of Health Services* 10:365–88.

———. 1984. A Cultural Account of Health: Self Control, Release and the Social Body. In *Issues in the Political Economy of Health Care,* ed. J. McKinlay. London: Tavistock.

Crick, Malcolm R. 1982. Anthropology of Knowledge. *Annual Review of Anthropology* 11:287–313.

Crigger, Bette. 1995. Negotiating the Moral Orders: Paradoxes of Ethics Consultation. *Kennedy Institute of Ethics Journal* 5(2):89–112.

Crosbie, Paul V. 1986. Rationality and Models of Reproductive Decision-Making. In *Culture and Reproduction,* ed. W. Penn Handwerker. Boulder, Colo.: Westview, 30–58.

Crosby, W. H. 1971. Food Pica and Iron Deficiency. *Archives of Internal Medicine* 127:960–61.

Cross, Alan W., and Larry R. Churchill. 1982. Ethical and Cultural Dimensions of Informed Consent: A Case Study and Analysis. *Annals of Internal Medicine* 96:110–13.

Csordas, Thomas J. 1983. The Rhetoric of Transformation in Ritual Healing. *Culture, Medicine, and Psychiatry* 7:333–75.

———. 1987. Health and the Holy in African and Afro-American Spirit Possession. *Social Science and Medicine* 24(1):1–11.

———. 1988a. Elements of Charismatic Persuasion and Healing. *Medical Anthropology Quarterly* 2:445–69.

———. 1988b. The Conceptual Status of Hegemony and Critique in Medical Anthropology. *Medical Anthropology* Quarterly 2:416–21.

———. 1990a. The 1988 Stirling Award Essay: Embodiment as a Paradigm for Anthropology. *Ethos* 18:5–47.

———. 1990b. Embodiment as a Paradigm for Anthropology. 1988 Stirling Award Essay. *Ethos* 18:5–47.

———. 1993a. *The Sacred Self: Cultural Phenomenology of a Charismatic World.* Berkeley: University of California Press.

———. 1993b. Somatic Modes of Attention. *Cultural Anthropology* 8:135–56.

———. 1994a. *The Sacred Self: A Cultural Phenomenology of Charismatic Healing.* Berkeley: University of California Press.

———. n.d. Talk to Them So They Understand: The Criterion of Success in Navajo Healing. Unpublished manuscript.

Csordas, Thomas J., ed. 1994. *Embodiment and Experience: The Existential Ground of Culture and Self.* Cambridge: Cambridge University Press.

Cunningham, Clark. 1973. Order in the Atoni House. In *Right and Left: On Dual Symbolic Classification,* ed. Rodney Needham. Chicago: University of Chicago Press, 204–38.

Currier, Richard. 1969. The Hot-Cold Syndrome and Symbolic Balance in Mexican and Spanish-American Folk Medicine. In *The Cross-Cultural Approach to Health Behavior,* ed. L. R. Lynch. Madison, N.J.: Fairleigh Dickinson University Press, 255–73.

Cuttmacher, S., and L. Garcia. 1975. Social Science and Health in Cuba: Ideology, Planning, and Health. In *Topias and Utopias in Health,* ed. S. Ingman and A. Thomas. The Hague: Mouton.

Dafni, A., and Z. Yaniv. 1994. Solanaceae as Medicinal Plants in Israel. *Journal of Ethnopharmacology* 44:11–18.

Danaher, Kevin, ed. 1994. *50 Years Is Enough.* Boston: South End Press.

D'Andrade, Roy G. 1976. A Propositional Analysis of U.S. American Beliefs about Illness. In *Meaning in Anthropology,* ed. K. H. Basso, and H. A. Selby. Albuquerque: University of New Mexico Press, 155–80.

———. 1984. Cultural Meaning Systems. In *Culture Theory: Essays on Mind, Emotion and Self,* ed. Richard A. Shweder and Robert Levine. Cambridge: Cambridge University Press, 88–119.

———. 1987. A Folk Model of the Mind. In *Cultural Models in Language and Thought,* ed. Dorothy Holland and Naomi Quinn. Cambridge: Cambridge University Press.

————. 1995. Moral Models in Anthropology. *Current Anthropology* 36(3):399–408.

D'Andrade, Roy G., Naomi R. Quinn, S. B. Nerlove, and A. K. Romney. 1972. Categories of Disease in American-English and Mexican-Spanish. In *Multidimensional Scaling: Theory and Applications in the Behavioral Sciences,* ed. A. K. Romney, R. N. Shephard, and S. B. Nerlove. New York: Seminar Press, 9–54.

Daniels, Norman. 1985. *Just Health Care.* New York: Cambridge University Press.

Dalton, P. R., and D. Pole. 1978. Water-Contact Patterns in Relation to Schistosoma Haematobium Infection. *Bulletin of the World Health Organization* 56:417–26.

Daly, Mary. 1978. Gyn/Ecology. Boston: Beacon Press.

Danzinger, R. 1994. The Social Impact of HIV/AIDS in Developing Countries. *Social Science and Medicine* 39(7):905–17.

Darity, W. A. 1965. Some Sociocultural Factors in the Administration of Technical Assistance and Training in Health. *Human Organization* 24(1):78–82.

Darnell, Regina. 1990. *Edward Sapir: Linguist, Anthropologist, Humanist.* Berkeley: University of California Press.

Davidson, William D. 1986. Psychiatry and Foreign Affairs: A Vision and a Commitment. *Psychoanalytic Inquiry* 6(2):223–42.

Davis, E. W., and J. A. Yost. 1983. The Ethnomedicine of the Waorani of Amazonian Ecuador. *Journal of Ethnopharmacology* 9:273–97.

Davis, Kingsley. 1959. The Myth of Functional Analysis as a Special Method in Sociology and Anthropology. *American Sociological Review* 24:752–71.

Davis, Kingsley, Mikhail S. Bernstam, and Rita Ricardo-Campbell, eds. 1986. Below-Replacement Fertility in Industrial Societies. *Population and Development Review* 12 (Suppl.).

Davis, Kingsley, and Judith Blake. 1956. Social Structure and Fertility. *Economic Development and Cultural Change* 4:211–35.

Davis, Shelton H. 1988. Introduction: Sowing the Seeds of Violence. In *Harvest of Violence: The Maya Indians and the Guatemalan Crisis,* ed. Robert Carmack. Norman: University of Oklahoma Press, 3–36.

Davis-Floyd, Robbie. 1992. *Birth as an American Rite of Passage.* Berkeley: University of California Press.

Davis-Floyd, Robbie, and Carolyn Sargent, eds. 1996. *Childbirth and Authoritative Knowledge: Cross-Cultural Perspectives.* Berkeley: University of California Press.

Davitz L. J., and J. R. Davitz. 1978. Black and White Nurses' Inferences of Suffering. *Nursing Times* 74:708–10.

Davitz, L. J., J. R. Davitz, and Y. Higuchi. 1977. Cross-cultural Inferences of Physical Pain and Psychological Distress—2. *Nursing Times* 73:536–58.

Davitz, L. J., Y. Sameshima, and J. R. Davitz. 1976. Suffering as Viewed in Six Different Cultures. *American Journal of Nursing* 76:1296–97.

Day, R., et al. 1987. Stressful Life Events Preceding the Acute Onset of Schizophrenia: A Cross-Cultural Study from the World Health Organization. *Culture, Medicine, and Psychiatry* 11: 123–205.

Day, S. 1988. Prostitute Women and AIDS: Anthropology. *AIDS* 2(6):421–28.

De Garine, Igor, and Sjors Koppert. 1990. Social Adaptation to Season and Uncertainty in Food Supply. In *Diet and Disease in Traditional and Developing Societies,* ed. G. A. Harrison and J. C. Waterlow. Cambridge: Cambridge University Press.

De Grazia, David. 1994. Autonomous Action and Autonomy-Subverting Psychiatric Conditions. *Journal of Medicine and Philosophy* 19(3):279–98.

Delaney, William, and Genevieve Ames. 1993. Intergration and Exchange in Multidisciplinary Alcohol Research. *Social Science and Medicine* 37(1):5–13.

Delaveau, P. 1981. Evaluation of Traditional Pharmacopoeias. In *Natural Products as Medicinal Agents,* ed. J. L. Beal and E. Reinhard. Stuttgart: Hippokrates Verlag, 395–404.

deMause, Lloyd. 1974. *The History of Childhood.* New York: Psychohistory Press.

———. 1977. Jimmy Carter and American Fantasy. In *Jimmy Carter and American Fantasy: Psychohistorical Explorations,* ed. Lloyd deMause and Henry Ebel. New York: Two Continents/ Psychohistory Press, 9–31.

———. 1982. *Foundations of Psychohistory.* New York: Creative Books.

———. 1984. *Reagan's America.* New York: Creative Books.

———. 1987. Schreber and the History of Childhood. *Journal of Psychohistory* 15(1):423–30.

———. 1988. What Incest Barrier? *Journal of Psychohistory* 15(3):273–77.

De Rosny, Eric. 1991. *L'Afrique des guerisons.* Paris: Karthala.

Dennis, Philip A. 1981. Grisi Siknis among the Miskito. *Medical Anthropology* 5:445–504.

Dentan, Robert Knox. 1988. Reply to Paul. *American Anthropologist* 90(2):420–21.

Department of Health, Education and Welfare. 1973. *Medical Malpractice: Secretary's Commission on Medical Malpractice.* Washington, D.C.: Department of Health, Education and Welfare.

De Rios, Marlene Dobkin. 1989. A Modern-Day Shamanistic Healer in the Peruvian Amazon: Pharmacopoeia and Trance. *Journal of Psychoactive Drugs* 21(1):91–99.

Dervin, Daniel. 1987. Abandonment: A Dominant Pattern in the Development of Creative Writers, Philosophers and Scientists since the Seventeenth Century. *Journal of Psychohistory* 15(2): 153–87.

———. 1988. Freud's Baby and Ours: Notes toward a Psychohistory of Psychoanalysis. *Journal of Psychohistory* 16(1):79–87.

Desjarlais, R. 1992. *Body and Emotion.* Philadelphia: University of Pennsylvania Press.

de Smet, Peter A. G. M. 1991. Is There Any Danger in Using Traditional Remedies? *Journal of Ethnopharmacology* 32:43–50.

Desowitz, R. S. 1981. *New Guinea Tapeworms and Jewish Grandmothers: Tales of Parasites and People.* New York: W. W. Norton.

Dettwyler, Katherine. 1994. *Dancing Skeletons: Life and Death in West Africa.* Prospect Heights, Ill.: Waveland Press.

Devereux, George. 1955. Charismatic Leadership and Crisis. *Psychoanalysis and the Social Sciences* 4:145–57.

———. 1956. Normal and Abnormal: The Key Problem of Psychiatric Anthropology. In *Some Uses of Anthropology: Theoretical and Applied,* ed. J. B. Casagrande, and T. Gladwin. Washington, D.C.: Anthropological Society of Washington, 3–48.

———. 1967. *From Anxiety to Method in the Behavioral Sciences.* The Hague: Mouton.

———. 1969. *Mohave Ethnopsychiatry.* Washington, D.C.: Smithsonian Institution Press.

———. 1976. *A Study of Abortion in Primitive Societies.* New York: International Universities Press.

———. 1978. *Ethnopsychoanalysis: Psychoanalysis and Anthropology as Complementary Frames of Reference.* Berkeley and Los Angeles: University of California Press.

———. 1980a. *Basic Problems of Ethno-Psychiatry,* trans. B. M. Gulati and G. Devereux. Chicago: University of Chicago Press.

———. 1980b. Female Juvenile Sex Delinquency in a Puritanical Society. In *Basic Problems of Ethnopsychiatry,* trans. B. M. Gulati and G. Devereux. Chicago: University of Chicago Press, 155–84.

———. 1980c. Normal and Abnormal. In *Basic Problems of Ethnopsychiatry,* trans. B. M. Gulati and G. Devereux. Chicago: University of Chicago Press, 3–71 (orig. 1962), 3–71.

———. 1980d. A Sociological Theory of Schizophrenia. In *Basic Problems of Ethno-Psychiatry,* trans. B. M. Gulati and G. Devereux. Chicago: University of Chicago Press, 185–213 (orig. 1939).

Devich, Renatt. 1985. Symbol and Psychosomatic Symptom in Bodily Space-Time: The Case of the Yaka of Zaire. *International Journal of Psychology* 20:589–616.

Devisch, René. 1993. *Weaving the Thread of Life: The Khita Gyn-Eco-Logical Healing Cult among the Yaka.* Chicago: University of Chicago Press.

De Vos, George A. 1973. *Socialization for Achievement.* Berkeley: University of California Press.

De Vos, George, and L. Bryce Boyer. 1988. *Symbolic Analysis Crossculturally: The Rorschach Test.* Berkeley and Los Angeles: University of California Press.

DeVos, George, Anthony Marsella, and Francis Hsu. 1985. Approaches to Culture and the Self. In *Culture and Self,* ed. Anthony Marsella, George DeVos, and Francis Hsu. London: Tavistock.

deVries, Martin. 1970. Heredity. *Encyclopedia Britannica* 11:419–27.

deVries, Martin, R. L. Berg, and M. Lipkin, eds. 1982. *The Use and Abuse of Medicine.* New York: Praeger.

Dewalt, Billie R., and Pertti J. Pelto, eds. 1985. *Micro and Macro Levels of Analysis in Anthropology.* Colorado: Westview Press.

DeWalt, Kathleen. 1981. Diet as Adaptation: The Search for Nutritional Strategies. *Federation Proceedings* 40:2606–10.

———. 1983. *Nutritional Strategies and Agricultural Change in a Mexican Community.* Ann Arbor: UMI Research Press.

DeWalt, Kathleen, and John Van Willigen. 1984. Research Priorities for Medical Anthropologists in the 1980's. *Social Science and Medicine* 18(10):845–46.

Dewey, Kathryn. 1989. Nutrition and the Commoditization of Food Systems in Latin America and the Caribbean. *Social Science and Medicine* 28(5):415–24.

de Zalduondo, B. 1991. Prostitution Viewed Cross-Culturally: Toward Recontextualizing Sex Work in AIDS Intervention Research. Special issue of *Journal of Sex Research* 28 (2)223–48.

Diener, P., K. Moore, and R. Mutaw. 1980. Meat Markets and Mechanical Materialism: The Great Protein Fiasco in Anthropology. *Dialectical Anthropology* 5:171–92.

Dillon-Malone, Clive. 1988. Matumwa Nchimi Healers and Wizardry Beliefs in Zambia. *Social Science and Medicine* 26:1159–72.

Dingwall, R., and P. Lewis, eds. 1983. *The Sociology of the Professions.* London: Macmillan.

Dobkin de Rios, Marlene. 1975. Man, Culture, and Hallucinogens: An Overview. In *Cannabis and Culture,* ed. Vera Rubin. The Hague: Mouton.

———. 1977. Plant Hallucinogens, Out-of-Body Experiences and New World Monumental Earthworks. In *Drugs, Rituals, and Altered States of Consciousness,* ed. Brian M. du Toit. Rotterdam: A. A. Balkema.

———. 1984. *Hallucinogens: Cross-Cultural Perspectives.* Albuquerque: University of New Mexico Press.

Dobzhansky, Theodosius. 1970. Heredity. *Encyclopedia Britannica* 11:419–27.

Dodge, Cole P., and Siddiq Abdel Rahman Ibrahim. 1988. The Civilians Suffer Most. In *War Wounds: Sudanese People Report on Their War.* London: Panos Institute, 45–52.

Dohrenwend, Barbara S., and Bruce P. Dohrenwend, eds. 1974. *Stressful Life Events: Their Nature and Effects.* New York: Wiley

———. 1981. *Stressful Life Events and Their Contexts.* New York: Prodist.

Doll, R., and A. Bradford Hill. 1950. Smoking and Carcinoma of the Lung: Preliminary Report. In *The Challenge of Epidemiology: Issues and Selected Readings,* ed. Carol Buck, Alvaro Llopis, Enrique Najera, and Milton Terris. Scientific Publication 505. Pan American Health Organization, 475–91.

———. 1964. Mortality in Relation to Smoking: Ten Years' Observations of British Doctors. In *The Challenge of Epidemiology: Issues and Selected Readings,* ed. Carol Buck et al. Scientific Publication 505. Pan American Health Organization, 631–67.

Dominguez, Virginia. 1994. A Taste for ''the Other'': Intellectual Complicity in Racializing Practices. *Current Anthropology* 35(4):333–48.

Dominguez, Xorge, and Janis B. Alcorn. 1985. Screening of Medicinal Plants Used by Huastec Mayans of Northeastern Mexico. *Journal of Ethnopharmacology* 13(2):139–56.

Donahue, John M. 1983. The Politics of Health Care in Nicaragua before and after the Revolution of 1979. *Human Organization* 42(3):264–72.

———. 1984. Studying the Transition to Socialism in the Nicaraguan Health System. *Medical Anthropology Quarterly* 15(3):70–71.

———. 1986a. *The Nicaraguan Revolution in Health.* South Hadley, Mass.: Bergin and Garvey.

———. 1986b. Planning for Primary Health Care in Nicaragua: A Study in Revolutionary Process. *Social Science and Medicine* 23:149–57.

Donaldson, Peter J. 1976. Foreign Intervention in Medical Education: A Case Study of the Rockefeller Foundation's Involvement in a Thai Medical School. *International Journal of Health Services* 6:251–70.

Donaldson, Sue K., and Dorothy M. Crowley. 1978. The Discipline of Nursing. *Nursing Outlook* 26:113–20.

Dorjahn, Vernon R. 1975. Migration in Central Sierra Leone. *Africa* 45:29–49.

Dougherty, Molly C. 1982. Southern Mid-wifery and Organized Health Care. *Medical Anthropology* 6(2):113–26.

———. 1985. Anthropologists in Nursing-Education Programs. In *Training Manual in Medical Anthropology,* ed. C. E. Hill. Washington, D.C.: American Anthropological Association, 58–70.

Dougherty, Molly C., and Toni Tripp-Reimer. 1985. The Interface of Nursing and Anthropology. *Annual Review of Anthropology* 14:219–41.

Doughty, Paul L. 1971. The Social Use of Alcoholic Beverages in a Peruvian Community. *Human Organization* 30(2):187–97.

Douglas, Mary. 1966. *Purity and Danger: An Analysis of the Concepts of Pollution and Taboo.* New York: Praeger.

———. 1970. *Natural Symbols.* New York: Vintage.

———. 1972. Deciphering a Meal. *Daedalus* 101:61–82.

———. 1984. Standard Social Usages of Food. In *Food and the Social Order: Studies of Food and Festivities in Three American Communities,* ed., Mary Douglas. New York: Russell Sage Foundation, 1–39.

Douglas, Mary, ed. 1987. *Constructive Drinking: Perspectives on Drink from Anthropology.* Cambridge: Cambridge University Press.

Douglas, Mary, and Aaron Wildavsky. 1982. *Risk and Culture: An Essay on the Selection of Technological and Environmental Dangers.* Berkeley: University of California Press.

Douglas, William. 1969. *Death in Murelaga: Funerary Ritual in a Spanish Basque Village.* Seattle: University of Washington Press.

Dow, James. 1986. Universal Aspects of Symbolic Healing: A Theoretical Synthesis. *American Anthropologist* 88:56–69.

Doyal, Lesley, and Imogen Pennel. 1979. *The Political Economy of Health.* Boston: South End Press.

Drane, James. 1988. *Becoming a Good Doctor.* Kansas City: Sheed and Ward.

Dreher, Melanie C. 1983. Marihuana and Work: Cannabis Smoking on a Jamaican Sugar Estate. *Human Organization* 42(1):1–8.

———. 1984a. Marijuana Use among Women—an Anthropological View. *Advances in Alcohol and Substance Abuse* 3(3):51–64.

———. 1984b. Schoolchildren and Ganja: Youthful Marijuana Consumption in Rural Jamaica. *Anthropology and Education Quarterly* 15:131–50.

———. 1984c. Anthropology and Cannabis Research. *Newsletter of the Alcohol and Drug Study Group,* American Anthropological Association, no. 12.

———. 1987. The Evolution of a Roots Daughter. *Journal of Psychoactive Drugs* 19(2):165–70.

Dressler, William W. 1979. Disorganization, Adaptation, and Arterial Blood Pressure. *Medical Anthropology* 3:225–48.

———. 1980. Coping Dispositions, Social Supports, and Health Status. *Ethos* 8:146–71.

———. 1982. *Hypertension and Culture Change: Acculturation and Disease in the West Indies.* South Salem, N.Y.: Redgrave Publishing Company.

———. 1984a. Hypertension and Perceived Stress: A St. Lucian Example. *Ethos* 12:265–83.

———. 1984b. Social and Cultural Influences in Cardiovascular Disease: A Review. *Transcultural Psychiatric Research Review* 21:5–42.

———. 1985a. Extended Family Relationships, Social Support, and Mental Health in a Southern Black Community. *Journal of Health and Social Behavior* 26:39–48.

———. 1985b. The Social and Cultural Context of Coping. *Social Science and Medicine* 21:499–506.

———. 1985c. Psychosomatic Symptoms, Stress, and Modernization: A Model. *Culture, Medicine, and Psychiatry* 9:257–86.

———. 1986a. Unemployment and Depressive Symptoms in a Southern Black Community. *Journal of Nervous and Mental Diseases* 174:639–45.

———. 1986b. Blood Pressure, Sex Roles, and Social Support. Abstracts of the 85th Annual Meeting of the American Anthropological Association, Philadelphia, December 3–7.

———. 1987. Building Models and Testing Theories in Specific Contexts. Abstracts of the 86th Annual Meeting of the American Anthropological Association, Chicago, November 18–22.

———. 1988. Social Consistency and Psychological Distress *Journal of Health and Social Behavior* 29:79–91.

———. 1989a. Type A Behavior and the Social Production of Cardiovascular Disease. *Journal of Nervous and Mental Disease* 177:181–90.

———. 1989b. Lifestyle, Stress, and Blood Pressure in a Southern Black Community. Paper presented at the 46th Annual Meeting of the American Psychosomatic Society, San Francisco, March 9–11.

———. 1989c. Cross-cultural Differences and Social Influences in Social Support and Cardiovascular Disease. In *Social Support and Cardiovascular Disease*, ed. Sally A. Shumaker and Susan M. Czajkowski. New York: Plenum Publishing.

———. 1991. *Stress and Adaptation in the Context of Culture: Depression in a Southern Black Community.* Albany, N.Y.: State University of New York Press.

———. 1993a. Social and Cultural Dimensions of Hypertension in Blacks: Underlying Mechanisms. In *Pathophysiology of Hypertension in Blacks,* ed. Janice G. Douglas and John C. S. Fray. New York: Oxford University Press.

———. 1993b. Type A Behavior: Contextual Effects within a Southern Black Community. *Social Science and Medicine* 36:289–95.

———. 1994. Cross-Cultural Differences and Social Influences in Social Support and Cardiovascular Disease. In *Social Support and Cardiovascular Disease*, ed. Sally A. Shumaker and Susan M. Czajkowski. New York: Plenum Publishing.

Dressler, William W., and Henrietta Bernal. 1982. Acculturation and Stress in a Low-Income Puerto Rican Community. *Journal of Human Stress* 8:32–38.

Dressler, William W., José Ernesto Dos Santos, Philip N. Gallagher, Jr., and Fernando Viteri. 1987. Arterial Blood Pressure and Modernization in Brazil. *American Anthropologist* 89:389–409.

Dressler, William W., Philip Evans, and Denis J. Pereira Gray. 1992. Status Incongruence and Serum Cholesterol in an English General Practice. *Social Science and Medicine* 34:757–62.

Dressler, William W., Gerald A. C. Grell, Philip N. Gallagher, Jr., and Fernando E. Viteri. 1988. Blood Pressure and Social Class in a Jamaican Community. *American Journal of Public Health* 78:714–16.

Dressler, William W., Alfonso Mata, Adolfo Chavez, and Fernando E. Viteri. 1987. Arterial Blood Pressure and Individual Modernization in a Mexican Community. *Social Science and Medicine* 24:679–87.

Dressler, William W., Alfonso Mata, Adolfo Chavez, Fernando E. Viteri, and Philip N. Gallagher. 1986. Social Support and Arterial Blood Pressure in a Central Mexican Community. *Psychosomatic Medicine* 48:338–50.

Dressler, William W., J. E. D. Santos, and Fernando E. Viteri. 1993. Social and Cultural Influences in the Risk of Cardiovascular Disease. In *Urban Health and Ecology in the Third World,* ed. Lawerence M. Schell, Malcolm T. Smith, and Alan Bilsborough. Cambridge: Cambridge University Press.

Dreyfus, H. F., and Dreyfus, S. E. 1992. What Is Moral Maturity? Towards a Phenomenology of Ethical Expertise. In *Revisioning Philosophy*. Albany, N.Y.: State University of New York Press, 111–31.

DuBois, Cora. 1944. *The People of Alor.* Minneapolis: University of Minnesota Press.

Dubos, Reñe. 1959. *Mirage of Health.* New York: Harper & Row.

———. 1965. *Man Adapting.* New Haven: Yale University Press.

DuBose, Edwin R., Ron Hamel, and Laurence J. O'Connell. 1994. *A Matter of Principles: Ferment in U.S. Bioethics.* Park Ridge, Ill.: Park Ridge Center for the Study of Health, Faith and Ethics.

Dufour, Darna L. 1987. Insects as Food: A Case Study from the Northwest Amazon. *American Anthropologist* 89(2):383–97.

Duku, Oliver M. 1988. Cut Off from Health Care. In *War Wounds: Sudanese People Report on Their War.* London: Panos Institute, 35–44.

Dula, Annette. 1991. Toward an African-American Perspective on Bioethics. *Journal of Health Care for the Poor and Underserved* 2(2):259.

———. 1994. African American Suspicion of the Health Care System Is Justified: What Do We Do about It? *Cambridge Quarterly of Healthcare Ethics* 3(3):347–58.

Dula, Annette, and Sara Goering. 1994. *"It Just Ain't Fair": The Ethics of Health Care for African Americans.* Westport, Conn.: Praeger.

Dundes, Alan. 1984. *Life Is Like a Chicken Coop Ladder: A Portrait of German Culture through Folklore.* New York: Columbia University Press.

———. 1985. The American Game of "Smear the Queer" and the Homosexual Component of Male Competitive Sport and Warfare. *Journal of Psychoanalytic Anthropology* 8(3):115–29.

Dunn, Fred L. 1968. Epidemiological Factors: Health and Disease in Hunter Gatherers. In *Man the Hunter,* ed. R. B. Lee and I. DeVore. Chicago: Aldine, 221–28.

———. 1976. Traditional Asian Medicine and Cosmopolitan Medicine as Adaptive Systems. In *Asian Medical Systems: A Comparative Study,* ed. C. Leslie. Berkeley and Los Angeles: University of California Press, 133–59.

———. 1979. Behavioural Aspects of the Control of Parasitic Diseases. *Bulletin of the World Health Organization* 57:499–512.

Dunn, F. L., and C. R. Janes. 1986. Introduction: Medical Anthropology and Epidemiology. In *Anthropology and Epidemiology,* ed. Craig Janes et al. Dordrecht: Reidel Publishing Co., 3–34.

Dunn, Richard S. 1972. *Sugar and Slaves.* Chapel Hill: University of North Carolina Press.

Durham, W. H. 1976. The Adaptive Significance of Cultural Behavior. *Human Ecology* 4:89–121.

———. 1982. Interactions of Genetic and Cultural Evolution: Models and Examples. *Human Ecology* 10:289–323.

———. 1983. Testing the Malaria Hypothesis in West Africa. In *Distribution and Evolution of Hemoglobin and Globin Loci,* ed. S. J. Bowman. Dordrecht: Elsevier Science, 45–72.

———. 1991. *Coevolution: Genes, Minds, and Human Diversity.* Palo Alto, Calif.: Stanford University Press.

Durkheim, E. 1951. *Suicide,* trans. J. Spaulding and G. Simpson. New York: Free Press (orig. 1897).

———. 1961. *The Elementary Forms of the Religious Life,* trans. Joseph Ward Swain. New York: Collier (orig. 1915).

Durkin-Longley, Maureen. 1984. Multiple Therapeutic Use in Urban Nepal. *Social Science and Medicine* 19:867–72.

Early, Evelyn A. 1982. The Logic of Well Being: Therapeutic Narratives in Cairo, Egypt. *Social Science and Medicine* 16:1491–97.

Eastwell, H. D. 1982. Voodoo Death and the Mechanism for Dispatch of the Dying in East Arnhem, Australia. *American Anthropologist* 84:5–18.

Eaton, Joseph, and Robert Weil. 1955. *Culture and Mental Disorders.* Glencoe, Ill.: Free Press.

Eaton, J. W., J. R. Eckman, E. Berger, and H. S. Jacob. 1976. Suppression of Malaria Infection by Oxidant Sensitive Erythrocytes. *Nature* 264:758–60.

Eaton, William W. 1978. Life Events, Social Supports, and Psychiatric Symptoms: A Reanalysis of the New Haven Data. *Journal of Health and Social Behavior* 19:230–34.

Eberstadt, Nicholas. 1994. Health and Mortality in Central and Eastern Europe: Retrospect and Prospect. In *The Social Legacy of Communism,* ed. J. R. Millar and S. Wochik. Cambridge: Cambridge University Press with the Woodrow Wilson Center Press, 196–225.

Ebin, V. 1982. Interpretations of Infertility: The Aowin People of Southwest Ghana. In *Ethnography of Fertility and Birth,* ed. Carol P. MacCormack, 2nd ed. New York: Academic Press, 131–49.

Edel, Mary, and Abraham Edel. 1968. *Anthropology and Ethics: The Guess for Moral Understanding.* Cleveland: Case Western Reserve University Press.

Edelmann, Robert J., and Kevin J. Connolly. 1986. Psychological Aspects of Infertility. *British Journal of Medical Psychology* 59(3):209–19.

Edgerton, Robert B. 1965. Cultural vs. Ecological Factors in the Expression of Values, Attitudes and Personality Factors. *American Anthropology* 67:442–47.

———. 1966. Conceptions of Psychosis in Four East African Societies. *American Anthropologist* 68:408–25.

———. 1967. *The Cloak of Competence.* Berkeley: University of California Press.

———. 1969. On the "Recognition" of Mental Illness. In *Changing Perspectives in Mental Illness,* ed. S. Plog and R. B. Edgerton. New York: Holt, Rinehart, and Winston.

———. 1971a. *The Individual in Cultural Adaptation.* Los Angeles: University of California Press.

———. 1971b. A Traditional African Psychiatrist. *Southwestern Journal of Anthropology* 27:259–78.

Edgerton, Robert. 1980. Traditional Treatment for Mental Illness in Africa: A Review. *Culture, Medicine and Psychiatry* 4:167–89.

———. 1985. *Rules, Exceptions, and Social Order.* Berkeley: University of California Press.

———. 1992. *Sick Societies: Challenging the Myth of Primitive Harmony.* New York: Free Press.

Edgerton, Robert B., and Alex Cohen. 1994. Culture and Schizophrenia: The DOSMD Challenge. *British Journal of Psychiatry* 164:222–31.

Edholm, Felicity, Olivia Harris, and Kate Young. 1977. Conceptualizing Women. *Critique of Anthropology* 3:101–30.

Edungbola, L. D. 1980. Water Utilization and Its Health Implications in Ilorin, Kwara State, Nigeria. *Acta Tropica* 37:73–81.

Edungbola, L. D., and S. J. Watts. 1985. Epidemiological Assessment of the Distribution and Endemicity of Guinea Worm Infection in Asa, Kwara State, Nigeria. *Tropical and Geographical Medicine* 37:22–28.

Edwards, S. E., R. W. S. Cheetham, E. Majozi, and A. J. Lasich. 1986. Zulu Culture-bound Psychiatric Syndromes. *South African Journal of Hospital Medicine* (April), 82–86.

Ehlers, Tracy B. 1987. A Guatemalan Town 10 Years Later. *Cultural Survival Quarterly* 11(3):25–29.

Ehrenreich, Barbara, and Dierdre English. 1978. *For Her Own Good: 150 Years of the Experts' Advice to Women.* New York: Anchor.

Ehrlich, P. R., A. H. Ehrlich, and J. P. Holdren. 1973. *Human Ecology.* San Francisco: W. H. Freeman.

Eisenberg, Leon. 1977. Disease and Illness: Distinctions between Professional and Popular Ideas of Sickness. *Culture, Medicine and Psychiatry* 1:9–23.

———. 1988. Science in Medicine: Too Much or Too Little and Too Limited in Scope? *American Journal of Medicine* 84:483–91.

Ekunwe, Ebun O., and Ross Kessell. 1984. Informed Consent in the Developing World. *Hastings Center Report* 145(3):22–24.

El-Bayoumi, Jehan A., and Soheir A. Morsy. 1993. HIV/AIDS: The Interfacing of Biomedicine and Anthropology. *Transforming Anthropology* 4(1 and 2): 1–8.

El-Mehairy, Theresa. 1984. *Medical Doctors: A Study of Role Concept and Job Satisfaction, the Egyptian Case.* Leiden: E. J. Brill.

El-Mofty, M. M. n.d. Review of Research Protocol. "Placebo-Controlled Double-Blind Study to

Determine the Efficacy of Topical Niclosamide 1% Lotion in the Prevention of Naturally Occurring *Schistosoma haematobium* Infection in Egyptian Farmers Engaged in Irrigation. Unpublished report.

El-Rafie, Muhammad, W. A. Hassouna, N. Loza Hirshorn, A. S. Nagaty, S. Nasser, and S. Riyad. 1990. Effect of Diarrheal Disease Control on Infant and Child Mortality in Egypt. *Lancet* 335(8586):334–38.

El-Sayed, Mustafa Kamel. 1986. Reflections on Dependency. Its Status and Theories. *Kadaya Fikriya* 2:18–29.

Elder, M. G. 1883. *Labor among Primitive Peoples*. St. Louis: J. H. Chambers and Co.

Elder, M. G. 1981. and Charles H. Hendrix, eds. *Preterm Labor. Obstetrics and Gynecology*. Vol. 1. London: Butterworth International Medical Reviews.

Elgood, C. 1962. Tibb-ul-Nabi. Medicine of the Prophet. *Osiris* 14:33–192.

Eliot, Charles W. 1914. *Some Roads toward Peace: A Report to the Trustees of the Endowment on Observations Made in China and Japan in 1912*. Washington, D.C.: Carnegie Endowment for International Peace.

Elkamel, Farag. 1991. Personal communication.

Ellen, R. 1982. *Environment, Subsistence and System*. Cambridge: Cambridge University Press.

Elling, Ray H. 1981. The Capitalist World-System and International Health. *International Journal of Health Services* 11:21–51.

Ellison, Peter T., Nadine R. Peacock, and Catherine Lager. 1986. Salivary Progesterone and Luteal Function in Two Low-Fertility Populations of Northeast Zaire. *Human Biology* 58:473–83.

Emanuel, Linda, Marion Danis, Robert Pearlman, and Peter Singer. 1995. Advance Care Planning as a Process: Structuring the Discussions in Practice. *Journal of the American Geriatrics Society* 43:440–46.

Endleman, Robert. 1981. *Psyche and Society: Explorations in Psychoanalytic Sociology*. New York: Columbia University Press.

Eng, Robert Y., and Thomas C. Smith. 1976. Peasant Families and Population Control in 18th Century Japan. *Journal of Interdisciplinary History* 11:417–45.

Engel, George L. 1977. The Need for a New Medical Model: A Challenge for Biomedicine. *Science* 196:129–36.

Englehardt, H. Tristram, Jr. 1975. The Concepts of Health and Disease. In *Evaluation and Explanation in the Biomedical Sciences*, ed. H. Tristram Engelhardt, Jr., and Stuart F. Spicker. Dordrecht: D. Reidel, 125–41.

———. 1986. *The Foundations of Bioethics*. New York: Oxford University Press.

———. 1991. *Bioethics and Secular Humanism: The Search for a Common Mortality*. Philadelphia: Trinity Press.

Engelmann, George J. 1883. *Labor among Primitive Peoples*. St. Louis: Chambers & Co.

Erickson, Erik H. 1950. *Childhood and Society*. New York: Norton.

———. 1974. *Dimensions of a New Identity*. New York: Norton.

Escobar, Arturo. 1985. Discourse and Power in Development: Michel Foucault and the Relevance of His Work to the Third World. *Alternatives* 10:377–400.

———. 1987. Power and Visibility: The Invention and Management of Development in the Third World. Ph.D. dissertation, University of California, Berkeley.

Escobar, G. J., E. Salazar, and M. Chung. 1983. Beliefs Regarding the Etiology and Treatment of Infantile Diarrhea in Lima, Peru. *Social Science and Medicine* 17:1257–69.

Estroff, Sue E. 1981. *Making It Crazy: An Ethnography of Psychiatric Clients in an American Community*. Berkeley: University of California Press.

———. 1988. Whose Hegemony? A Critical Commentary on Critical Medical Anthropology. *Medical Anthropology Quarterly* n.s. 2(4):421–26.

Etkin, Nina L. 1979a. Introduction to *Biomedical Evaluation of Indigenous Medical Practices*, ed. Etkin. Special edition of *Medical Anthropology* 3(4):393–400.

———. 1979b. Indigenous Medicine among the Hausa of Northern Nigeria: Laboratory Evaluation for Potential Therapeutic Efficacy of Antimalarial Plant Medicinals. Special edition of *Medical Anthropology* 3(4):401–29.

―――. 1980. Indigenous Medicine in Northern Nigeria. I. Oral Hygiene and Medical Treatment. *Journal of Preventive Dentistry* 6:143–49.

―――. 1981. A Hausa Herbal Pharmacopoeia: Biomedical Evaluation of Commonly Used Plant Medicines. *Journal of Ethnopharmacology* 4(1):75–98.

―――. 1986. Multidisciplinary Perspectives in the Interpretation of Plants Used in Indigenous Medicine and Diet. In *Plants in Indigenous Medicine and Diet: Biobehavioral Approaches,* ed. N. L. Etkin. Bedford Hills, N.Y.: Redgrave, 2–29.

―――. 1988a. Cultural Constructions of Efficacy. In *The Context of Medicines in Developing Countries: Studies in Pharmaceutical Anthropology,* ed. S. van der Geest and S. R. Whyte. Dordrecht: Kluwer, 299–326.

―――. 1988b. Ethnopharmacology: Biobehavioral Approaches in the Anthropological Study of Indigenous Medicines. *Annual Review of Anthropology* 17:23–42.

―――. 1990. Ethnopharmacology: Biological and Behavioral Perspectives in the Study of Indigenous Medicines. In *Medical Anthropology: A Handbook of Theory and Method,* ed. Thomas M. Johnson and Carolyn F. Sargent. Westport, Conn.: Greenwood Press, 149–58.

―――. 1993. Anthropological Methods in Ethnopharmacology. *Journal of Ethnopharmacology* 38: 93–104.

―――. 1994a. Consuming a Therapeutic Landscape: A Multicontextual Framework for Assessing the Health Significance of Human-Plant Interactions. *Journal of Home and Consumer Horticulture* 1(2/3):61–81.

―――. 1994b. The Negotiation of ''Side'' Effects in Hausa (Northern Nigeria) Therapeutics. In *Medicines: Meanings and Contexts,* ed. N. L. Etkin and M. L. Tan. Amsterdam: University of Amsterdam, 17–32.

―――. In press. Ethnopharmacology. In *The Encyclopedia of Cultural Anthropology.* New York: Human Relations Area Files and Henry Holt Publishers.

Etkin N. L., ed. 1986. *Plants in Indigenous Medicine and Diet: Biobehavioral Approaches.* Bedford Hills, N.Y.: Redgrave Publishing Co.

―――. 1994. *Eating on the Wild Side: The Pharmacologic, Ecologic, and Social Implications of Using Noncultigens.* Tucson: University of Arizona Press.

Etkin N. L., and P. J. Ross, 1982a. Malaria, Medicine, and Meals: Plant Use among the Hausa and Its Impact on Disease. In *The Anthropology of Medicine: From Culture to Method,* ed. L. Romanucci-Ross, D. E. Moerman, and L. R. Trancredi. New York: Praeger, 231–59.

―――. 1982b. Food as Medicine and Medicine as Food: An Adaptive Framework for the Interpretation of Plant Utilization among the Hausa of Northern Nigeria. *Social Science and Medicine* 16:1559–73.

―――. 1991a. Should We Set a Place for Diet in Ethnopharmacology? *Journal of Ethnopharmacology* 32:25–36.

―――. 1991b. Recasting Malaria, Medicine and Meals: A Perspective on Disease Adaptation. In *The Anthropology of Medicine,* ed. L. Romanucci-Ross, D. E. Moerman, and L. R. Tancredi. 2d ed. New York: Praeger Publishers, 230–58.

Etkin, Nina L., Paul J. Ross, and Ibrahim Muazzamu. 1990. The Indigenization of Pharmaceuticals: Therapeutic Innovations in Rural Hausaland. *Social Science and Medicine* 30(8):919–28.

Evaneshko, V., and E. E. Bauwens. 1976. Cognitive Analysis and Decision-making in Medical Emergencies. In *Health Care Dimensions: Transcultural Health Care Issues and Conditions,* ed. M. Leininger. Philadelphia: Davis, 83–102.

Evaneshko, V., and M. A. Kay. 1982. The Ethnoscience Research Technique. *Western Journal of Nursing Research* 4:49–64.

Evans, A. S. 1982a. Epidemiological Concepts and Methods. In *Bacterial Infections of Humans: Epidemiology and Control,* ed. A. S. Evans and H. A. Feldman. New York: Plenum Press, 1–48.

———. 1982b. Epidemiological Concepts and Methods. In *Viral Infections of Humans: Epidemiology and Control,* ed. A. S. Evans. New York: Plenum Press, 3–42.

———. 1986. Epidemic Investigation. In *Methods in Observational Epidemiology,* ed. J. L. Kelsey, W. D. Thompson, and A. S. Evans. New York: Oxford University Press, 212–53.

Evans-Pritchard, E. E. 1937. *Witchcraft, Oracles and Magic among the Azande.* Oxford: Clarendon.

———. 1940. *The Nuer.* Oxford: Oxford University Press.

Everett, Michael W., Jack O. Waddell, and Dwight B. Heath, eds. 1976. *Cross-Cultural Approaches to the Study of Alcohol: An Interdisciplinary Perspective.* The Hague: Mouton.

Ewald, Paul W. 1994. *Evolution of Infectious Disease.* New York: Oxford University Press.

Fabrega, Horacio, Jr. 1970a. Dynamics of Medical Practice in a Folk Community. *Milbank Memorial Fund Quarterly* 48:391–412.

———. 1970b. On the Specificity of Folk Illnesses. *Southwestern Journal of Anthropology* 26:305–14.

———. 1972. Medical Anthropology. In *Biennial Review of Anthropology, 1971,* ed. Bernard J. Siegel. Stanford: Stanford University Press.

———. 1974. *Disease and Social Behavior: An Interdisciplinary Perspective.* Cambridge: MIT Press.

———. 1975. The Need for an Ethnomedical Science. *Science* 189:969–75.

———. 1976. The Function of Medical Care Systems: A Logical Analysis. *Perspectives in Biology and Medicine* 20:108–19.

———. 1977. Group Difference in the Structure of Illness. *Culture, Medicine and Psychiatry* 1:379–94.

———. 1979. The Ethnography of Illness. *Social Science and Medicine* 13A:565–75.

———. 1982. Culture and Psychiatric Illness: Biomedical and Ethnomedical Aspects. In *Cultural Conceptions of Mental Health and Therapy,* ed. A. Marsella and G. White. Dordrecht, Holland: D. Reidel.

———. 1989a. The Self and Schizophrenia. *Schizophrenia Bulletin* 15:277–90.

———. 1989b. Cultural Relativism and Psychiatric Illness. *Journal of Nervous and Mental Disease* 177:415–24.

———. 1990a. A Plea for a Broader Ethnomedicine. *Culture, Medicine and Psychiatry* 14:129–32.

———. 1990b. *An Ethnomedical Perspective of Medical Ethics.* New York: Oxford University Press.

Fabrega, Horacio, Jr., and Daniel B. Silver. 1973. *Illness and Shamanistic Curing in Zinacantan.* Stanford: Stanford University Press.

Fahim, Hussein. 1982. *Indigenous Anthropology in Non-Western Countries.* Durham, N.C.: Carolina Academic Press.

———. 1987. Anthropology and Contemporary Arab Thought. Paper presented at the Symposium, The Arab Intelligentsia, Cairo, Arab Republic of Egypt, March 26–31.

Fairbairn, W. Ronald D. 1954. *An Object-Relations Theory of the Personality.* New York: Basic Books.

Fairbank, D. T., and R. L. Hough. 1981. Cross-cultural Differences in Perceptions of Life Events. In B. S. Dohrenwend and B. P. Dohrenwend, eds., *Stressful Life Events and Their Contexts.* New York: Prodist.

Farias, Pablo. 1991. The Social-Political Dimensions of Trauma in Salvadoran Refugees: Analysis of a Clinical Sample. *Culture, Medicine and Psychiatry* 15:167–92.

Farmer, Paul. 1988. Bad Blood, Spoiled Milk: Bodily Fluids as Moral Barometers in Rural Haiti. *American Ethnologist* 15:62–83.

———. 1992. *AIDS and Accusation: Haiti and the Geography of Blame.* Berkeley: University of California Press.

———. 1995. Commentary: AIDS and the Political Economy of Brutality. *Anthropology Newsletter,* April, p. 25.

Farnsworth, Norman R., and Djaja Soejarto. 1991. Global Importance of Medicinal Plants. In *Con-*

servation of Medicinal Plants, ed. O. Akerele, V. Heywood, and H. Synge. Cambridge: Cambridge University Press, 25–51.

Farooq, M. 1966. Importance of Determining Transmission Sites in Planning Bilharziasis Control. *American Journal of Epidemiology* 83:603–12.

Farooq, M., and M. B. Mallah. 1966. The Behavioural Pattern of Social and Religious Water-Contact Activities in the Egypt-49 Bilharziasis Project Area. *Bulletin of the World Health Organization* 35:377–387.

Farooq, M., J. Nielsen, S. A. Samaan, M. B. Mallah, and A. A. Allam. 1966. The Epidemiology of *Schistosoma haematobium* and *S. mansoni* Infections in the Egypt-49 Project Area. 2. Prevalence of Bilharziasis in Relation to Personal Attributes and Habits. *Bulletin of the World Health Organization* 35:293–318.

Farooq, M., and S. A. Samaan. 1967. The Relative Potential of Different Age-Groups in the Transmission of Schistosomiasis in the Egypt-49 Project Area. *Annals of Tropical Medicine and Parasitology* 61:315–20.

Fawcett, J. 1980. A Framework for Analysis and Evaluation of Conceptual Models of Nursing. *Nursing Education* 5:10–14.

Feder, Ernest. 1981. The Deterioration of the Food Situation in the Third World and the Capitalist System. *International Journal of Health Services* 11:247–62.

Fee, Elizabeth, ed. 1983. *Women and Health: The Politics of Sex in Medicine.* Farmingdale, N.Y.: Baywood Publishing Company.

Fee, Elizabeth, and Nancy Krieger. 1994. *Women's Health, Politics and Power: Essays on Sex/ Gender, Medicine, and Public Health.* Farmingdale, N.Y.: Baywood Publishing Company.

Feher, Michel, Ramona Naddaff, and Nadia Tzi, eds. 1989. *Fragments for a History of the Human Body.* MIT: Zone Books.

Feierman, S. 1986. Popular Control over the Institutions of Health: A Historical Study. In *The Professionalisation of African Medicine,* ed. M. Last and G. L. Chavunduka. Manchester: Manchester University Press for the International African Institute, 205–20.

Feierman, Steven, and John M. Janzen, eds. 1992. *The Social Basis of Health and Healing in Africa.* Berkeley: University of California Press.

Feinstein, Alvan R. 1977. A Critical Overview of Diagnosis in Psychiatry. In *Psychiatric Diagnosis,* ed. Vivian M. Rakoff, Harvey C. Stancer, and Henry B. Kedward. New York: Brunner/ Mazel, 189–206.

Feld, Steven. 1982. *Sound and Sentiment: Birds, Weeping, Poetics and Song in Kaluli Expression.* Philadelphia: University of Pennsylvania Press.

Feldman, Allen. 1991. *Formations of Violence: The Narrative of the Body and Political Terror in Northern Ireland.* Chicago: University of Chicago Press.

Feldman, D. A., and T. M. Johnson, eds. 1986. *The Social Dimensions of AIDS: Method and Theory.* New York: Praeger.

Feldman, Jamie. 1992. The French Are Different: French and American Medicine in the Context of AIDS. *Western Journal of Medicine* 157(30):5–9.

Fenner, F. 1980. Sociocultural Change and Environmental Diseases. In *Changing Disease Patterns and Human Behavior,* ed. N. F. Stanley and R. A. Joske. London: Academic Press, 7–26.

Fenner, F., and F. N. Ratcliffe. 1965. *Myxomatosis.* Cambridge: Cambridge University Press.

Fenwick, A., A. K. Cheesmond, and M. A. Amin. 1981. The Role of Field Irrigation Canals in the Transmission of *Schistosoma mansoni* in the Gezira Scheme, Sudan. *Bulletin of the World Health Organization* 59:777–86.

Fenwick, A., A. K. Cheesmond, M. Kardaman, M. A. Amin, and B. K. Manjing. 1982. Schistosomiasis among Labouring Communities in the Gezira Irrigated Area, Sudan. *Journal of Tropical Medicine and Hygiene* 85:3–11.

Ferguson, Anne. 1981. Commercial Pharmaceutical Medicine and Medicalization: A Case Study from El Salvador. *Culture, Medicine and Psychiatry* 5(2):105–34.

———. 1986. Class Differences in Women's Roles as Health Care Managers: A Case Study from

El Salvador. Paper presented at the National Women's Studies Association Meetings, Champagne-Urbana, June 11–15.

Ferreira, Antonio J. 1963. Family Myth and Homeostasis. *Archives of General Psychiatry* 9:55–61.

Ferro-Luzzi, G. E. 1980. Food Avoidances at Puberty and Menstruation in Tamilnad. In *Food, Ecology, and Culture: Readings in the Anthropology of Dietary Practice,* ed. J. Robson. New York: Gordon and Breach, 101–8.

Field, M. G. 1976a. Comparative Sociological Perspectives on Health Care Systems. In *Medicine in Chinese Cultures,* ed. Arthur Kleinman et al. Washington, D.C.: U.S. Government Printing Office.

———. 1976b. The Modern Medical System: The Soviet Variant. In *Asian Medical Systems,* ed. C. Leslie. Berkeley: University of California Press, 82–102.

———. 1991. The Hybrid Profession: Soviet Medicine. In *Professions and the State,* ed. A. Jones. Philadelphia: Temple University Press, 43–62.

———. 1994. Post-Communist Medicine: Morbidity, Mortality and the Deteriorating Health Situation. In *The Social Legacy of Communism,* ed. J. R. Millar and S. Wolchik. Cambridge: Cambridge University Press with the Woodrow Wilson Center Press, 178–195.

Fielding, N. G., and J. L. Fielding. 1986. *Linking Data.* Beverly Hills, Calif.: Sage.

Fields, A. Belden. 1988. In Defense of Political Economy and Systematic Analysis: A Critique of Prevailing Theoretical Approaches to the New Social Movements. In *Marxism and the Interpretation of Culture,* ed. Cary Nelson and Lauren Grossberg. Urbana and Chicago: University of Illinois Press, 141–58.

Fildes, Valerie. 1986. *Breasts, Bottles and Babies: A History of Infant Feeding.* Edinburgh: University of Edinburgh.

Finkler, Kaja. 1981. Non-medical Treatments and Their Outcomes. *Culture, Medicine, and Psychiatry* 5:65–103.

———. 1985. *Spiritualist Healers in Mexico: Successes and Failures in Alternative Therapeutics.* South Hadley, Mass.: Bergin & Garvey Publishers.

———. 1986. The Social Consequences of Wellness: A View of Healing Outcomes from Micro and Macro Perspectives. *International Journal of Health Services* 16(4):627–42.

———. 1991. *Physicians at Work, Patients in Pain.* Boulder, Colo.: Westview Press.

———. 1994. Sacred Healing and Biomedicine Compared. *Medical Anthropology Quarterly* n.s. 8(2):178–97.

Finlinson, H. Ann, Refaela R. Robles, Hector M. Colon, and J. Byran Page. 1993. Recruiting and Retaining Out-of-Treatment Injecting Drug Users in the Puerto Rico AIDS Prevention Project. *Human Organization* 52:169–75.

Firth, Raymond. 1975. The Sceptical Anthropologists? Social Anthropology and Marxist Views of Society. In *Marxist Analysis and Social Anthropology,* ed. Maurice Block. New York: John Wiley, 29–60.

———. 1981. Engagement and Detachment: Reflections on Applying Social Anthropology to Public Affairs. *Human Organization* 40:193–201.

Fisher, A. D. 1987. Alcoholism and Race: The Misapplication of Both Concepts to North American Indians. *Canadian Review of Sociology and Anthropology* 24(1):81–98.

Fisher, S., and S. Cleveland. 1958. *Body Image and Personality.* Princeton, N.J.: D. Van Nostrand.

Fitzgerald, Thomas, ed. 1976. *Nutrition and Anthropology in Action.* Amsterdam: Van Gorcum.

Flack, Harley E., and Edmund D. Pellegrino. 1992. *African-American Perspectives on Biomedical Ethics.* Washington, D.C.: Georgetown University Press.

Flaskerud, J. H. 1979. Use of Vignettes to Elicit Responses toward Broad Concepts. *Nursing Research* 28:210–12.

———. 1980a. Perceptions of Problematic Behavior by Appalachians, Mental Health Professions, and Lay Non-Appalachians. *Nursing Research* 29:140–49.

———. 1980b. Tool for Comparing the Perceptions of Problematic Behavior by Psychiatric Professionals and Minority Groups. *Nursing Research* 29:4–9.

Flaskerud, J. H., and E. Halloran. 1980. Areas of Agreement in Nursing Theory Development. *Advances in Nursing Science* 3(1):1–7.

Fletcher, John C., Norman Quist, and Albert R. Jonsen. 1989. *Ethics Consultation in Health Care.* Ann Arbor, Mich.: Health Administration.

Fletcher, Joseph. 1954. *Morals and Medicine.* Princeton, N.J.: Princeton University Press.

Fletcher, Robert H., Suzanne W. Fletcher, and Edward H. Wagner. 1982. *Clinical Epidemiology—The Essentials.* Baltimore, Md.: Williams & Wilkins.

Flick, L. H. n.d. Analysis of adolescent pregnancy rates. Personal communication.

Flint, M. 1975. The Menopause: Reward or Punishment? *Psychosomatics* 16:161–63.

Flowers, Michael J., and Deborah Heath. 1993. Micro-Anatomic Politics: Mapping the Human Genome Project. *Culture, Medicine, and Psychiatry* 17:27–41.

Flynn, Patricia. 1992. Legitimation and Power: Whose Discourse Trumps in Bioethics and Why? Paper presented at the American Anthropological Association Annual Meeting, San Francisco.

Folkman, Susan. 1984. Personal Control and Stress and Coping Processes: A Theoretical Analysis. *Journal of Personality and Social Psychology* 46:839–52.

Folkman, Susan, and Richard S. Lazarus. 1988. The Relationship between Coping and Emotion: Implications for Theory and Research. *Social Science and Medicine* 26:309–17.

Fong, Carolyn Mae. 1985. Ethnicity and Nursing Practice. *Topics in Clinical Nursing* 7(3):1–11.

Fontenot, Wonda L. 1994. *Secret Doctors: Ethnomedicine of African Americans.* Westport, Conn.: Bergin and Garvey.

Forbes, R. 1948. *Sixty Years of Medical Defence.* London: Medical Defence Union, Ltd.

Ford, Clellan Stearns. 1945. *A Comparative Study of Human Reproduction.* Yale University Publications in Anthropology. New Haven: Human Relations Area File Press.

Ford T. R., and D. D. Stephenson. 1954. *Institutional Nurses: Roles, Relationships and Attitudes in Three Alabama Hospitals.* Tuscaloosa: University of Alabama Press.

Forsythe, Diana. 1992. Blaming the User in Medical Information: The Cultural Blame of Scientific Practice. In *The Anthropology of Science and Technology,* ed. D. Hess and L. Layne. Greenwich, Conn.: JAI Press, 95–111.

Fortes, Meyer. 1959. *Oedipus and Job in West African Religion.* Cambridge: Cambridge University Press.

Foster, George M. 1953. Relationships between Spanish and Spanish-American Folk Medicine. *Journal of American Folklore* 66:201–17.

———. 1958. *Problems of Intercultural Health Programs.* New York: Social Science Research Council.

———. 1965. Peasant Society and the Image of the Limited Good. *American Anthropologist* 67: 293–315.

———. 1974. Medical Anthropology: Some Contrasts with Medical Sociology. *Medical Anthropology Newsletter* 6(1):1–6.

———. 1978a. Hippocrates' Latin American Legacy: "Hot" and "Cold" in Contemporary Folk Medicine. In *Colloquia in Anthropology,* ed. R. K. Wetherington. Dallas: Southern Methodist University, 3–19.

———. 1978b. Humoral Pathology in Spain and Spanish America. In *Homenaje a Julio Caro Baroja,* ed. A. Carreira, J. A. Cid, M. Gutierrez Esteve, and R. Rubio. Madrid: Centro de Investigaciones Sociologicas, 357–70.

———. 1984a. The Concept of "Neutral" in Humoral Medical Systems. *Medical Anthropology* 8: 181–94.

———. 1984b. Anthropological Research Perspectives on Health Problems in Developing Countries. *Social Science and Medicine* 18(10):847–54.

———. 1987a. World Health Organization Behavioral Science Research: Problems and Prospects. *Social Science and Medicine* 24:709–15.

———. 1987b. Bureaucratic Aspects of International Health Agencies. *Social Science and Medicine* 25:1039–48.

Foster, George M., and Barbara Gallatin Anderson. 1978. *Medical Anthropology.* New York: John Wiley and Sons.

Foucault, Michel. 1973. *Madness and Civilization: A History of Insanity in the Age of Reason.* New York: Vintage.

———. 1975. *The Birth of the Clinic: An Archeology of Medical Perception.* New York: Vintage.

———. 1979. *Discipline and Punish: The Birth of the Prison.* New York: Vintage.

———. 1980a. *The History of Sexuality.* Vol. 1: *An Introduction.* New York: Vintage.

———. 1980b. *Power/Knowledge: Selected Interviews and Other Writings.* New York: Pantheon.

———. 1980c. Body/Power. In *Power/Knowledge: Selected Interviews and Other Writings 1972– 1977,* ed. C. Gordon. New York: Pantheon, 55–62.

———. 1984. Politics and Ethics: An Interview. In *The Foucault Reader,* ed. P. Rabinow. New York: Pantheon, 373–90.

———. 1988. Truth, Power, Self: An Interview with Michel Foucualt. In *Techologies of the Self,* ed. L. Martin, H. Gutman and P. Hutton. Amherst: University of Massachusetts Press, 9– 16.

Fourastié, Jean. 1972. From the Traditional to the ''Tertiary Life Cycle.'' In *Readings in Population,* ed. William Petersen. New York: Macmillan.

Fox, K. F. 1988. Social Marketing of ORT and Contraceptives in Egypt. *Studies in Family Planning* 19(2):95–108.

Fox, Renee C. 1959. *Experiment Perilous.* New York: Free Press.

———. 1974. Ethical and Existential Developments in Contemporaneous American Medicine: Their Implications for Culture and Society. *Milbank Memorial Fund Quarterly* 52:445–83.

———. 1976. Advanced Medical Technology—Social and Ethical Implications. *Annual Review of Sociology* 2:231–68.

———. 1990. The Evolution of American Bioethics: A Sociological Perspective. In *Social Science Perspectives on Medical Ethics,* ed. George Weisz. Philadelphia: University of Pennsylvania Press, 201–20.

Fox, Renee C., and Judith P. Swazey. 1974. *Courage to Fail.* Chicago: University of Chicago Press.

———. 1984. Medical Mortality Is Not Bioethics: Medical Ethics in China and the United States. *Perspectives in Biology and Medicine* 27:336–60.

———. 1992. *Spare Parts.* New York: Oxford University Press.

Frake, Charles O. 1961. The Diagnosis of Disease among the Subanum of Mindanao. *American Anthropologist* 63:113–32.

Franco, Jean. 1988. Beyond Ethnocentrism: Gender, Power, and the Third World Intelligentsia. In *Marxism and the Interpretation of Culture,* ed. Cary Nelson and Lawrence Grossberg. Urbana: University of Illinois Press, 508–15.

Franco-Agudelo, Saul. 1983. The Rockefeller Foundation's Antimalarial Program in Latin America: Donating or Dominating? *International Journal of Health Services* 13:51–67.

Frank, André G. 1975. Anthropology = Ideology, Applied Anthropology = Politics. *Race and Class* 15(1):57–68.

———. 1977. Dependence Is Dead, Long Live Dependence and the Class Struggle: An Answer to Critics. *World Development* 5(4):355–70.

Frank, Gelya. 1986. On Embodiment: A Case Study of Congenital Limb Deficiency in American Culture. *Culture, Medicine and Psychiatry* 10:189–219.

Frank, G., L. Blackhall, and S. Murphy. 1994. Ethnicity and Attitudes toward Patient Autonomy: From Cultural Pluralism to Structuration in End of Life Decision-Making. Paper presented at the Annual Meetings of the American Anthropological Association, December.

Frank, Jerome. 1973. *Persuasion and Healing.* Rev. ed. Baltimore: Johns Hopkins University Press.

———. 1978. *Psychotherapy and the Human Predicament.* New York: Schocken.

Frank, Jerome, and Julia Frank. 1991. *Persuasion and Healing.* 3d rev. ed. Baltimore: Johns Hopkins University Press.

Frankel, Mark S., and Albert H. Teich, eds. 1994. *The Genetic Frontier: Ethics, Law, and Policy.* Washington, D.C.: American Association for the Advancement of Science.

Frankel, Stephen, and Gilbert Lewis, eds. 1989. *A Continuing Trial of Treatment: Medical Pluralism in Papua New Guinea.* Dordrecht: Kluwer Academic Publishers.

Frankena, William K. 1973. *Ethics.* 2d ed. Englewood Cliffs, N.J.: Prentice-Hall.

Frankenberg, Ronald. 1974. Functionalism and After? Theory and Developments in Social Science Applied to the Health Field. *International Journal of Health Services* 4(3):411–27.

———. 1978. Economic Anthropology or Political Economy? The Barotose Social Formation: A Cast Study. In *The New Economic Anthropology,* ed. J. Clammer. New York: St. Martin's Press, 32–57.

———. 1980. Medical Anthropology and Development: A Theoretical Perspective. *Social Science and Medicine* 14b (4):197–207.

———. 1986. Sickness as Cultural Performance: Drama, Trajectory, and Pilgrimage. Root Metaphors and the Making Social of Disease. *International Journal of Health Services* 16:603–26.

———. 1988a. "Your Time or Mine?" An Anthropological View of the Tragic Temporal Contradictions of Biomedical Practice. *International Journal of Health Services* 18(1):11–34.

———. 1988b. Gramsci, Culture and Medical Anthropology: Kundry and Parsifal? Or Rat's Tail to Sea Serpent? *Medical Anthropology Quarterly* 2:324–37.

———. 1988c. Rejoinder. *Medical Anthropology Quarterly* n.s. 2(4):454–59.

Frankenburg, Ronald, ed. 1988. Gramsci, Marxism, and Phenomenology: Essays for the Development of Critical Medical Anthropology. *Medical Anthropology Quarterly* 2.

Franklin, Sarah. 1990. Deconstructing "Desperateness": The Social Construction of Infertility. In *Popular Representations of New Reproductive Technologies,* ed. M. McNeil, I. Varcoc, and S. Yearley. New York: St. Martin's Press, 200–29.

Frazer, James George. 1911. *The Golden Bough.* Vol. 1–2, pt. 1. 3d ed. London: Macmillan.

Freedman, A., H. Kaplan, and B. Sadock. 1976. *Modern Synopsis of Comprehensive Textbook of Psychiatry II.* Baltimore, Md.: Williams and Wilkins Co.

Freeland, W. J., P. H. Calcott, and Lisa R. Anderson. 1985. Tannins and Saponin: Interaction in Herbivore Diets. *Biochemical Systematics and Ecology* 13(2):189–93.

Freidson, Eliot. 1970. *Profession of Medicine: A Study of the Sociology of Applied Knowledge.* New York: Dodd, Mead.

———. 1972. Client Control and Medical Practice. In *Patients, Physicians, and Healers,* ed. E. Gartly Jaco. New York: Free Press, 214–21.

———. 1986. *Professional Powers: A Study of the Institutionalization of Formal Knowledge.* Chicago: University of Chicago Press.

Freidson, Eliot, and J. Lorber, eds. 1972. *Medical Men and Their Work: A Sociological Reader.* Chicago: Aldine.

Frelick, B. 1994. The Year in Review. In *World Refugee Survey.* Washington, D.C.: U.S. Committee for Refugees Mandate.

French, C. M., and G. S. Nelson. 1982. Hydatid Disease in the Turkana District of Kenya. Part II. A Study in Medical Geography. *Annals of Tropical Medicine and Parasitology* 76:439–57.

French, C. M., G. S. Nelson, and M. Wood. 1982. Hydatid Disease in the Turkana District of Kenya. Part I. The Background to the Problem with Hypotheses to Account for the Remarkably High Prevalence of the Disease in Man. *Annals of Tropical Medicine and Parasitology* 76:425–37.

French, John R. P., Jr., W. Rodgers, and Sidney Cobb. 1974. Adjustment as Person-Environment Fit. In *Coping and Adaptation,* ed. George V. Coelho, David A. Hamburg, and John E. Adams. New York: Basic Books.

Freud, Anna. 1936. *The Ego and the Mechanisms of Defense.* New York: International Universities Press.

Freud, Sigmund. 1920. *Beyond the Pleasure Principle.* Standard Edition of the Complete Psychological Works of Sigmund Freud (SE). London: Hogarth Press, 1955, 18:3–64.

———. 1923. *The Ego and the Id.* SE. London: Hogarth Press, 1961, 19:3–66.

———. 1927. *The Future of an Illusion.* SE. London: Hogarth Press, 1961, 21:5–56.

Freund, Paul, and Mac Marshall. 1977. Research Bibliography of Alcohol and Kava Studies in Oceania: Update and Additional Items. *Micronesia* 13:313–17.

Fridja, Nico. 1987. *The Emotions.* Cambridge: Cambridge University Press.

Friedan, Betty. 1993. *Fountain of Age.* New York: Simon & Schuster.

Friede, A., J. A. Reid, and P. W. O'Carroll. 1993. *CDC Wonder/PC, Version 2: User's Guide.* Atlanta: Public Health Service. A-45.

Friede, A., J. A. Reid, and H. W. Ory. 1993. CDC WONDER: A Comprehensive Online Public Health Information System of the Centers for Disease Control and Prevention. *American Journal of Public Health* 83 (3).

Friedl, John. 1982. Explanatory Models of Black Lung: Understanding the Health-Related Behavior of Appalachian Coal Miners. *Culture, Medicine and Psychiatry* 6:3–10.

Friedlander, Myrna L., Theodore J. Ksul, and Carolyn A. Stimel. 1984. Abortion: Predicting the Complexity of the Decision-Making Process. *Women and Health* 9(1):43–54.

Friedman, G. D. 1987. *Primer of Epidemiology.* New York: McGraw-Hill.

Friedman, Howard S., and Stephanie Booth-Kewley. 1988. Validity of the Type A Construct. *Psychological Bulletin* 104:381–84.

Friedman, Paul. 1983. The Relevance of Anthropology for Clinical Work: The Observations of a Physician–Social Scientist. In *Clinical Anthropology,* ed. Demitri Shimkin and Peggy Golde. Lanham, Md.: University Press of America, 239–45.

Frisancho, A. Roberto. 1993. *Human Adaptation and Accommodation.* Enl. and rev. ed. of *Human Adaptation.* Ann Arbor: University of Michigan Press.

Frisch, R. E., and R. Revelle. 1971. Height and Weight at Menarche and a Hypothesis of Menarche. *Archives of Diseases of Children* 46:695–701.

Frisch, R. E., R. Revelle, and S. Cook. 1973. Components of the Critical Weight at Menarche and at Initiation of the Adolescent Growth Spurt: Estimated Total Water, Lean Body Mass, and Fat. *Human Biology* 48:469–83.

Frohock, Fred M. 1986. *Special Care: Medical Decisions at the Beginning of Life.* Chicago: University of Chicago Press.

Fuchs, Fritz, and Phillip G. Stubblefield, eds. 1984. *Preterm Birth: Causes, Prevention, and Management.* New York: Macmillan.

Fujita, Chihiro. 1986. *Morita Therapy: A Psychotherapeutic System for Neurosis.* Tokyo and New York: Igaku-Shoin.

Fuller, G. K., and D. C. Fuller. 1981. Hydatid Disease in Ethiopia: Epidemiological Findings and Ethnographic Observations of Disease Transmission in Southwestern Ethiopia. *Medical Anthropology* 5:293–311.

Furbee, L., R. A. Benfer. 1983. Cognitive and Geographic Maps: Study of Individual Variation among Tojolabal Mayans. *American Anthropologist* 85:305–34.

Furer-Haimendorf, C. von. 1967. *Morals and Merit.* London: Weidenfeld & Nicolson.

Furst, Peter T. 1976. *Hallucinogens and Culture.* San Francisco: Chandler and Sharp.

Furst, Peter T., ed. 1972. *Flesh of the Gods: The Ritual Use of Hallucinogens.* New York: Praeger.

Gadamer, H. G. 1984. *Truth and Method.* New York: Crossroad.

Gailey, Christine Ward. 1987. *Kinship to Kingship.* Austin: University of Texas Press.

Gaines, Atwood D. 1982. Knowledge and Practice: Anthropological Ideas and Psychiatric Practice. In Noel J. Chrisman and Thomas W. Maretzki, eds., *Clinically Applied Anthropology: Anthropologists in Health Science Settings.* Dordrecht: D. Reidel, 243–75.

————. 1991. Cultural Constructivism: Sickness Histories and the Understanding of Ethnomedicines beyond Critical Medical Anthropologies. In *Anthropologies of Medicine: A Colloquium on Western European and American Perspectives,* ed. Beatrix Pfiederer and Gilles Bibeau. Wiesbaden: Verlag Vieweg, 221–58.

————. 1992. From DSM-I to II-R: Voices of Self, Mastery and the Other: A Cultural Constructivist Reading of a U.S. Psychiatric Classification. *Social Science and Medicine* 35(1):3–24.

Gaines, Atwood, ed. 1992. *Ethnopsychiatry: The Cultural Construction of Professional and Folk Psychiatries.* Albany, N.Y.: State University of New York Press.

Gaines, Atwood, and Paul Farmer. 1986. Visible Saints: Social Cynosures and Dysphoria in the Mediterranean Tradition. *Culture, Medicine and Psychiatry* 10(4):295–330.

Galaty, J. G., Dan Aronson, P. C. Salzman, and Amy Chouinard, eds. 1981. *The Future of Pastoral Peoples.* Ottawa: International Development Research Center.

Galazka, S., and J. K. Eckert. 1986. Clinically Applied Anthropology: Concepts for the Family Physician. *Journal of Family Practice* 22(2):159–65.

Gallagher, Catherine. 1986. The Body Versus the Social Body in the Works of Thomas Malthus and Henry Mayhew. *Representations* 14:83–106.

Galloway, Patrick R. 1986. Long-Term Fluctuations in Climate and Population. *Population and Development Review* 12:1–24.

GAP (Group for the Advancement of Psychiatry). 1987. *Us and Them: The Psychology of Ethnonationalism.* GAP Report 123 by the Committee on International Relations, with H. F. Stein. New York: Brunner/Mazel.

Garcia, Jorge L. A. 1992. African-American Perspectives, Cultural Relativism and Normative Issues: Some Conceptual Problems. In *African-American Perspectives on Biomedical Ethics,* ed. Harley Flack and Edmund D. Pellegrino. Washington, D.C.: Georgetown University Press, 11–65.

Garfield, Sol L. 1986. Problems in Diagnostic Classification. In *Contemporary Directions in Psychopathology toward the DSM-IV,* ed. Theodore Millon and Gerald L. Klerman. New York: Guilford Press, 99–114.

Garn, S., N. J. Smith, and D. C. Clark. 1975. The Magnitude and Implication of Apparent Race Differences in Hemoglobin Values. *American Journal of Clinical Nutrition* 28:563–68.

Garnsey, Peter. 1988. *Famine and Food Supply in the Graeco-Roman World.* Cambridge: Cambridge University Press.

Garrett, J., et al. 1993. Life-Sustaining Treatments during Terminal Illness: Who Wants What? *Journal of General Internal Medicine* 8:361–68.

Garrett, Laurie. 1994. *The Coming Plague: Newly Emerging Diseases in a World Out of Balance.* New York: Farrar, Straus and Giroux.

Garrison, Vivian. 1977a. Doctor, Espiritista, or Psychiatrist: Health Seeking Behavior in a Puerto Rican Neighborhood of New York City. *Medical Anthropology* 1:65–191.

————. 1977b. The "Puerto Rican Syndrome" in Psychiatry and Espiritismo. In *Case Studies in Spirit Possession,* ed. V. Crapanzano and V. Garrison. New York: John Wiley and Sons, 383–449.

Garro, Linda C. 1986. Intracultural Variation in Folk Medical Knowledge: A Comparison between Curers and Noncurers. *American Anthropologist* 88:351–70.

————. 1988. Explaining High Blood Pressure: Variation in Knowledge about Illness. *American Ethnologist* 15:98–119.

Gbeassor, M., Y. Kossou, K. Amegbo, C. de Souza, K. Koumaglo, and A. Denke. 1989. Antimalarial Effects of Eight African Medicinal Plants. *Journal of Ethnopharmacology* 25:115–18.

Gebrian, B. 1989. Haitian Health Foundation Primary Health Care Program. Unpublished annual report.

————. 1993. Community Participation in Primary Health Care in Rural Haiti: An Ecological Approach. Ph.D. dissertation, University of Connecticut.

Geertz, Clifford. 1973a. *The Interpretation of Cultures: Selected Essays.* New York: Basic Book.

————. 1973b. Ideology as a Cultural System. In *The Interpretation of Cultures,* ed. C. Geertz. New York: Basic Books, 193–234.

―――. 1973c. Religion as a Cultural System. In *The Interpretation of Cultures,* ed. C. Geertz. New York: Basic Books, 87–126.

―――. 1980. *Negara: The Theatre-State in Nineteenth Century Bali.* Princeton: Princeton University Press.

―――. 1984a. From the Native's Point of View: On the Nature of Anthropological Understanding. In *Culture Theory,* ed. Richard Shweder and Robert LeVine. Cambridge: Cambridge University Press, 123–36.

―――. 1984b. Anti-Relativism. *American Anthropologist* 86:263–78.

―――. 1994. The Strange Estrangement: Taylor and the Natural Sciences. In *Philosophy and an Age of Pluralism,* ed. James Tully. Cambridge: Cambridge University Press, 83–95.

Geertz, Hildred. 1959. The Vocabulary of Emotion: A Study of Javanese Socialization Processes. *Psychiatry* 22:225–37.

Gefou-Madianou, Dimitra, ed. 1992. *Alcohol, Gender and Culture.* London and New York: Routledge.

Gehrie, Mark J. 1976. Childhood and Community: On the Experience of Young Japanese Americans in Chicago. *Ethos* 4(3):353–83.

Geison, Gerald L., ed. 1984. *Professions and the French State, 1700–1900.* Philadelphia: University of Pennsylvania Press.

Gelfand, T. 1980. *Professionalizing Modern Medicine: Paris Surgeons and Medical Science and Institutions in the 18th Century.* Westport, Conn.: Greenwood Press.

Gelso, Charles, and Jean Canter. 1985. The Relationship in Counseling and Psychotherapy: Components, Consequences, and Theoretical Antecedents. *Counseling Psychologist* 13:155–243.

George, Susan. 1977. *How the Other Half Dies: The Real Reasons for World Hunger.* Montclair, N.J.: Allanheld, Osmun and Co.

―――. 1981. *Feeding the Few: Corporate Control of Food.* Washington, D.C.: Institute for Policy Studies.

Germain, C. 1979. *The Cancer Unit: An Ethnography.* Wakefield, Mass.: Nursing Resources.

Geschiere, Peter. 1988. Sorcery and the State. *Critique of Anthropology* 6(1):35–63.

―――. 1995. *Sorcellerie et Politique en Afrique: La Viande des Autres.* Paris: Karthala.

Geser, A., N. Charney, and N. E. Day. 1978. Environmental Factors in the Etiology of Nasopharyngeal Carcinoma: Report on a Case-Control Study in Hong Kong. In *NPC: Etiology and Control,* ed. G. de-The and Y. Ito. Lyon: IARC, 213–29.

Gessain, M. 1963. Coniagui Women, Guinea. In *Women of Tropical Africa,* ed. D. Paulme. London: Routledge and Kegan Paul, 17–46.

Gezira Board. 1987. *The Gezira Scheme: Past, Present and Future.* Wad Medani, Sudan: Gezira Scheme Board.

Gibb, G. D. 1984. A Comparative Study of Recidivists and Contraceptors along the Dimensions of Control and Impulsivity. *International Journal of Psychiatry* 19(6):581–91.

Gilbert, M. Jean. 1980. Los Parientes: Social Structural Factors and Kinship Relations among Second Generation Mexican Americans. Ph.D. dissertation, University of California, Santa Barbara.

―――. 1990–91. The Anthropologist as Alcohologist: Qualitative Perspectives and Methods in Alcohol Research. *International Journal of Addictions* 25(2A):127–48.

Gilbert, M. Jean, and Richard C. Cervantes. 1987. *Mexican Americans and Alcohol.* Monograph 11. Los Angeles: Spanish Speaking Mental Health Research Center.

Gilbert, Robert I., and James H. Mielke, eds. 1985. *The Analysis of Prehistoric Diets.* Orlando, Fla.: Academic Press.

Gilligan, Carol, Janie Victoria Ward, and Jill McLean Taylor, eds. 1988. *Mapping the Moral Domain.* Cambridge, Mass.: Harvard University Press.

Ginsburg, Faye. 1989. *Contested Lives: The Abortion Debate in an American Community.* Berkeley: University of California Press.

Ginsburg, Faye, and Rayna Rapp. 1991. The Politics of Reproduction. *Annual Review of Anthropology* 20:311–43.

Gish, Oscar, and Martin Godfrey. 1979. A Reappraisal of the "Brain Drain" with Special Reference to the Medical Profession. *Social Science and Medicine* 18C:1–44.

Gittelsohn, J. 1989. Intrahousehold Food Distribution in Rural Nepal. Ph.D dissertation, University of Connecticut.

———. 1991. Opening the Box: Intrahousehold Food Allocation in Rural Nepal. *Social Science and Medicine* 33(10):1141–54.

Glander, K. E. 1982. The Impact of Plant Secondary Compounds on Primate Feeding Behavior. *Year-book of Physical Anthropology* 25:1–18.

———. 1994. Nonhuman Primate Self-Medication with Wild Plant Foods. In *Eating on the Wild Side: The Pharmacologic, Ecologic and Social Implications of Using Noncultigens,* ed. N. L. Etkin. Tucson: University of Arizona Press, 227–39.

Glass, James M. 1989. *Private Terror/Public Life.* Ithaca: Cornell University Press.

Glick, Leonard B. 1967. Medicine as an Ethnographic Category: The Gimi of the New Guinea Highlands. *Ethnology* 6:31–56.

Glittenberg, J. E. 1981. Variations in Stress and Coping in Three Migrant Settlements—Guatemala City. *Image* 13:43–46.

Gluckman, Max. 1965. Foreword to *Sorcery in Its Social Setting,* by Max Marwick. Manchester: Manchester University Press.

Gluckman, Max, ed. 1964. *Closed Systems and Open Minds: The Limits of Naiveté in Social Anthropology.* Chicago: Aldine Publishing Company.

Goforth, Lynnel. 1988. Household Structure and Birth Attendant Choice in a Yucatec Maya Community. Ph.D. dissertation, University of California, Los Angeles.

Golde, Peggy. 1983a. Foreword: Clinical Anthropology as a Committed Profession. In *Clinical Anthropology,* ed. Demitri Shimkin and Peggy Golde. Lanham, Md.: University Press of America, 27–37.

———. 1983b. Anthropological Contributions to Psychotherapy: An Overview. In *Clinical Anthropology,* ed. Demetri Shimkin and Peggy Golde. Lanham, Md.: University Press of America, 75–86.

Golde, Peggy, and Demitri B. Shimkin. 1980. Clinical Anthropology—An Emerging Health Profession? *Medical Anthropology Newsletter* 12(1):15–16.

Goldsmith, Douglas S., Dana E. Hunt, Douglas S. Lipton, and David L. Strug. 1984. Methadone Folklore: Beliefs about Side Effects and Their Impact on Treatment. *Human Organization* 43(4):330–40.

Golladay, Frederick, and Bernhard Liese. 1980. *Health Problems and Policies in Developing Countries.* Washington, D.C.: World Bank.

Golomb, Lewis. 1986. Rivalry and Diversity among Thai Curer-Magicians. *Social Science and Medicine* 22:691–97.

Gonen, Jay Y. 1975. *A Psychohistory of Zionism.* New York: Mason Charter.

Good, Byron J. 1977. The Heart of What's the Matter: The Semantics of Illness in Iran. *Culture, Medicine and Psychiatry* 1:25–58.

———. 1992. Culture and Psychopathology: Directions for Psychiatric Anthropology. In *New Directions for Psychological Anthropology,* ed. T. Schwartz, G. White, and C. Lutz. Cambridge: Cambridge University Press.

———. 1994. *Medicine, Rationality and Experience: An Anthropological Perspective.* Cambridge: Cambridge University Press.

Good, Byron J., and Mary-Jo DelVecchio Good. 1981. The Meaning of Symptoms: A Cultural Hermeneutic Model for Clinical Practice. In *The Relevance of Social Science for Medicine,* ed. L. Eisenberg and A. Kleinman. Dordrecht: D. Reidel, 165–97.

———. 1982. Toward a Meaning Centered Analysis of Popular Illness Categories. In *Cultural Conceptions of Mental Health and Therapy,* ed. A. Marsella and G. White. Dordrecht, Holland: D. Reidel.

————. 1993. "Learning Medicine": The Constructing of Medical Knowledge at Harvard Medical School. In *Knowledge, Power and Practice: The Anthropology of Medicine and Everyday Life,* ed., Shirley Lindenbaum and Margaret Lock. Berkeley: University of California Press, 81–107.

Good, Byron J., Mary Jo DelVecchio Good, and Robert Moradi. 1985. The Interpretation of Iranian Depressive Illness and Dysphoric Affect. In *Culture and Depression,* ed. Arthur Kleinman and Byron Good. Berkeley: University of California Press.

Good, Byron J., and Arthur Kleinman 1985. Epilogue to *Culture and Depression,* ed. Arthur Kleinman and Byron Good. Berkeley: University of California Press.

Good, C. M. 1987. *Ethnomedical Systems in Africa: Patterns of Traditional Medicine in Urban and Rural Kenya.* New York: Guilford Press.

Good, Mary-Jo DelVecchio. 1991. The Practice of Biomedicine and the Discourse on Hope: A Preliminary Investigation into the Culture of American Oncology. In *Anthropologies of Medicine: A Colloquium on West European and North American Perspectives,* ed. Beatrix Pfleiderer and Gilles Bibeau. Heidelberg, Germany: Vieweg, Bertelsmann Publishing Group International, 121–36.

————. 1995. *American Medicine: The Quest for Competence.* Berkeley and Los Angeles: University of California Press.

Good, Mary-Jo DelVecchio, and Byron J. Good. 1988. Ritual, the State, and the Transformation of Emotional Discourse in Iranian Society. *Culture, Medicine and Psychiatry* 12:43–63.

Good, Mary-Jo DelVecchio, Byron J. Good, Paul E. Brodwin, and Arthur Kleinman. 1992. *Pain as Human Experience: An Anthropological Perspective.* Berkeley: University of California Press.

Good, Mary-Jo DelVecchio, et al. 1990. American Oncology and the Discourse on Hope. *Culture, Medicine and Psychiatry* 14:59–79.

Goodenough, Ward. 1963. *Cooperation in Change.* New York: Russell Sage Foundation.

Goodgame, Richard W. 1990. AIDS in Uganda—Clinical and Social Factors. *New England Journal of Medicine* 323(6):383–89.

Goodman, Alan, and Thomas Leatherman, eds. 1996. *Building a New Biocultural Synthesis: Political-Economic and Critical Perspectives on Human Biology.* Ann Arbor: University of Michigan Press.

Goodman, Steven M., and Joseph J. Hobbs. 1988. The Ethnobotany of the Egyptian Eastern Desert: A Comparison of Common Plant Usage between Two Culturally Distinct Bedouin Groups. *Journal of Ethnopharmacology* 23:73–89.

Goody, Jack. 1977. *The Domestication of the Savage Mind.* Cambridge: Cambridge University Press.

Goonatilake, S. 1984. *Aborted Discovery: Science and Creativity in the Third World.* London: Zed Press.

Gordon, Andrew J., ed. 1978. Ethnicity and Alcohol Use. *Medical Anthropology* 2(4): entire issue.

Gordon, Daniel. 1991. Female Circumcision and Genital Operations in Egypt and the Sudan: A Dilemma for Medical Anthropology. *Medical Anthropology Quarterly* 5(1):3–14.

Gordon, Deborah. 1988a. Tenacious Assumptions in Western Medicine. In *Biomedicine Examined,* ed. Margaret Lock and Deborah Gordon. Dordrecht: D. Reidel.

————. 1988b. Clinical Science and Clinical Expertise: Changing Boundaries between Art and Science in Medicine. In *Biomedicine Examined,* ed. Margaret Lock and Deborah R. Gordon. Boston: Kluwer Academic Publishers, 257–95.

————. 1990. Embodying Illness, Embodying Cancer. *Culture, Medicine and Psychiatry* 14:275–97.

————. 1991. Culture, Cancer, and Communication in Italy. In *Anthropologies of Medicine: A Colloquium on West European and North American Perspectives,* ed. Beatrix Pfleiderer and

Gilles Bibeau. Heidelberg, Germany: Vieweg, Bertelsmann Publishing Group International, 137–56.

———. 1994. The Ethics of Ambiguity and Concealment. In *Interpretive Phenomenology,* ed. Patricia Benner. Thousand Oaks, Calif.: Sage.

Gordon, J. E., J. B. Wylon, and W. Ascoli. 1967. The Second Year Death Rate in Less Developed Countries. *American Journal of Medical Sciences* 254:357–80.

Gordon, Kathleen, D. 1987. Evolutionary Perspectives on Human Diet. In *Nutritional Anthropology,* ed. Francis E. Johnston. New York: Alan R. Liss, Inc., 3–39.

Gore, Susan. 1985. Social Support and Styles of Coping with Stress. In *Social Support and Health,* ed. S. Cohen and S. L. Syme. Orlando, Fla.: Academic Press.

Gorman, M. E. 1986. The AIDS Epidemic in San Francisco: Epidemiological and Anthropological Perspectives. In *Anthropology and Epidemiology,* ed. C. R. Janes, R. Stall, and S. M. Gifford. Dordrecht: Reidel, 157–74.

Gough, Kathleen. 1968. World Revolution and the Science of Man. In *The Dissenting Academy,* ed. Theodore Rosak. London: Chatton and Windus.

Gough, Kathleen, and H. Sharma, eds. 1975. *Imperialism and Revolution in South Asia.* New York: Monthly Review Press.

Gould, Carol C. 1983. *Beyond Domination: New Perspectives on Women and Philosophy.* Totowa, N.J.: Rowman and Littlefield Publishers.

Gould, Harold. 1965. Modern Medicine and Folk Cognition in Rural India. *Human Organization* 24:201–8.

Gove, S., and G. Pelto. 1994. Focused Ethnographic Studies in the WHO Programme: The Control of Acute Respiratory Infections. *Medical Anthropology* 15(4):409–24.

Graham, Joe S. 1976. The Role of Curanderos in the Mexican-American Folk System in West Texas. In *American Folk Medicine,* ed. W. D. Hand. Berkeley: University of California Press, 175–89.

Gran, Peter. 1979. Medical Pluralism in Arab and Egyptian History: An Overview of Class Structure and Philosophies of the Main Phase. *Social Science and Medicine* 13b:339–48.

Grant, James P. 1988. *The State of the World's Children 1988.* Oxford: Oxford University Press.

———. 1993. Jumpstarting Development. *Foreign Policy* 91:124–137.

———. 1994. *The State of the World's Children 1994.* Oxford: Oxford University Press/ UNICEF.

Graver, Ellen. 1988. Factors Affecting Maternal Compliance to a Nutrition Education Program for Fat Infants. Master's thesis, University of Arizona.

Graves, Theodore D. 1967. Acculturation, Access, and Alcohol in a Tri-Ethnic Community. *American Anthropologist* 69: 306–21.

Graves, Theodore D., and Nancy B. Graves. 1979. Stress and Health: Modernization in a Traditional Polynesian Society. *Medical Anthropology* 3:23–59.

———. 1980. Kinship Ties and the Preferred Adaptive Strategies of Urban Migrants. In *The Versatility of Kinship,* ed. Linda S. Cordell and Stephen J. Beckerman. New York: Academic Press.

———. 1985. Stress and Health among Polynesian Migrants to New Zealand. *Journal of Behavioral Medicine* 8:1–19.

Graves, Theodore D., Nancy B. Graves, Vineta N. Semu, and Iulai Ah Sam. 1982. Patterns of Public Drinking in a Multiethnic Society: A Systematic Observational Study. *Journal of Studies on Alcohol* 43:990–1009.

Gray, R. H. 1974. The Decline of Mortality in Ceylon and the Demographic Effects of Malaria Control. *Population Studies* 28:205–29.

Gray, Ronald. 1983. The Impact of Health and Nutrition on Natural Fertility. In *Determinants of Fertility in Developing Countries,* ed. R. A. Bulatao and R. D. Lee. Vol. 1. New York: Academic Press, 139–63.

Green, Edward C. 1985. Traditional Healers, Mothers and Childhood Diarrheal Disease in Swaziland: The Interface of Anthropology and Health Education. *Social Science and Medicine* 20(3):277–85.

Greenberg, Joel. 1988. U.S. Doctors Find "Epidemic of Army Violence" in Areas. *Jerusalem Post,* February 12:1, 4.

Greenberg, R. S., and M. A. Ibrahim. 1985. Epidemiological Techniques and Planned Investigation: The Case-Control Study. In *Oxford Textbook of Public Health.* Vol. 3:*Investigative Methods in Public Health,* ed. Walter W. Holland, Roger Detels, and George Knox. Oxford: Oxford University Press.

Greene, L. S. 1973. Physical Growth and Development, Neurological Maturation, and Behavioral Functioning in Two Ecuadorian Andean Communities in Which Goiter Is Endemic. I. Outline of the Problem of Endemic Goiter and Cretinism. Physical Growth and Neurological Maturation in the Adult Population of La Esperanza. *American Journal of Physical Anthropology* 41:139–52.

———. 1977. Hyperendemic Goiter, Cretinism, and Social Organization in Highland Ecuador. In *Malnutrition, Behavior, and Social Organization,* ed. L. S. Green. New York: Academic Press, 55–94.

———. 1980. Social and Biological Predictors of Physical Growth and Neurological Development in an Area Where Iodine and Protein-Energy Malnutrition Are Endemic. In *Social and Biological Predictors of Nutritional Status, Physical Growth and Neurological Development,* ed. L. S. Greene and F. E. Johnston. New York: Academic Press, 223–56.

Greene, Owen, Barry Rubin, Neil Turok, Philip Webber, and Graeme Wilkinson. 1982. *London after the Bomb: What a Nuclear Attack Really Means.* Oxford: Oxford University Press.

Greenhalgh, Susan. 1985a. Is Inequality Demographically Induced? *American Anthropologist* 87: 571–94.

———. 1985b. Sexual Stratification: The Other Side of "Growth with Equity" in East Asia. *Population and Development Review* 11:265–314.

———. 1989. New Directions in Fertility Research: Anthropological Perspectives. Paper prepared for the General Conference of the IUSSP, New Delhi, September 20–27.

———. 1990. Toward a Political Economy of Fertility: Anthropological Contributions. *Population and Development Review* 16:85–106.

Greep, R. O., M. A. Koblinsky, and F. S. Jaffe. 1976. *Reproduction and Human Welfare: A Challenge to Research.* Cambridge, Mass.: MIT Press.

Grey-Turner, E., and F. M. Sutherland. 1982. *History of the British Medical Association.* Vol. 2: *1932–1981.* London: British Medical Association.

Griaule, Marcel. 1965. *Conversations with Ogotemmeli.* Oxford: Oxford University Press.

Groger, Lisa. 1992. Tied to Each Other Through Ties to the Land: Informal Support of Black Elders in Southern U.S. Community. *Journal of Cross-Cultural Gerontology* 7:205–20.

Grossinger, Richard. 1980. *Planet Medicine: From Stone Age Shamanism to Post-Industrial Healing.* Garden City, N.Y.: Doubleday.

Gruenbaum, Ellen. 1981. Medical Anthropology, Health Policy and the State: A Case Study of Sudan. *Review* 1:47–65.

———. 1983. Struggling with the Mosquito: Malaria Policy and Agricultural Development in Sudan. *Medical Anthropology* 7(2):51–62.

———. 1989. The Islamic Movement, Development, and Health Education: Recent Changes in Clitoridectomy and Infibulation Practices of Rural Women in Central Sudan. Revised draft of paper presented to the Symposium on Medical Anthropology in the Arab World, American Anthropological Association Meeting, Washington, D.C., November 17.

Guarnaccia, P., B. Good, and Arthur Kleinman. 1990. A Critical Review of Epidemiological Studies of Puerto Rican Mental Health. *American Journal of Psychiatry* 147(11):1449–56.

Guillemin, Jeanne Harley, and Linda Lytle Holmstrom. 1986. *Mixed Blessings: Intensive Care for Newborns.* New York: Oxford University Press.

Gulliver, Philip H. 1957. Nyakyusa Labour Migration. *Journal of the Rhodes-Livingstone Institute* 21:32–63.

———. 1958. *Land Tenure and Social Change among the Nyakyusa.* Kampala: East African Institute of Social Research.

Gupta, Akhil, and James Ferguson. 1992. Beyond "Culture:" Space, Identity and the Politics of Difference. *Cultural Anthropology* 7:6–23.

Gussler, Judith. 1987. Culture, Community, and the Course of Infant Feeding. In *Nutritional Anthropology*, ed. F. E. Johnston. New York: Alan R. Liss, 155–72.

Gussler, Judith, and Nancy Mock. 1983. A Comparative Description of Infant Feeding Practices in Zaire, the Philippines and St. Kitts–Nevis. *Ecology of Food and Nutrition* 13:75–85.

Gussow, Zachary W. 1960. "Piblotoq" (Hysteria) among the Polar Eskimo: An Ethno-Psychiatric Study. In *Psychoanalysis and the Social Sciences*, ed. W. Muensterberger and S. Axelrod. New York: International Universities Press.

———. 1989. *Leprosy, Racism, and Public Health: Social Policy and Chronic Disease Control.* Boulder, Colo.: Westview Press.

Gutmann, Amy. 1992. Introduction to *Multiculturalism and "The Politics of Recognition."* Princeton, N.J.: Princeton University Press.

Guttentag, Marcia, and Paul F. Secord. 1983. *Too Many Women?* Beverly Hills, Calif.: Sage.

Guttmacher, Sally, and L. Garcia. 1975. Social Science and Health in Cuba. Ideology, Planning, and Health. In *Topias and Utopias*, ed. S. Ingman and A. Thomas. The Hague: Mouton.

Guyer, J. 1988. Changing Nuptiality in Nigerian Community: Observations from the Field. Paper presented at IUSSP workshop on Nuptiality in Sub-Saharan Africa: Current Changes and Impact on Policy, Paris.

Hackenberg, Robert A., Beverly H. Hackenberg, Henry F. Mogalit, Esperonza I. Cabral, and Santiago V. Guzman. 1983. Migration, Modernization, and Hypertension. *Medical Anthropology* 7:45–71.

Hagey, R. S. 1980. Healing Entrepreneurship in the Philippines. Ph.D. dissertation, Case Western Reserve.

Hahn, Robert A. 1983a. Biomedical Practice and Anthropological Theory: Frameworks and Directions. *Annual Review of Anthropology* 12:305–33.

———. 1983b. Culture and Informed Consent. In *Making Choices. Report of the President's Commission for Ethical Problems in Medicine and Biomedical and Behavioral Research.* Washington, D.C.: Government Printing Office, 37–62.

———. 1984. Rethinking "Illness" and "Disease." *Contributions to Asian Studies* 18:1–23.

———. 1985. Culture-Bound Syndromes Unbound. *Social Science and Medicine* 21:165–71.

———. 1995. *Sickness and Healing: An Anthropological Perspective.* New Haven: Yale University Press.

Hahn, Robert A., and Atwood D. Gaines, eds. 1985. *Physicians of Western Medicine: Anthropological Approaches to Theory and Practice.* Dordrecht: D. Reidel.

Hahn, Robert, and Arthur Kleinman. 1983a. Belief as Pathogen, Belief as Medicine. *Medical Anthropology Quarterly* 14(4):3,16–19.

———. 1983b. Biomedical Practice and Anthropological Theory. *Annual Review of Anthropology* 12:305–33.

———. 1984. Rethinking "Illness" and "Disease." *Contributions to Asian Studies* 18:1–23.

Haldane, J. B. S. 1949. Disease and Evolution. *La Ricerca Scientifica* 19:68–76.

Hale, Sondra. 1981. History, Development, and Liberation: Northern Sudanese Women. Paper presented at the African Studies Association Annual Meeting, Los Angeles, November.

Halifax, Joan, and H. Weidman. 1973. Religion as a Mediating Institution in Acculturation. In *Religious Systems and Psychotherapy*, ed. Richard Cox. Springfield, Ill.: Charles C. Thomas.

Hall, R. L., V. M. Hesselbrock, and J. R. Stabenau. 1983. Familial Distribution of Alcohol Use: I Assortative Mating in the Parents of Alcoholics. *Behavior Genetics* 13:361–72.

Hall, Roberta A. 1986. Alcohol Treatment in American Indian Populations: An Indigenous Treatment Modality Compared with Traditional Approaches. In *Alcohol and Culture*, ed. Thomas F. Babor. New York: New York Academy of Sciences.

Hallowell, A. Irving. 1934. Culture and Mental Disorder. *Journal of Abnormal and Social Psychology* 29:1–9.

———. 1938. Fear and Anxiety as Cultural and Individual Variables in a Primitive Society. *Journal of Social Psychology* 147(11):1449–56.

————. 1955. The Self on Its Behavioral Environment. In *Culture and Experience*. Philadelphia: University of Pennsylvania Press.

Halmos, P. 1973. *Professonalisation and Social Change*. Keele, England: Sociological Review.

Hammady, Iman. 1979. Islamic Medical Centers in Egypt: A Case Study. Unpublished abstract.

Hammel, E. A. 1983. *The China Lectures*. Program in Population Research Working Paper, no. 10. University of California, Berkeley.

Hammel, E. A., and Nancy Howell. 1987. Research in Population and Culture: An Evolutionary Framework. *Current Anthropology* 28:141–60.

Hammerschmidt, Dale E. 1986. Chinese Diet and Traditional Materia Medica: Effects on Platelet Function and Atherogenesis. In *Plants in Indigenous Medicine and Diet,* ed. N. L. Etkin. Beford Hills, N.Y.: Redgrave, 171–85.

Hammond, E. C., Selikoff, I. J., and H. Seidman. 1979. Asbestos Exposure, Cigarette Smoking and Death Rates. *Annals of the New York Academy of Science* 330:473–90.

Hanhart, J. 1993. Women's Views on Norplant: A Study from Lombok, Indonesia. In *Norplant: Under Her Skin,* ed. B. Minzes, A. Hardon, and J. Hanhart. Amsterdam: Women's Health Action Foundation, 27–46.

Handlin, Oscar. 1951. *The Uprooted*. Boston: Little, Brown.

Handwerker, Lisa. 1994. Medical Risk: Implicating Poor Pregnant Women. *Social Science and Medicine* 38(5):665–75.

————. 1995. Social and Ethical Implications of In Vitro Fertilization in Contemporary China. *Cambridge Quarterly of Healthcare Ethics* 4:355–63.

Handwerker, W. Penn. 1974. Changing Household Organization in the Origins of Market Places in Liberia. *Economic Development and Cultural Change* 22:229–48.

————. 1979. Daily Markets and Urban Economic Development. *Human Organization* 40:27–39.

————. 1980. Market Places, Travelling Traders, and Shops: Commercial Structural Variation in the Liberian Interior prior to 1940. *African Economic History* 9:3–26.

————. 1983. The First Demographic Transition. *American Anthropologist* 85:5–27.

————. 1986. The Modern Demographic Transition. *American Anthropologist* 88:400–17.

————. 1988. Sampling Variability in Microdemographic Estimation of Fertility Parameters. *Human Biology* 60:305–18.

————. 1989a. *Women's Power and Social Revolution*. Newbury Park, Calif.: Sage Publications.

————. 1989b. The Origins and Evolution of Culture. *American Anthropologist* 91(2):313–27.

————. 1989c. *Population, Power, and Evolution*. Manuscript.

————. 1990. Demography. In *Medical Anthropology: Contemporary Theory and Method,* ed. Thomas M. Johnson and Carolyn F. Sargent. Westport, Conn.: Praeger Publishers.

Hanks, L. M., and J. R. Hanks. 1955. Diphtheria Immunization in a Thai Community. In *Health, Culture, and Community,* ed. B. D. Paul. New York: Russell Sage Foundation, 155–85.

Hanna, Joel M., Gary D. James, and Joann M. Martz. 1986. Hormonal Measures of Stress. In *The Changing Samoans: Behavior and Health in Transition,* ed. Paul T. Baker, Joel M. Hanna, and Thelma S. Baker. New York: Oxford University Press.

Haraway, Donna. 1988. The Biopolitics of Postmodern Bodies: Determinations of Self in Immune System Discourse. Manuscript prepared for the Wenner-Gren Foundation in Anthropology.

————. 1991. *Simians, Cyborgs and Women: The Reinvention of Nature*. New York: Routledge.

Hardy, M. 1983. Metaparadigms and Theory Development. In *The Nursing Profession: A Time to Speak,* ed. N. L. Chaska. New York: McGraw-Hill, 421–37.

Haring, Douglas, ed. 1956. *Personal Character and Cultural Milieu*. Syracuse: Syracuse University Press.

Harrell, B. B. 1981. Lactation and Menstruation in Cultural Perspective. *American Anthropology* 83:796–823.

Harris, Grace. 1978. *Casting Out Anger: Religion among the Taita of Kenya*. Cambridge: Cambridge University Press.

Harris, H. W., and J. H. McClement. 1983. Pulmonary Tuberculosis. In P. D. Hoeprich, ed., *Infectious Diseases*. New York: Harper & Row.

Harris, Marvin. 1974. *Cows, Pigs, Wars and Witches*. New York: Vintage.

————. 1979. *Cultural Materialism: The Struggle for a Science of Culture.* New York: Random House.

Harris, Marvin, and Eric B. Ross, eds. 1987a. *Death, Sex, and Fertility.* New York: Columbia University Press.

————. 1987b. *Food and Evolution: Toward a Theory of Human Food Habits.* Philadelphia: Temple University Press.

Harris, Olivia, and Kate Young. 1981. Engendered Structures: Some Problems in the Analysis of Reproduction. In *The Anthropology of Pre-Capitalist Societies,* ed. Joel Kahn and Josep Llobera. London: Macmillan, 109–47.

Harrison, Faye V. 1991. *Decolonizing Anthropology: Moving further toward an Anthropology of Liberation.* Washington, D.C. American Anthropological Association.

Harrison, Gail G. 1975. Primary Adult Lactose Deficiency: A Problem in Anthropological Genetics. *American Anthropologist* 77:812–35.

Harrison, Lawrence. 1985. *Underdevelopment Is a State of Mind.* Lanham, Md.: University Press of America.

Hart, Donn V. 1969. *Bisayan Filipino and Malayan Humoral Pathologies: Folk Medicine and History in Southeast Asia.* Southeast Asia Data Paper. Cornell University.

Hart, Keith. 1982. *The Political Economy of West African Agriculture.* Cambridge: Cambridge University Press.

Hartmann, Betsy. 1987. *Reproductive Rights and Wrongs: The Global Politics of Population Control and Contraceptive Choice.* New York: Harper & Row.

Hartmann, Heinz, Ernest Kris, and Rudolph M. Loewenstein. 1969. Some Psychoanalytic Comments on "Culture and Personality." In *Man and His Culture,* ed. Warner Muensterberger. New York: Taplinger (orig. 1951), 239–270.

Hartog, Joseph, and Elizabeth Ann Hartog. 1983. Cultural Aspects of Health and Illness Behavior in Hospitals. *Western Journal of Medicine* 139(6):910–17.

Harwood, Alan. 1971. The Hot-Cold Theory of Disease: Implications for Treatment of Puerto Rican Patients. *Journal of the American Medical Association* 216:1153–58.

————. 1977a. Puerto Rican Spiritism Part I—Description and Analysis of an Alternative Psychotherapeutic Approach. *Culture, Medicine and Psychiatry* 1:69–95.

————. 1977b. Puerto Rican Spiritism Part 2—An Institution with Preventive and Therapeutic Functions in Community Psychiatry. *Culture, Medicine and Psychiatry* 1:135–53.

————. 1977c. *RX: Spiritist As Needed. A Study of a Puerto Rican Community Mental Health Resource.* New York: John Wiley and Sons.

Harwood, Alan, ed. 1981. *Ethnicity and Medical Care.* Cambridge: Harvard University Press.

Hasan, Khwaja A. 1975. What Is Medical Anthropology? *Medical Anthropology Newsletter* 6(3): 7–10.

Hatch, Elvin. 1983. *Culture and Morality: The Relativity of Values in Anthropology.* New York: Columbia University Press.

Head, Henry. 1920. *Studies in Neurology.* 2 vols. London: Hodder Stoughton.

Heath, Deborah, and Paul Rabinow. 1993. An Introduction to Bio-Politics: The Anthropology of the New Genetics and Immunology. *Culture, Medicine, and Psychiatry* 17:27–41.

Heath, Dwight B. 1958. Drinking Patterns of the Bolivian Camba: *Quarterly Journal of Studies on Alcohol* 19:491–508.

————. 1971. Peasants, Revolution, and Drinking: Interethnic Drinking Patterns in Two Bolivian Communities. *Human Organization* 30(2):179–86.

————. 1975. A Critical Review of Ethnographic Studies of Alcohol Use. In *Research Advances in Alcohol and Drug Problems,* vol 2, ed. R. Gibbins et al. New York: John Wiley and Sons.

————. 1976. Anthropological Perspectives on Alcohol: An Historical Review. In *Cross-Cultural Approaches to the Study of Alcohol: An Interdisciplinary Approach,* ed. M. Everett et al. The Hague: Mouton.

———. 1983. Alcohol Use among North American Indians: A Cross-cultural Survey of Patterns and Problems. In *Research Advances in Alcohol and Drug Problems,* vol. 7, ed. R. Smart, et al. New York: Plenum.

———. 1984. Cross-cultural Studies of Alcoholism. In *Recent Developments in Alcoholism,* vol. 2, ed. Marc Galanter. New York: Plenum.

———. 1985. American Experiences with Alcohol: Commonalities and Contrasts. In *The American Experience with Alcohol,* ed. L. Bennett and G. Ames. New York: Plenum.

———. 1986. Concluding Remarks. In *Alcohol and Culture: Comparative Perspectives from Europe and America,* vol. 472, ed. Thomas F. Babor. New York: New York Academy of Sciences, 234–36.

———. 1987a. A Decade of Development in the Anthropological Study of Alcohol Use, 1970–1980. In *Constructive Drinking,* ed. Mary Douglas. Cambridge: Cambridge University Press.

———. 1987b. Anthropology and Alcohol Studies: Current Issues. *Annual Review of Anthropology* 16: 99–120.

———. 1988. Alcohol Control Policies and Drinking Patterns: An International Game of Politics against Science. *Journal of Substance Abuse* 1:121–25.

———. 1991. Women and Alcohol: Cross-Cultural Perspectives. *Journal of Substance Abuse* 3: 175–85.

Heath, Dwight B., ed. 1985. Alcohol Studies and Anthropology: Methodological and Practical Issues. Abstracts published in *Drinking and Drug Practices Surveyor* 20:48–53.

Heath, Dwight B., and A. M. Cooper. 1981. *Alcohol Use and World Cultures: A Comprehensive Bibliography of Anthropological Sources.* Bibliographic Series 15. Toronto: Addiction Research Foundation.

Heath, Dwight B., Jack O. Waddell, and Martin D. Topper, eds. 1981. Cultural Factors in Alcohol Research and Treatment of Drinking Problems. *Journal of Studies on Alcohol* Suppl. 9.

Hefferty, F., and J. McKinley. 1993. *The Changing Medical Profession: An International Perspective.* New York: Oxford University Press.

Heggenhougen, H. K. 1984a. Traditional Medicine and the Treatment of Drug Addicts: Three Examples from Southeast Asia. *Medical Anthropology Quarterly* 16(1):3–7.

———. 1984b. Will Primary Health Care Efforts Be Allowed to Succeed? *Social Science and Medicine* 19(3):217–24.

Heidegger, Martin. 1962. *Being and Time.* New York: Harper & Row.

Heinrich, M., H. Rimpler, and N. Antonio Barrera. 1992. Indigenous Phytotherapy of Gastrointestinal Disorders in a Lowland Mixe Community (Oaxaca, Mexico): Ethnopharmacologic Evaluation. *Journal of Ethnopharmacology* 36:63–80.

Heitman, Elizabeth. 1994. Cultural Diversity and the Clinical Encounter: Intercultural Dialogue in Multi-Ethnic Patient Care. In *Theological Analysis of the Clinical Encounter,* ed. G. P. McKenny and J. R. Sande. Kluwer Academic Publishers, 203–23.

Helitzer-Allen, D., M. Makhambera, and A. M. Wangel. 1994. *Obtaining Sensitive Information: The Need for More Than Focus Groups.* Reproductive Health Matters 3. Delhi, India, 75–82.

Helman, Cecil. 1978. Feed a Cold, Starve a Fever: Folk Models of Infection in an English Suburban Community and Their Relation to Medical Treatment. *Culture, Medicine and Psychiatry* 2: 107–37.

———. 1984a. Interpreting the Evidence on Social Support. *Social Psychiatry* 19:49–52.

———. 1984b. *Culture, Health and Illness.* Bristol: John Wright & Sons Ltd.

———. 1985. Psyche, Soma and Society: The Social Construction of Psychosomatic Disorders. *Culture, Medicine and Psychiatry* 9:1–26.

———. 1987. Heart Disease and the Cultural Construction of Time: The Type A Behaviour Pattern as a Western Culture-Bound Syndrome. *Social Science and Medicine* 25(9):969–79.

Henderson, A. S. 1984a. Heart Disease and the Cultural Construction of Time. *Social Science and Medicine* 25:969–79.

————. 1984b. Interpreting the Evidence on Social Support. *Social Psychiatry* 9:49–52. Henderson, B. E., et al. 1976. Risk Factors Associated with Nasopharyngeal Carcinoma. *New England Journal of Medicine* 295:1101–6.

Henderson, P. 1975. Population Policy, Social Structure and the Health System in Puerto Rico: The Case of Female Sterilization. Ph. D. dissertation, University of Connecticut.

Hennekens, Charles H., and J. E. Buring. 1987. *Epidemiology in Medicine.* Boston: Little, Brown.

Henry, J. P., and J. C. Cassel. 1969. Psychosocial Factors in Essential Hypertension. *American Journal of Epidemiology* 90:171–200.

Henry, Jules. 1963. *Culture against Man.* New York: Random House.

Henry, Jules, and Melford E. Spiro. 1953. Psychological Techniques: Projective Tests in Field Work. In *Anthropology Today,* ed. A. L. Kroeber. Chicago: University of Chicago Press, 417–29.

Herman, Elizabeth. n.d. Personal communication.

Herrick, James. 1983. The Symbolic Roots of Three Potent Iroquois Medicinal Plants. In *The Anthropology of Medicine,* ed. Lola Romanucci-Ross, Daniel Moerman, and L. Tancredi. New York: Bergin & Garvey, 134–55.

Herskovits, M. 1972. *Cultural Relativism: Perspectives in Cultural Pluralism.* New York: Random House.

Herz, Barbara, and Anthony Measham. 1987. *The Safe Motherhood Initiative: Proposals for Action.* Washington, D.C.: World Bank.

Hess, David J. 1995. *Science and Technology in a Multicultural World: The Cultural Politics of Facts and Artifacts.* New York: Columbia University Press.

Hess, David J., and Linda Layne, eds. 1992. *The Anthropology of Science and Technology.* Knowledge and Society, vol. 9. Greenwich, Conn.: JAI Press.

Heurtin-Roberts, Suzanne. 1995. Exiting the Ivory Tower for the Real World: A Comment on Critical Praxis. *Medical Anthropology Quarterly* 9(1):110–12.

Heyneman, D. 1971. Mis-Aid to the Third World: Disease Repercussions Caused by Ecological Ignorance. *Canadian Journal of Public Health* 62:303–13.

————. 1979. Dams and Disease. *Human Nature* 2(2):50–57.

————. 1983. Development and Disease: A Dual Dilemma. *Journal of Parasitology* 70:3–17.

Heywood, Arthur. 1991. *Primary Health Care in the Atatcora, Benin.* Amsterdam: Royal Tropical Institute.

Hill, Carole E. 1988. Review of *Culture, Politics and Medicine in Costa Rica* by Setha Low. *American Ethnologist* 15(1):173.

Hill, Carole E., ed. 1985. *Training Manual in Medical Anthropology.* Washington, D.C.: American Anthropological Association.

Hill, Polly. 1986. *Development Economics on Trial: The Anthropological Case for the Prosecution.* Cambridge: Cambridge University Press.

Hill, Thomas W. 1978. Drunken Comportment of Urban Indians: "Time-out" Behavior? *Journal of Anthropological Research* 34(3):442–67.

————. 1984. Ethnohistory and Alcohol Studies. In *Recent Developments in Alcoholism,* vol. 2, ed. Marc Galanter. New York: Plenum.

Hillier, S. M., and J. A. Jewell. 1983. *Health Care and Traditional Medicine in China, 1800–1982.* London: Routledge & Kegan Paul.

Himes, Norman. 1970. *Medical History of Contraception.* New York: Schocken Books.

Hippler, Arthur E. 1974. The North Alaska Eskimos: A Culture and Personality Perspective. *American Ethnologist* 1(3):449–69.

————. 1977. Discussion and Debate: On Stein and Kleinman, and the Crucial Issues in Medical Anthropology. *Medical Anthropology Newsletter* 9(1):18–19.

Ho, H. C. 1972. Current Knowledge of the Epidemiology of NPC: A Review. In *Oncogenesis and Herpesviruses.* Lyon: IARC, 357–66.

Hoben, Allan. 1982. Anthropologists and Development. *Annual Review of Anthropology* 11:349–75.

Hofferth, Sandra J., and Cheryl D. Hayes, eds. 1987. *Risking the Future: Adolescent Sexuality, Pregancy, and Childbearing.* Washington, D.C.: National Research Council, National Academy Press.

Hoffmaster, Barry. 1990. Morality and the Social Sciences. In *Social Science Perspectives on Medical Ethics,* ed. George Weiss. Philadelphia: University of Pennsylvania Press, 241–60.

———. 1992. Can Ethnography Save the Life of Medical Ethics? *Social Science and Medicine* 35(12):1421–32.

Hogarth, Robin M., and Melvin W. Reder, eds. 1987. *Rational Choice.* Chicago: University of Chicago Press.

Hogle, Linda F. Standardization across Non-Standard Domains: The Case of Organ Procurement. *Science, Technology and Human Values* (in press).

Hollan, Douglas. 1988. Staying "Cool" in Toraja: Informal Strategies of the Management of Anger and Hostility in a Nonviolent Society. *Ethos* 16:52–72.

———. 1994. Suffering and the Work of Culture: A Case of Magical Poisoning in Toraja. *American Ethnologist* 21:74–87.

Hollan, Douglas, and Jane Wellenkamp. 1994. *Contentment and Suffering: Culture and Experience in Toraja.* New York: Columbia University Press.

Holland, Celia V. 1989. Man and His Parasites: Integration of Biomedical and Social Approaches to Transmission and Control. *Social Science and Medicine* 29:403–11.

Holland, Dorothy. 1992. How Cultural Systems Become Desire: A Case Study of American Romance. In *Human Motives and Cultural Models,* ed. Roy D'Andrade and Claudia Strauss. Cambridge: Cambridge University Press.

Holland, William R. 1963a. *Medicina Maya en los Altos de Chiapas.* Mexico: Instituto Nacional Indigenista.

———. 1963b. Mexican-American Medical Beliefs: Science or Magic? *Arizona Medicine* 89 102.

Holmberg, Allan R. 1971. The Rhythms of Drinking in a Peruvian Coastal Mestizo Community. *Human Organization* 30(2):198–202.

Holmes, Helen B., and Laura M. Purdy. 1992. *Feminist Perspectives in Medical Ethics.* Bloomington: Indiana University Press.

Holmes T. H., and R. H. Rahe. 1967. The Social Readjustment Rating Scale. *Journal of Psychosomatic Research* 11:213–18.

Honigmann, John J. 1947. Witch-Fear in Post-Contact Kaska Society. *American Anthropologist* 49: 222–43.

———. 1956. Toward a Distinction between Psychiatric and Social Abnormality. In *Personal Character and Cultural Milieu,* ed. Douglas G. Haring. Syracuse, N.Y.: Syracuse University Press, 429–45.

Hook, E. B. 1978. Dietary Cravings and Aversions during Pregnancy. *American Journal of Clinical Nutrition* 31:1355–62.

———. 1980. Influence of Pregnancy on Dietary Selection. *International Journal of Obesity* 4: 338–40.

Hook, R. H. 1979. Phantasy and Symbol: A Psychoanalytic Point of View. In *Fantasy and Symbol: Studies in Anthropological Interpretation,* ed. R. H. Hook. New York: Academic Press, 267–91.

Hooley, J., J. Orley, and J. D. Teasedale. 1986. Levels of Expressed Emotion and Relapse in Depressed Patients. *British Journal of Psychiatry* 148:642–47.

Hopkins, D. R. 1983. *Princes and Peasants: Small Pox in History.* Chicago and London: Chicago University Press.

Hopkins, Lawrence, and Immanual Wallerstein. 1967. The Comparative Study of National Societies. Social Science Information n. 6:25–58.

Hopper, Kim. 1975. Of Language and the Sorcerer's Appendix: A Critical Appraisal of Horacio Fabrega's *Disease and Social Behavior. Medical Anthropology Newsletter* 19(3):9–14.

———. 1982. Discussant comments following the organized session, The Lure and Haven of Illness, 81st Annual Meeting of the American Anthropological Association, Washington, D.C.

———. 1988. More Than Passing Stranger: Homelessness and Mental Illness in New York City. *American Ethnologist* 15(1):155–67.

———. 1991. Some Old Questions for the New Cross-Cultural Psychiatry. *Medical Anthropology Quarterly* 5(4):299–330.

———. 1992. Cervantez's Puzzle—A Commentary on Alex Cohen's Prognosis for Schizophrenia in the Third World: A Re-evaluation of Cross-Cultural Research. *Culture, Medicine, and Psychiatry* 16(1):89–100.

Horn, G. H. 1986a. Hepatitis B, a Serious Health Concern in Egypt. *Cairo Today* 8(1):53–55.

———. 1986b. Feeding Egypt. *Cairo Today* 7(2):24–27.

Horn, James J. 1985. Brazil: The Health Care Model of the Military Modernizers and Technocrats. *International Journal of Health Services* 15(1):47–68.

Horowitz, M. J. 1966. Body Image. *Archives of General Psychiatry* 14:456–61.

Horton, Donald J. 1943. The Functions of Alcohol in Primitive Societies: A Cross-Cultural Study. *Quarterly Journal of Studies on Alcohol* 4:199–320.

House, James S., and Robert L. Kahn. 1985. Measures and Concepts of Social Support. In *Social Support and Health,* ed. Sheldon Cohen and S. Leonard Syme. Orlando, Fla.: Academic Press.

Howell, Nancy. 1979. *The Demography of the Dobe !Kung.* New York: Academic Press.

———. 1986. Demographic Anthropology. *Annual Review of Anthropology* 15:219–46.

Howell, Signe. 1984. *Society and Cosmos: Chewong of Peninsular Malaysia.* New York: Oxford University Press.

Howes, David. 1991. *The Varieties of Sensory Experience: A Sourcebook in the Anthropology of the Senses.* Toronto: University of Toronto Press.

Hrdy, D. 1987. Cultural Practices Contributing to the Transmission of Human Immunodeficiency Virus in Africa. *Reviews of Infectious Disease* 9(6):1109–19.

Huang, D. P., J. H. C. Ho, and T. A. Gough. 1978. Analysis for Volatile Nitrosamines in Salt-Preserved Foodstuffs Traditionally Consumed by Southern Chinese. In *NPC: Etiology and Control,* ed. G. de-The and Y. Ito. Lyon: IARC, 309–14.

Hudelson, P. 1989. Management of Diarrhea in Managua, Nicaragua. Ph.D. dissertation, University of Connecticut.

Huffman, S. L., A. K. M. A. Chowdhury, and W. H. Mosley. 1978. Postpartum Amenorrhea: How Is It Affected by Maternal Nutritional Status? *Science* 200:1155–57.

Hufford, David J. 1988. Review: Simons, Ronald C. and Charles C. Hughes, *The Culture-Bond Syndromes: Folk Illnesses of Psychiatric and Anthropological Interest. Culture, Medicine, and Psychiatry* 12:503–12.

Hugh-Jones, C. 1979. *From the Milk of the River: Spatial and Temporal Process in Northwest Amazonia.* Cambridge: Cambridge University Press.

Hughes, Charles C. 1968. Ethnomedicine. In *International Encyclopedia of the Social Sciences,* ed. David Sills. Vol. 10. New York: Crowell Collier and Macmillan, 87–92.

———. 1985a. Culture-Bound or Construct-Bound? In *The Culture-Bound Syndromes: Folk Illnesses of Psychiatric and Anthropological Interest,* ed. Ronald C. Simons and Charles C. Hughes. Dordrecht: D. Reidel, 3–24.

———. 1985b. Glossary of 'Culture-Bound' or Folk Psychiatric Syndromes. In *The Culture-Bound Syndromes: Folk Illnesses of Psychiatric and Anthropological Interest,* ed. Ronald C. Simons and Charles C. Hughes. Dordrecht: D. Reidel, 469–505.

———. 1989. On Fabrega and "Cultural Relativism." *Journal of Nervous and Mental Disease* 177(7):426–30.

———. 1993. Culture in Clinical Psychiatry. In *Culture, Ethnicity, and Mental Illness,* ed. Albert C. Gaw. Washington, D.C.: American Psychiatric Press, 3–41.

Hughes, Charles, and John Hunter. 1970. Disease and "Development" in Africa. *Social Science and Medicine* 3:443–93.

————. 1971. Disease and "Development" in Africa. In *The Social Organization of Health*, ed. H. Dreitzel. New York: Macmillan, 150–214.

Hughes, Charles C., and Donald A. Kennedy. 1983. Beyond the Germ Theory: Reflections on Relations between Medicine and the Behavioral Sciences. In *Advances in Medical Social Science,* ed. Julio L. Ruffini. New York: Gordon and Breach Science Publishers, 321–99.

Hull, Diana. 1979 Migration, Adaptation, and Illness: A Review. *Social Science and Medicine* 13A: 25–36.

Humphrey, Derek. 1991. *Final Exit.* Eugene, Ore.: Hemlock Society.

Hunscher, H., and I. Macy. 1951. Dietary Study Methods. I. Uses and Abuses of Dietary Study Methods. *Journal of the American Dietetic Association* 27:558–63.

Hunt, E. E. 1978. Ecological Frameworks and Hypothesis Testing in Medical Anthropology. In *Health and the Human Condition,* ed. M. H. Logan and E. E. Hunt. North Scituate, Mass.: Duxbury Press, 84–100.

Hunt, Linda M. 1985. Relativism in the Diagnosis of Hypoglycemia. *Social Science and Medicine* 20:1289–94.

————. 1992. To Save a Life at All Costs: Ethical Issues in the Context of Mexican Biomedicine. Paper Presented to the 91st Annual Meeting of the American Anthropological Association, San Francisco.

Hunt, Linda M., Brigitte Jordan, Susan Irwin, and Carole H. Browner. 1989. Compliance and the Patient's Perspective. *Culture, Medicine and Psychiatry* 13(38):315–39.

Hunter, John M. 1973. Geophagy in Africa and in the United States: A Cultural Nutrition Hypothesis. *Geographical Review* 63:170–95.

Hunter, Kathryn Montgomery. 1989. A Science of Individuals: Medicine and Casuistry. *Journal of Medicine and Philosophy* 14:193–212.

————. 1991. *Doctors' Stories: The Narrative Structure of Medical Knowledge.* Princeton: Princeton University Press.

Husting, E. L. 1970. Sociological Patterns and Their Influence on the Transmission of Bilharziasis. *Central African Journal of Medicine* (July Suppl.):5–10.

————. 1983. Human Water Contact Activities Related to the Transmission of Bilharziasis (Schistosomiasis). *Journal of Tropical Medicine and Hygiene* 86:23–35.

Hutchinson, Janis. 1986. Association between Stress and Blood Pressure Variation in a Caribbean Population. *American Journal of Physical Anthropology* 71:69–79.

Hutchinson, S. A. 1984. Creating Meaning Out of Horror. *Nursing Outlook* 32(2):86–90.

Huxtable, Ryan J. 1992. The Pharmacology of Extinction. *Journal of Ethnopharmacology* 37:1–11.

Hymes, Dell. 1969. *Re-Inventing Anthropology.* New York: Random House.

Iamo, Wari. 1987. One of the Things That Brings Good Name is Betel: A Keakalo Conception of Betel Use. In *Drugs in Western Pacific Societies,* ASAO Monograph No. 11., ed. Lamont Lindstrom. Lanham, Md. University Press of America, 135–48.

————. 1972. The Use of Anthropology: Critical, Political, Personal. In *Re-Inventing Anthropology.* New York: Holt, Reinhart and Winston, 3–83.

ICD-9. 1980. International Classification of Diseases, 9th rev. In *Clinical Modification,* vol. 1. 2d ed. DHHS Publication no. (IPHS) 801260. Washington, D.C.: U.S. Department of Health and Human Services, Public Health Service—Health Care Financing Administration.

IFDA (International Forum for Development Alternatives). 1980. Building Blocks for Alternative Development Strategies: A Progress Report from the Third System Project. *Dossier 17* (May–June).

Ijsselmuiden, Carel B., and Ruth Faden. 1992. Research and Informed Consent in Africa—Another Look. *New England Journal of Medicine* 326(12):830–34.

Ilfeld, Frederic W. 1977. Current Social Stressors and Symptoms of Depression. *American Journal of Psychiatry* 134:161–66.

Illich, I. 1975. *Medical Nemesis: The Expropriation of Health.* London: Calder and Boyars.

————. 1976. *Medical Nemesis: The Expropriation of Health.* New York: Bantam.

Imhof, Arthur. 1985. From the Old Mortality Pattern to the New: Implications of a Radical Change from the Sixteenth to the Twentieth Century. *Bulletin of the History of Medicine* 59:1–29.

Inglis, B. 1964. *Fringe Medicine.* London: Faber.

Inhorn, Marcia. 1994. *Quest for Conception: Gender, Infertility, and Egyptian Medical Traditions.* Philadelphia: University of Pennsylvania Press.

Inhorn, Marcia C., and Peter J. Brown. 1990. The Anthropology of Infectious Disease. *Annual Review of Anthropology* 19:89–117.

Inhorn, Marcia C., and Kimberly A. Buss. 1993. Infertility, Infection, and Iatrogenesis in Egypt: The Anthropological Epidemiology of Blocked Tubes. *Medical Anthropology* 15:217–44.

———. 1994. Ethnography, Epidemiology and Infertility in Egypt. *Social Science and Medicine* 39(5):671–86.

Institute of Medicine. 1991. *Nutrition during Lactation.* Washington, D.C.: National Academy Press.

———. 1992. *Emerging Infections: Microbial Threats to Health in the United States.* Washington, D.C.: National Academy Press.

International Bank for Reconstruction and Development. 1988. *Social Indicators of Development.* Baltimore: Johns Hopkins University Press.

International Conference on Population. 1984. *New Hope in Dark Times: UNICEF's Assessment of Past Experience with a Child Survival Package: Its Effectiveness and Its Social and Economic Feasibility.* United Nations Children's Fund, Expert Group on Mortality and Health Policy. Rome, May 30–June 3, 1983.

Iris, Madelaine Anne. 1990. Uses of Guardianship as a Protective Intervention for Frail Older Adults. *Journal of Elder Abuse and Neglect* 2(3–4):57–71.

———. 1995. The Ethics of Decision Making for the Critically Ill Elderly. *Cambridge Quarterly of Healthcare Ethics* 4(2):135–41.

Irwin, K., et al. 1991. Knowledge, Attitudes and Beliefs about HIV Infection and AIDS among Health Factory Workers and Their Wives in Kinshasa, Zaire. *Social Science and Medicine* 32(8):917–30.

Irwin, Susan, and Brigitte Jordan. 1987. Knowledge, Practice, and Power: Court-Ordered Cesarean Sections. *Medical Anthropology Quarterly* n.s. 1(3):319–34.

Isaacs, Hope. 1983. On Teaching Medical Anthropology to Clinicians: Is It Clinical Anthropology? In *Clinical Anthropology,* ed. Demitri Shimkin and Peggy Golde. Lanham, Md.: University Press of America, 259–67.

Ishikawa, Eisei, and David L. Swain, trans. 1981. *The Committee on the Compilation of Materials on Damage Caused by the Atomic Bombs in Hiroshima and Nagasaki.* New York: Basic Books.

Jachimowicz, Edith, 1975. Islamic Cosmology. In *Ancient Cosmologies,* ed. Carmen Blacker and Michael Lowe. London: George Allen and Unwin.

Jackson, I. M. D. 1984. That Thyroid Nodule: Is It Cancer? *Modern Medicine* 52:88–94.

Jackson, J. A., ed. 1970. *Professions and Professionalisation.* Cambridge: Cambridge University Press.

Jacob, J. 1988. *Doctors and Rules: A Sociology of Professional Values.* London: Routledge.

Jacobson, David. 1986. Types and Timing of Support. *Journal of Health and Social Behavior* 27: 250–64.

———. 1987. The Cultural Context of Social Support and Support Networks. *Medical Anthropology Quarterly* 1:42–67.

Jacobson, Gaynor. 1977. The Refugee Movement: An Overview. *International Migration Review* 11:514–23.

James, Sherman A. 1994. John Henryism and the Health of African-Americans. *Culture, Medicine and Psychiatry* 18:163–82.

James, Sherman A., Sue A. Hartnett, and William D. Kalsbeek. 1983. John Henryism and Blood Pressure Differences among Black Men. *Journal of Behavioral Medicine* 6:259–78.

James, Sherman A., David S. Strogatz, Steven B. Wing, and Diane L. Ramsey. 1987. Socioeconomic Status, John Henryism, and Hypertension in Blacks and Whites. *American Journal of Epidemiology* 126:664–73.

James, W. P. T., and P. Trayhurn. 1976. An Integrated View of the Metabolic and Genetic Basis for Obesity. *Lancet* 770–73.

James, Wendy. 1973. The Anthropologist as Reluctant Imperialist. In Talal Asad, ed., *Anthropology and the Colonial Encounter.* New London: Ithaca Press, 41–70.

James, William. 1884. What Is Emotion? *Mind* 9:188–205.

Jamison, Dean, et al. 1993. *World Development Report. Investing in Health. World Development Indicators.* Oxford: Oxford University Press World Bank.

Jamison, Dean T., Alberto M. Torres, Lincoln C. Chen, and Joseph L. Melnick. 1991. Poliomyelitis: What Are the Prospects for Eradication and Rehabilitation? *Health Policy and Planning* 6(2):107–18.

Jamous, H., and B. Peloille. 1970. Changes in the French University-Hospital System. In *Professions and Professionalisation,* ed. J. A. Jackson. Cambridge: Cambridge University Press, 111–53.

Janes, Craig R. 1986. Migration and Hypertension: An Ethnography of Disease Risk in an Urban Samoan Community. In *Anthropology and Epidemiology,* ed. C. Janes, et al. Dordecht: D. Reidel, 175–212.

———. 1990. *Migration, Social Change, and Health: A Samoan Community in Urban California.* Stanford: Stanford University Press.

———. 1995. The Transformations of Tibetian Medicine. *Medical Anthropology Quarterly* 9(1): 6–39.

Janes, Craig R., and Ivan G. Pawson. 1986. Migration and Biocultural Adaptation: Samoans in California. *Social Science and Medicine* 22:821–34.

Janes, Craig R., Ron Stall, and Sandra M. Gifford. 1986. *Anthropology and Epidemiology.* Dordecht: D. Reidel.

Janet, Pierre. 1924. *The Major Symptoms of Hysteria.* Harvard University Lectures. New York: Macmillan.

Janzen, John M. 1978a. The Comparative Study of Medical Systems as Changing Social Systems. *Social Science and Medicine* 12:121–29.

———. 1978b. *The Quest for Therapy In Lower Zaire.* Berkeley: University of California Press.

———. 1981. The Need for a Taxonomy of Health in the Study of African Therapeutics. *Social Science and Medicine* 15B:185–94.

———. 1982a. Drums Anonymous. In *Use and Abuse of Medicine,* ed. M. de Vries, R. L. Berg, and M. Lipkin. New York: Praeger, 154–66.

———. 1982b. *Lemba 1650–1930: A Drum of Affliction in Africa and the New World.* New York: Garland Publishing Co.

———. 1987. Therapy Management: Concept, Reality, Process. *Medical Anthropology Quarterly* 1:68–84.

———. 1992. *Ngoma: Discourses of Healing in Central and Southern Africa.* Berkeley: University of California Press.

Jecker, Nancy S., Joseph A. Carrese, and Robert Pearlman. 1995. Caring for Patients in Cross-Cultural Settings. *Hasting Center Report* 25(1):6–14.

Jeffery, R. 1988. *The Politics of Health in India.* Berkeley: University of California Press.

Jelliffe, Derrick B. 1957. Social Culture and Nutrition Culture Blocks and Protein Malnutrition in Early Childhood in Rural West Bengal. *Pediatrics* 20:128–38.

———. 1966. Diarrhoea in Childhood. In *Medical Care in Developing Countries,* ed. Maurice King. Nairobi: Oxford University Press, 15:2–15:6.

Jelliffe, D. B., and E. F. P. Jelliffe. 1975. Human Milk, Nutrition, and the World Resource Crisis. *Science* 188:557–60.

———. 1977. The Infant Food Industry and International Health. *International Journal of Health Services* 7:249–54.

Jellinek, E. M. 1952. Phases of Alcohol Addiction. *Quarterly Journal of Studies on Alcohol* 13: 673–84.

———. 1960. *The Disease Concept of Alcoholism.* Highland Park, N.J.: Hillhouse.

Jenkins, Janis H. 1988. Ethnopsychiatric Interpretations of Schizophrenic Illness: The Problem of Nervios within Mexican-American Families. *Culture, Medicine and Psychiatry* 12(3):303–31.

———. 1991a. The State Construction of Affect: Political Ethos and Mental Health among Salvadoran Refugees. *Culture, Medicine, and Psychiatry* 15:139–65.

———. 1991b. Anthropology, Expressed Emotion, and Schizophrenia. *Ethos: The Journal of the Society for Psychological Anthropology* 19:387–431.

———. 1994. Culture, Emotion and Psychopathology. In *Emotion and Culture: Empirical Studies of Mutal Influence,* ed. Shinobu Kitayama and Hazel Arkus. Washington, D.C.: American Psychiatric Association.

Jenkins, J. H., and M. Karno. 1992. The Meaning of "Expressed Emotion": Theoretical Issues Raised by Cross-Cultural Research. *American Journal of Psychiatry* 149:9–21.

Jenkins, J. H., A. Kleinman, and B. J. Good. 1991. Cross-Cultural Aspects of Depression. In *Advances in Affective Disorders: Theory and Research, Psychosocial Aspects,* ed. L. Becker and A. Kleinman. Vol. 1. Hillsdale, N.J.: Erlbaum.

Jenkins, Janis, and Martha Valienta. 1994. Bodily Transactions of the Passions: El Calor among Salvadoran Women Refugees. In *Emodiment and Experience: The Existeutial Ground of Culture and Self,* ed. Thomas Gordas. Cambridge: Cambridge University Press.

Jennings, Bruce. 1990. Ethics and Ethnography in Neonatal Intensive Care. In *Social Science Perspectives on Medical Ethics,* ed. George Weisz. Philadelphia: University of Pennsylvania Press, 261–72.

Jerome, Norge W., Randy F. Kandel, and Gretel Pelto, eds. 1980. *Nutritional Anthropology.* Pleasantville, N.Y.: Redgrave.

Jobin, W. R., and E. Ruiz-Tiben. 1968. Bilharzia and Patterns of Human Contact with Water in Puerto Rico. *Boletin Asociación Medica de Puerto Rico* 60:279–84.

Jocobsen, Rick. 1986. Using Organization to Pursue Political Economic Analysis: The Case for Primary Health Care for the Poor. *Medical Anthropology Quarterly* 17(5):131–32.

Johannes, Adell. 1986. Medicinal Plants of the New Guinea Highlands: An Ethnopharmacologic and Phytochemical Update. In *Plants in Indigenous Medicine and Diet,* ed. N. L. Etkin. Bedford Hills, N.Y.: Redgrave, 186–210.

Johansson, Sten, and Ola Nygren. 1991. The Missing Girls of China: A New Demographic Account. *Population and Development Review* 17:35–51.

Johns, Timothy A. 1986. Chemical Selection in Andean Domesticated Tubers as a Model for the Acquisition of Empirical Plant Knowledge. In *Plants in Indigenous Medicine and Diet: Biobehavioral Approaches,* ed. N. L. Etkin. Bedford Hills, N.Y.: Redgrave, 266–88.

———. 1990. *With Bitter Herbs They Shall Eat It: Chemical Ecology and the Origins of Human Diet and Medicine.* Tucson: University of Arizona Press.

Johns, Timothy, John O. Kokwaro, and Ebi K. Kimanani. 1990. Herbal Remedies of the Luo of Siaya District, Kenya: Establishing Quantitative Criteria for Consensus. *Economic Botany* 44:369–81.

Johns, Timothy, and Isao Kubo. 1988. A Survey of Traditional Methods Employed for the Detoxification of Plant Foods. *Journal of Ethnobiology* 8:81–129.

Johnson, Adeline, and Stanislaus Szurek. 1952. The Genesis of Antisocial Acting Out in Children and Adults. *Psychoanalytic Quarterly* 21:323–43.

Johnson, F. E., A. F. Roche, L. M. Schell, and H. N. B. Wettenhall. 1975. Critical Weight at Menarche: Critique of a Hypothesis. *American Journal of Diseases of Children* 129:19–23.

Johnson, Frank. 1985. The Western Conception of Self. In *Culture and Self,* ed. A. Marsella, George DeVos, and F. Hsu. London: Tavistock.

Johnson, Lyndon. 1965. Transcript of the President's Message to Congress on the State of the Union. *New York Times,* January 5.

Johnson, Terrence. 1972. *Professions and Power.* London: Macmillan.

———. 1973. Imperialism and the Professions. In *Professionalisation and Social Change,* ed. P. Halmos. Keele, England: Sociological Review, 281–309.

Johnson, Thomas M. 1981. The Anthropologist as a Role Model for Medical Students. *Practicing Anthropology* 4:8–10.

———. 1987a. Premenstrual Syndrome as a Western Culture-Specific Disorder. *Culture, Medicine, and Psychiatry* 11(3):337–56.

———. 1987b. Practicing Medical Anthropology: Clinical Strategies for Work in the Hospital. In *Applied Anthropology in America*, ed. Elizabeth Eddy and William Partridge. 2d ed. New York: Columbia University Press, 316–39.

———. 1987c. Consultation Psychiatry as Applied Medical Anthropology. In *Encounters with Biomedicine: Case Studies in Medical Anthropology*, ed. Hans A. Baer. New York: Gordon and Breach Science Publishers, 269–93.

———. 1991a. Anthropologists in Medical Education: Ethnographic Prescriptions. In *Training Manual in Applied Medical Anthropology*, ed. Carole E. Hill. 2d ed. Washington, D.C.: American Anthropological Association, 125–60.

———. 1991b. Anthropology and the World of Physicians. *Anthropology Newsletter* 32(8):20 and 32(9):16.

———. 1994. Presidential Message: On Paradigm Shifts in Medical Anthropology. *Anthropology Newsletter* (April): 31.

———. 1995. Critical Praxis beyond the Ivory Tower: A Critical Commentary. *Medical Anthropology Quarterly* 9(1):107–10.

Johnson, Thomas, ed. 1984. Perspectives on Post Doctoral Public Health Training for Medical Anthropologists. *Medical Anthropological Quarterly* 15(4):90–101.

Johnson, Thomas M., and Carolyn F. Sargent, eds. 1990. *Medical Anthropology: Contemporary Theory and Method.* New York: Praeger.

Johnston, Francis E., ed. 1987. *Nutritional Anthropology.* New York: Alan R. Liss.

Johnston, M., and M. E. Sarty. 1978. Maternal Beliefs about Vitamin Efficacy in Four U.S. Subcultures. *Journal of Cross-Cultural Psychology* 9:327–37.

Jones, Elise F., Jacqueline Darroch Forrest, Noreen Goldman, Stanley Henshaw, Richard Lincoln, Jeanie I. Rosoff, Charles F. Westoff, and Deirdre Wulf. 1986. *Teenage Pregnancy in Industrialized Countries.* New Haven: Yale University Press.

Jones, James. 1981. *Bad Blood: The Scandalous Story of the Tuskegee Experiment.* New York: Free Press.

Jong, J. T. V. M. de. 1987. *A Descent into African Psychiatry.* Amsterdam: Royal Tropical Institute.

Jonsen, Albert, and Stephen Toulmin. 1988. *The Abuse of Casuistry.* Berkeley: University of California Press.

———. 1991. Of Balloons and Bicycles—or—The Relationship between Ethical Theory and Practical Judgment. *Hastings Center Report* 21(5):14–16.

Joralemon, Donald. 1985. Altar Symbolism in Peruvian Ritual Healing. *Journal of Latin American Lore* 11:3–29.

———. 1995. Organ Wars: The Battle for Body Parts. *Medical Anthropology Quarterly* 9(3).

Jordan, Brigitte. 1977. The Self-Diagnosis of Early Pregnancy: An Investigation of Competence. *Medical Anthropology* 1(2):1–38.

———. 1978. *Childbirth in Four Cultures.* Montreal: Eden Press Women's Publications.

———. 1989. Cosmopolitical Obstetrics: Insights on the Training of Traditional Midwives. *Social Science and Medicine* 28(9):937–45.

———. 1993. Birth in Four Cultures: A Crosscultural Investigation of Childbirth in the Yucatan, Holland, Sweden, and the United States. Prospect Heights, IL: Waveland Press.

Jordan, Peter. 1985. *Schistosomiasis: The St. Lucia Project.* Cambridge: Cambridge University Press.

Joyce, C. R. B., and R. M. C. Welldon. 1965. The Objective Efficacy of Prayer: A Double-Blind Clinical Trial. *Journal of Chronic Diseases* 18:367–77.

Justice, Judithanne. 1983. The Invisible Worker: The Role of the Peon in Nepal's Health Service. *Social Science and Medicine* 17:967–70.

———. 1984. Can Socio-Cultural Information Improve Health Planning? A Case Study of Nepal's Assistant Nurse-Midwife. *Social Science and Medicine* 19:193–98.

————. 1986. *Policies, Plans and People: Culture and Health Development in Nepal.* Berkeley: University of California Press.

————. 1987. The Bureaucratic Context of International Health: A Social Scientist's View. *Social Science and Medicine* 25:1301–6.

Kahn, H. A., and C. T. Sempos. 1989. *Statistical Methods in Epidemiology.* New York: Oxford University Press.

Kakar, Sudhir. 1982. *Shamans, Mystics, and Doctors: A Psychological Inquiry into India and Its Healing Traditions.* New York: Alfred A. Knopf.

Kanner, Allen D., James C. Coyne, Catherine Schaefer, and Richard S. Lazarus. 1980. Comparison of Two Modes of Stress Measurement: Daily Hassles and Uplifts Versus Major Life Events. *Journal of Behavioral Medicine* 4:1–39.

Kao, F. F., and J. J. Kao, eds. 1979. *Recent Advances in Acupuncture Research.* Garden City, N.Y.: Institute for Advanced Research on Asian Science and Medicine.

Kapferer, Bruce. 1979a. Emotion and Feeling in Sinhalese Exorcism. *Social Analysis* 1:177–98.

————. 1979b. Entertaining Demons: Comedy, Interaction, and Meaning in a Sinhalese Healing Rite. *Social Analysis* 1:108–76.

————. 1983. A Celebration of Demons: Exorcism and the Aesthetics of Healing in Sri Lanka. Bloomington: University of Indiana Press.

Kaplan, Bert, ed. 1961. *Studying Personality Cross-Culturally.* Evanston, Ill.: Row Peterson.

Kaplan, David, and Robert A. Manners. 1972. *Culture and Theory.* Englewood Cliffs, N.J.: Prentice-Hall.

Kaplan, R. M. 1985. Behavioral Epidemiology, Health Promotion, and Health Services. *Medical Care* 23(5):564–83.

Kapur, M., ed. 1979. *Psychotherapeutic Processes: Proceedings of the Seminar Held at NIMHANS in October 1978.* Bangalore: National Institute of Mental Health and Neuro Sciences.

Kapur, R. L. 1987. Commentary on Culture Bound Syndromes and International Disease Classifications. *Culture, Medicine, and Psychiatry* 11:43–48.

Kardiner, A. 1939. *The Individual and His Society.* New York: Columbia University Press.

————. 1945. *The Psychological Frontiers of Society.* New York: Columbia University Press.

Karno, M., and J. H. Jenkins. 1995. Culture and the Diagnosis of Schizophrenia and Related Disorders. In *Considerations for DSM-IV: A Sourcebook,* ed. J. E. J. Mezzich et al. NIMH-Sponsored Group on Culture and Diagnosis. Washington, D.C.: American Psychiatric Association.

Karno, M., J. H. Jenkins, A. de la Selva, A. Santana, F. Telles, C. Lopez, and J. Mintz. 1987. Expressed Emotion and Schizophrenic Outcome among Mexican-American Families. *Journal of Nervous and Mental Disorders* 175(3):143–51.

Kasiske, B. L., et al. 1991. The Effect of Race on Access and Outcome in Transplantation. *New England Journal of Medicine* 324:302–7.

Kasl, S. V. 1979. Mortality and the Business Cycle: Some Questions about Research Strategies When Utilizing Macro-social and Ecological Data. *American Journal of Public Health* 69: 784.

Katon, Wayne, and Arthur Kleinman. 1980. Clinical Social Science Interventions in Primary Care: A Review of Doctor-Patient Negotiation and Other Relevant Social Science Concepts and Strategies. In *The Relevance of Social Science for Medicine,* ed. L. Eisenberg and A. Kleinman. Dordrecht: D. Reidel, 253–78.

Katz, M., D. Despommier, and R. Gwadz. 1982. *Parasitic Diseases.* New York: Springer-Verlag.

Katz, Pearl. 1990. Ritual in the Operating Room. In *American Culture: Essays on the Familiar and Unfamiliar,* ed. Leonard Plonicov. Pittsburgh: University of Pittsburgh Press, 279–94.

Katz, Richard. 1982. *Boiling Energy.* Cambridge: Harvard University Press.

Katz, Solomon H. 1982. Food, Behavior and Biocultural Evolution. In *The Psychobiology of Human Food Selection,* ed. L. M. Barker. Westport, Conn.: AVI, 171–88.

————. 1987. Food and Biocultural Evolution: A Model for the Investigation of Modern Nutritional Problems. In *Nutritional Anthropology,* ed. F. E. Johnston. New York: Alan R. Liss, 41–63.

Katz, M., D. Despommier, and R. Gwadz. 1982. *Parasitic Diseases.* New York: Springer-Verlag.

Katz, S. H., M. Hediger, and L. Valleroy. 1974. Traditional Maize Processing Techniques in the New World: Anthropological and Nutritional Significance. *Science* 184:765–73.

Katz, S. V., and J. Schall. 1979. Fava Bean Consumption and Biocultural Evolution. *Medical Anthropology* 3:459–76.

Kaufert, Joseph M., and John D. O'Neil. 1990. Biomedical Rituals and Informed Consent: Native Canadians and the Negotiation of Clinical Trust. In *Social Science Perspectives on Medical Ethics,* ed. George Weisz. Philadelphia: University of Pennsylvania Press.

Kaufert, Patricia A. 1982. Myth and the Menopause. *Sociology Health Illness* 4(2):141–66.

———. 1985. Midlife in the Midwest: Canadian Women in Manitoba. In *In Her Prime: A New View of Middle-Aged Women,* ed. Judith K. Brown and Virginia Kerns. South Hadley, Mass.: Bergin and Garvey, 181–97.

———. 1988. Inuit and Obstetricians: Analysis of a Dialogue on Risks in Childbirth. Paper prepared for participants in Conference on Analysis in Medical Anthropology, sponsored by the Wenner-Gren Foundation for Anthropological Research, Lisbon, Portugal, March 5–13.

Kaufman, Lorraine. 1980. Thoughts on Clinical Anthropology. *Medical Anthropology Newsletter* 12(1):17–18.

Kaufman, Sharon R. 1988. Toward a Phenomenology of Boundaries in Medicine: Chronic Illness Experience in the Case of Stroke. *Medical Anthropology Quarterly* 2:338–52.

———. 1993. *The Healer's Tale: Transforming Medicine and Culture.* Madison: University of Wisconsin.

———. 1994. Old Age, Disease and the Discourse on Risk: Geriatric Assessment in U.S. Health Care. *Medical Anthropology Quarterly* 8(4):430–447.

Kawashiri, N., et al. 1986. Effects of Traditional Crude Drugs on Fibrinolysis by Plasmin: Antiplasmin Principles in Eupolyphaga. *Chemical Pharmaceutical Bulletin* 34:2512–17.

Kay, Margarita A. 1977a. Health and Illness in a Mexican American Barrio. In *Ethnic Medicine in the Southwest,* ed. Edward H. Spicer. Tucson: University of Arizona Press, 99–166.

———. 1977b. The Florilegio Medicinal: Source of Southwest Ethnomedicine. *Ethnohistory* 24:251–59.

———. 1979. Lexemic Change and Semantic Shift in Disease Names. *Culture, Medicine and Psychiatry* 3:73–94.

Kay, Margarita A., ed. 1982. *Anthropology of Human Birth.* Philadelphia: F. A. Davis Co.

Kayser-Jones, J. S. 1979. Care of the Institutionalized Aged in Scotland and the United States: A Comparative Study. *Western Journal of Nursing Research* 1:190–200.

———. 1982. Institutional Structures: Catalysts of or Barriers to Quality Care for the Institutionalized Aged in Scotland and the U.S. *Social Science and Medicine* 16:935–44.

———. 1995. Decision Making in the Treatment of Acute Illness in Nursing Homes: Framing the Decision Problem, Treatment Plan and Outcome. *Medical Anthropology Quarterly* 9(2):235–56.

Kayser-Jones, Jeanie, and Barbara A. Koenig. 1994. Ethical Issues in Qualitative Research with the Aged. In *Qualitative Research Methods in Aging,* ed. J. F. Gubrium and A. Sankar. Newbury Park, Calif.: Sage Publications, 15–32.

Kearney, Michael. 1986. From the Invisible Hand to Visible Feet. *Annual Review of Anthropology* 15:331–61.

Keesing, Roger. 1978. *Review of Meaning in Anthropology,* by K. H. Basso and H. A. Selby. *American Anthropologist* 80:132–33.

———. 1981. *Cultural Anthropology: A Contemporary Perspective.* New York: Holt, Rinehart and Winston.

Kekes, John. 1993. *The Morality of Pluralism.* Princeton, N.J.: Princeton University Press.

Kelsey, J. L., W. D. Thompson, and A. S. Evans. 1986. *Methods in Observational Epidemiology.* New York: Oxford University Press.

Kendall, Carl. 1988. The Implementation of a Diarrheal Disease Control Program in Honduras: Is it "Selective Primary Health Care" or "Integrated Primary Health Care"? Special issue of *Social Science and Medicine* 27(1):17–24.

Kendall, Carl, et al. 1988. Dengue Control: The Challenge to the Social Sciences. Agenda and readings for a workshop, Johns Hopkins University, School of Hygiene and Public Health.

Kendall, Carl, Dennis Foote, and Reynaldo Martorel. 1983. Anthropology, Communications, and Health: The Mass Media and Health Practices Program in Honduras. *Human Organization* 42:353–60.

————. 1984. Ethnomedicine and Oral Rehydration Therapy: A Case Study of Ethnomedical Investigation and Program Planning. *Social Science and Medicine* 19:253–60.

Kennedy, John. 1967. Nubian Zar Ceremonies as Psychotherapy. *Human Organization* 26:185–94.

Kennedy, John G. 1974. Cultural Psychiatry. In *Handbook of Social and Cultural Anthropology,* ed. John J. Honigmann. Chicago: Rand McNally, 1119–98.

————. 1987. *The Flower of Paradise: The Institutionalized Use of the Drug Qat in North Yemen.* Dordrecht: D. Reidel.

Kennedy, Mark. 1988. An Inquiry into the Role of the Nation State in Development: Rethinking Dependency. Paper prepared for the 10th International Colloquium on the World Economy, Cairo, A.R.E., February 11–13.

Kenny, Michael. 1978. Latah: The Symbolism of a Putative Mental Disorder. *Culture, Medicine, and Psychiatry* 2:209–23.

Kepel, Gilles. 1985. *The Prophet and the Pharaoh: Muslim Extremism in Egypt.* London: Al Saqi Books.

Kernberg, Otto. 1975. *Borderline Conditions and Pathological Narcissism.* New York: Jason Aronson.

Kessler, Ronald C., and Paul D. Cleary. 1980. Social Class and Psychological Distress. *American Sociological Review* 45:463–78.

Kessler, Ronald C., and Marilyn Essex. 1982. Marital Status and Depression. The Importance of Coping Resources. *Social Forces* 61:484–507.

Keyes, C., and E. Daniel, eds. 1983. *Karma: An Anthropological Inquiry.* Berkeley and Los Angeles: University of California Press.

Keyes, John. 1993. *The Morality of Pluralism.* Princeton, N.J.: Princeton University Press.

Keyfitz, Nathan. 1972. Population Theory and Doctrine: An Historical Survey. In *Readings in Population,* ed. William Petersen. New York: Macmillan.

————. 1977. *An Introduction to the Mathematics of Population.* Reading, Mass.: Addison-Wesley.

Kiefer, Christie W. 1976. Review of Morita Psychotherapy. *Medical Anthropology Newsletter* 7(4): 11–12.

Kiev, Ari, ed. 1964. *Magic, Faith, and Healing: Studies in Primitive Psychiatry Today.* London: Free Press of Glencoe, Collier-Macmillan Ltd.

Kilborne, Benjamin. 1988. *George Devereux: In Memoriam.* Psychoanalytic Study of Society, vol. 12. Hillsdale, N.J.: Analytic Press, xi–xxxix.

Kim, Eun-Shil. 1993. The Making of the Modern Female Gender: The Politics of Gender in Reproductive Practices in Korea. Ph.D. dissertation, University of California, Berkeley.

Kimball, B. A. 1992. *The "True Professional Ideal" in America: A History.* Cambridge, Mass.: Blackwell.

King, J., and A. Ashworth. 1987. Historical Review of the Changing Patterns of Infant Feeding in Developing Countries: The Case of Malaysia, the Caribbean, Nigeria and Zaire. *Social Science and Medicine* 25:1307–20.

Kinzie, D., R. Frederickson, B. Rath, J. Fleck, and W. Karls. 1984. Posttraumatic Stress Disorder among Survivors of Cambodian Concentration Camps. *American Journal of Psychiatry* 141: 645–50.

Kiple, Kenneth F., ed. 1993. *The Cambridge World History of Human Disease.* Cambridge: Cambridge University Press.

Kirmayer, Laurence. 1984. Culture, Affect and Somatization. Parts 1 and 2. *Transcultural Psychiatry Review* 21(3):159–88; (4):237–62.

————. 1988. Mind and Body as Metaphors: Hidden Values in Biomedicine. In *Biomedicine Examined,* ed. M. Lock and D. R. Gordon. Dordrecht: Kluwer Academic Publishers, 57–93.

————. 1992. The Body's Insistence on Meaning: Metaphor as Presentation and Representation in Illness Experience. *Medical Anthropology Quarterly* 6(4):323–46.

Kitayama, Shinobu, and Hazel Markus. 1994. *Emotion and Culture: Empirical Studies of Mutual Influence.* Washington, D.C.: American Psychological Association Press.

Kittay, Eva Fader, and Diana T. Meyers, eds. 1987. *Women and Moral Theory.* Savage, Md.: Rowman and Littlefield.

Kitzinger, Sheila. 1978. *Women as Mothers.* New York: Random House.

Klee, Linnea, and Genevieve Ames. 1987. Re-evaluating Risk Factors for Women's Drinking: A Study of Blue-collar Wives. *American Journal of Preventive Medicine* 3(1):31–41.

Klein, H. E., M. M. Mosberger, T. B. Person, and R. E. Vandivort. 1978. Transcultural Nursing Research with Schizophrenics. *International Journal for Nursing Studies* 15:135–42.

Klein, Melanie. 1955. On Identification. In *New Directions in Psychoanalysis,* ed. M. Klein, P. Heimann, and R. Money-Kyrle. New York: Basic Books, 309–45.

Klein, Melanie, Paula Heimann, and Roger Money-Kyrle, eds. 1955. *New Directions in Psychoanalysis.* New York: Basic Books.

Kleinman, Arthur M. 1973. Medicine's Symbolic Reality. *Inquiry* 16:206–13.

————. 1977. Depression, Somatization, and the New Cross-Cultural Psychiatry. *Social Science and Medicine* 11:3–10.

————. 1980. *Patients and Healers in the Context of Culture.* Berkeley: University of California Press.

————. 1982a. Clinically Applied Anthropology on a Psychiatric Consultation-Liaison Service. In N. Chrisman and T. Maretzkied., eds., *Clinically Applied Anthropology: Anthropologists in Health Science Settings.* Boston: Reidel, 83–115.

————. 1982b. Neurasthenia and Depression: A Study of Somatization and Culture in China. *Culture, Medicine and Psychiatry* 6:117–190.

————. 1983. Editor's Note. *Culture, Medicine and Psychiatry* 7:97–99.

————. 1985. Interpreting Illness Experience and Clinical Meanings: How I See Clinically Applied Anthropology. *Medical Anthropology Quarterly* 16(3):69–71.

————. 1986. *Social Origins of Distress and Disease: Depression and Neurasthenia in Modern China.* New Haven, Conn.: Yale University Press.

————. 1987. Anthropology and Psychiatry: The Role of Culture in Cross-cultural Research on Illness. *British Journal of Psychiatry* 151:447–54.

————. 1988a. *Rethinking Psychiatry.* New York: Free Press.

————. 1988b. *The Illness Narratives: Suffering, Healing and the Human Condition.* New York: Free Press.

————. 1993. What Is Specific to Western Medicine. In W. B. Bynum and R. Porter, eds., *Companion Encyclopedia for the History of Medicine.* London and New York: Routledge.

————. 1995. Anthropology of Bioethics. In *Encyclopedia of Bioethics,* ed. Warren Reich. New York: Macmillan.

————. In press. What is Specific to Western Medicine? In *Encyclopedia of the History of Medicine,* ed. W. F. Bynum and Roy Porter. New York: Routledge.

Kleinman, Arthur M., et al. 1975. *Medicine in Chinese Cultures: Comparative Studies of Health Care in Chinese and Other Societies.* DHEW Publication No. (NIH) 75-653. Washington, D.C.: U.S. Government Printing Office.

————. 1995. The Social Course of Epilepsy: Chronic Illness as Social Experience in Interior China. *Social Science and Medicine* 40(10):1319–30.

Kleinman, Arthur M., L. Eisenberg, and B. J. Good. 1978. Culture, Illness and Care: Clinical Lessons from Anthropologic and Cross-cultural Research. *Annals of Internal Medicine* 88: 251–58.

Kleinman, Arthur M., and J. Gale. 1982. Patients Treated by Physicians and Folk Healers: A Comparative Outcome Study in Taiwan. *Culture, Medicine, and Psychiatry* 6:405–23.

Kleinman, Arthur M., and Byron Good, eds. 1985. *Culture and Depression: Studies in the Anthropology and Cross-Cultural Psychiatry of Affect and Disorder.* Berkeley: University of California Press.

Kleinman, Arthur M., and Joan Kleinman. 1985. Somatization: The Interconnections in Chinese Society among Culture, Depressive Experiences, and Meanings of Pain. In *Culture and Depression: Studies in the Anthropology and Cross-Cultural Psychiatry of Affect and Disorder,* ed. Arthur Kleinman and Byron Good. Berkeley: University of California Press, 429–90.

———. 1991. Suffering and Its Professional Transformation: Toward an Ethnography of Interpersonal Experience. *Culture, Medicine, and Psychiatry* 15(3):275–301.

———. 1995. Transformations of Health and Suffering. In *Morality and Health,* ed. Allen Brandt and P. Roazin. New York: Routledge.

Kleinman, Arthur M., and L. Sung. 1979. Why Do Indigenous Practitioners Successfully Heal? *Social Science and Medicine* 138:7–26.

Klessig, Jill. 1992. The Effect of Values and Culture on Life-Support Decisions. *Western Journal of Medicine* 157:316–22.

Kloos, H. 1977. Schistosomiasis and Irrigation in the Awash Valley of Ethiopia. Ph.D. dissertation, University of California, Davis.

———. 1985. Water Resources Development and Schistosomiasis Ecology in the Awash Valley, Ethiopia. *Social Science and Medicine* 20:609–25.

Kloos, H., G. I. Higashi, J. A. Cattani, V. D. Schinski, N. S. Mansour, and K. D. Murrell. 1983. Water Contact Behavior and Schistosomiasis in an Upper Egyptian Village. *Social Science and Medicine* 17:545–62.

Kloos, H., G. I. Higashi, V. D. Schinski, N. S. Mansour, A. M. Polderman, A. Lemma, and K. D. Murrell. 1980–1981. Human Behavior and Schistosomiasis in an Ethiopian Town and an Egyptian Village: Tensae Berhan and El Ayaisha. *Rural Africana* 8–9:35–63.

Kloos, H., and A. Lemma. 1977. Schistosomiasis in Irrigation Schemes in the Awash Valley, Ethiopia. *American Journal of Tropical Medicine and Hygiene* 26:899–908.

Kloos, H., A. Lemma, and G. De Sole. 1978. *Schistosoma mansoni* Distribution in Ethiopia: A Study in Medical Geography. *Annals of Tropical Medicine and Parasitology* 72:461–70.

Kloos, H., and F. S. McCullough. 1982. Planta Molluscicides. *Planta Medica* 46:195–209.

Kloos, H., A. M. Polderman, G. De Sole, and A. Lemma. 1977. Haematobium Schistosomiasis among Seminomadic and Agricultural Afar in Ethiopia. *Tropical and Geographical Medicine* 29:399–406.

Kloos, H., and K. Thompson. 1979. Schistosomiasis in Africa: An Ecological Perspective. *Journal of Tropical Geography* 48:31–46.

Kluckhohn, Clyde. 1944. The Influence of Psychiatry on Anthropology in America during the Last 100 Years. In *One Hundred Years of American Psychiatry,* ed. J. K. Hall, G. Zilboorg, and H. A. Bunker. New York: Columbia University Press.

Knauft, B. M. 1987. Divergence between Cultural Success and Reproductive Fitness in Preindustrial Societies. *Cultural Anthropology* 2:94–114.

Knodel, John. 1983. Natural Fertility. In *The Determinants of Fertility in Developing Countries,* ed. R. A. Bulatao and R. D. Lee. Vol 1. New York: Academic Press, 61–102.

Koblinsky, Marge, Judith Timyan, and Jill Gay, eds. 1993. *The Health of Women: A Global Perspective.* Boulder, Colo.: Westview Press.

Koenig, Barbara A. 1988. The Technological Imperative in Medical Practice: The Social Creation of ''Routine'' Treatment. In *Biomedicine Examined,* ed. Margaret Lock and Deborah R. Gordon. Boston: Kluwer Academic Publishers, 19–57.

———. 1993. Cultural Diversity in Decision-Making about Care at the End-of-Life. In *Dying, Decision-Making, and Appropriate Care.* Washington, D.C.: Institute of Medicine/National Academy of Sciences.

Koenig, Barbara, and Margaret Clark. 1989. Examining Orthodoxies: The Role of Anthropology in Bioethics. American Anthropological Association Annual Meeting, Washington, D.C.

Koenigsberg, Richard A. 1975. *Hitler's Ideology: A Study in Psychoanalytic Sociology.* New York: Library of Social Science.

Kohut, Heinz. 1971. *The Analysis of the Self.* New York: International Universities Press.
———. 1977. *Restoration of the Self.* New York: International Universities Press.
Kolasa, Kathryn M. 1981. Nutritional Anthropologists and Nutrition Educators—Potentials for a Multi-dimensional World View. *Journal of Nutritional Education* 13(1, Suppl.):s9–s15.
Komlos, John, ed. 1994. *Stature, Living Standards, and Economic Development: Essays on Anthropometric History.* Chicago and London: University of Chicago Press.
Konner, Melvin. 1993. *Medicine at the Crossroads: The Crisis in Health Care.* New York: Pantheon.
Konrad, G., and I. Szelenyi. 1979. *The Intellectuals on the Road to Class Power.* Brighton: Harvester Press.
Kopelman, Loretta M. 1994. Case Method and Casuistry; The Problem of Bias. *Theoretical Medicine* 15(1):21–38.
Koptiuch, Kristin. 1985. Fieldwork in the Postmodern World: Notes on Ethnography in an Expanded Field. Paper presented at the 84th Annual Meeting of the American Anthropological Association, Washington, D.C.
Korbin, Jill. 1987. Child Sexual Abuse: Implications from the Cross-Cultural Record. In *Child Survival,* ed. Nancy Scheper-Hughes. Dordrecht: D. Reidel.
Koshi, P. T. 1972. Role of Prejudice in Rejection of Health Care. *Nursing Research* 21:53–58.
Koshi, P. T., ed. 1977. Foreword. *Nursing Clinics of North America* 12(1):1–3.
Koss, Joan. 1975. Therapeutic Aspects of Puerto Rican Cult Practices. *Psychiatry* 28:160–71.
Kracke, Waud H. 1978. *Force and Persuasion: Leadership in an Amazonian Society.* Chicago: University of Chicago Press.
Krech, S. 1978. Disease, Starvation and Northern Athapaskan Social Organization. *American Ethnologist* 5:710–32.
Kreier, R., and R. Baron. 1987. *Health Consequences of War in Nicaragua, 1985–86.* New York: National Central American Health Rights Network.
Krieger, Judith. 1994. Women, Men and Household Food in Cameroon. Ph.D. dissertation, University of Kentucky.
Krieger, N. 1994. Epidemiology and the Web of Causation: Has Anyone Seen the Spider. *Social Science and Medicine* 39(7):887–903.
Krieger, Nancy. 1993. Analyzing Socioeconomic and Racial/Ethnic Patterns in Health and Health Care. *American Journal of Public Health* 83:1086–87.
Krieger, N., and M. Bassett. 1986. The Health of Blackfolk: Disease, Class and Ideology in Science. *Monthly Review* 38(3):74–85.
Kris, Ernst. 1956. The Personal Myth—A Problem in Psychoanalytic Technique. *Journal of the American Psychoanalytic Association* 4:653–81.
Kristal, A. R., A. L. Shattuck, H. J. Henry, and A. S. Fowler. 1990. Rapid Assessment of Dietary Intake of Fat, Fiber, and Saturated Fat: Validity of an Instrument Suitable for Community Intervention Research and Nutritional Surveillance. *American Journal of Health Promotion* 4:288–95.
Kroeber, Alfred L. 1917. *The Superorganic. American Anthropologist* 19:163–213.
———. 1947. *Cultural and Natural Areas of Native North America.* Berkeley and Los Angeles: University of California Press.
———. 1948. *Anthropology.* New York: Harcourt, Brace and World.
Kuhn, Thomas. 1970. *The Structure of Scientific Revolutions.* Chicago: University of Chicago Press.
Kundera, Milan. 1984. The Novel and Europe. *New York Review of Books* 31:15–19.
Kunitz, Stephen J. 1994. *Disease and Social Diversity: The European Impact on the Health of Non-Europeans.* New York: Oxford University Press.
Kunitz, Stephen J., and Jerrold Levy. 1981. Navajos. In *Ethnicity and Medical Care,* ed. Alan Harwood. Cambridge: Harvard University Press.
———. 1986. The Prevalence of Hypertension among Elderly Navajos: A Test of the Acculturative Stress Hypothesis. *Culture, Medicine, and Psychiatry* 10:97–121.

————. 1994. *Drinking Careers: A Twenty-five Year Study of Three Navajo Populations.* New Haven: Yale University Press.

Kunstadter, Peter. 1975. Do Cultural Differences Make Any Difference? Choice Points in Medical Systems Available in North-Western Thailand. In *Medicine in Chinese Cultures: Comparative Studies of Health Care in Chinese and other Cultures,* ed. A. Kleinman et al. Washington, D.C.: U.S. Government Printing Office for Fogarty International Center, NIH.

————. 1980. Medical Ethics in Cross-Cultural and Multi-Cultural Perspectives. *Social Science and Medicine* 14B:289–96.

————. 1986. Ethnicity, Ecology, and Mortality Transitions in Northwestern Thailand. In *Anthropology and Epidemiology,* C. Janes et al. Dordrecht: D. Reidel, 125–56.

Kunzle, David. 1981. *Fashion and Fetishism: A Social History of the Corset, Tight-Lacing, and Other Forms of Body-Sculpture in the West.* London: Rowan and Littlefield.

Kuo, Wen. 1976. Theories of Migration and Mental Health: An Empirical Testing on Chinese-Americans. *Social Science and Medicine* 10:297–306.

Kurtz, E. 1979. *Not-God: A History of Alcoholics Anonymous.* Center City, Minn.: Hazelden Educational Services.

La Barre, Weston. 1954. *The Human Animal.* Chicago: Chicago University Press, 1968.

————. 1956. Social Cynosure and Social Structure. In *Personal Character and Cultural Milieu,* ed. Douglas G. Haring. Syracuse, N.Y.: Syracuse University Press, 535–46.

————. 1958. The Influence of Freud on Anthropology. *American Imago* 15:275–328.

————. 1962. Transference Cures in Religious Cults and Social Groups. *Journal of Psychoanalysis in Groups* 1(1):66–75.

————. 1968. Personality from a Psychoanalytic Viewpoint. In *The Study of Personality,* ed. Edward Norbeck. New York: Holt, Rinehart and Winston, 65–87.

————. 1969. *They Shall Take Up Serpents: Psychology of the Southern Snake-Handling Cult.* New York: Schocken.

————. 1970. *The Peyote Cult.* New York: Shocken Books.

————. 1971a. Anthropological Perspectives on Sexuality. In *Sexuality: A Search for Perspective,* ed. D. Grumman and A. M. Barclay. New York: Van Nostrand Reinhold Co., 38–53.

————. 1971b. Materials for a History of Studies of Crisis Cults: A Bibliographic Essay. *Current Anthropology* 12:3–44.

————. 1972. *The Ghost Dance: The Origins of Religion.* New York: Dell.

————. 1978. The Clinic and the Field. In *The Making of Psychological Anthropology,* ed. G. D. Spindler. Berkeley and Los Angeles: University of California Press, 258–99.

————. 1980. *Cultures in Context.* Durham, N.C.: Duke University Press.

————. 1984. *Muelos: A Stone Age Superstition.* New York: Columbia University Press.

————. 1987. An Integrated Approach to the Pharmacological Evaluation of Traditional Materia Medica. *Journal of Ethnopharmacology* 20:191–207.

Labov, William, and D. Fanshel. 1977. *Therapeutic Discourse.* New York: Academic Press.

Laderman, Carol. 1983. *Wives and Midwives: Childbirth and Nutrition in Rural Malaysia.* Berkeley: University of California Press.

————. 1984. Food Ideology and Eating Behavior. *Social Science and Medicine* 19(5):547–60.

————. 1987a. The Ambiguity of Symbols in the Structure of Healing. *Social Science and Medicine* 24(4):293–301.

————. 1987b. Destructive Heat and Cooling Prayer: Malay Humoralism in Pregnancy, Childbirth and the Postpartum Period. *Social Science and Medicine* 25(4):357–67.

————. 1991. *Taming the Wind of Desire: Psychology, Medicine and Aesthetics in Malay Shamanistic Performance.* Berkeley: University of California Press.

Laderman, Carol, and Marina Roseman, eds. 1995. *The Performance of Healing.* London: Routledge.

LaFarque, J. R. 1972. Role of Prejudice in Rejection of Health Care. *Nursing Research* 21:53–58.

LaFontaine, J. S. 1985. Person and Individual. In *The Category of the Person: Anthropology, Philosophy, History,* ed. M. Carrithers, S. Collins, and S. Lukes. Cambridge: Cambridge University Press, 123–40.

Lagache, Daniel. 1973. Introduction. In *The Language of Psycho-Analysis,* trans. J. Laplanche, J. B. Pontalis, and Donald Nicholson-Smith. New York: Norton, vii–ix.

Lakoff, George, and Zoltan Kovecses. 1987. The Cognitive Model of Anger Inherent in American English. In *Human Motives and Cultural Models,* ed. Roy D'Andrade and Claudia Strauss. Cambridge: Cambridge University Press.

Lamphere, Louise. 1992. *Structuring Diversity: Ethnographic Perspectives on the New Immigration.* Chicago: University of Chicago Press.

Lancaster, Roger Nelson. 1983. What AIDS Is Doing to Us. *Christopher Street* 73:48–52.

Landy, David. 1977. Anthropological Approaches to the Study of Human Adaptation to Health and Disease. In *Culture, Disease, and Healing: Studies in Medical Anthropology,* ed. D. Landy. New York: Macmillan, 11–13.

———. 1983a. Medical Anthropology: A Critical Appraisal. In *Advances in Medical Science,* Vol. 1, ed. Julio Ruffini. New York: Gordon and Breach, 184–314.

———. 1983b. Pibloktoq (Hysteria) and Inuit Nutrition: Possible Implication of Hypervitaminosis A. New Approaches to Culture-Bound Syndromes Symposium at the International Congress of Anthropological and Ethnological Sciences and at the Society for the Study of Psychiatry and Culture, August 1983, October 1983, Vancouver B.C., and Newport, R.I.

Landy, David, ed. 1977. *Culture, Disease, and Healing: Studies in Medical Anthropology.* New York: Macmillan.

Lane, Sandra D. 1985. Health Systems Assessment in Damanhour, Egypt. University of California San Francisco: Program on Medical Anthropology, Research Report, Unpublished.

———. 1987. A Biocultural Study of Trachoma in an Egyptian Hamlet. Ph.D. dissertation, University of California at San Francisco.

———. 1988. A Bitter Smile: The Political Epidemiology of Neonatal Tetanus in Egypt. Paper presented at the Annual Meeting of the American Anthropological Association, Phoenix, Arizona, November 16–20.

———. 1994. Research Ethics in Egypt. In *Principles of Health Care Ethics,* ed. Raanan Gillon. New York: John Wiley.

Lang, Gretchen. 1974. Adaptive Strategies of Urban Indian Drinkers: Chippewa in Minneapolis. Ph.D. dissertation, University of Minnesota.

Lang, S. D., and M. I. Millar. 1987. The "Hierarchy of Resort" Reexamined: Status and Class Differentials as Determinants of Therapy for Eye Disease in the Egyptian Delta. *Urban Anthropology* 16:151–82.

Langdon, Jean Matteson, and Gerhard Baer. 1992. *Portal of Power: Shamanism in South America.* Albuquerque N.M.: University of New Mexico Press.

Langer, Suzanne K. 1957. *Philosophy in a New Key.* Cambridge: Harvard University Press.

Langner, Thomas S., and Stanley T. Michael. 1963. *Life Stress and Mental Health.* New York: Free Press.

Lanoix, J. N. 1958. Relation between Irrigation Engineering and Bilharziasis. *Bulletin of the World Health Organization* 18:1011–35.

Laplanche, J., and J.-B. Pontalis. 1973. *The Language of Psycho-Analysis,* trans. Donald Nicholson-Smith. New York: Norton.

La Puma, John, and David L. Schiedermayer. 1994. *Ethics Consultation: A Practical Guide.* Boston: Jones and Bartlett Publishers.

La Puma, John, and Stephen Toulmin. 1989. Ethics Consultants and Ethics Committees. *Archives of Internal Medicine* 149:1109–12.

Laqueur, Thomas. 1986. Orgasm, Generation, and the Politics of Reproductive Biology. *Representations* 14:1–41.

Larkin, G. 1983. *Occupational Monopoly and Modern Medicine.* London: Tavistock.

LaRocco, James M., James S. House, and John R. P. French, Jr. 1980. Social Support, Occupational Stress, and Health. *Journal of Health and Social Behavior* 21:202–18.

LaRoche, C., et al. 1984. Grief Reactions to Perinatal Death: A Follow-up Study. *Canadian Journal of Psychiatry* 29(1):14–19.

Larson, A. 1989. Social Context of Human Immunodeficiency Virus Transmission in Africa: Historical and Cultural Bases of East and Central Africa Sexual Relations. *Reviews of Infectious Disease* 11(5):716–31.

Larson, David, and Susan S. Larson. 1994. The Forgotten Factor in Physical and Mental Health: What Does the Research Show? John Templeton Foundation, Seminar Text.

Larson, M. S. 1977. *The Rise of Professionalism.* Berkeley: University of California Press.

Lasker, Judith. 1977. The Role of Health Services in Colonial Rule: The Case of the Ivory Coast. *Culture, Medicine and Psychiatry* 1:277–97.

Last, M., and G. L. Chavunduka, eds. 1986. *The Professionalisation of African Medicine.* Manchester: Manchester University Press for the International African Institute.

Laughlin, Charles, Jr., and Ivan Brady, eds. 1978. *Extinction and Survival in Human Populations.* New York: Columbia University Press.

Laurell, Asa Cristina. 1989. Social Analysis of Collective Health in Latin America. *Social Science and Medicine* 11:1183–91.

Laurell, Asa Cristina, J. B. Gil, T. Machetoo, J. Palomo, C. P. Rulfo, M. R. de Chavez, M. Urbina, and N. Velazquez. 1977. Disease and Rural Development: A Sociological Analysis of Morbidity in Two Mexican Villages. *International Journal of Health Services* 7(3):401–23.

Lauritzen, Paul. 1993. *Pursuing Parenthood: Ethical Issues in Assisted Reproduction.* Indianapolis: Indiana University Press.

Lawler, Ronald O. 1988. Moral Reflections on the New Technologies: A Catholic Analysis. *Women and Health* 13(1):167–77.

Lazarus, Ellen S. 1987. What Women Want: Women and Obstetricians. Paper prepared for presentation at the 86th Annual Meeting of the American Anthropological Association, Chicago, November 18–22.

———. 1988a. Theoretical Considerations for the Study of the Doctor-Patient Relationship: Implications of a Perinatal Study. *Medical Anthropology Quarterly* n.s. 2(1):34–59.

———. 1988b. Poor Women, Poor Outcomes: Social Class and Reproductive Health. In *Childbirth in America: Anthropological Perspectives,* ed. Karel L. Michaelson. South Hadley, Mass.: Bergin and Garvey.

———. 1988c. ''I'm Just a Clerk'': Medical Workers and Prenatal Care (Some Thoughts on Critical Medical Perspectives in Childbirth Studies). Paper prepared for presentation at the 87th Annual Meeting of the American Anthropological Association, Phoenix, Arizona, November 16–20.

———. 1994. What Do Women Want: Issues of Choice, Control, and Class in Pregnancy and Childbirth. *Medical Anthropology Quarterly* 8(1):25–46.

Lazarus, Ellen, and Gregory Pappas. 1986. Categories of Thought and Critical Theory: Anthropology and the Social Science of Medicine. *Medical Anthropology Quarterly* 17(5):136–37.

Lazarus, Richard S. 1966. *Psychological Stress and the Coping Process.* New York: McGraw-Hill.

Lazarus, Richard S., and Susan Folkman. 1986. Cognitive Theories of Stress and the Issue of Circularity. In *Dynamics of Stress: Physiological, Psychological, and Social Perspectives,* ed. Mortimer H. Appley and Richard Trumbull. New York: Plenum Press.

Leacock, Eleanor. 1972. Introduction to *The Origin of the Family, Private Property and the State.* New York: International Publishers.

———. 1982. Marxism and Anthropology. In *The Left Academy: Scholarship on American Campuses.* New York: McGraw-Hill.

Leader, Arthus, Patrick J. Taylor, and Judith C. Daniluk. 1984. Infertility: Clinical and Psychological Aspects. *Psychiatric Annals* 14(6):461–62, 465–67.

Learmonth, Andrew. 1988. *Disease Ecology.* Oxford: Basil Blackwell.

Leatherman, Thomas, J., Alan Goodman, and R. Brooke Thomas. 1993. On Seeking Common Ground between Medical Ecology and Critical Medical Anthropology. *Medical Anthropology Quarterly* 7(2):202–7.

Leatherman, Thomas, J., Susan Luerssen, Lisa Marowitz, and R. Brooke Thomas. 1986. Illness and Political Economy: The Andean Dialectic. *Cultural Survival Quarterly* 10(3):19–22.

Leavitt, Judith Walzer. 1986. *Brought to Bed: Childbearing in America 1750–1950.* New York: Oxford University Press.

———. 1987. The Growth of Medical Authority: Technology and Morals in Turn-of-the-Century Obstetrics. *Medical Anthropology Quarterly* n.s. 1(3):230–55.

Lebot, Vincent, Mark Merlin, and Lamont Lindstrom. 1992. *Kava: The Pacific Drug.* New Haven: Yale University Press.

Lebra, Takie Sugiyama. 1976. *Japanese Patterns of Behavior.* Honolulu: University Press of Hawaii.

———. 1982. Self-Reconstruction in Japanese Religious Psychotherapy. In Anthony Marsella and Geoffrey White, eds., *Cultural Conceptions of Mental Health and Therapy.* Dordrecht: D. Reidel, 269–84.

Leder, Drew. 1990. Clinical Interpretation: The Hermeneutics of Medicine. *Theoretical Medicine* 11(1):9–24.

Lederberg, Joshua, Robert E. Shope, and Stanley C. Oaks, eds. 1992. *Emerging Infections: Microbial Threats to Health in the United States.* Washington, D.C.: National Academy Press.

Lederer, Wolfgang. 1959. Primitive Psychotherapy. *Psychiatry* 22:255–65.

Lee, Nancy. 1964. *The Search for an Abortionist.* Chicago: University of Chicago Press.

Lee, Richard. 1978. Towards a Marxist Methodology for Anthropology. Paper presented at the symposium Ways of Knowing in Anthropology, American Anthropological Association Annual Meetings, Los Angeles, November 16.

———. 1992. Art, Science, or Politics: The Crisis in Hunter-Gatherer Studies. *American Anthropologist* 94:31–54.

Lee, Richard B. 1979. *The !Kung San.* New York: Cambridge University Press.

Lee, Ronald. 1982. From Rome to Manila: How Demography Has Changed in Three Decades. Program in Population Research Working Paper, no. 4. University of California, Berkeley.

———. 1984. Malthus and Boserup: A Dynamic Synthesis. Program in Population Research Working Paper, no. 15. University of California, Berkeley.

Leeman, Larry. 1986. Pueblo Models of Communal Sickness and Wellbeing. Paper read at the Kroeber Anthropological Society Meetings, Berkeley, March 8.

Leeson, Joyce. 1974. Social Science and Health Policy in Preindustrial Society. *International Journal of Health Services* 4(3):429–40.

Leff, J. 1981. *Psychiatry around the Globe.* New York: M. Dekker.

Leighton, Alexander H., T. Adeoye Lambo, Charles C. Hughes, Dorothea C. Leighton, Jane M. Murphy, and David B. Macklin. 1963. *Psychiatric Disorder among the Yoruba: A Report from the Cornell-Aro Mental Health Research Project in the Western Region, Nigeria.* Ithaca: Cornell University Press.

Leighton, Alexander, and Dorothea Leighton. 1941. Elements of Psychotherapy in Navajo Religion. *Psychiatry* 4:515–24.

Leighton, Dorothea C. 1983. Anthropology in Medicine—A Personal History: How Can the Health Professionals Use Anthropology? In *Clinical Anthropology,* ed. Demetri Shimkin and Peggy Golde. Lanham, Md: University Press of America, 229–38.

Leighton, Dorothea C., J. S. Harding, D. B. Macklin, A. M. Macmillan, and Alexander H. Leighton. 1963. *The Character of Danger.* New York: Basic Books.

Leininger, M. 1970. *Nursing and Anthropology: Two Worlds to Blend.* New York: Wiley.

———. 1977. Transcultural Nursing and a Proposed Conceptual Framework. In *Transcultural Nursing Care of Infants and Children: Proceedings of the First Transcultural Nursing Conference,* ed. M. Leininger. Salt Lake City: University of Utah, College of Nursing, 1–18.

————. 1978. Culturalogical Assessment Domains for Nursing Practices. In *Transcultural Nursing: Concepts, Theories and Practices,* ed. M. Leininger. New York: Wiley, 85–106.

————. 1981. The Phenomenon of Caring: Importance, Research Questions and Theoretical Considerations. In *Caring: An Essential Human Need: Proceedings of Three National Caring Conferences,* ed. M. Leininger. Thorofare, N.J.: Slack, 3–15.

Leininger, M., ed. 1978b. *Transcultural Nursing: Concepts, Theories and Practices.* New York: Wiley.

Leland, Joy. 1976. *Firewater Myths.* New Brunswick, N.J.: Rutgers Center of Alcohol Studies.

Lemert, Edwin M. 1965. Forms and Pathology of Drinking in Three Polynesian Societies. *American Anthropologist* 66(2):361–75.

Leng, Chee Heng. 1982. Health Status and the Development of Health Services in a Colonial State: The Case of British Malaya. *International Journal of Health Services* 12:397–416.

Leonard, William R. 1991. Household Level Strategies for Protecting Children from Seasonal Food Scarcity. *Social Science and Medicine* 33(10):1127–33.

Leridon, Henri. 1977. *Human Fertility.* Chicago: University of Chicago Press.

Leridon, Henri, and Jane Menken, eds. 1979. *Natural Fertility.* Liege: Ordina.

Leslie, Charles M. 1972. The Professionalization of Ayurvedic and Unani Medicine. In *Medical Men and Their Work: A Sociological Reader,* ed. E. Freidson and E. J. Lorber. Chicago: Aldine, 39–54.

————. 1975. Pluralism and Integration in the Indian and Chinese Medical Systems. In *Medicine in Chinese Cultures,* ed. E. Alexander, A. Kleinman, and P. Kunstadter. Washington, D.C.: John E. Fogerty International Center, NIH.

————. 1976. Introduction to *Asian Medical Systems: A Comparative Study,* ed. C. Leslie. Berkeley and Los Angeles: University of California Press, 133–58.

Leslie, Charles, M., ed. 1980. Medical Pluralism. *Social Science and Medicine* 14B.

Leslie, Charles M., and E. Taylor. 1973. Asian Medical Systems: A Symposium on the Role of Comparative Sociology in Improving Health Care. *Social Science and Medicine* 7:307–18.

Leslie, Charles, and Allan Young, eds. 1992. *Path to Asian Medical Knowledge.* Berkeley: University of California Press.

Lett, James. 1987. *The Human Enterprise: A Critical Introduction to Anthropological Theory.* Boulder, Colo.: Westview Press.

Levi-Strauss, Claude. 1963a. The Effectiveness of Symbols. In *Structural Anthropology.* New York: Basic Books.

————. 1963b. The Sorcerer and His Magic. In *Structural Anthropology.* New York: Basic Books.

————. 1963c. *Structural Anthropology.* New York: Basic Books.

Levine, Nancy E. 1987. Differential Child Care in Three Tibetan Communities: Beyond Son Preference. *Population and Development Review* 13:282–304.

Levin, Betty Wolder. 1986. Caring Choices: Decision Making about Treatment for Catastrophically Ill Newborns. Ph.D. dissertation, Columbia University.

Levin, Betty Wolder, John M. Driscoll, and Alan Fleischman. 1991. Treatment Choice for Infants in the NICU at Risk for AIDs. *Journal of the American Medical Association* 265(22):2976–81.

Levin, Jeffrey, and H. Vanderpool. 1987. Is Frequent Religious Attendance Really Conducive to Better Health? Toward an Epidemiology of Religion. *Social Science and Medicine* 24:589–600.

Levine, J. D., N. C. Gordon, and H. L. Fields. 1978. The Mechanism of Placebo Analgesia. *Lancet* ii: 656–57.

————. 1965. Le Triangle Colinaire. *L'Arc* 26:19–29.

LeVine, Robert A. 1973. *Culture, Behavior, and Personality.* Chicago: Aldine.

————. 1974. *Culture and Personality: Contemporary Readings.* Chicago: Aldine Publishing Co.

————. 1990. Infant Environments in Psychoanalysis: A Cross-Cultural View. In *Cultural Psy-*

chology: Essays on Comparative Human Development, ed. J. Stigler, R. Shweder, and G. Herdt. New York: Cambridge University Press.

Levine, Robert J. 1991. Informed Consent: Some Challenges to the Universal Validity of the Western Model. *Law, Medicine, and Health Care* 19(3–4).

Levy, Jerrold E., and Steven J. Kunitz. 1974. *Indian Drinking: Navajo Practices and Anglo-American Theories.* New York: John Wiley and Sons.

———. 1981. Economic and Political Factors Inhibiting the Use of Basic Research Findings in Indian Alcoholism Programs. *Journal of Studies on Alcohol (suppl. 9).*

Levy, Robert. 1973. *Tahitians.* Chicago: University of Chicago Press.

———. 1983. Introduction: Self and Emotion. *Ethos* 11:128–34.

———. 1984. Emotion, Knowing and Culture. In *Culture Theory: Essays on Mind, Self, and Emotion,* ed. R. Shweder and R. LeVine. Cambridge: Cambridge University Press.

Levy, Robert, and Michelle Rosaldo, eds. 1983. Self and Emotion. *Ethos* 113.

Lewin, Ellen. 1974. *Mothers and Children: Latin American Immigrants in San Francisco.* New York: Arno Press.

———. 1985. By Design: Reproductive Strategies and the Meaning of Motherhood. In *The Sexual Politics of Reproduction,* ed. Hilary Homans. London: Gower, 123–38.

Lewis, G. A. 1977. Fear of Sorcery and the Problem of Death by Suggestion. In *The Anthropology of the Body,* ed. J. Blacking. ASA Monograph 15. London: Academic Press, 111–43.

Lewis, Gilbert. 1975. *Knowledge of Illness in a Sepik Society.* London: Athlone.

Lewis, I. M. 1971. *Ecstatic Religion: An Anthropological Study of Spirit Possession and Shamanism.* London: Penguin.

———. 1983. Spirit Possession and Biological Reductionism: A Rejoinder to Kehoe and Giletti. *American Anthropologist* 85:412–13.

Lewis, Walter H., and Memory P. F. Elvin-Lewis. 1977. *Medical Botany.* New York: Wiley.

Lewontin, R. C. 1978. Adaptation. *Scientific American* 239:212–30.

Lex, Barbara. 1974. Voodoo Death: New Thoughts on an Old Explanation. *American Anthropologist* 76:818–23.

Lex, Barbara, Margaret L. Griffin, Nancy K. Mello, and Jack H. Mendelson. 1986. Concordant Alcohol and Marihuana Use in Women. *Alcohol* 3:193–200.

Lex, Barbara W., Jack H. Mendelson, Samuel Bavli, Kathy Harvey, and Nancy K. Mello. 1984. Effects of Acute Marijuana Smoking on Pulse Rate and Mood States in Women. *Psychopharmacology* 84:178–87.

Lex, Barbara W., Susan L. Palmieri, Nancy K. Mello, and Jack H. Mendelson. 1988. Alcohol Use, Marihuana Smoking, and Sexual Activity in Women. *Alcohol* 5:21–25.

Lieban, Richard W. 1967. *Cebuano Sorcery.* Berkeley and Los Angeles: University of California Press.

———. 1973. Medical Anthropology. In *Handbook of Social and Cultural Anthropology,* ed. J. Honigmann Chicago: Rand-McNally, 1031–73.

———. 1990. Medical Anthropology and the Comparative Study of Medical Ethics. In *Social Science Perspectives on Medical Ethics,* ed. George Weisz. Philadelphia: University of Pennsylvania Press, 221–40.

Liebow, Elliot. 1967. *Tally's Corner.* Boston: Little, Brown.

Light, Donald and Sol Levine. 1989. The Changing Character of the Medical Profession. Unpublished manuscript.

Like, Robert C., and J. Ellison. 1981. Sleeping Blood, Tremor and Paralysis: A Trans-cultural Approach to an Unusual Conversion Reaction. *Culture, Medicine and Psychiatry* 5:49–63.

Like, Robert C., and R. Prasaad Steiner. 1986. Medical Anthropology and the Family Physician. *Family Medicine* 18(2):87–92.

Lilienfeld, A. M. 1976. *Foundations of Epidemiology.* New York: Oxford University Press.

Lilienfeld, D. E., and P. D. Stolley. 1994. *Foundations of Epidemiology.* 3d ed. New York: Oxford University Press.

Lindenbaum, Shirley. 1979. *Kuru Sorcery: Disease and Danger in the New Guinea Highland.* Palo Alto, Calif.: Mayfield.

Lindenbaum, Shirley, and Margaret Lock, eds. 1993. *Knowledge, Power, and Practice.* Berkeley: University of California Press.

Lindstrom, Lamont. 1987. *Drugs in Western Pacific Societies: Relations of Substance.* ASAO Monograph 11. Lanham, Md.: University Press of America.

Linke, Uli. 1986. Where Blood Flows, a Tree Grows: A Study of Root Metaphors and German Culture. Ph.D. dissertation, University of California, Berkeley.

Little, Kenneth. 1973. *African Women in Towns.* Cambridge: Cambridge University Press.

Littlewood, Roland. 1990. From Categories to Texts: A Decade of the "New Cross-Cultural Psychiatry." *British Journal of Psychiatry* 156:308–27.

Littlewood, Roland, and Maurice Lipsedge. 1985. Culture-bound Syndromes. In *Recent Advances in Clinical Psychiatry,* ed. Kenneth Granville-Grossman. Edinburgh: Churchill Livingstone, 105–42.

Liu, K., J. Stamler, A. Dyer, J. McKeever, and P. McKeever. 1978. Statistical Methods to Assess and Minimize the Role of Intra-Individual Variability in Obscuring the Relationship between Dietary Lipids and Serum Cholesterol. *Journal of Chronic Diseases.* 31:399–418.

Livingstone, Frank B. 1958. Anthropological Implications of Sickle Cell Gene Distribution in West Africa. *American Anthropologist* 60:533–62.

———. 1971. Malaria and Human Polymorphisms. *Annual Review of Genetics* 5:33–64.

———. 1976. Hemoglobin History in West Africa. *Human Biology* 48:487–500.

———. 1985. *Frequencies of Hemoglobin Variants: Thallassemia, the Glucose-6-Phosphate Dehydrogenase Deficiency, G6PD Variants and Ovalocytosis in Human Populations.* New York: Oxford University Press.

Llewellyn-Jones, Derek, ed. 1986. Abortion. In *Fundamentals of Obstetrics and Gynaecology.* Vol. 1: *Obstetrics.* London: Faber and Faber, 191–201.

Lloyd, J. W. 1971. Long-Term Mortality Study of Steelworkers: V. Respiratory Cancer in Coke Plant Workers. *Journal of Occupational Medicine* 13:53–58.

Lloyd, J. W., F. E. Lundin, Jr., C. K. Redmond, and P. B. Geiser. 1970. Long-Term Mortality Study of Steelworkers. IV. Mortality by Work Area. *Journal of Occupational Medicine* 12:151–57.

Lock, Margaret. 1980. *East Asian Medicine in Urban Japan: Varieties of Medical Experience.* Berkeley: University of California Press.

———. 1982. On Revealing the Hidden Curriculum. *Medical Anthropology Quarterly* 14(1):19–21.

———. 1986a. Plea for Acceptance: School Refusal Syndrome in Japan. *Social Science and Medicine* 23:99–112.

———. 1986b. The Anthropological Study of the American Medical System: Center and Periphery. *Social Science and Medicine* 22(9):931–32.

———. 1987. DSM-III as a Culture-Bound Construct: Culture-Bound Syndromes and International Disease Classifications. *Culture, Medicine, and Psychiatry* 11(1):35–42.

———. 1988a. Introduction to *Biomedicine Examined,* ed. M. Lock and D. Gordon. Dordrecht: Kluwer Academic Publishers.

———. 1988b. New Japanese Mythologies: Faltering Discipline and the Ailing Housewife. *American Ethnologist* 15:43–61.

———. 1988c. The Making of a Nation: Interpretations of School Refusal in Japan. In *Biomedicine Examined,* ed. M. Lock and D. R. Gordon. Dordrecht: Kluwer Academic Publishers.

———. 1988d. Mind, Matter, and Menopause: Medical Knowledge and Ideology. In *Analysis in Medical Anthropology,* ed. S. Lindenbaum and M. Lock. Dordrecht: Kluwer Academic Publishers.

———. 1988e. Nerves and Nostalgia: Medical Care for Greek-Canadian Immigrants in Quebec.

Paper given at Anthropologies of Medicine: A Colloquium on Western European and North American Perspectives, Hamburg, December.

———. 1990. On Being Ethnic: The Politics of Identity Breaking and Making in Canada, or Nevra on Sunday. *Culture, Medicine and Psychiatry* 14:237–51.

———. 1993a. Cultivating the Body: Anthropology and Epistemologies of Bodily Practice and Knowledge. *Annual Reviews of Anthropology* 22:133–56.

———. 1993b. *Encounters with Aging: Mythologies of Menopause in Japan and North America.* Berkeley: University of California Press.

———. 1993c. The Politics of Mid-Life and Menopause: Ideologies for the Second Sex in North America and Japan. In Shirley Lindenbaum and Margaret Lock, eds., *Knowledge, Power and Practice: The Anthropology of Medicine and Everyday Life.* Berkeley: University of California Press.

———. 1995. Contesting the Natural in Japan: Moral Dilemmas and Technologies of Dying. *Culture, Medicine, and Psychiatry* 19(1):1–38.

Lock, Margaret, and Pamela Dunk. 1987. My Nerves Are Broken: The Communication of Suffering in a Greek-Canadian Community. In *Health in Canadian Society: Sociological Perspectives,* ed. D. Coburn, C. D'Arcy, P. New, and G. Torrence. Toronto: Fitzhenry and Whiteside, 295–313.

Lock, Margaret, and Deborah R. Gordon, eds. 1988. *Biomedicine Examined.* Dordrecht: Kluwer Academic Publishers.

Lock, Margaret, and Christina Honde. 1990. Reaching Consensus about Death: Heart Transplants and Cultural Identity in Japan. In *Social Science Perspectives on Medical Ethics,* ed. George Weisz. Philadelphia: University of Philadelphia Press, 99–120.

Loewy, Erich. 1991. *Suffering and the Beneficent Community:-Beyond Libertarianism.* Albany: State University of New York Press.

Logan, Michael H. 1977. Anthropological Research on the Hot-Cold Theory of Disease: Some Methodological Suggestions. *Medical Anthropology* 1:87–108.

———. 1979. Variations Regarding Susto Causality among the Cakchiquel of Guatemala. *Culture, Medicine and Psychiatry* 3:153–66.

———. 1983. The Role of Pharmacists and Over-the-Counter Medications in the Health Care System of a Mexican City. *Medical Anthropology* 7(3):69–87.

———. 1988. Plant Attributes, Selection, and the Discovery of Medical Knowledge. Presented at the 87th Annual Meetings of the American Anthropological Association, Phoenix, November.

Logan, Michael, and Edward E. Hunt. 1978. *Health and the Human Condition.* North Scituate, Mass.: Duxbury Press.

Lohiya, N. K., R. B. Goyal, D. Jayaprakash, A. S. Ansari, and S. Sharma. 1994. Antifertility Effects of Aqueous Extract of Carica Papaya Seeds in Male Rats. *Planta Medica* 60:400–4.

Lopez Austin, A. 1967. Cuarenta Clases de Magos del Mundo Nahuatl. *Estudios de Cultura Nahuatl* 7:87–117

———. 1975. *Textos de Medicina Nahuatl.* Mexico City: Universidad Nacional Autonoma de Mexico.

———. 1980. *Cuerpo Humano e Ideologica. Las Concepciones de los Antiguous Nahuas.* Mexico City: Universidad Nacional Autonoma de Mexico.

Lorimer, Frank. 1954. *Culture and Human Fertility: A Study of the Relation of Cultural Conditions to Fertility in Nonindustrial and Transitional Societies.* Paris: UNESCO.

Louie, Kem B. 1985. Providing Health Care to Chinese Clients. *Topics in Clinical Nursing* 7(3): 18–26.

Lovejoy, Owen. 1981. The Origin of Man. *Science* 211:341–50.

Low, Setha. 1985a. Culturally Interpreted Symptoms or Culture-Bound Syndromes: A Cross-Cultural Review of Nerves. *Social Science and Medicine* 21:187–97.

———. 1985b. *Culture, Politics and Medicine in Costa Rica.* Bedford Hills, N.Y.: Redgrave Publishing.

———. 1988. Medical Practice in Response to a Folk Illness: The Diagnosis and Treatment of Nervios in Costa Rica. In *Biomedicine Examined,* ed. M. Lock and D. R. Gordon. Dordrecht: Kluwer Academic Publishers, 415–38.

Lozoff, B., K. R. Kamath, and R. A. Feldman. 1975. Infection and Disease in South Indian Families: Beliefs about Childhood Diarrhea. *Human Organization* 34:353–58.

Luborsky, Lester. 1986. Do Therapists Vary Much in Their Success: Findings from Four Outcome Studies. *American Journal of Orthopsychiatry* 56:501–12.

Luborsky, Lester, et al. 1985. Therapeutic Success and Its Determinants. *Archives of General Psychiatry* 42:602–11.

Ludwig, Emil. 1937. *The Nile: The Life Story of a River.* New York: Viking Press.

Luker, Christine. 1975. *Taking Chances: Abortion and the Decision Not to Contracept.* Berkeley: University of California Press.

Luria, A. R. 1972. *The Man with a Shattered Sword.* New York: Basic Books.

Lurie, Sue. 1994. Ethical Dilemmas and Professional Roles in Occupational Medicine. *Social Science and Medicine* 38(10):1367–74.

Lutz, Catherine. 1982. The Domain of Emotion Words on Ifaluk. *American Ethnologist* 9: 113–28.

———. 1985a. Depression and the Translation of Emotional Worlds. In *Culture and Depression,* ed. Arthur Kleinman and Byron Good. Berkeley: University of California Press.

———. 1985b. Ethnopsychology Compared to What? Explaining Behavior and Consciousness among the Ifaluk. In *Person, Self and Experience: Exploring Pacific Ethnopsychologies,* ed. Geoffrey M. White and John Kirkpatrick. Berkeley and Los Angeles: University of California Press.

———. 1988. *Unnatural Emotions: Everyday Sentiments on a Micronesian Atoll and Their Challenge to Western Theory.* Chicago: University of Chicago Press.

———. 1990. Engendered Emotions: Gender, Power, and the Rhetoric of Emotional Control in American Discourse. In *Language and the Politics of Emotion,* ed. Catherine Lutz and Lila Abu-Lughod. Cambridge: Cambridge University Press.

Lutz, Catherine, and Lila Abu-Lughod, eds. 1990. *Language and the Politics of Emotion.* Cambridge: Cambridge University Press.

Lutz, Catherine, and Geoffrey White. 1986. The Anthropology of Emotions. *Annual Review of Anthropology* 15:405–36.

Lyon, Margot L. 1990. Order and Healing: The Concept of Order and Its Importance in the Conceptualization of Healing. *Medical Anthropology* 12:249–68.

MacAndrew, Craig, and Robert B. Edgerton. 1969. *Drunken Comportment: A Social Explanation.* New York: Aldine.

MacIntyre, Alasdair. 1984. *After Virtue.* Notre Dame, Ind.: Notre Dame University Press.

Macintyre, Sally. 1986. The Patterning of Health by Social Position in Contemporary Britain. *Social Science and Medicine* 23:393–415.

MacCormack, C. P. 1984. Human Ecology and Behaviour in Malaria Control in Tropical Africa. *Bulletin of the World Health Organization* 62:81–87.

———. 1985. Anthropology and the Control of Tropical Disease. *Anthropology Today* 1(3): 14–16.

MacCormack, C. P., ed. 1982. *Ethnography of Fertility and Birth.* London: Academic Press.

MacCormack, C. P., and Alizon Draper. 1987. Social and Cognitive Aspects of Female Sexuality in Jamaica. In *The Cultural Construction of Sexuality,* ed. Pat Caplan. London: Tavistock, 143–65.

MacCormack, C. P., and M. Strathern, eds. 1980. *Nature, Culture and Gender.* Cambridge: Cambridge University Press.

MacLennan, Carol A. 1988. From Accident to Crash: The Auto Industry and the Politics of Injury. *MAQ* n.s. 2(3):233–50.

Macleod, R., and M. Lewis, eds. 1988. *Disease, Medicine, and Empire: Perspectives on Western Medicine and Experience of European Expansion.* London: Routledge.

MacLeod, Robert B. 1969. Phenomenology and Crosscultural Research. In *Interdisciplinary Relationships in the Social Sciences,* ed. Muzafer Sherif and Carolyn W. Sherif. Chicago: Aldine Publishing Company, 177–96.

MacNab, E. 1970. A *Legal History of Health Professions in Ontario.* Toronto: Committee on the Healing Arts.

Macrae, W. D., J. B. Hudson, and G. H. N. Towers. 1988. Studies on the Pharmacological Activity of Amazonian Euphorbiaceae. *Journal of Ethnopharmacology* 22:143–72.

Mafeje, Archie. 1976. The Problem of Anthropology in Historical Perspective: An Inquiry into the Growth of the Social Sciences. *Revue canadienne des études africaines/Canadian Journal of African Studies* 10(2):307–33.

Magubane, B. 1971. A Critical Look on the Indices Used in the Study of Social Change in Modern Africa. *Current Anthropology* 12:153–70.

———. 1979. *The Political Economy of Race and Class in South Africa.* New York: Monthly Press.

Mahler, Halfdan. 1981. The Meaning of "Health for All by the Year 2000." *World Health Forum* 3(1):5–22.

Maida, Carl A. 1984. Social-Network Considerations in the Alcohol Field. In *Recent Developments in Alcoholism,* vol. 2, ed. Marc Galanter. New York: Plenum.

Mail, Patricia D., and David R. McDonald. 1980. *Tulapi to Tokay: A Bibliography of Alcohol Use and Abuse among Native Americans of North America.* New Haven: HRAF Press.

Malinowski, Bronislaw. 1929. Practical Anthropology. *Africa* 2(1):22–38.

———. 1932. *The Sexual Life of Savages in Northwestern Melanesia.* London: Routledge and Kegan Paul.

Malone, Marvin H., and Ana Rother. 1994. *Heimia salicifolia:* A Phytochemical and Phytopharmacologic Review. *Journal of Ethnopharmacology* 42:135–59.

Malthus, Thomas. 1972. Population. The First Essay. In *Population Crisis: An Interdisciplinary Perspective,* ed. S. T. Reid and D. L. Lyon. Glenview, Ill.: Scott Foresman, 10–11.

Mandelbaum, David G. 1965. Alcohol and Culture. *Current Anthropology* 6:281–94.

———. 1966. *Edward Sapir: Culture, Language and Personality.* Berkeley and Los Angeles: University of California Press (orig. 1949).

Mandell, G. L., R. G. Douglas, and J. E. Bennett. 1985. *Principles and Practice of Infectious Diseases.* 2d ed. New York: John Wiley.

Mandl, P. E. 1983. Growth Charts, Oral Rehydration Therapy, Breast-feeding, and Immunization on a Wider Scale. *Assignment Children* 61/62:11–18.

Manning, Peter, and Horatio Fabrega. 1973. The Experience of Self and Body: Health and Illness in the Chiapas Highlands. In *Phenomenological Sociology,* ed. George Psathas. New York: Wiley, 59–73.

Manson, Spero, James H. Shore, and Joseph D. Bloom. 1985. The Depressive Experience in American Indian Communities: A Challenge for Psychiatric Theory and Diagnosis. In *Culture and Depression: Studies in the Anthropology and Cross-Cultural Psychiatry of Affect and Disorder,* ed. Arthur Kleinman and Byron Good. Berkeley: University of California Press.

Mapother, E. D. 1968. *The Medical Profession and Its Educational and Licensing Bodies.* Dublin: Fannin & Co.

Marchione, T. 1980. A History of Breastfeeding Practices in the English Speaking Caribbean in the Twentieth Century. *Food and Nutrition Bulletin* 2:9–18.

———. 1981. *Ethnographic Study: Phase I. Field Manual.* Infant Feeding Practices Study. Population Council, Columbia University, Cornell University.

Marcus, George. 1986. Contemporary Problems of Ethnography in the Modern World System. In *Writing Culture,* ed. J. Clifford and G. Marcus. Berkeley: University of California Press.

Marcus, George, and Michael Fischer. 1986. *Anthropology as Cultural Critique: An Experimental Moment in the Human Sciences.* Chicago: University of Chicago Press.

Maretzki, Thomas W. 1980. Reflections on Clinical Anthropology. *Medical Anthropology Newsletter* 12(1):19–21.

———. 1982. A Postdoctoral Training Program for Anthropologists in Clinical Research. *Medical Anthropology Quarterly* 14(1):21–23.

Mariner, W. K. 1993. Distinguishing "Exploitable" from "Vulnerable" Populations: When Consent Is Not the Issue. In *Ethics and Research on Human Subjects: International Guidelines,* ed. Z. Bankowski and R. J. Levine. Geneva: Council for International Organizations of Medical Sciences, 44–55.

Marino, Anthony. 1970. Family, Fertility, and Sex Ratios in the British Caribbean. *Population Studies* 24:159–72.

Marmot, M. G., and S. L. Syme. 1976. Acculturation and Coronary Heart Disease in Japanese-Americans. *American Journal of Epidemiology* 104:225–47.

Marmot, M. G, and J. N. Morris. 1984. The Social Environment. In *Oxford Textbook of Public Health,* Vol. 1 *History, Determinants, Scope, and Strategies,* ed. Walter W. Holland, Roger Detels, and George Knox. Oxford: Oxford University Press, 97–118.

Marmot, Michael, and Tores Theorell. 1988. Social Class and Cardiovascular Disease: The Contribution of Work. *International Journal of Health Services* 18:659–74.

Mars, Gerald. 1987. Longshore Drinking, Economic Security, and Union Politics in Newfoundland. In *Constructive Drinking,* ed. Mary Douglas. Cambridge: Cambridge University Press, 91–101.

Marsella, Anthony J. 1982. Culture and Mental Health: An Overview. In *Cultural Conceptions of Mental Health and Therapy,* ed. Anthony J. Marsella and Geoffrey M. White. Dordrecht: D. Reidel, 359–88.

Marsella, Anthony J., George DeVos, and Francis L. K. Hsu, eds. 1985. *Culture and Self: Asian and Western Perspectives.* New York: Tavistock Publications.

Marshall, John F. 1977. Acceptability of Fertility Regulating Methods: Designing Technology to Fit People. *Preventive Medicine* 6(1):65–73.

Marshall, Leslie. 1985. *Infant Care and Feeding: Cases from the South Pacific.* New York: Gordon & Breach Science Publishers.

Marshall, Lorna. 1965. The Kung Bushman of the Kalahari Desert. In *Peoples of Africa,* ed. J. L. Gibbs. New York: Rinehart & Winston.

Marshall, Mac. 1976. A Review and Appraisal of Alcohol and Kava Studies in Oceania. In *Cross-Cultural Approaches to the Study of Alcohol,* ed. M. Everett et al. The Hague: Mouton.

———. 1979. *Weekend Warriors: Alcohol in a Micronesian Culture.* Palo Alto: Mayfield.

———. 1982. *Through a Glass Darkly: Beer and Modernization in Papua New Guinea.* Monograph 18. Boroko, Papua New Guinea: Institute for Applied Social and Economic Research.

———. 1983. Alcohol and Drug Studies in Anthropology: Where Do We Go From Here? *Newsletter of the Alcohol and Drug Studies Group, American Anthropological Association* 9:6–13.

———. 1985. Social Thought, Cultural Belief and Alcohol. *Journal of Drug Issues* (Winter): 63–71.

———. 1987. An Overview of Drugs in Oceania. In *Drugs in Western Pacific Societies,* ed. Lamont Lindstrom. Lanham, Md.: University Press of America.

———. 1988. Alcohol Consumption as a Public Health Problem in Papua New Guinea. *International Journal of the Addictions* 23(6):573–89.

———. 1990a. "Problem Deflation" and the Ethnographic Record: Interpretation and Introspection in Anthropological Studies of Alcohol. *Journal of Substance Abuse* 2:353–67.

———. 1990b. Combining Insights from Epidemiological and Ethnographic Data to Investigate Substance Use in Truk, Federated States of Micronesia. *British Journal of Addiction* 85: 1457–68.

Marshall, Mac, ed. 1979. *Beliefs, Behaviors, and Alcoholic Beverages: A Cross-Cultural Survey.* Ann Arbor: University of Michigan Press.

Marshall, Patricia Loomis. 1982. Rural and Urban Factors in Alcohol Use in an Appalachian Setting. Ph.D. dissertation, University of Kentucky.

———. 1991. Research Ethics in Applied Medical Anthropology. In *Training Manual in Medical Anthropology,* ed. Carole Hill. 2d ed. Washington, D.C.: American Anthropological Association and Society for Applied Anthropology.

———. 1992. Anthropology and Bioethics. *Medical Anthropology Quarterly* 6(1):49–73.

Marshall, Patricia, David C. Thomasma, and Juritt Bergsma. 1994. Intercultural Reasoning: The Challenge for International Bioethics. *Cambridge Quarterly of Healthcare Ethics* 3:321–328.

Martin, Emily. 1987. The *Woman in the Body: A Cultural Analysis of Reproduction.* Boston: Beacon Press.

———. 1988. The Cultural Construction of Gendered Bodies: Biology Metaphors of Production and Destruction. Paper presented at the Meeting of the American Anthropological Association, Phoenix, Arizona, November 16–20.

———. 1994. *Flexible Bodies: Tracking Immunity in American Culture from the Days of Polio to the Age of AIDS.* Boston: Beacon Press.

Martinez, H., et al. 1988. *Uso de Alimentos Y Bebidas en El Hogar en El Manejo de La Diarrea Aguda del Nino.* Mexico City: Instituto Nacional de la Nutricion 'Salvador Zubiran.'

Marwick, Max G. 1964. Witchcraft as a Social Strain Gauge. *Australian Journal of Science* 26: 263–68.

———. 1965. Some Problems in the Sociology of Sorcery and Witchcraft. In *African Systems of Thought,* ed. M. Fortes and G. Dieterlen. London: Oxford University Press for the International African Institute, 171–91.

Marx, Karl, and Frederick Engels. 1970. *The German Ideology.* New York: International Publishers.

Mascolo, N., R. Sharma, S. C. Jain, and F. Capasso. 1988. Ethnopharmacology of *Calotropis procera* flowers. *Journal of Ethnopharmacology* 22:211–21.

Mason, Douglas. 1988. *Licensed to Live.* London: Adam Smith Institute.

Mason, John W. 1975. A Historical View of the Stress Field. *Journal of Human Stress* 1:6–12, 22–36.

Massara, E. B. 1980. Obesity and Cultural Weight Evaluations. *Appetite* 1:291–98.

Massey, Douglas S., and Felipe Garcia España. 1987. The Social Process of International Migration. *Science* 237:733–38.

Masson, Jeffrey M. 1984. The *Assault on Truth: Freud's Suppression of the Seduction Theory.* New York: Farrar, Strauss and Giroux.

Mata, L. J. 1978. *The Children of Santa Maria Cauque: A Prospective Field Study of Health and Growth.* Cambridge: MIT Press.

Mata, L. J., J. J. Urrutia, and A. Lechtig. 1971. Infection and Nutrition of Children of a Low Socioeconomic Rural Community. *American Journal of Clinical Nutrition* 24:249–59.

Mathews, Dale, David Larson, and Constance Barry. 1993. *The Faith Factor: An Annotated Bibliography of Clinical Research on Spiritual Subjects.* Betheseda: National Institute for Healthcare Research.

Mathias-Mundy, Evelyn, and Constance M. McCorckle. 1989. *Ethnoveterinary Medicine: An Annotated Bibliography.* Ames: Iowa State University Research Foundation.

Mathieu, Arline. 1993. The Medicalization of Homelessness and the Theater of Repression. *Medical Anthropology Quarterly* 7(2):170–84.

Matossian, R. M., M. D. Rickard, and J. D. Smith. 1977. Hydatidosis: A Global Problem of Increasing Importance. *Bulletin of the World Health Organization* 55:499–507.

Matthews, Holly. 1992. The Directive Force of Morality Tales in a Mexican Community. In *Human Motives and Cultural Models,* ed. R. D'Andrade and C. Strauss. Cambridge: Cambridge University Press.

Matthews, Mervyn. 1978. *Privilege in the Soviet Union.* London: Allan & Unwin.

Mattingly, Cheryl. 1991. The Narrative Nature of Clinical Reasoning. *American Journal of Occupational Therapy* 45(11):998–1005.

Mausner, J. S., and S. Kramer. 1985. *Mausner and Bahn Epidemiology—An Introductory Text.* Philadelphia: W. B. Saunders Company.

Mauss, Marcel. 1979 (1950). *Sociology and Psychology: Essays.* London: Routledge & Kegan Paul.

———. 1985 (1938). A Category of the Human Mind: The Notion of the Person, the Notion of the Self. In *The Category of the Person: Anthropology, Philosophy, History,* ed. M. Carrithers, S. Collins, and S. Lukes. Cambridge: Cambridge University Press, 1–25.

Mauss, M., and H. Beuchat. 1904. Essai sur les variations saisonnieres des sociétés. Eskimoes-Etudes de morphologie sociale. *L'Annee sociologique* 9:39.

May, J. M. 1958. *The Ecology of Human Disease.* New York: MD Publications.

———. 1960. The Ecology of Human Disease. *Annals of the New York Academy of Science* 84: 789–94.

———. 1961. *Studies in Disease Ecology.* New York: Hafner.

Maybury-Lewis, David H. P. 1967. *Akwe-Shavante Society.* Oxford: Clarendon Press.

Mayr, Ernst. 1982. *The Growth of Biological Thought: Diversity, Evolution, and Inheritance.* Cambridge: Belknap Press of Harvard University Press.

Mburu, F. M. 1981. Implications of the Ideology and Implementation of Health Policy in a Developing Country. *Social Science and Medicine* 15:17–24.

McClain, Carol. 1975. Ethno-obstetrics in Ajijic. *Anthropological Quarterly* 48(1):38–56.

———. 1982. Toward a Comparative Framework for the Study of Childbirth: A Review of the Literature. In *Anthropology of Human Birth,* ed. Margarita Artschwager Kay. Philadelphia: F. A. Davis Co., 25–59.

———. 1985. Why Women Choose Trial of Labor or Repeat Cesarean Section. *Journal of Family Practice* 21(3):210–16.

McClain, Carol, ed. 1989. *Women as Healers.* New Brunswick, N.J.: Rutgers University Press.

McClelland, C. E. 1991. *The German Experience of Professionalisation: Modern Learned Professions and Their Organizations from the Early 19th Century to the Hitler Era.* Cambridge: Cambridge University Press.

McCracken, R. D. 1971. Lactose Deficiency: An Example of Dietary Evolution. *Current Anthropology* 12:479–517.

McDonald, Catherine. 1981. Political-Economic Structures—Approaches to Traditional and Modern Medical Systems. *Social Science and Medicine* 15A:101–8.

McDonald, Maryon, ed. 1994. *Gender, Drink and Drugs.* Oxford: Berg Publishers.

McElroy, Ann, ed. 1990. Steps toward an Integrative Medical Anthropology. *Medical Anthropology Quarterly* n.s. 4(3).

McElroy, A., and P. K. Townsend. 1989. *Medical Anthropology in Ecological Perspective.* Boulder, Colo.: Westview Press.

———. 1990. Biocultural Models in Studies of Human Health and Adaption. *Medical Anthropology Quarterly* 4(3):243–65.

McEvoy, Frederick D. 1971. *History, Tradition and Kinship as Factors in Modern Sabo Labor Migration.* Ann Arbor: University Microfilms.

McFarlane, Allan H., Geoffrey R. Norman, David L. Streiner, Ranjan Roy, and Deborah J. Scott. 1980. A Longitudinal Study of the Influence of the Psychosocial Environment on Health Status: A Preliminary Report. *Journal of Health and Social Behavior* 21:124–33.

McGarvey, Stephen T., and Diana E. Schendel. 1986. Blood Pressure of Samoans. In *The Changing Samoans: Behavior and Health in Transition,* ed. Paul T. Baker, Joel M. Hanna, and Thelma S. Baker. New York: Oxford University Press.

McGrath, J. 1990. AIDS in Africa: A Bioanthropological Perspective. *American Journal of Human Biology* 2:381–96.

McGrath, J., et al. 1993. Anthropology and AIDS: The Cultural Context of Sexual Risk Behavior among Urban Bagandan Women in Kampala, Uganda. *Social Science and Medicine* 36(4): 429–39.

McGuire, Meredith. 1987. *Ritual Healing in Suburban America.* New Brunswick: Rutgers University Press.

McKeown, T. 1976a. *The Modern Rise of Population.* Cambridge: Cambridge University Press.

———. 1976b. *The Role of Medicine: Dream, Mirage, or Nemesis?* Princeton: Princeton University Press, and London: Nuffield Provincial Hospitals Trust.

McKinlay, John B. 1981. Social Network Influences on Morbid Episodes and the Career of Help Seeking. In *The Relevance of Social Science for Medicine,* ed. Leon Eisenberg and Arthur Kleinman. Dordrecht: D. Reidel Publishing Company, 77–107.

McLaren, Angus. 1984. *Reproductive Rituals: The Perception of Fertility in England from the Sixteenth to the Nineteenth Century.* London: Methuen.

McLuhan, Marshall. 1964. *Understanding Media: The Extensions of Man.* New York: McGraw-Hill.

McMillen, Marilyn M. 1979. Differential Mortality by Sex in Fetal and Neonatal Deaths. *Science* 204:89.

McNeill, W. H. 1976. *Plagues and Peoples.* Garden City, N.Y.: Doubleday.

———. 1980. Migration Patterns and Infection in Traditional Societies. In *Changing Disease Patterns and Human Behavior.* London: Academic Press, 27–36.

McQuestion, Michael, ed. 1983. *Oral Rehydration Therapy: An Annotated Bibliography.* Scientific Publication 445. Washington, D.C.: World Health Organization.

McSpadden, Lucia Ann. 1987. Ethiopian Refugee Resettlement in the Western United States: Social Context and Psychological Well-being. *International Migration Review* 21:796–819.

Mead, Margaret. 1935. *Sex and Temperament in Three Primitive Societies.* New York: William Morrow and Co.

———. 1943. The Problem of Changing Food Habits. In *The Problem of Changing Food Habits,* National Research Council Bulletin, no. 108. Washington, D.C.: National Academy of Sciences-National Research Council, 20–31.

———. 1947. The Concept of Culture and the Psychosomatic Approach. *Psychiatry* 10:57–76.

———. 1977. Contemporary Implications of the State of the Art. In *Malnutrition, Behavior and Social Organization,* ed. L. S. Greene. New York: Academic Press.

Mead, Margaret, and Niles Newton. 1967. Cultural Patterning of Perinatal Behavior. In *Childbearing—Its Social and Psychological Aspects,* ed. S. Richardson and A. Guttmacher. Baltimore: Williams and Wilkins Co., 142–244.

Mechanic, D. M. 1968. *Medical Sociology.* New York: Free Press.

Mejia, Alfonso. 1980. World Physician Migration. Paper presented at the Seminar on the Arab Brain Drain, UN Economic and Social Council, Economic Commission for Western Asia, Beirut, Lebanon, February 4–8.

Meleis, Afaf I., and Albert R. Jonsen. 1983. Ethical Crises and Cultural Differences. *Western Journal of Medicine* 138:889–93.

Mellor, John W., and Sarah Gavian. 1987. Famine: Causes, Prevention, and Relief. *Science* 235: 539–45.

Melman, Seymour. 1965. *Our Depleted Society.* New York: Delta.

———. 1988. *The Demilitarized Society: Disarmament and Conversion.* Montreal: Harvest House.

Menken, Jane, James Trussell, and Ulla Carsen. 1986. Age and Infertility. *Science* 233:1389–94.

Merchant, Carolyn. 1980. *The Death of Nature: Women, Ecology, and the Scientific Revolution.* New York: Harper & Row.

Merchant, James. 1980. Coal Workers, Pneumoconiosis. In *Maxy-Rosenau Public Health and Preventive Medicine,* ed. John M. Last. 11th ed. New York: Appleton-Century-Crofts, 610–29.

Merson, M. 1993. The HIV/AIDS Pandemic: Global Spread and Global Response. Paper presented at the IX International Conference on AIDS, Berlin, June.

Messerschmidt, D. A., ed. 1981. *Anthropologists at Home in North America: Methods and Issues in the Study of One's Own Society.* Cambridge: Cambridge University Press.

Messing, Simon. 1958. Group Therapy and Social Status in the Zar Cult of Ethiopia. In M. Opler, ed., *Culture and Mental Health.* New York: Macmillan.

Metzger, D., and Gerlad Williams. 1963. Tenejapa Medicine I: The Curer. *Southwestern Journal of Anthropology* 19:216–34.

Michaels, David. 1988. Waiting for the Body Count: Corporate Decision Making and Bladder Cancer in the U.S. Dye Industry. *Medical Anthropology Quarterly* n.s. 2(3):215–32.

Michaelson, K., et al. 1988. *Childbirth in America: Anthropological Perspectives.* South Hadley, Mass.: Bergin and Garvey.

Miles, Stephen H. 1992. Medical Futility. *Law, Medicine, and Health Care* 20(4):310–15.

Milingo, E. 1984. *The World Is Between: Christian Healing and the Struggle for Spiritual Survival.* London: C. Hurst & Co.

Millar, M. I., and S. D. Lane. 1988. Ethno-Ophthalmology in the Egyptian Delta: An Historical Systems Approach to Ethnomedicine in the Middle East. *Social Science and Medicine* 26: 651–57.

Miller, Barbara Diane, ed. 1993. *Sex and Gender Hierarchies.* Cambridge: Cambridge University Press.

Minkowski, Eugene. 1958. Findings in a Case of Schizophrenic Depression. In *Existence: A New Dimension in Psychiatry and Psychology,* ed. Rollo May, Ernest Angel, and Henri Ellenberger. New York: Simon & Schuster, 127–38.

Mintzes, B., A. Hardon, and J. Hanhart, eds. 1993. *Norplant: Under Her Skin.* Amsterdam: Women's Health Action Foundation.

Mitchell, J. Clyde. 1961. Wage Labour and African Population Movements in Central Africa. In *Essays on African Populations,* ed. K. Barbour and R. L. Prothero. London: Routledge and Kegan Paul.

Modell, Judith. 1989. Last Chance Babies: Interpretations of Parenthood in an In Vitro Fertilization Program. *Medical Anthropology* 3(2):124–38.

Moerman, Daniel E. 1979a. Symbols and Selectivity. *Journal of Ethnopharmacology* 1:111–19.

———. 1979b. Anthropology of Symbolic Healing. *Current Anthropology* 20:59–80.

———. 1983a. Physiology and Symbols: The Anthropological Implications of the Placebo Effect. In *The Anthropology of Medicine: From Culture to Method,* ed. Lola Romanucci-Ross, Daniel E. Moerman, and Laurence R. Tancredi. New York: Praeger, 156–67.

———. 1983b. General Medical Effectiveness and Human Biology: Placebo Effects in the Treatment of Ulcer Disease. *Medical Anthropology Quarterly* 14:3–16.

———. 1986. *Medicinal Plants of Native America.* Ann Arbor: University of Michigan Museum of Anthropology.

———. 1989. Poisoned Apples and Honeysuckles: The Medicinal Plants of Native America. *Medical Anthropology Quarterly* 3(1):52–61.

Moghissi, K. S., and T. N. Evans, eds. 1977. *Nutritional Impacts on Women.* New York: Harper & Row.

Molgaard, C. A., and E. L. Byerly. 1981. Applied Ethnoscience in Rural America: New Age Health and Healing. In *Anthropologists at Home in America: Methods and Issues in the Study of One's Own Culture,* ed. D. Messerschmidt. Cambridge: Cambridge University Press, 153–66.

Molina-Guzman, Gustavo. 1979. Third World Experiences in Health Planning. *International Journal of Health Services* 9:139–50.

Mollica, R., G. Wyshak, and J. Lavalle. 1987. The Psychosocial Impact of War Trauma and Torture on Southeast Asian Refugees. *American Journal of Psychiatry* 144:1567–72.

Monod, Théodore, ed. 1975. *Pastoralism in Tropical Africa.* London: Oxford University Press.

Monroe, Scott M., Donald F. Imhoff, Beverly D. Wise, and Joyce E. Harris. 1983. Prediction of

Psychological Symptoms under High Risk Psychosocial Circumstances: Life Events, Social Support, and Symptom Specificity. *Journal of Abnormal Psychology* 92:338–50.

Montagu, M. F. Ashley. 1949. Embryology from Antiquity to the End of the 18th Century. *Ciba Symposia* 10(4):994–1008.

Montague, J., and J. Lamstein. 1988. Private Sector and Family Planning: Hitting Full Stride. *Family Planning Enterprise* 1(1):1–3.

Montasser, Kamal M. 1994. The Impact of Privatization of Egyptian Health Care Services on Urban Women's Health. Unpublished research proposal.

Montgomery, Edward. 1976. Systems and the Medical Practitioners of a Tamil Town. In *Asian Medical Systems: A Comparative Study,* ed. C. Leslie. Berkeley and Los Angeles: University of California Press, 272–84.

Montgomery, E., and J. Bennett. 1979. Anthropological Studies of Food and Nutrition: The 1940s and the 1970s. In *Uses of Anthropology,* ed. E. Goldschmidt. Special publication, no. 11. Washington, D.C.: American Anthropological Association, 124–43.

Moran, Emilio, ed. 1990. *The Ecosystem Concept in Anthropology: From Concept to Practice.* Ann Arbor: University of Michigan Press.

Moran, M., and B. Wood. 1992. *States, Regulation and the Medical Profession.* Buckingham: Open University Press.

Moreno, Jonathan D. 1995. *Deciding Together: Bioethics and Moral Consensus.* New York: Oxford University Press.

Morey Nancy E., and Robert V. Morey. 1994. Organizational Culture: The Management Approach. In *Practicing Anthropology in Corporate America: Consulting on Organizational Culture,* ed. Ann T. Jordan. Washington, D.C.: American Anthropological Association, 17–24.

Morgan, Lynn M. 1987. Dependency Theory in the Political Economy of Health: An Anthropological Critique. *Medical Anthropology Quarterly* 1(2):131–55.

———. 1989. When Does Life Begin? In *Abortion Rights and "Fetal Personhood,"* ed. Edd Doer and James W. Prescott. Long Beach, Calif.: Centerline Press, 97–114.

———. 1989b. The Importance of the State in Primary Health Care in Costa Rica, Guatemala, Nicaragua, and El Salvador. *Medical Anthropology Quarterly* 3(3):227–31.

———. 1993a. Comments on Wiley's *Adaptation and the Biocultural Paradigm in Medical Anthropology:* A Critical Review. *Medical Anthropology Quarterly* 7(2):199–201.

———. 1993b. *Community Participation in Health: The Politics of Primary Care in Costa Rica.* Cambridge: Cambridge University Press.

Morgan, Lynn A., ed. 1989. The Political Economy of Primary Health Care Initiatives. *Medical Anthropology Quarterly* 3 (3).

Morgan, W. T. W. 1981. Ethnobotany of the Turkana: Use of Plants by a Pastoral People and Their Livestock in Kenya. *Economic Botany* 35(1):96–130.

Morgen, Sandra. 1986. The Dynamics of Co-optation in a Feminist Health Clinic. *Social Science and Medicine* 23(2):201–10.

Morgenstern, H. 1980. The Changing Association between Social Status and Coronary Heart Disease in a Rural Population. *Social Science and Medicine* 14A:191–201.

Morice, R. 1978. Psychiatric Diagnosis in a Transcultural Setting: The Importance of Lexical Categories. *British Journal of Psychiatry* 182:87–95.

Morikawa, Isao. 1994. Patients' Rights in Japan: Progress and Resistance. *Kennedy Institute of Ethics Journal* 4(4):337–44.

Morley, Peter. 1988. Review of Special Journal Issues. *Transcultural Psychiatric Research Review* 25(2):112–18.

Morowitz, Harold J. 1991. Balancing Species Preservation and Economic Considerations. *Science* 253:752–54.

Morreim, E. Havvi. 1995. *Balancing Act: The New Medical Ethics of Medicine's New Economics.* Washington, D.C.: Georgetown University Press.

Morse, Stephen S., ed. 1993. *Emerging Viruses.* New York: Oxford University Press.

Morsy, Soheir A. 1978. Sex Roles, Power, and Illness in an Egyptian Village. *American Ethnologist* 5:137–50.

———. 1979. The Missing Link in Medical Anthropology: The Political Economy of Health. *Reviews in Anthropology* 6:349–63.

———. 1980. Reorientation in Capitalist Development: A Note on Sadat's Infitah. Paper presented at the Central States Meeting of the American Anthropological Association, Ann Arbor, Mich., April 9–11.

———. 1981. Towards a Political Economy of Health: A Critical Note on the Medical Anthropology of the Middle East. *Social Science and Medicine* 15(b):159–63.

———. 1982. Childbirth in an Egyptian Village. In *An Anthropology of Human Birth,* ed. M. Kay. Philadelphia: F. A. Davis, 147–74.

———. 1986a. "Indigenous" Anthropology in the Context of Intellectual Dependency. Paper presented at the Annual Central States Meeting of the American Anthropological Association, Chicago, March 27–29.

———. 1986b. Reflections on the Politics of Health. *Al-Talica* (February): 49–59. (in Arabic)

———. 1986c. U.S. Aid to Egypt: An Illustration and Account of U.S. Foreign Assistance Policy. *Arab Studies Quarterly* 8(4):358–89.

———. 1986d. Subdermal Implant Contraception, Women and Power in Egypt: How Is a Woman to Know: What Is an Anthropologist to Tell? Paper presented at the Society for Medical Anthropology, invited session on Knowledge and Power in the Management of Reproduction, AES Annual Spring Meeting of the American Anthropological Association, Wrightsville, North Carolina, April 24–27.

———. 1988a. Discussant's Commentary on "Reproductive Technology, Medical Practice, Public Expectations and New Representations of the Human Body," invited session, Society for Medical Anthropology, Annual Meeting of the American Anthropological Association, Phoenix, Arizona, November 16–20.

———. 1988b. Islamic Clinics in Egypt: The Cultural Elaboration of Biomedical Hegemony. *Medical Anthropology Quarterly* n.s. 2(4):355–67.

———. 1988c. Spirit Possession in Egyptian Ethnomedicine: Origins, Comparison, and Historical Specificity. Paper presented at the Workshop on "Contributions of the Zar Cult in African Traditional Medicine," Institute of African and Asian Studies, Khartoum, Sudan, January 11–13.

———. 1989a. Drop the Label: An "Emic" View of Critical Medical Anthropology. *Anthropology Newsletter* 30(2):13–16.

———. 1989b. Biotechnology and the International Politics of Population Control: Long-Term Contraception in Egypt. Manuscript:

———. 1991. Spirit Possession in Egyptian Ethnomedicine: Origins, Comparisons and Historical Specificity. In *Women's Medicine: The Zar-Bori Cult in Africa and Beyond,* ed. I. M. Lewis, Ahmed Al-Safi, and Sayyid Hurreiz. Edinburgh: Edinburgh University Press for the International African Institute, 189–208.

———. 1993a. *Gender, Sickness, and Healing in Rural Egypt: Ethnography in Historical Context.* Boulder, Colo.: Westview Press.

———. 1993b. Bodies of Choices: Norplant Experimental Trials on Egyptian Women. In *Norplant under Her Skin,* ed. Barbara Mintzes, Anita Hardon, and Jannemieke Hanhart. Amsterdam: Eduron, 89–114.

———. 1993c. Sociomedical Discourse and Critical Scholarship: Modernism, Post-Modernism, and the Pursuit of Relevance. Paper presented at the SSRC/ACLS Conference on Questions of Modernity: Strategies for Post-Orientalist Scholarship in the Middle East and South Asia, Cairo, A.R.E., May 28–30.

———. 1995. Deadly Reproduction among Egyptian Women: Maternal Mortality and the Medicalization of Population Control. In *Conceiving the New World Order: Local/Global Inter-*

sections in the Politics of Reproduction, ed. Faye Ginsberg and Rayna Rapp. Berkeley: University of California Press.

Morsy, Soheir A., and Jehan A. El-Bayoumi. 1993. Risk as an Analytical Construct: Implication for Children's Health in Arab Societies. *Childhood: A Global Journal of Child Research* 1 (2).

Morsy, Soheir A., Cynthia Nelson, Reem Saad Luka, and Hania Shokamy. 1986. Anthropology and the Call for Indigenization of Social Science in the Arab World. Paper presented at the International Conference on "Contemporary Arab Studies," American University in Cairo, October 15–17. (Forthcoming in The State of the Art in Contemporary Arab Studies. Tarek Ismail, ed.) Alberta: University of Alberta Press.

Morton, R. F., J. R. Helbel, and R. J. McCarter. 1990. *A Study Guide to Epidemiology and Biostatistics.* Rockville, Md.: Aspen Publishers.

Moses, Yolanda T. 1977. Female Status, the Family, and Male Dominance in a West Indian Community. *Signs: Journal of Women in Culture and Society* 3(1):142–53.

Mosley, W. Henry. 1983. Will Primary Health Care Reduce Infant and Child Mortality? A Critique of Some Current Strategies, with Special Reference to Africa and Asia. Paper presented at the IUSSP Seminar on Social Policy, Health Policy and Mortality Prospects, Paris, February 28–March 4.

Mosley, W. Henry, ed. 1978. *Nutrition and Human Reproduction.* New York: Plenum.

Mosley, W. Henry, and Lincoln C. Chen, eds. 1984. *Child Survival: Strategies for Research. Population and Development Review* 10 (Suppl.)

Muecke, M. A. 1979. An Exploration of "Wind Illness" in Northern Thailand. *Culture, Medicine and Psychiatry* 3:267–300.

Muensterberger, Werner, ed. 1969. *Man and His Culture.* New York: Taplinger.

Mulkay, Michael. 1979. *Science and the Sociology of Knowledge.* London: George Allen and Unwin.

Muller, Charlotte. 1990. *Health Care and Gender.* New York: Russell Sage Foundation.

Muller, Jessica H. 1992. Shades of Blue: The Negotiation of Limited Codes by Medical Residents. *Social Science and Medicine* 8:885–98.

———. 1994. Anthropology, Bioethics, and Medicine: A Provocative Trilogy. *Medical Anthropology Quarterly* 8(4):448–67.

Muller, Jessica H., and Brian Desmond. 1992. Ethical Dilemmas in a Cross-Cultural Context—A Chinese Example. *Western Journal of Medicine* 157:323–27.

Muller, Jessica H., and Barbara A. Koenig. 1988. On the Boundary of Life and Death: The Definition of Dying by Medical Residents. In *Biomedicine Examined,* ed. Margaret Lock and Deborah R. Gordon. Boston: Kluwer Academic Publishers, 19–57.

Mullings, Leith. 1984. *Therapy, Ideology and Social Change: Mental Healing in Urban Ghana.* Berkeley: University of California Press.

Murase, Takao. 1982. Sunao: A Central Value in Japanese Psychotherapy. In Anthony Marsella and Geoffrey White, eds., *Cultural Conceptions of Mental Health and Therapy.* Dordrecht: D. Reidel, 217–32.

Murphy, Henry B. M. 1961. Social Change and Mental Health. *Milbank Memorial Quarterly* 39: 385–434.

———. 1977. Transcultural Psychiatry Should Begin at Home. *Psychological Medicine* 7:369–71.

———. 1982a. Blood Pressure and Culture: The Contribution of Cross-cultural Comparisons to Psychosomatics. *Psychotherapeutics and Psychosomatics* 38:244–55.

———. 1982b. *Comparative Psychiatry: The International and InterCultural Distribution of Mental Illness.* New York: Springer-Verlag

Murphy, Henry B. M., et al. 1963. A Cross-Cultural Survey of Schizophrenic Symptomatology. *International Journal of Social Psychiatry* 9:237–49.

Murphy, Jane. 1964. Psychotherapeutic Aspects of Shamanism on St. Lawrence Island, Alaska. In *Magic, Faith, and Healing,* ed. Ari Kiev. New York: Macmillan.

Murray, R. F., Jr. 1992. Minority Perspectives on Biomedical Ethics. In *Transcultural Dimensions in Medical Ethics,* ed. E. Pellegrino, P. Mazzrella, and P. Corsi. Frederick, Md.: University Publishing Group.

Myers, Fred. 1979. Emotions and the Self: A Theory of Personhood and Political Order among Pintupi Aborigines. *Ethos* 7:343–70.

———. 1986. *Pintupi Country, Pintupi Self: Sentiment, Place and Politics among Western Desert Aborigines.* Washington, D.C.: Smithsonian Press.

Myers, L. 1982. *The Socialization of Neophyte Nurses.* Ann Arbor: University Microfilms International.

Myntti, Cynthia. 1988. Hegemony and Healing in Rural North Yemen. *Social Science and Medicine* 27(5):515–20.

Nadel, S. F. 1952. Witchcraft in Four African Societies: An Essay in Comparison. *American Anthropologist* 54:18–29.

Nader, Laura. 1969. Up the Anthropologist—Perspectives Gained from Studying Up. In *Reinventing Anthropology,* ed. Dell Hymes. New York: Random House.

Nag, Moni. 1966. *Factors Affecting Human Fertility in Non-Industrial Societies.* Yale University Publications in Anthropology 66. New Haven: Yale University Press.

Nag, Moni, Benjamin F. White, and R. Creighton Peet. 1978. An Anthropological Approach to the Study of the Economic Value of Children in Java and Nepal. *Current Anthropology* 19(2): 293–306.

Nagel, Thomas. 1972. War and Massacre. *Philosophy and Public Affairs* 1:19–36.

Naim, Samir. 1978. Towards a Demystification of Arab Social Reality: A Critique of Anthropological and Political Writings on Arab Society. *Review of Middle East Studies* 3:48–62.

Namboodiri, Krishnan, and C. M. Suchindran. 1987. *Life Table Techniques and Their Applications.* New York: Academic Press.

Nardi, Bonnie. 1983. Goals in Reproductive Decision Making. *American Ethnologist* 10(4):697–714.

Naroll, Raoul. 1983. *The Moral Order: An Introduction to the Human Situation.* Beverly Hills, Calif.: Sage.

Nash, June. 1979. *We Eat the Mines and the Mines Eat Us: Dependency and Exploitation in Bolivian Tin Mines.* New York: Columbia University Press.

———. 1981. Ethnographic Aspects of the World Capitalist System. *Annual Review of Anthropology* 10:393–423.

Nash, June, and Max Kirsch. 1986. Polychlorinated Biphenyls in the Electrical Machinery Industry: An Ethnological Study of Community Action and Corporate Responsibility. *Social Science and Medicine* 23(2):131–38.

———. 1988. The Discourse of Medical Science in the Construction of Consensus between Corporation and Community. *Medical Anthropology Quarterly* n.s. 2(2):158–171.

National Commission for the Protection of Biomedical and Behavioral Research. 1978. *The Belmont Report: Ethical Principles and Guidelines for the Protection of Human Subjects of Research.* Washington, D.C.: U.S. Government Printing Office.

Nations, Marilyn K. 1982. *Illness of the Child: The Cultural Context of Child Diarrhea.* Ann Arbor: University Microfilms International.

———. 1986. Epidemiological Research on Infectious Disease: Quantitative Rigor or Rigormortis? Insights from Ethnomedicine. In *Anthropology and Epidemiology: Interdisciplinary Approaches to the Study of Health and Disease,* ed. C. R. Janes, R. Stall, and S. M. Gifford. Dordrecht: D. Reidel, 97–123.

Nations, Marilyn K., and L. A. Rebhun. 1988. Angels with Wet Wings Won't Fly: Maternal Sentiment in Brazil and the Image of Neglect. *Culture, Medicine and Psychiatry* 12(2):141–200.

Navarro, Vicente. 1974. The Underdevelopment of Health or the Health of Underdevelopment: An Analysis of the Distribution of Human Health Resources in Latin America. *International Journal of Health Services* 4(1):5–27.

———. 1976. *Medicine under Capitalism.* New York: Prodist.

———. 1977. Social Class, Political Power, and the State and Their Implications in Medicine. *International Journal of Health Services* 7(2):255–92.

———. 1984. A Critique of the Ideological and Political Position of the Brandt Report and the Alma Ata Declaration. *International Journal of Health Services* 14:159–72.

———. 1985. U.S. Marxist Scholarship in the Analysis of Health and Medicine. *International Journal of Health Services* 15(4):525–44.

———. 1986. *Crisis, Health and Medicine: A Social Critique.* London: Tavistock.

Navarro, Vicente, ed. 1981. *Imperialism, Health and Medicine.* Farmingdale, N.Y.: Baywood Publishing Co.

Needham, Rodney, ed. 1967. Percussion and Transition. *Man* 2:606–14.

———. 1973. *Right and Left: Essays on Dual Symbolic Classification.* Chicago: University of Chicago Press.

Nelson, M., A. E. Black, J. A. Morris, and T. J. Cole. 1989. Between- and Within-Subject Variation in Nutrient Intake from Infancy to Old Age: Estimating the Number of Days Required to Rank Dietary Intakes with Desired Precision. *American Journal of Clinical Nutrition* 50:155–67.

Nerlove, S. B. 1974. Women's Workload and Infant Feeding Practices: A Relationship with Demographic Implications. *Ethnology* 13:125–214.

Ness, Robert C. 1980. The Impact of Indigenous Healing Activity: An Empirical Study of Fundamentalist Churches. *Social Science and Medicine* 14B:167–80.

———. 1982. Medical Anthropology in a Preclinical Curriculum. In *Clinically Applied Anthropology: Anthropologists in Health Science Settings,* ed. Noel J. Chrisman and Thomas W. Maretzki. Dordrecht: D. Reidel, 35–61.

Nesse, Randolph M., and George C. Williams. 1994. *Why We Get Sick: The New Science of Darwinian Medicine.* New York: Random House.

Netting, R. M. 1965. Trial Model of Cultural Ecology. *Anthropological Quarterly* 38:81–96.

———. 1985. Population Pressure and Intensification: Some Anthropological Reflections on Malthus, Marx, and Boserup. Paper prepared for the symposium on Anthropological Demography, annual meetings of the American Anthropological Association.

Neu, Jerome. 1977. *Emotion, Thought, and Therapy.* London: Routledge and Kegan Paul.

New, Peter K., and M. L. New. 1975. The Links between Health and the Political Structure in New China. *Human Organization* 34.

Newman, Lucille, ed. 1985. *Women's Medicine.* New Brunswick, N.J.: Rutgers University Press.

Newton, Lisa H. 1990. Ethical Imperialism and Informed Consent. *IRB: A Review of Human Subjects Research* 12(3):10–11.

Newton, Niles, and Michael Newton. 1972. Childbirth in Crosscultural Perspective. In *Modern Perspectives in Psycho-Obstetrics,* ed. J. Howells. Edinburgh: Oliver and Boyd, 150–72.

Newton, Paul. 1991. The Use of Medicinal Plants by Primates: A Missing Link? *Trends in Ecology and Evolution* 6:297–99.

Newton, Paul, and Toshisada Nishida. 1990. Possible Administration of Herbal Drugs by Wild Chimpanzees, Pan troglodytes. *Animal Behavior* 39:798–801.

Ngokwe, Ndolamb. 1987. Varieties of Palm Wine among the Lele of the Kasai. In *Constructive Drinking,* ed. Mary Douglas. Cambridge: Cambridge University Press.

Ngubane, Harriet. 1977. *Body and Mind in Zulu Medicine: An Ethnography of Health and Disease in Nyuswa-Zulu Thought and Practice.* New York: Academic Press.

Nichols, Philip. 1988. *Homeopathy and the Medical Profession.* London: Routledge.

Nichter, Mark. 1981. Idioms of Distress. *Culture, Medicine and Psychiatry* 5:379–408.

———. 1988. From Aralu to ORS: Sinhalese Perceptions of Digestion, Diarrhea, and Dehydration. *Social Science and Medicine* 27(1):39–52.

———. 1989. *Anthropology and International Health: South Asian Case Studies.* Dordrecht: Kluwer Academic Publications.

Nichter, Mark, ed. 1992. *Anthropological Approaches to the Study of Ethnomedicine.* Philadelphia: Gordon and Breach Science Publishers.

Nichter, Mark, and Elizabeth Cartwright. 1991. Saving the Children for the Tobacco Industry. *Medical Anthropology Quarterly* 5(3):236–56.

Nichter, Mark, and M. Nichter. 1983. The Ethnophysiology and Folk Dietetics of Pregnancy: A Case Study from South India. *Human Organization* 42(3):235–46.

———. 1986. A Tale of Simeon: Reflections on Raising a Child While Conducting Fieldwork in Rural South India. In *Family Album: Anthropological Fieldwork with Children,* ed. J. Kassel. Philadelphia: Temple University Press.

Nichter, Mark, Gordon Trockman, and Jean Grippen. 1985. Clinical Anthropologist as Therapy Facilitator: Role Development and Clinician Evaluation in a Psychiatric Training Program. *Human Organization* 44(1):72–80.

Niederland, William G. 1974. *The Schreber Case: Psychoanalytic Profile of a Paranoid Personality.* New York: Quadrangle/New York Times Book Co.

Nietschmann, Bernard. 1987. Militarization and Indigenous People. *Cultural Survival Quarterly* 11(3):1–16.

Nogami, M., T. Moriura, M. Kubo, and T. Tani. 1986. Studies on the Origin, Processing and Quality of Crude Drugs. *Chemical and Pharmaceutical Bulletin* 34:3854–60.

Noguchi, M. 1978. Studies on the Pharmaceutical Quality Evaluation of Crude Drug Preparations Used in the Oriental Medicine "Kampoo." II. Precipitation Reaction of Berberine and Glycyrrhizin in Aqueous Solution. *Chemical and Pharmaceutical Bulletin* 26:2624–29.

Nolan, Michael F. 1989. Foreword to *Ethnoveterinary Medicine: An Annotated Bibliography,* ed. E. Matias-Mundy and C. M. McCorckle. Ames: Iowa State University Research Foundation, v–vii.

Nolen-Hoeksema, S. 1990. *Sex Differences in Depression.* Stanford: Stanford University Press.

Noll, Richard. 1983. Shamanism and Schizophrenia: A State-Specific Approach to the "Schizophrenic Metaphor" of Shamanic States. *American Ethnologist* 10:443–59.

Nolte, Sharon, and Sally Ann Hastings. 1991. The Meiji State's Policy toward Women, 1890–1910. In *Recreating Japanese Women, 1600–1945,* ed. G. L. Berstein. Berkeley: University of California Press, 151–74.

Nordstrom, Carolyn, and JoAnn Martin. 1992. *The Paths to Domination, Resistance and Terror.* Berkeley and Los Angeles: University of California Press.

Notes and Queries. 1951. *Notes and Queries on Anthropology.* 6th ed. Committee of the Royal Anthropological Institute of Great Britain and Ireland. London: Routledge and Kegan Paul.

Nunberg, Herman. 1955. *Principles of Psychoanalysis.* New York: International Universities Press.

Nyazema, N. Z. 1986. Herbal Toxicity in Zimbabwe. *Transactions of the Royal Society of Tropical Medicine and Hygiene* 80:448–50.

Nzimiro, Ikenna. 1977. *The Crisis in the Social Sciences: The Nigerian Situation.* Third World Forum Occasional Paper # 2. Mexico: Third World Forum Coordinating Secretariat.

O'Brien, Bernie. 1984. *Patterns of European Diagnoses and Prescribing.* London: Office of Health Economics.

O'Laughlin, Bridget. 1974. Mediation of Contradiction: Why Mbum Women Do Not Eat Chicken. In *Women, Culture and Society,* ed. M. Z. Rosaldo and L. Lamphere. Stanford: Stanford University Press.

———. 1975. Marxist Approaches in Anthropology. *Annual Review of Anthropology* 5:341–70.

O'Neill, John. 1985. *Five Bodies: The Human Shape of Modern Society.* Ithaca: Cornell University Press.

———. 1989. The Cultural and Political Context of Patient Dissatisfaction in Cross-Cultural Clinical Encounters: A Canadian Inuit Study. *Medical Anthropology Quarterly* 3(4):323–44.

O'Nell, Carl W., and Henry A. Selby. 1968. Sex Differences in the Incidence of Susto in Two Zapotec Pueblos: An Analysis of the Relationships between Sex Role Expectations and a Folk Illness. *Ethnology* 7:95–105.

Oakley, Ann. 1972. *Sex, Gender and Society.* London: Maurice Temple Smith.

———. 1976. Wisewoman and Medicine Man: Changes in the Management of Childbirth. In *The*

Rights and Wrongs of Women, ed. J. Mitchell and A. Oakley. Harmondsworth: Penguin Books, 17–58.

———. 1977. Cross-cultural Practices. In *Benefits and Hazards of the New Obstetrics,* ed. Tim Chard and M. Richards. London: William Heinemann Medical Books.

———. 1979a. A Case of Maternity: Paradigms of Women as Maternity Cases. *Signs: Journal of Women in Culture and Society* 7(10):607–32.

———. 1979b. *Becoming a Mother.* London: Martin Robertson and Co.

———. 1980. *Women Confined: Towards a Sociology of Childbirth.* New York: Schocken Books.

———. 1986. *The Captured Womb: A History of the Medical Care of Pregnant Women.* Oxford: Basil Bernstein.

Oaks, Stanley C., Violaine Mitchell, Greg Pearson, and Charles Carpenter, eds. 1991. *Malaria: Obstacles and Opportunities.* Washington, D.C.: National Academy Press.

Obbo, C. 1993. HIV Infection through Social and Geographic Networks in Uganda. *Social Science and Medicine* 36(7):949–55.

Obeyesekere, Gananath. 1978. The Impact of Ayurvedic Ideas on the Culture and the Individual in Sri Lanka. In *Asian Medical Systems: A Comparative Study,* ed. C. Leslie. Berkeley: University of California Press, 201–27.

———. 1981. *Medusa's Hair: An Essay on Personal Symbols and Religious Experience.* Chicago: University of Chicago Press.

Ochs, Elinor, and Bambi Schieffelin, eds. 1986. *Language Socialization across Cultures.* Cambridge: Cambridge University Press.

———. 1989. Language Has a Heart. *Text* 9:7–25.

Odell, Mary E. 1986. Price or Production? Domestic Economies, Household Structure, and Fertility in a Guatemalan Village. In *Culture and Reproduction,* ed. W. Penn Handwerker. Boulder, Colo.: Westview, 125–43.

Odum, E. P. 1971. *Fundamentals of Ecology.* 3d ed. Philadelphia: Saunders.

Ohnuki-Tierney, E. 1994. Brain Death and Organ Transplantation: Cultural Bases of Medical Technology. *Current Anthropology* 25 (3).

Okuyama, T., et al. 1986. Effect of Oriental Plant Drugs on Platelet Aggregation. III. *Planta Medica* 52:171–75.

Olesen, V., and E. Whittaker. 1968. *The Silent Dialogue: A Study in the Psychology of Professional Socialization.* San Francisco: Jossey-Bass.

Omery, A. 1983. Phenomenology: A Method for Nursing Research. *Advances in Nursing Science* 5(2):49–63.

Omvedt, Gail. 1975. The Political Economy of Starvation. *Race and Class* 17(2):111–30.

Ong, Aihwa. 1988. The Production of Possession: Spirits and the Multinational Corporation in Malaysia. *American Ethnologist* 15:28–42.

Onoge, Omafume. 1975. Capitalism and Public Health: A Neglected Theme in the Medical Anthropology of Africa. In *Topias and Utopias of Health,* ed. S. R. Ingman and A. E. Thomas. The Hague: Mouton, 219–32.

Ooms, Theodora, ed. 1981. *Teenage Pregnancy in a Family Context.* Philadelphia: Temple University Press.

Opler, Marvin K. 1957. Schizophrenia and Culture. *Scientific American* 197: 103–10.

———. 1959. Cultural Differences in Mental Disorders: An Italian and Irish Contrast in the Schizophrenias—U.S.A. In *Culture and Mental Health,* ed. M. K. Opler. New York: Macmillan.

Opler, Morris E. 1936. Some Points of Comparison and Contrast between the Treatment of Functional Disorders by Apache Shamans and Modern Psychiatric Practice. *American Journal of Psychiatry* 92:1371–87.

Orlove, B. S. 1980. Ecological Anthropology. *Annual Review of Anthropology* 9:235–338.

Ornstein, R. E. 1973. Right and Left Thinking. *Psychology Today* (May) 87–92.

Orona, Celia J., Barbara A. Koenig, and Anne J. Davis. 1994. Cultural Issues in Non-Disclosure. *Cambridge Quarterly for Health Care Ethics* 3 (3).

Orr, Robert D., Patricia A. Marshall, and Jamie Osborn. 1995. Cross-Cultural Considerations in Clinical Ethics Consultations. *Archives in Family Medicine* 4:159–164.

Orth-Gomer, Kristina, and Anna-Lena Unden. 1987. The Measurement of Social Support in Population Surveys. *Social Science and Medicine* 24:83–94.

Ortner, Sherry B. 1974. Is Female to Male as Nature Is to Culture? In *Woman, Culture, and Society,* ed. Michelle Zimbalist Rosaldo and Louise Lamphere. Stanford: Stanford University Press, 67–89.

———. 1984. Anthropological Theory since the Sixties. *Comparative Studies in Society and History* 26(1):126–66.

Ortner, Sherry B., and Harriet Whitehead, eds. 1981. *Sexual Meanings.* Cambridge: Cambridge University Press.

Ortiz de Montellano, Bernard. 1986. Aztec Medicinal Herbs: Evaluation of Etherapeutic Effectiveness. In *Plants in Indigenous Medicine and Diet: Biobehavioral Approaches,* ed. N. L. Etkin. New York: Gordon and Breach Science Publishers, 113–27.

———. 1987. "Caida de Mollera" Aztec Sources for a Mesoamerican Disease of Alleged Spanish Origin. *Ethnohistory* 34:381–99.

———. 1992. Syncretism in Mexican and Mexican-American Folk Medicine." Working Papers no. 5. College Park, M.d.: Department of Spanish and Portuguese, University of Maryland.

Orubuloye, I., J. Caldwell, and P. Caldwell. 1991. Sexual Networking in Ekiti District of Nigeria. *Studies in Family Planning* 22(2):61–73.

———. 1992. Sexual Networking and the Risk of AIDS in Southwest Nigeria. In *Sexual Behavior and Networking: Anthropological and Socio-Cultural Studies on the Transmission of HIV,* ed. T. Dyson. Liege, Belgium: International Union for the Scientific Study of Population, 283–302.

———. 1993. African Women's Control over Their Sexuality in the Era of AIDS: A Study of the Yoruba of Nigeria. *Social Science and Medicine* 37(7):859–72.

Osborne, N. G., and M. D. Feit. 1992. The Use of Race in Medical Research. *Journal of the American Medical Association* 267:275–79.

Osborne, O. 1972. Social Structure and Health Care Systems: A Yoruba Example. *Rural Africana* 17:80–86.

Osherson, Samuel, and Lorna Amarasingham. 1981. The Machine Metaphor in Medicine. In *Social Contexts of Health, Illness and Patient Care,* ed. E. Mishler. Cambridge: Cambridge University Press, 218–49.

Ots, Thomas. 1990. The Angry Liver, the Anxious Heart and the Melancholy Spleen. *Culture, Medicine and Psychiatry* 14:21–58.

Ott, Eleanor. 1993. Ethics and the Neo-Shaman. Paper presented to the International Society for Shamanic Research, Budapest, July.

Overall, Christine. 1987. *Ethics and Human Reproduction.* Boston: Allen and Unwin.

———. 1993. *Human Reproduction: Principles, Practices, and Policies.* Toronto: Oxford University Press.

Owen, Roger. 1969. *Cotton and the Egyptian Economy, 1820–1914: A Study in Trade and Development.* Oxford: Oxford University Press.

Oyebola, D. D. O. 1981. Professional Associations, Ethics, and Discipline among Yoruba Traditional Healers of Nigeria. *Social Science and Medicine* 15B:87–92.

———. 1986. National Medical Politics in Nigeria. In *The Professionalisation of African Medicine,* ed. M. Last and G. L. Chavunduka. Manchester: Manchester University Press for the International African Institute, 221–36.

Oyeneye, O. Y. 1985. Mobilizing Indigenous Resources for Primary Health Care in Nigeria: A Note on the Place of Traditional Medicine. *Social Science and Medicine* 20:67–69.

Pacey, Arnold. 1982. Taking Soundings for Development and Health. *World Health Forum* 3:40–44.

———. 1983. *The Culture of Technology.* Cambridge: MIT Press.

Packard, R., and P. Epstein. 1991. Epidemiologists, Social Scientists and the Structure of Medical Research on AIDS in Africa. *Social Science and Medicine* 33(7):771–94.

Padgett, Deborah, and Thomas Johnson. 1987. Patients and Physicians in Distress: The Role of Critical Perspectives in Clinically Applied Medical Anthropology. Paper presented at the American Anthropological Association Meeting, Chicago, November.

Page, J. Bryan. 1977. The Study of San Jose, Costa Rica, Street Culture: Codes and Communication in Lower-class Society. In *Drugs, Rituals and Altered States of Consciousness,* ed. Brian M. du Toit. Rotterdam: A. A. Balkema.

———. 1987. Prevention of Alcohol and Drug Abuse: What Anthropologists Can Learn and What We Can Teach. *Newsletter of the Alcohol and Drug Study Group, American Anthropological Association,* no. 19.

Page, J. Bryan, Dale D. Chitwood, Prince C. Smith, Normie Kane, and Duane C. McBride. 1990. Intravenous Drug Use and HIV Infection in Miami. *Medical Anthropology Quarterly* 4(1): 56–71.

Page, J. Bryan, Jack Fletcher, and William R. True. 1988. Psychosociocultural Perspectives on Chronic Cannabis Use: The Costa Rican Follow-up. *Journal of Psychoactive Drugs* 20:57–65.

Palinkas, Lawerence A., Michael A. Downs, John S. Petterson, and John Russell. 1993. Social, Cultural, and Psychological Impacts of the Exxon Valdez Oil Spill. *Human Organization* 52:1–13.

Palinkas, Lawrence A., John Russell, Michael A. Downs, and John S. Petterson. 1992. Ethnic Differences in Coping and Depressive Symptoms after the Exxon Valdez Oil Spill. *Journal of Nervous and Mental Disease* 180:287–95.

Pandolfi, Mariella. 1992. Beyond Gramsci and De Martino: Medical Anthropology in Contemporary Italy. *Medical Anthropology Quarterly* 6(2):162–65.

Panos Institute. 1988. *AIDS and the Third World.* London: Panos Publications.

Pardo, F., F. Perich, L. Villarroel, and R. Torres. 1993. Isolation of Verbascoside, An Antimicrobial Constituent of *Buddleja globosa* Leaves. *Journal of Ethnopharmacology* 39:31–38.

Parin, Paul. 1988. The Ego and the Mechanism of Adaptation. In *The Psychoanalytic Study of Society,* ed. L. B. Boyer and S. A. Grolnick. Vol. 12. Hillsdale, N.J.: Analytic Press, 97–130.

Parin, Paul, and Goldy Parin-Matthey. 1978. The Swiss and Southern German Lower-Middle Class: An Ethnopsychoanalytic Study. *Journal of Psychological Anthropology* 1(1):101–19.

Parker, R. 1987. Acquired Immunodeficiency Syndrome in Urban Brazil. *Medical Anthropology Quarterly* 1(2):155–75.

———. 1992. Sexual Diversity, Cultural Analysis, and AIDS Education in Brazil. In *The Time of AIDS: Social Analysis, Theory and Method,* ed. G. Herdt and S. Lindenbaum. Newbury Park, Calif.: Sage, 225–42.

Parker, Seymour. 1988. Rituals of Gender: A Study of Etiquette Symbols and Cognition. *American Anthropologist* 90:372–84.

Parkes, Colin Murray. 1988. Bereavement as a Psychosocial Transition: Processes of Adaptation to Change. *Journal of Social Issues* 44:53–65.

Parry, N., and J. Parry. 1976. *The Rise of the Medical Profession.* London: Croom Helm.

Parsons, Talcott. 1951. *The Social System.* Glencoe, Ill.: Free Press.

———. 1958. Definitions of Health and Illness in the Light of American Values and Social Structure. In *Patients, Physicians, and Illness,* ed. E. G. Jaco. Glencoe: Free Press.

Partridge, William L. 1977. Transformation and Redundancy in Ritual: A Case from Colombia. In *Drugs, Rituals and Altered States of Consciousness,* ed. Brian M. du Toit. Rotterdam: A. A. Balkema.

Patcher, Lee M. 1994. Culture and Clinical Care: Folk Illness Belief and Behaviors and Their Implications for Health Care Delivery. *Journal of the American Medical Association* 271(9): 690–94.

Patterson, C. H. 1985. What Is the Placebo in Psychotherapy? *Psychotherapy* 22:163–69.

Pattison, E. Mansell, N. Lapins, and F. Doerr. 1973. Faith Healing: A Study of Personality and Function. *Journal of Nervous and Mental Disorders* 157:397–409.

Paul, Benjamin, ed. 1955. *Health, Culture, and Community.* New York: Russell Sage Foundation.

Paul, J. 1987. *Medicine and Imperialism.* New York.

Paul, Lois. 1975. Recruitment to a Ritual Role. The Midwife in a Maya Community. *Ethos* 3(3): 449–67.

———. 1978. Careers of Midwives in a Mayan Community. In *Women in Ritual and Symbolic Roles,* ed. J. Hoch-Smith and A. Spring New York: Plenum, 129–49.

Paul, Robert A. 1976. The Sherpa Temple as a Model of the Psyche. *American Ethnologist* 3:131–46.

———. 1978. Instinctive Aggression in Man: The Semai Case. *Journal of Psychological Anthropology* 1(1):65–79.

———. 1985. Freud and the Seduction Theory: A Critical Examination of Masson's The Assault on Truth. *Journal of Psychoanalytic Anthropology* 8(3):161–87.

———. 1988. Commentary Response to Robarchek and Dentan. *American Anthropologist* 90(2): 418–20.

Paulme, Denise, ed. 1960. *Women of Tropical Africa.* Berkeley and Los Angeles: University of California Press.

Payer, Lynn. 1988. *Medicine and Culture: Varieties of Treatment in the United States, England, West Germany, and France.* New York: Henry Holt.

Payne, D., B. Grab, R. E. Fontaine, and J. Hempel. 1976. Impact of Control Measures on Malaria Transmission and General Mortality. *Bulletin of the World Health Organization* 54:369–77.

Pearce, Tola O. 1980. Political and Economic Changes in Nigeria and the Organization of Medical Care. *Social Science and Medicine* 14B:91–98.

———. 1986. Professional Interests and the Creation of Medical Knowledge in Nigeria. In M. Last and G. L. Chavunduka, eds., *The Professionalisation of African Medicine.* Manchester: Manchester University Press for the International African Institute, 237–58.

Pearlin, Leonard I. 1982. The Social Contexts of Stress. In *Handbook of Stress: Theoretical and Clinical Aspects,* ed. Leo Goldberger and Shlomo Breznitz. New York: Free Press.

Pearlin, Leonard I., and Carmi Schooler. 1978. The Structure of Coping. *Journal of Health and Social Behavior* 19:2–21.

Pearlman, Robert, et al. 1993. Contributions of Empirical Research to Medical Ethics. *Theoretical Medicine* 14:197–210.

Pearson, Maggie. 1982. Social Factors and Leprosy in Lamjung, West Central Nepal: Implications for Disease Control. *Ecology of Disease* 1:229–36.

Peattie, Lisa. 1968. *The View from the Barrio.* Ann Arbor: University of Michigan Press.

Peel, Sir John, ed. 1985. *Test Tube Babies: A Christian View.* Oxford: Becket Publications.

Peiris, Ralph. 1969. The Implantation of Sociology in Asia. *International Social Science Journal* 21 (3).

Pelaez, U., and F. Uribe. 1986. La Gran Ilusion de la Objectividad. *Boletin Antropologico* 6:163–78.

Pelligrino, Edmund D. 1988. Clinical Ethics: Biomedical Ethics at the Bedside. *Journal of the American Medical Association* 260:837–39.

———. 1992. Intersections of Western Biomedical Ethics and World Culture: Problematic and Possibility. *Cambridge Quarterly of Health Care Ethics* 3:191–96.

———. 1993. The Metamorphosis of Medical Ethics: A 30-Year Retrospective. *Journal of the American Medical Association* 2699:1158–62.

Pellegrino, Edmund D., Mazzarella P., and P. Corsi. 1992. *Transcultural Dimensions in Medical Ethics.* Frederick, Md.: University Publishing Group.

Pellegrino, Edmund D., and David C. Thomasma. 1981. *A Philosophical Basis of Medical Practice:*

  Toward a Philosophy and Ethic of the Healing Professions. New York: Oxford University Press.

———. 1989. *For the Patient's Good: The Restoration of Beneficence in Health Care.* New York: Oxford University Press.

———. 1993. *The Virtues in Medical Practice.* New York: Oxford University Press.

Pelto, G. H. 1984. Ethnographic Studies of the Effects of Food Availability and Feeding Practices. *Food and Nutrition Bulletin* 6(1):33–43.

———. 1987. Cultural Issues in Maternal and Child Health and Nutrition. *Social Science and Medicine* 25:553–59.

Pelto, G. H., and P. J. Pelto. 1989. Small But Healthy? An Anthropological Perspective. *Human Organization* 48(1):11–15.

Pelto, G. H., P. J. Pelto, and E. Messer, eds. 1989. *Methods in Nutritional Anthropology.* Tokyo: United Nations University.

Perkin, Harold. 1990. *The Rise of Professional Society.* London: Routledge.

Perry, Helen Swick. 1982. *Psychiatrist of America: The Life of Harry Stack Sullivan.* Cambridge: Belknap Press of Havard University Press.

Petchesky, Rosalind Pollack. 1984. *Abortion and Woman's Choice: The State, Sexuality, and Reproductive Freedom.* New York: Longman.

Peters, Edward. 1985. *Torture.* London: Basil Blackwell.

Peters, Larry. 1981. *Ecstasy and Healing in Nepal: An Ethnopsychiatric Study of Tamang Shamanism.* Malibu: Undena Publications.

Peters, Larry, and D. Price-Williams. 1980. Towards an Experiential Analysis of Shamanism. *American Ethnologist* 7:398–418.

Peterson, Jane A. 1995. The Hour of Departure: Force that Create Refugees and Migrants. *World Watch Paper* 125. Washington, D.C.: World Watch Institute.

Petrovic, Gajo. 1988. Philosophy and Revolution: Twenty Sheaves of Questions. In *Marxism and the Interpretation of Culture,* ed. C. Nelson and L. Grossberg. Chicago: University of Illinois Press, 235–48.

Pharaon, H. M., W. J. Darby, H. A. Shammout, E. B. Bridgeforth, and C. S. Wilson. 1965. A Year-Long Study of the Nurture of Infants and Pre-school Children in Jordan. *Journal of Tropical Pediatrics and African Child Health* 2.

Phillips, J. 1955. The Hookworm Campaign in Ceylon. In *Hands Across Frontiers: Case Studies in Technical Cooperation,* ed. H. M. Teaf, Jr., and P. G. Franck. Ithaca: Cornell University Press, 265–305.

Phillips, Michael R. 1985. Can "Clinically Applied Anthropology" Survive in Medical Care Settings? *Medical Anthropology Quarterly* 16(2):31–36.

Phillipson, J. David, and Linda A. Anderson. 1989 Ethnopharmacology and Western Medicine. *Journal of Ethnopharmacology* 25:61–72.

Phipps-Yonas, Susan. 1980. Teenage Pregnancy and Motherhood: A Review of the Literature. *American Journal of Orthopsychiatry* 50(3):403–31.

Physicians for Human Rights. 1988. *The Casualties of Conflict: Medical Care and Human Rights in the West Bank and Gaza Strip.* Somerville, Mass.: Physicians for Human Rights.

———. 1989. *Winds of Death: Iraq's Use of Poison Gas against Its Kurdish Population.* Somerville, Mass.: Physicians for Human Rights.

Piault, C., ed. 1975. *Prophestisme et therapeutique: Albert Atcho et la communauté Bregbo.* Paris: Hermann.

Pilisuk, Marc, and Susan Hillier Parks. 1986. *The Healing Web: Social Networks and Human Survival.* Hanover, N. H.: University Press of New England.

Pinxten, Rik. 1986. The Developmental Dynamics of Peace. In *Peace and War: Cross-Cultural Perspectives,* ed. Mary LeCron Foster and Robert A. Rubinstein. New Brunswick, N.J.: Transaction Books.

Pirie, Peter. 1972. The Effects of Treponematosis and Gonorrhaea on the Populations of the Pacific Islands. *Human Biology in Oceania* 1:187–206.

Plattner, S., et al. 1989. Ethnographic Method. *Anthropology Newsletter* 30:32.

Plorde, James J. 1980. Schistosomaisis (Bilharziasis). In *Harrison's Principles of Internal Medicine,* ed. K. Isselbacher, R. Adams, E. Braunwald, R. Petersdorf, and Jean Wilson. New York: McGraw-Hill, 909–11.

Plowman, Timothy. 1986. Coca Chewing and the Botanical Origins of Coca (*Erythroxylum* spp.) in South America. In *Coca and Cocaine,* ed. D. Pacini and C. Franquemont. Cambridge, Mass.: Cultural Survival, 5–33.

Plutchik, Robert. 1980. A Language for the Emotions. *Psychology Today* 13(9):68–78.

Poirier, Suzanne, and Daniel J. Brauner. 1990. The Voices of the Medical Record. *Theoretical Medicine* 11(1):29–40.

Poland, Marilyn L. 1985. Importance of Cross-Training and Research Strategies in Clinical Medicine. *Medical Anthropology Quarterly* 16(3):61–63.

Polanyi, M. 1958. *Personal Knowledge.* Chicago: University of Chicago Press.

———. 1969. *Knowing and Being.* Chicago: University of Chicago Press.

Polderman, A. M. 1979. Transmission Dynamics of Endemic Schistosomiasis. *Tropical and Geographical Medicine* 31:465–75.

Polgar, Steven. 1962. Health and Human Behavior: Areas of Interest Common to the Social and Medical Sciences. *Current Anthropology* 3:159–205.

Polgar, Steven, ed. 1971. *Culture and Population: A Collection of Current Studies.* Cambridge, Mass.: Schenkmann Publishing Company.

Polgar, Steven, and John Marshall. 1976. The Search for Culturally Acceptable Fertility Regulating Methods. In *Culture Natality and Family Planning,* ed. John Marshall and Steven Polgar. Chapel Hill, N.C.: Carolina Population Center, 204–18.

Pollitt, K. 1982. The Politically Correct Body. *Mother Jones* May:66–67.

Pond, C. M. 1978. Morphological Aspects and the Ecological and Mechanical Consequences of Fat Deposition in Wild Vertebrates. *Annual Review of Ecological Systems* 9:519–70.

Popkin, Barry M. 1994. The Nutritional Transition in Low-Income Countries: An Emerging Crisis. *Nutritional Reviews* 52:285–98.

Porter, Euginia. 1990. Social Context and Historical Emergence: The Underlying Dimension of Medical Ethics. *Theoretical Medicine* 11(2):145–66.

Pottier, Johan, ed. 1993. *Practicing Development: Social Science Perspectives.* New York: Routledge.

Potts, M., and A. Resenfield. 1991. The Fifth Freedom Revisited: I, Background to Existing Programs. *Lancet* 336:1227–31.

Powell, Dorian. 1982. Network Analysis: A Suggested Model for the Study of Women and the Family in the Caribbean. In *Women and the Family,* ed. Jocelyn Massiah. ISER, Cave Hill, Barbados: University of the West Indies, 131–62.

Powell, D. E. 1994. The Religious Renaissance in the Soviet Union and Its Successor States. In *The Social Legacy of Communism,* ed. J. R. Millar and S. Wolchik. Cambridge: Cambridge University Press with the Woodrow Wilson Center Press, 271–305.

Powers, Marla N. 1980. Menstruation and Reproduction: An Oglala Case. *Signs* 6(1):54–65.

Pratt, Mary Louise. 1986. Fieldwork in Common Places. In J. Clifford and G. E. Marcus, eds., *Writing Culture: The Poetics and Politics of Ethnography.* Berkeley: University of California Press, 27–50.

Preble, E., and J. J. Casey, Jr. 1969. Taking Care of Business: The Heroin User's Life on the Street. *International Journal of the Addictions* 4:1–24.

Prentice, A. M., Susan B. Roberts, Ann Prentice, Alison A. Paul, M. Watkinson, Anne A. Watkinson, and R. G. Whitehead. 1982a. Dietary Supplementation of Lactating Gambian Women. I. Effect on Breast-Milk Volume and Quality. *Human Nutrition: Clinical Nutrition* 37c:53–64.

Prentice, A. M., Roger G. Whitehead, Michael Watkinson, William H. Lamb, and Tim J. Cole. 1982b. Prenatal Dietary Supplementation of African Women and Birth-Weight. *Lancet* 489–92.

President's Commission for the Study of Ethical Problems in Medicine and Biomedical and Behavioral Research. 1981. *Defining Death: Medical, Legal and Ethical Issues in the Determination of Death.* Washington, D.C.: U.S. Government Printing Office.

———. 1983. *Deciding to Forgo Life-Sustaining Treatment.* Washington, D.C.: Government Printing Office.

Press, Irwin. 1985. Speaking Hospital Administration's Language: Strategies for Anthropological Entree in the Clinical Setting. *Medical Anthropology Quarterly* 16(30):67–69.

———. 1990. Levels of Explanation and Cautions for a Critical Clinical Anthropology. *Social Science and Medicine* 30(9):1001–9.

Press, Nancy, and Carole Browner. 1995. Risk, Autonomy, and Responsibility: Informed Consent for Prenatal Testing. *Hastings Center Report* 25(3):S9–S12.

Press, Nancy, W. Burke, and S. J. Durfy. In press. Women's Knowledge, Medicine's Hope: Genetic Susceptibility Testing for Breast Cancer. In *Setting Priorities in Genetic Services,* ed. P. Boyle, D. Callahan, and K. Nolan. Washington, D.C.: Georgetown University Press.

Pressat, R. 1962. *Demographic Analysis.* Chicago: Aldine.

Price, Max. 1988. The Consequences of Health Service Privatisation for Equality and Equity in Health Care in South Africa. *Social Science and Medicine* 27(7):703–16.

Price-Williams, Douglas. 1987. The Waking Dream in Ethnographic Perspective. In Barbara Tedlock, ed., *Dreaming: Anthropological and Psychological Perspectives.* Cambridge: Cambridge University Press.

Prince, A. M. 1990. Control of Hepatitis B Infection in Third World Countries. *Transfusion Medicine Review* 4(3):187–90.

Prince, Raymond. 1964. Indigenous Yoruba Psychiatry. In *Magic, Faith, and Healing,* ed. Ari Kiev. New York: Free Press, 84–120.

———. 1969. Psychotherapy and the Chronically Poor. In *Culture Change, Mental Health and Poverty,* ed. Joseph C. Finney. Lexington: University of Kentucky Press, 20–41.

———. 1976. Psychotherapy as the Manipulation of Endogenous Healing Mechanisms: A Transcultural Survey. *Transcultural Psychiatric Research Review* 13:115–33.

———. 1977. Foreword to *Case Studies in Spirit Possession,* ed. Vincent Crapanzano and Vivian Garrison. New York: John Wiley and Sons, xi–xvi.

———. 1980. Variations in Psychotherapeutic Procedures. In *Handbook of Cross-Cultural Psychology: Psychopathology,* ed. Harry C. Triandis and Juris G. Draguns. Vol. 6. Boston: Allyn and Bacon, 291–309.

———. 1982. Shamans and Endorphins: Hypothesis for a Synthesis. *Ethos* 10:409–23.

Prince, Raymond, ed. 1968. *Trance and Possession States.* Montreal: R. M. Bucke Memorial Society.

Prince, Raymond, and Françoise Tcheng-Laroche. 1987. Culture-Bound Syndromes and International Disease Classifications. *Culture, Medicine, and Psychiatry* 11:3–19.

Prior, Marcia. 1993. Matrifocality, Power and Gender Relations in Jamaica. In *Gender in Cross-Cultural Perspective,* ed. Caroline B. Brettell and Carolyn F. Sargent. Englewood Cliffs, N.J.: Prentice-Hall 310–18.

Prochaska, J. O., and C. C. DiClemente. 1984. *The Transtheoretical Approach: Crossing the Traditional Boundaries of Therapy.* Homewood, Ill.: Dow-Jones/Irwin.

Pugh, R. N. H., and H. M. Gilles. 1978. Malumfashi Endemic Diseases Research Project. III. Urinary Schistosomiasis: A Longitudinal Study. *Annals of Tropical Medicine and Parasitology* 72: 471–82.

Pyramarn, Kosum. 1989. New Evidence on Plant Exploitation and Environment during the Hoabinhian (Late Stone Age) from Ban Kao Caves, Thailand. In *Foraging and Farming: The Evolution of Plant Exploitation,* ed. D. R. Harris and G. C. Hillman. London: Unwin Hyman, 289–91.

Quandt, Sara. 1983. Changes in Maternal Postpartum Adiposity and Infant Feeding Patterns. *American Journal of Physical Anthropology* 60:455–61.

———. 1984. Nutritional Thriftiness and Human Reproduction: Beyond the Critical Body Composition Hypothesis. *Social Science and Medicine* 19:177–82.

———. 1985. Biological and Behavioral Predictors of Exclusive Breastfeeding Duration. *Medical Anthropology* 9:139–51.

———. 1986a. Nutritional Anthropology: The Individual Focus. In *Training Manual in Nutritional Anthropology*, ed. Sara Quandt and Cheryl Ritenbaugh. Special publication 20. Washington, D.C.: American Anthropological Association.

———. 1986b. Patterns of Variation in Breastfeeding Behaviors. *Social Science and Medicine* 23: 445–53.

———. 1987a. Methods for Determining Dietary Intake. In *Nutritional Anthropology*, ed. F. E. Johnston. New York: Alan R. Liss, 67–84.

———. 1987b. Variation in Nutrient Intake of Infants and Its Implications for Collecting Reliable Dietary Intake Data. *American Journal of Physical Anthropology* 73(4):515–23.

———. 1988. *Guyana Food Marketing and Nutrition Education Project.* Newton, Mass.: Education Development Center.

Quandt, Sara A., Kathleen M. DeWalt, and Joan B. Popyach. n.d. Effects of Food Acquisition Patterns on Dietary Status of the Rural Elderly: Seasonal and Gender Differences. Unpublished manuscript.

Quandt, Sara A., J. B. Popyach, and Kathleen DeWalt. 1994. Home Gardening and Food Preservation Practices of the Elderly in Rural Kentucky. *Ecology of Food and Nutrition* 31:183–99.

Quandt, Sara A., and Cheryl Ritenbaugh, eds. 1986. *Training Manual in Nutritional Anthropology.* Special Publication 20. Washington, D.C.: American Anthropological Association.

Quirk, Gregory J., and Leonel Casco. 1994. Stress Disorders of Families of the Disappeared: A Controlled Study in Honduras. *Social Science and Medicine* 39:1675–79.

Qureshi, S., A. H. Shah, and A. M. Ageel. 1992. Toxicity Studies on *Alpinia galanga* and *Curcuma longa. Plant Medica* 58:124–27.

Rabinow, Paul. 1986. Representations Are Social Facts: Modernity and Post-Modernity in Anthropology. In *Writing Culture: The Poetics and Politics of Ethnography*, ed. J. Clifford and G. E. Marcus. Berkeley: University of California Press.

Rabkin, Judith G., and Elmer L. Struening. 1976. Life Events, Stress, and Illness. *Science* 144: 1013–20.

Rachels, James. 1975. Active and Passive Euthanasia. *New England Journal of Medicine* 292:78–80.

Ragoné, Helena. 1994. *Surrogate Motherhood: Conception in the Heart.* Boulder, Colo.: Westview Press.

Ragucci, A. T. 1981. Italian Americans. In *Ethnicity and Medical Care*, ed. R. R. Reiter. Cambridge: Harvard University Press, 211–63.

Rahe, Richard H., and Ransom J. Arthur. 1978. Life Change and Illness Studies: Past History and Future Directions. *Journal of Human Stress* 4:3–15.

Rahnema, Majid. 1986. Under the Banner of Development. *Development* 3:47–67.

———. 1988. A New Variety of AIDS and Its Pathogens: Homo Economicus, Development and Aid. *Alternatives* 13:117–36.

Rajasekaran, M., J. S. Bapna, S. Lakshmanan, A. G. R. Nair, A. J. Veliath, and M. Panchanadam. 1988. Antifertility Effect in Male Rats of Oleanolic Acid, A Triterpene from Eugenia Jambolana Flowers. *Journal of Ethnopharmacology* 24:115–21.

Ramsey, Mathew. 1984. The Politics of Medical Monopoly in Nineteenth-Century Medicine: The French Model and Its Rivals. In *Professions and the French State, 1700–1900*, ed. G. L. Geison. Philadelphia: University of Pennsylvania Press, 225–305.

———. 1988. *Professionalisation and Popular Medicine in France: The Social World of Medical Practice.* Cambridge: Cambridge University Press.

Ramsey, Paul. 1970. *The Patient as Person.* New Haven, Conn.: Yale University Press.

———. 1978. *Ethics at the Edges of Life.* New Haven: Yale University Press.

Rankin-Hill, Lesley M., and Michael L. Blakey. 1994. W. Montague Cobb (1904–1990): Physical Anthropologist, Anatomist, and Activist. *American Anthropologist* 96(1):74–96.

Raphael, D., and F. Davis. 1985. *Only Mothers Know: Patterns of Infant Feeding in Traditional Cultures.* Westport, Conn.: Greenwood Press.

Rapp, Rayna. 1987. Reproduction and Gender Hierarchy: Amniocentesis in Contemporary America. Paper presented at Wenner-Gren Conference #103, Mijas, Spain.

———. 1988a. Chromosomes and Communication: The Discourse of Genetic Counselling. *Medical Anthropology Quarterly* 2(2):143–57.

———. 1988b. The Power of ''Positive'' Diagnosis: Medical and Maternal Discourses on Amniocentesis. In *Childbirth in America: Anthropological Perspectives,* ed. Karen Michaelson. New York: Bergin and Garvey, 103–16.

———. 1989. Chromosomes and Communication: The Discourse of Genetic Counseling. *Medical Anthropology Quarterly* 2(2):143–57.

———. 1993. Accounting for Amniocentesis. In *Knowledge, Power and Practice,* ed. Shirley Lindenbaum and Margaret Lock. Berkeley: University of California Press, 55–79.

———. n.d. Constructing Amniocentesis. Unpublished manuscript.

Rappaport, R. A. 1976. Adaptation and Maladaptation in Social Systems. In *The Ethical Basis of Economic Freedom,* ed. I. I. Hill. Chapel Hill, N.C.: American Viewpoint.

———. 1979. *Ecology, Meaning, and Religion.* Richmond, Calif.: North Atlantic.

Rashad, Hoda. 1989. ORT and Its Effect on Child Mortality in Egypt. *Journal of Biosocial Science* 10 (Suppl.):105–13.

Ratcliffe, John. 1978. Social Justice and the Demographic Transition: Lessons from India's Kerala State. *International Journal of Health Services* 8:123–44.

———. 1985. The Influence of Funding Agencies on International Health Policy, Research and Programs. *Mobius* 5:93–115.

Ratcliffe, John, and Amalia Gonzalez-del-Valle. 1988. Rigor in Health-Related Research: Toward an Expanded Conceptualization. *International Journal of Health Services* 18(3):361–92.

Ratner, Mitchell S., ed. 1993. *Crack Pipe as Pimp: An Ethnographic Investigation of Sex-for-Crack Exchanges.* New York: Lexington Books.

Raup, David M. 1986. Biological Extinction in Earth History. *Science* 231:1528–33.

Rayner, Mary. 1987. Turning a Blind Eye?—Medical Accountability and the Prevention of Torture in South Africa. Washington, D.C.: American Association for the Advancement of Science.

Read, Kenneth E. 1955. Morality and the Concept of the Person among the Gahuka-Gama. *Oceania* 25:253–82.

Redfield, Robert, Ralph Linton, and Melville J. Herskovits. 1936. Memorandum on the Study of Acculturation. *American Anthropologist* 38:149–52.

Redl, K., W. Breu, B. Davis, and R. Bauer. 1994. Anti-Inflammatory Active Polyacetylenes from *Bidens campyloteca. Plant Medica* 60:62.

Reed, D., D. McGee, J. Cohen, K. Yano, S. L. Syme, and M. Feinleib. 1982. Acculturation and Coronary Heart Disease among Japanese Men in Hawaii. *American Journal of Epidemiology* 115:894–905.

Reich, Warren. 1987. Caring for Life in the First of It: Moral Dilemmas for Perinatal and Neonatal Ethics. *Seminars in Perinatology* 11(30:279–87.

Reichel-Dolmatoff, G. 1971. *Amazonian Cosmos: The Sexual and Religious Symbolism of the Tukanao Indians.* Chicago: University of Chicago Press.

Reid, Janice, and Lyn Reynolds. 1990. Requiem for RSI: The Explanation and Control of an Occupational Epidemic. *Medical Anthropology Quarterly* 4(2):162–91.

Reinhard, Karl J., J. Richard Ambler, and Magdalene McGuffie. 1985. Diet and Parasitism at Dust Devil Cave. *American Antiquity* 50:819–924.

Reinhard, Karl J., Donny L. Hamilton, and Richard H. Hevly. 1991. Use of Pollen Concentration in Paleopharmacology: Coprolite Evidence of Medicinal Plants. *Journal of Ethnobiology* 11: 117–32.

Reischauer, Edwin O. 1977. *The Japanese.* Cambridge, Mass.: Harvard University Press.

Reiter, Rayna, ed. 1981. *Toward an Anthropology of Women.* New York: Monthly Review Press.

Renteln, A. D. 1988. Relativism and the Search for Human Rights. *American Anthropologist* 90: 56–72.

Reports, Population. 1992. *the Environment and Population Growth: Decade for Action.* Population Reports Series M(10):1–35.

Rey, Joseph M., Gavin W. Steward, Jon M. Plapp, Marie R. Bashir, and Ian N. Richards. 1988. DSM-III Axis IV Revisited. *American Journal of Psychiatry* 145(3):286–92.

Reynolds, David K. 1989. *Flowing Bridges, Quiet Waters: Japanese Psychotherapies, Morita and Naikan.* Albany: State University of New York Press.

Richards, Audrey I. 1932. *Hunger and Work in a Savage Tribe: A Functional Study of Nutrition among the Southern Bantu.* London: G. Routledge and Sons.

————. 1939. *Land, Labour, and Diet in Northern Rhodesia: An Economic Study of the Bemba Tribe.* London: Oxford University Press.

Richardson, Bonham. 1985. *Panama Money in Barbados, 1900–1920.* Knoxville: University of Tennessee Press.

Richman, Judith A., Moises Gavira, Joseph A. Flaherty, Susan Birz, and Ronald M. Wintrob. 1987. The Process of Acculturation: Theoretical Perspectives and an Empirical Investigation in Peru. *Social Science and Medicine* 25:839–47.

Ricoeur, Paul. 1965. *Freedom and Nature.* Evanston: Northwestern University Press.

Rios, J. L., M. C. Recio, and A. Villar. 1988. Screening Methods for Natural Products with Antimicrobial Activity: A Review of the Literature. *Journal of Ethnopharmacology* 23:127–49.

Ripp, Joseph L. 1984. Revolutionary Nicaragua: An Arena for Research in Medical Anthropology. *Medical Anthropology Quarterly* 15(3):68–69.

Ritenbaugh, Cheryl. 1978. Human Foodways: A Window on Evolution. In *The Anthropology of Health,* ed. Eleanor E. Bauwens. St. Louis: Mosby, 111–20.

————. 1982. Obesity as a Culture-Bound Syndrome. *Culture, Medicine, and Psychiatry* 6:347–61.

Rivers, W. H. R. 1924. *Medicine, Magic, and Religion.* London: Kegan, Paul, Trench, Trubner & Co.

Robarchek, Clayton A., and Robert K. Dentan. 1987. Blood Drunkenness and the Bloodthirsty Semai. *American Anthropologist* 89(2):356–65.

Robbins, Michael C., and Annette M. Kline. 1988. To Smoke or Not to Smoke: A Decision Theory Perspective. Paper presented at the meetings of the American Anthropological Association.

Roberts, George, and S. Sinclair. 1978. *Women in Jamaica.* New York: KTO Press.

Robertson, John A. 1994. The Question of Human Cloning. *Hastings Center Report* 24(20):6–14.

Robey, B., S. Rutstein, and L. Morris. 1993. The Fertility Decline in Developing Countries. *Scientific American* December: 60–67.

Robson, E. 1991. The Curative Power of Egyptian TV. *Source* (March):6–8.

Rodenbeck, Max. 1988. The Success and Failures of US Aid to Egypt. *MEI* (September):17–18.

Rodriguez, E., et al. 1985. Thiarubrine A, a Bioactive Constituent of Aspilia (Asteraceae) Consumed by Wild Chimpanzees. *Experientia* 41:419–20.

Rogers, Carl, et al. 1967. *The Therapeutic Relationship and Its Impact: A Study of Psychotherapy with Schizophrenics.* Madison: University of Wisconsin Press.

Rohde, Jon E. 1983. Why the Other Half Dies: The Science and Politics of Child Mortality in the Third World. *Assignment Children* 61/62:35–67.

Rohde, Jon, and Robert Northrup. 1976. Taking Science Where the Diarrhea Is. In *Acute Diarrhea in Childhood.* New York: North-Holland, 341.

Roheim, Gezai. 1943. *The Origin and Function of Culture.* Nervous Mental Disease Monographs, no. 69. New York: Nervous and Mental Disease Pub.

Romalis, Coleman. 1981. Taking Care of the Little Woman: Father-Physician Relations during Pregnancy and Childbirth. In *Childbirth: Alternatives to Medical Control,* ed. Shelly Romalis. Austin: University of Texas Press, 92–122.

Romalis, Shelly, ed. 1981. *Childbirth: Alternatives to Medical Control.* Austin: University of Texas Press.

Romanucci-Ross, Lola. 1969. The Hierarchy of Resort in Curative Practices: The Admiralty Islands, Melanesia. *Journal of Health and Social Behavior* 10:201–9.

Romanucci-Ross, Lola, and Daniel E. Moerman. 1988. The Extraneous Factor in Western Medicine. *Ethos* 16:146–66.

Romanucci-Ross, Lola, Daniel E. Moerman, and Laurence R. Tancredi, eds. 1983. *The Anthropology of Medicine: From Culture to Method.* New York: Praeger.

Romney, A. K. 1972. Categories of Disease in American-English and Mexican-Spanish. In *Multidimensional Scaling: Theory and Applications in the Behavioral Sciences,* ed. A. K. Romney, R. N. Shepard, and S. B. Nerlove. New York: Seminar Press, 9–54.

Romney, A. K., S. C. Weller, and W. H. Batchelder. 1986. Culture As Consensus: A Theory of Culture and Informant Accuracy. *American Anthropologist* 88:313–38.

Room, Robin. 1983. *Sociological Aspects of the Disease Concept of Alcoholism. Recent Advances in Alcohol and Drug Problems,* Vol. 7. New York: Plenum.

———. 1984. Alcohol and Ethnography: A Case of Problem Deflation? *Current Anthropology* 25(2):169–91.

Roos, Gun, Sara A. Quandt, and Kathleen M. DeWalt. 1993. Meal Patterns of the Elderly in Rural Kentucky. *Appetite* 21:295–98.

Rosaldo, Michelle Z. 1974. Woman, Culture, and Society: A Theoretical Overview. In *Woman, Culture, and Society,* ed. Michelle Zimbalist Rosaldo and Louise Lamphere. Stanford: Stanford University Press, 67–89.

———. 1980a. The Use and Abuse of Anthropology: Reflections on Feminism and Cross-Cultural Understanding. *Signs: Journal of Woman in Culture and Society* 5(3):389–417.

———. 1980b. *Knowledge and Passion: Ilongot Notions of Self and Social Life.* Cambridge: Cambridge University Press.

———. 1984. Toward an Anthropology of Self and Feeling. In *Culture Theory,* ed. Richard Shweder and Robert LeVine. Cambridge: Cambridge University Press.

Rosaldo, Michelle Zimbalist, and Louise Lamphere, eds. 1974. *Woman, Culture, and Society.* Stanford: Stanford University Press.

Rosaldo, Renato. 1984. Grief and the Headhunter's Rage: On the Cultural Force of Emotions. In *Text, Play and Story,* ed. Edward Bruner. Washington, D.C.: American Ethnological Society, 178–95.

Rose, Geoffrey, and D. J. P. Barker. 1978. What Is a Case? Dichotomy or Continuum? *British Medical Journal,* September 23, 873–74.

Rose, G., and M. G. Marmot. 1981. Social Class and Coronary Heart Disease. *British Heart Journal* 45:13–19.

Roseberry, William. 1988. Political Economy. *Annual Review of Anthropology* 17:161–185.

———. 1989. *Anthropologies and Histories: Essays in Culture, History, and Political Economy.* New Brunswick: Rutgers University Press.

Roseman, Marina. 1991. *Healing Sounds from the Malaysian Rainforest: Temiar Music and Medicine.* Berkeley and Los Angeles: University of California Press.

Rosenfield, Patricia L. n.d. The Contribution of Social and Political Factors to Good Health. Man-
uscript.
Rosenstock, Irwin M. 1990. The Health Belief Model: Explaining Health Behavior Through Ex-
pectancies. In *Health Behavior and Health Education,* ed. Karen Glanz, Marcus Lewis, and
Barbara K. Rimer. San Francisco: Jossey-Bass.
Rosenthal, M. M. 1987. *Dealing with Medical Malpractice: The British and Swedish Experience.*
London: Tavistock.
Ross, Colin A., Shaun Joshi, and Raymond Currie. 1990. Dissociative Experiences in the General
Population. *American Journal of Psychiatry* 147(11):1547–52.
Ross, Eric B. 1986. Potatoes, Population, and the Irish Famine: The Political Economy of Demo-
graphic Change. In *Culture and Reproduction,* ed. W. Penn Handwerker. Boulder, Colo.:
Westview, 196–220.
Roth, Julius. 1957. Ritual and Magic in the Control of Contagion. *American Sociology Review* 22:
310–14.
———. 1972. Some Contingencies of the Moral Evaluation and Control of Clientele: The Case of
the Hospital Emergency Service. *American Journal of Sociology* 77:840–55.
Rothman, Barbara K. 1986. *The Tentative Pregnancy.* New York: Viking/Penguin
———. 1988. The Decision to Have or Not to Have Amniocentesis for Prenatal Diagnosis. In
Childbirth in America, Anthropological Perspectives, ed. Karen L. Michaelson. South Had-
ley, Mass.: Bergin and Garvey, 90–102.
———. 1989. *Recreating Motherhood. Ideology and Technology in a Patriarchal Society.* New
York: W. W. Norton & Co.
Rothman, David. 1990. Human Experimentation and the Orgins of Bioethics in the United States.
In *Social Science Perspectives on Medical Ethics,* ed. George Weisz. Newton, Mass.: Kluwer
Press, 185–200.
———. 1991. *Strangers at the Bedside: A History of How Law and Bioethics Transferred Medical
Decision-Making.* New York: Basic Books.
Rothman, K. J. 1986. *Modern Epidemiology.* Boston: Little, Brown.
———. 1988. *Causal Inference.* Chestnut Hill, Mass.: Epidemiology Resources.
Rouget, Gilbert. 1980. *Music and Trance.* Chicago: University of Chicago Press.
Royal College of Physicians. 1948. *The Nomenclature of Disease.* 7th ed. London: His Majesty's
Stationery Office.
Rubel, Arthur J. 1960. Concepts of Disease in Mexican-American Culture. *American Anthropologist*
62:795–814.
———. 1964. The Epidemiology of a Folk Illness: Susto in Hispanic America. *Ethnology* 3:268–
83.
———. 1966a. *Across the Tracks: Mexican-Americans in a Texas City.* Austin: University of Texas
Press.
———. 1966b. The Role of Social Science Research in Recent Health Programs in Latin America.
Latin American Research Review 2:37–56.
———. 1983a. Mexican American Folk Healing. *Reviews in Anthropology* 65–71.
———. 1983b. Review of Robert T. Trotter II and Juan Antonio Chavira, *Curanderismo: Mexican
American Folk Healing. Reviews in Anthropology* 65–71.
Rubel, Arthur J., Carl W. O'Nell, and Rolando Collado Ardon. 1984. *Susto: A Folk Illness.* Berkeley
and Los Angeles: University of California Press.
Rubel, Arthur J., Karen Weller-Fahey, and Mimi Trosdal. 1975. Conception, Gestation, and Delivery
According to Some Mananabang of Cebu. *Philippine Quarterly of Culture and Society* 3:
131–45.
Rubenstein, R. A. 1984 Epidemiology and Anthropology: Notes on Science and Scientism. *Com-
munication and Cognition* 17(2/3):163–85.
Rubenstein, R. A., and J. D. Perloff. 1986. Identifying Psychosocial Disorders in Children: On
Integrating Epidemiological and Anthropological Understandings. In *Anthropology and Ep-*

idemiology: Interdisciplinary Approaches to the Study of Health and Disease, ed. Craig R. Janes, Ron Stall and Sandra M. Gifford. Dordrecht: D. Reidel, 303–32.

Rubin, Susan, et al. 1994. Increasing the Completion of the Durable Power of Attorney for Health Care. *Journal of the American Medical Association,* January 19, 209–12.

Rubin, Vera, ed. 1975. *Cannabis and Culture.* The Hague: Mouton.

Rubin, Vera, and Lambros Comitas. 1975. *Ganja in Jamaica.* The Hague: Mouton.

Rubinstein, Robert A. 1984. Epidemiology and Anthropology: Notes on Science and Scientism. *Communication and Cognition* 17:163–85.

———. 1988. Anthropology and International Security. In *The Social Dynamics of Peace and Conflict: Culture in International Security,* ed. R. A. Rubinstein and M. L. Foster. Boulder, Colo.: Westview Press, 17–34.

Rubinstein, Robert L. 1995. Narratives of Elder Parental Death: A Structural and Cultural Analysis. *Medical Anthropology Quarterly* 9(2):257–76.

Rubinstein, Robert A., and Ronald T. Brown. 1984. An Evaluation of the Validity of the Diagnostic Category of Attention Deficit Disorder. *American Journal of Orthopsychiatry* 543:398–414.

Ruiz, M. C. 1981. Open-closed Mindedness, Intolerance of Ambiguity and Nursing Faculty Attitudes toward Culturally Different Patients. *Nursing Research* 30:177–81.

Russell, James. 1991. Culture and the Categorization of Emotions. *Psychological Bulletin* 110(3): 426–50.

Ryan, F. 1993. *The Forgotten Plague: How the Battle against Tuberculosis Was Won—and Lost.* Boston: Little, Brown.

Ryan, Michael. 1978. *The Organisation of Soviet Medical Care.* Oxford: B. Blackwell.

Rycroft, Charles. 1968. *A Critical Dictionary of Psychoanalysis.* Harmondsworth, England: Penguin.

Ryder, R., et al. 1989. Perinatal Transmission of HIV-1 to Infants of Seropositive Women in Zaire. *New England Journal of Medicine* 320:1637.

Saa, Louis. 1986. Anthropology's Native Problem. *Harper's Magazine* (May):49–57.

Sacks, Oliver. 1973 (1970). *Migraine: The Evolution of a Common Disorder.* Berkeley: University of California Press.

———. 1985. *The Man Who Mistook His Wife for a Hat and Other Clinical Tales.* New York: Summit Books.

Sahlins, M. D., and E. Service. 1960. *Evolution and Culture.* Ann Arbor: University of Michigan Press.

Said, Edward W. 1979. *The Question of Palestine.* New York: Random House.

Saks, M. P. 1994. *Professions and the Public Interest: Medical Power, Altruism, and Alternative Medicine.* London: Routledge.

Salame, Ghassan. 1990. ''Strong'' and ''Weak'' States: A Qualified Return to the Muqaddimah. In *The Arab State,* ed. Gicomo Luciani. Berkeley: University of California Press, 29–64.

Saleh, Saneya A. W. 1979. *The Brain Drain in Egypt.* Cairo Papers in Social Science, vol. 2, monograph 3. Cairo: American University in Cairo.

Salmon, J. W., ed. 1984. *Alternative Medicines: Popular and Policy Perspectives.* London: Tavistock.

Salmond, Clare E., Jill G. Joseph, I. M. Prior, D. G. Stanley, and Albert F. Wessen. 1985. Longitudinal Analysis of the Relationship between Blood Pressure and Migration: The Tokelau Island Migrant Study. *American Journal of Epidemiology* 122:291–301.

Sandelowski, Margarete. 1993. *With Child in Mind: Studies of the Personal Encounter with Infertility.* Philadelphia: University of Pennsylvania Press.

Sander, Fred. 1979. *Individual and Family Therapy: Toward an Integration.* New York: Jason Aronson.

Sanders, Cheryl J. 1994. European-American Ethos and Principlism: An African American Challenge. In *A Matter of Principles: Ferment in U.S. Bioethics,* ed. Edwin R. DuBose, Ron Hamel, and Laurence J. O'Connell. Park Ridge, Ill.: Park Ridge Center for the Study of Health, 148–63.

Sanders, David. 1982. Nutrition and the Use of Food as a Weapon in Zimbabwe and Southern Africa. *International Journal of Health Services* 12:201–13.

———. 1985. *The Struggle for Health: Medicine and the Politics of Underdevelopment.* London: Macmillan.

Sanders, Lee, Susan Kelly, Patricia Marshall, and Barbara Koenig. 1994. Multiple Perspectives on the Ethics of Pilot Ethnography. Unpublished manuscript.

Sandner, Donald. 1979. *Navajo Symbols of Healing.* New York: Harcourt Brace Jovanovich.

Sandoval, Mercedes. 1979. Santeria as a Mental Health Care System: An Historical Overview. *Social Science and Medicine* 13B:137–51.

Santos, Jose Luis dos. 1981. Homeopathy in Campinas (Brazil): A Study of a Socio-Symbolic Field. Ph.D Dissertation, University of London.

Sapir, Edward. 1917. Do We Need a Superorganic? *American Anthropologist* 19:441–47.

———. 1949. Cultural Anthropology and Psychiatry. In *Selected Writings of Edward Sapir in Language, Culture and Personality,* ed. David G. Mandelbaum. Berkeley: University of California Press, 507–21.

———. 1961. *Culture, Language, and Personality: Selected Essays,* ed. D. G. Mandelbaum. Berkeley: University of California Press.

Sapolsky, Robert M. 1994. *Why Zebras Don't Get Ulcers: A Guide to Stress, Stress-Related Diseases and Coping.* New York: Freeman

Sarason, Barbara R., and Irwin G. Sarason. 1994. Assessment of Social Support. In *Social Support and Cardiovascular Disease,* ed. Sally A. Shumaker and Susan M. Czakowski. New York: Plenum Press.

Sargent, Carolyn. 1982. *The Cultural Context of Therapeutic Choice: Obstetrical Decisions among the Bariba of Benin.* Dordrecht: D. Reidel.

———. 1986. Prospects for the Professionalisation of Indigenous Midwifery in Benin. In *The Professionalisation of African Medicine,* ed. M. Last and G. L. Chavunduka. Manchester: Manchester University Press for the International African Institute, 137–50.

———. 1989. *Maternity, Medicine and Power: Reproductive Decisions in Urban Benin.* Berkeley: University of California Press.

Sargent, C., and J. Marcucci. 1988. Khmer Prenatal Health Practices and the American Clinical Experience. In *Childbirth in America: Anthropological Perspectives,* ed. K. Michaelson et al. South Hadley, Mass.: Bergin and Garvey, 79–89.

Sargent, Carolyn, and Nancy Stark. 1989. Childbirth Education and Childbirth Models: Parental Perspectives on Control, Anesthesia, and Technological Intervention in the Birth Process. *Medical Anthropology Quarterly* 3(1):36–51.

Sartorius, N., A. Japlensky, and R. Shapiro. 1978. Cross-Cultural Differences in the Short-Term Prognosis of Schizophrenic Psychosis. *Schizophrenia Bulletin* 4:102–13.

Scarry, Elaine. 1985. *The Body in Pain: The Making and Unmaking of the World.* Oxford: Oxford University Press.

Schaefer, James M. 1976. Drunkenness and Culture Stress: A Holocultural Test. In *Cross-Cultural Approaches to the Study of Alcohol,* ed. M. Everett et al. The Hague: Mouton.

———. 1981. Firewater Myths Revisited: Review of Findings and Some New Directions. *Journal of Studies on Alcohol* (Suppl. 9).

Schafer, Roy. 1983. *The Analytic Attitude.* New York: Basic Books.

Schantz, P. M. 1983. Human Behavior and Parasitic Zoonoses in North America. In *Human Ecology and Infectious Disease,* ed. N. A. Croll and J. H. Cross. New York: Academic Press, 21–48.

Schatzman, Morton. 1973. Paranoia or Persecution: The Case of Schreber. *Journal of Psychohistory* 1(1):62–88.

Scheder, C. 1988. A Sickly-Sweet Harvest: Farmworker Diabetes and Social Equality. *Medical Anthropology Quarterly* n.s. 2(3):251–77.

Scheff, Thomas. 1979. *Catharsis in Healing, Ritual, and Drama.* Berkeley: University of California Press.

Schensul, S., and M. G. Borrero, eds. 1982. Action Research and Health Systems Change in an Inner-City Puerto Rican Community. Special issue of *Urban Anthropology.*

Schensul, S., J. Schensul, G. Dudit, U. Bhowon, and S. Ragobur. 1994. Sexual Intimacy and Changing Lifestyles in an Era of AIDS: Young Women Workers in Mauritius. *Reproductive Health Matters* 3:83–93.

Scheper-Hughes, Nancy. 1979. *Saints, Scholars, and Schizophrenics: Mental Illness in Rural Ireland.* Berkeley: University of California Press.

———. 1984a. Maternal Detachment and Infant Survival in a Brazilian Shantytown. *Social Science and Medicine* 19:535–46.

———. 1984b. Infant Mortality and Infant Care: Cultural and Economic Constraints on Nurturing in Northeast Brazil. *Social Science and Medicine* 19(5):535–46.

———. 1988. The Madness of Hunger: Sickness, Delirium and Human Needs. In *Analysis in Medical Anthropology,* ed. S. Lindenbaum and M. Lock. Dordrecht: Kluwer Academic Publishers.

———. 1990. Three Propositions for a Critical Applied Medical Anthropology. *Social Science and Medicine* 30(2):189–97.

———. 1992. *Death without Weeping: The Violence of Everyday Life in Brazil.* Berkeley: University of California Press.

———. 1993. Embodied Knowledge: Thinking with the Body in Critical Medical Anthropology. In Robert Borofsky, ed., *Assessing Cultural Anthropology.* New York: McGraw-Hill, 229–42.

Scheper-Hughes, Nancy, ed. 1984. Demographic Transition in a Sicilian Rural Town. *Journal of Family History* 9:245–72.

———. 1987. *Child Survival: Anthropological Perspectives on the Treatment and Maltreatment of Children.* Boston: D. Reidel.

Scheper-Hughes, Nancy, and Margaret Lock. 1986. Speaking ''Truth'' to Illness: Metaphors, Reification, and a Pedagogy for Patients. *Medical Anthropology Quarterly* 17(5):137–40.

———. 1987. The Mindful Body: A Prolegomenon to Future Work in Medical Anthropology. *Medical Anthropology Quarterly* 1:6–41.

Scheper-Hughes, Nancy, and Anne M. Lovell. 1986. Breaking the Circuit of Social Control: Lessons in Public Psychiatry from Italy and Franco Basaglia. *Social Science and Medicine* 23(2):159–78.

Scheper-Hughes, Nancy, and Howard Stein. 1987. Child-Abuse and the Unconscious. In *Child Survival: Anthropological Approaches to the Treatment and Maltreatment of Children,* ed. Nancy Scheper-Hughes. Dordrecht: D. Reidel.

Scheper-Hughes, Nancy, and D. Stewart. 1983. Curanderismo in Taos County, New Mexico: A Possible Case of Anthropological Romanticism? *Western Journal of Medicine* 139(6):71–80.

Schertz, Lyle. 1972. The Success of Agriculture in Meeting World Food Needs. *Ecology of Food and Nutrition* 1:207–12.

Schieffelin, Edward L. 1976. *The Sorrow of the Lonely and the Burning of the Dancers.* New York: St. Martin's Press.

———. 1979. Mediatros as Metaphors: Moving a Man to Tears on Papua New Guinea. In *The Imagination of Reality: Essays in Southeast Asian Communication Systems,* ed. A. L. Becker and A. Yengoyan. Norwood, N.J.: Ablex Publishing.

———. 1983. Anger and Shame in the Tropical Forest: On Affect as a Cultural System in Papua New Guinea. *Ethos* 11:181–91.

———. 1985. Performance and the Cultural Construction of Reality. *American Ethnologist* 12:707–24.

Schiffer, R. L. 1988. The Exploding City. *Populi* 15(2):49–54.

Schilder, Paul. 1970 (1950). *The Image and Appearance of the Human Body.* New York: International Universities Press.

Schiller, N., S. Crystal, and D. Lewellen. 1994. Risky Business: The Cultural Construction of AIDS Risk Groups. *Social Science and Medicine* 38(10):1337–46.

Schiller, Nina Glick. 1992. What's Wrong with This Picture? The Hegemonic Construction of Culture in AIDS Research in the United States. *Medical Anthropology Quarterly* 6(3):237–54.

Schlesselman, J. J. 1982. *Case-Control Studies: Design, Conduct, Analysis.* New York: Oxford University Press.

Schneider, Jane. 1978. Peacocks and Penguins: The Political Economy of European Cloth and Colors. *American Anthropologist* 5.

Schneider, Jane, and Peter Schneider. 1984. Demographic Transition in a Sicilian Town. *Journal of Family History* 9:245–72.

Schneiderman, Lawrence J., and Nancy S. Jecker. 1995. *Wrong Medicine: Doctors, Patients, and Futile Treatment.* Baltimore: Johns Hopkins University Press.

Schoepf, Brooke. 1975. Breaking through the Looking Glass: The View from Below. In *The Politics of Anthropology,* ed. G. Huizer and B. Mannheim. The Hague: Mouton.

———. 1981. Ethical, Methodological and Political Issues of AIDS Research in Central Africa. *Social Science and Medicine* 33(7):749–63.

———. 1988. Women, AIDS and Economic Crisis in Zaire. *Canadian Journal of African Studies* 22(3):625–44.

———. 1991a. Ethical, Methodological and Political Issues in AIDS Research in Central Africa. *Social Science and Medicine* 33(7):749–63.

———. 1991b. Political Economy, Sex and Cultural Logics: A View from Zaire. *African Urban Quarterly* 6(1,2):94–106.

———. 1992a. Sex, Gender and Society in Zaire. In *Sexual and Behavioral Networking: Anthropological and Sociocultural Studies on the Transmission of HIV,* ed. T. Dyson. Liege, Belgium: International Union for the Scientific Study of Population, 353–76.

———. 1992b. Women at Risk: Case Studies from Zaire. In *The Time of AIDS: Social Analysis, Theory and Method,* ed. G. Herdt and S. Lindenbaum. Newbury Park, Calif.: Sage, 259–86.

———. 1992c. AIDS, Sex and Condoms: African Healers and the Reinvention of Tradition in Zaire. *Medical Anthropology* 14:225–42.

———. 1992d. Ethical, Methodological and Political Issues of AIDS Research in Central Africa. *Social Science and Medicine* 33(7):749–63.

———. 1993. AIDS Action—Research with Women in Kinshasa, Zaire. *Social Science and Medicine* 37(11):1401–13.

Schoepf, B., E. Walu, W. Rukarangiru, N. Payanzo, and C. Schoepf. 1991. Gender, Power and Risk of AIDS in Central Africa. In *Women and Health in Africa,* ed. M. Turshen. Trenton, N.J.: Africa World Press, 187–203.

Scholte, B. 1983. Cultural Anthropology and the Paradigm Concept: A Brief History of Their Recent Convergence. In *Functions and Uses of Disciplinary Histories,* ed. Loren Graham et al., Dordrecht: D. Reidel.

Schooler, C., and W. Caudill. 1964. Symptomology in Japanese and American Schizophrenics. *Ethnology* 3:172–78.

Schram, Ralph. 1971. *A History of the Nigerian Health Services.* Ibadan: Ibadan University Press.

Schreiber, Janet M., and John P. Homiak. 1981. Mexican Americans. In *Ethnicity and Medical Care,* ed. A. Harwood. Cambridge: Harvard University Press, 264–336.

Schrimshaw, N. S., C. E. Taylot, and J. E. Gordon. 1976. *Interactions of Nutrition and Infection.* Monograph Series, no. 57 Geneva: World Health Organization.

Schroyer, Trent. 1970. Marx and Habermas. *Continuum* 8 (1).

Schueler, Elizabeth, and George Armelagos. 1989. Biological Consequences of a Nuclear War. In

The Anthropology of War and Peace: Perspectives on the Nuclear Age, ed. Paul Turner and David Pitt. Granby, Mass.: Bergin and Garvey, 103–13.

Schuftan, Claudio. 1985. The Role of Health and Nutrition in Development. *Dossier* 49:41–56.

Schulman, S. 1958. Basic Functional Roles in Nursing: Mother Surrogate and Healer. In *Patients, Physicians and Illness,* ed. E. G. Jaco. Glencoe, Ill.: Free Press, 528–37.

Schumann, Debra A. 1986. Fertility and Historical Variation in Economic Strategy among Migrants to the Lacandon Forest, Mexico. In *Culture and Reproduction,* ed. W. Penn Handwerker. Boulder, Colo.: Westview, 144–58.

Schwartz, Theodore. 1992. Anthropology and Psychology: An Unrequited Relationship. In *New Directions in Psychological Anthropology,* ed. Theodore Schwartz, Geoffrey White, and Catherine Lutz. Cambridge: Cambridge University Press.

Schwartz, Theodore, and Lola Romanucci-Ross. 1974. Drinking and Inebriate Behavior in the Admiralty Islands, Melanesia. *Ethos* 2:213–31.

Schwartz, Theodore, Geoffrey White, and Catherine Lutz, eds. 1992. *New Directions in Psychological Anthropology.* Cambridge: Cambridge University

Schweder, Richard A., and Robert A. LeVine. 1984. *Culture and Theory: Essays on Mind, Self, and Emotion.* Cambridge: Cambridge University Press.

Scotch, Norman A. 1963. Medical Anthropology. In *Biennial Review of Anthropology, 1963,* ed. Bernard J. Siegel. Stanford University Press, 30–68.

Scott, Clarissa. 1975. The Relationship between Beliefs about the Menstrual Cycle and Choice of Fertility Regulating Methods within Five Ethnic Groups. *International Journal of Gynecology and Obstetrics* 13:105–9.

Scott, James. 1985. *Weapons of the Weak: Everyday Forms of Peasant Resistance.* New Haven: Yale University Press.

Scott, Robert, and Alan Howard. 1970. Models of Stress. In *Social Stress,* ed. Sol Levine and Norman A. Scotch. Chicago: Aldine.

Scrimshaw, N. S., C. E. Taylor, and J. E. Gordon. 1968. *Interactions of Nutrition and Infection.* Monograph Series, no. 57. Geneva: World Health Organization.

Scrimshaw, Nevin. 1974. Myths and Realities in International Health Planning. *American Journal of Public Health* 64:792–98.

Scrimshaw, Susan C. M. 1978. Infant Mortality and Behavior in the Regulation of Family Size. *Population and Development Review* 4:383–404.

———. 1980. Acceptability of New Contraceptive Technology. In *Research Frontiers in Fertility Regulation,* ed. Gerald I. Zatuchni, Mariam H. Labbok, and John J. Sciarra. New York.: Harper & Row, 72–82.

———. 1985. Bringing the Period Down: Government and Squatter Settlement Confront Induced Abortion in Ecuador. In *Micro and Macro Levels of Analysis in Anthropology: Issues in Theory and Research,* ed. B. R. DeWalt and P. J. Pelto. Boulder, Colo.: Westview Press.

Scrimshaw, S. C. M., and E. Hurtado. 1987. *Rapid Assessment Procedures: For Nutrition and Primary Health Care: Anthropological Approaches to Improving Programme Effectiveness.* Tokyo: United Nations University; UNICEF; and UCLA Latin American Center.

———. 1988. Anthropological Involvement in the Central American Diarrheal Disease Control Program. Special issue of *Social Science and Medicine* 27(1):97–106.

Scudder, Thayer. 1973. The Human Ecology of Big Projects: River Basin Development and Resettlement. *Annual Review of Anthropology* 2:45–67.

———. 1975. Resettlement. In *Man-Made Lakes and Health,* ed. N. F. Stanley and M. P. Alpers, New York: Academic Press, 453–71.

Scudder, Thayer, and Elizabeth Colson. 1982. From Welfare to Development: A Conceptual Framework for the Analysis of Dislocated People. In *Involuntary Migration and Resettlement: The Problems and Responses of Dislocated People,* ed. Art Hansen and Anthony Oliver-Smith. Boulder, Colo.: Westview Press, 267–87.

Scull, Andrew. 1977. *Decarceration: Community Treatment and the Deviant.* Englewood Cliffs, N.J.: Prentice-Hall.

———. 1979. *Museums of Madness: The Social Organization of Insanity in Nineteenth-Century England.* London: Allen Lane.

Secunda, Victoria. 1984. *By Youth Possessed: The Denial of Age in America.* Indianapolis: Bobbs-Merrill.

Segall, M. E. 1965. Blood Pressure and Culture Change. *Nursing Science* 3:373–82.

Seidel, G. 1993. The Competing Discourses of HIV/AIDS in Sub-Saharan Africa: Discourses of Rights and Empowerment vs. Discourses of Control and Exclusion. *Social Science and Medicine* 36(3):175–94.

Seligmann, C. G. 1911. *The Melanesians of British New Guinea.* Cambridge: Cambridge University Press.

Selikoff, I. J., et al. 1968. Asbestos Exposure, Smoking, and Neoplasia. *Journal of the American Medical Association* 204:106–14.

Sell, Ralph, and Stephen Kunitz. 1986. Debt, Dependency and Death in the 1970's: The Political Economy of Mortality in the Capitalist World System. Paper prepared for presentation at the Annual Meeting of the International Sociological Association, New Delhi, India, August.

Selye, Hans. 1956. *The Stress of Life.* New York: McGraw-Hill.

———. 1975. Confusion and Controversy in the Stress Field. *Journal of Human Stress* 1:37–44.

Sen, Amartya K. 1979. Rational Fools: A Critique of the Behavioral Foundations of Economic Theory. In *Philosophy and Economic Theory,* ed. Frank Hahn and Martin Hollis Oxford: Oxford University Press, 87–109.

Sevenet, T., L. Allorge, B. David, K. Awang, A. Hamid, A. Hadi, C. Kan-Fan, J. C. Quirion, F. Remy, H. Schaller, and L. E. Teo. 1994. A Preliminary Chemotaxonomic Review of Kopsia (Apocynaceae). *Journal of Ethnopharmacology* 41:147–83.

Shahid, N. S., A. S. M. Rahman, K. M. A. Azia, A. S. G. Faruque, and M. A. Bari. 1983. Beliefs and Treatment Related to Diarrhoeal Episodes Reported in Association with Measles. *Tropical and Geographical Medicine* 35:151–56.

Shariati, Ali. 1979. *On the Sociology of Islam,* trans. Hamid Algar. Berkeley: Mixan Press.

Sharman, A., J. Thephano, K. Curtis, and E. Messer, eds. 1991. *Diet and Domestic Life in Society.* Philadelphia: Temple University Press.

Sharp, Lesley. 1993. *The Possessed and the Dispossessed: Spirits, Identity, and Power in a Madagascar Migrant Town.* Berkeley: University of California Press.

Sharp, Lesley A. 1995. Organ Transplantation as a Transformative Experience: Anthropological Insights into the Restructuring of the Self. *Medical Anthropological Quarterly* 9(3).

Sharpe, Ella Freeman. 1948. An Examination of Metaphor. In *The Psychoanalytic Reader,* ed. Robert Fliess. New York: International Universities Press (orig. 1940), 273–86.

Shedlin, Michelle, and Paula E. Hollerbach. 1978. *Modern and Traditional Fertility Regulation in a Mexican Community: Factors in the Process of Decision-Making.* New York: The Population Council.

———. 1981. Modern and Traditional Fertility Regulation in a Mexican Community: The Process of Decision Making. *Studies in Family Planning* 12(6/7): 278–96.

Sheldon, H. 1984. *Boyd's Introduction to the Study of Disease.* 9th ed. Philadelphia: Lea & Febiger.

Sheldon, T. A., and H. Parker. 1992. Race and Ethnicity in Health Research. *Journal of Public Health Medicine* 14:104–10.

Sheps, M. C., and Jane A. Menken. 1973. *Mathematical Models of Conception and Birth.* Chicago: University of Chicago Press.

Sheridan, Allan. 1980. *Michel Foucault: The Will to Truth.* London: Tavistock.

Sherwin, Susan. 1992. *No Longer Patient: Feminist Ethics and Health Care.* Philadelphia: Temple University Press.

Shiloh, Ailon. 1968. The Interaction between the Middle Eastern and Western Systems of Medicine. *Social Science and Medicine* 2:235–48.

———. 1977. Therapeutic Anthropology: The Anthropologist as Private Practitioner. *American Anthropologist* 79:443–45.

————. 1980. Therapeutic Anthropology. *Medical Anthropology Newsletter* 12(1):14.

Shimkin, Demitri B., et al. 1983. The Social Sciences and Medicine in Community Health: The Community Control of Hypertension in Central Mississippi. In *Clinical Anthropology,* ed. Demitri Shimkin and Peggy Golde. Lanham, Md.: University Press of America, 155–221.

Shimkin, Demitri, and Peggy Golde. 1983. *Clinical Anthropology: A New Approach to American Health Problems?* Lanham, Md.: University Press of America.

Shore, Chris. 1992. Virgin Births and Sterile Debates: Anthropology and the New Reproductive Technologies. *Current Anthropology* 33:295–314 (including commentaries).

Shryock, H. S., and J. S. Seigel. 1973. *The Methods and Materials of Demography.* Washington, D. C.: Bureau of the Census.

Shrylock, R. H. 1967. *Medical Licensing in America, 1650–1965.* Baltimore: Johns Hopkins University Press.

Shukri, Ghali. 1985. Conceptual Problems on the Arab Road towards a Sociology of Knowledge. *Al-Mustaqbal Al-Arabi* 77(7):126–36. (in Arabic)

Shutler, Mary Elizabeth. 1979. Disease and Curing in a Yaqui Community. *In Ethnic Medicine in the Southwest,* ed. E. Spicer. Tucson: University of Arizona Press.

Shweder, Richard A. 1965. Aspects of Cognition in Zinacanteco Shamans: Experimental Results. In *Reader in Comparative Religion: An Anthropological Approach,* ed. W. A. Lessa and E. Z. Vogt. New York: Harper & Row, 407–12.

————. 1985. Menstrual Pollution, Soul Loss and the Comparative Study of Emotions. In *Culture and Depression: Studies in the Anthropology and Cross-Cultural Psychiatry of Affect and Disorder,* ed. Arthur Kleinman and Byron Good. Berkeley: University of California Press.

————. 1990a. Cultural Psychology: What Is It? In *Cultural Psychology: Essays on Comparative Human Development,* ed. James Stigler, Richard Shweder, and Gilbert Herdt. Cambridge: Cambridge University Press.

————. 1990b. Ethical Relativism: Is There a Defensible Version? *Ethos* 18(2):219–23.

Shweder, Richard, and Edmund J. Bourne. 1982. Does the Concept of the Person Vary Cross-Culturally? In *Cultural Conceptions of Mental Health and Therapy,* ed. Anthony J. Marsella and Geoffrey M. White. Dordrecht: Kluwer Academic Publishers, 97–137.

Shweder. Richard A., and Robert Le Vine, eds. 1984. *Culture Theory: Essays on Mind, Self, and Emotion.* Cambridge: Cambridge University Press.

Sibisi, Harriet. 1981. Aspects of Clinical Practice and Traditional Organisation of Indigenous Healers in South Africa. *Social Science and Medicine* 15B:3.

Sider, Gerald. 1974. *The Shaping of American Anthropology, 1883–1911, A Franz Boas Reader.* New York: Basic Books.

Siegel, D., R. Baron, and J. Eitel. 1985. *Health Consequences of War in Nicaragua.* San Francisco: San Francisco Bay Area Committee for Health Rights in Central America.

Siegel, D., R. Baron, and F. Epstein. 1985. The Epidemiology of Aggression. *Lancet* 1:1492–93.

Siegler, Mark, Edmund D. Pellegrino, and Peter A. Singer. 1990. Clinical Medical Ethics. *Journal of Clinical Ethics* 1(1):5–9.

Sigerist, Henry E. 1951. *A History of Medicine: (I) Primitive and Archaic Medicine.* New York: Oxford University Press

Silva, M., and D. Rothbart. 1984. An Analysis of Changing Trends in Philosophies of Science on Nursing Theory Development and Testing. *Advances in Nursing Science* 6(2):1–13.

Silverberg, James. 1986. The Anthropology of Global Integration: Some Grounds for Optimism about World Peace. In *The Social Dynamics of Peace and Conflict: Culture in International Security,* ed. R. A. Rubinstein and M. L. Foster. Boulder, Colo.: Westview Press, 281–91.

Silverman, M., P. Lee, and M. Lydecker. 1982. *Prescriptions for Death: The Drugging of the Third World.* Berkeley: University of California Press.

Simmons, Ozzie G. 1968. The Sociocultural Integration of Alcohol Use. *Quarterly Journal of Studies on Alcohol* 29:152–71.

Simon, Julian L. 1977. *The Economics of Population Growth.* Princeton: Princeton University Press.

————. 1986. *Theory of Population and Economic Growth.* Oxford: Basil Blackwell.

Simonelli, Jeanne J. 1990. The Politics of Below-Replacement Fertility: Policy and Power in Hungary. In *Births and Power: Social Change and the Politics of Reproduction,* ed. W. Penn Handwerker. Boulder, Colo.: Westview Press, 101–11.

Simons, Ronald C. 1985a. The Resolution of the Latah Paradox. In *The Culture-Bound Syndromes: Folk Illnesses of Psychiatric and Anthropological Interest,* ed. R. Simons and C. Hughes. Dordrecht: D. Reidel.

———. 1985b. Sorting the Culture-Bound Syndromes. In *The Culture-Bound Syndromes: Folk Illnesses of Psychiatric and Anthropological Interest,* ed. Ronald C., Simons and Charles C. Hughes. Dordrecht: D. Reidel, 25–38.

Simons, Ronald C., and Charles C. Hughes. 1985. *The Culture-Bound Syndromes: Folk Illnesses of Psychiatric and Anthropological Interest.* Dordrecht: D. Reidel.

———. 1993. The Culture-Bound Syndromes. In *Culture, Ethnicity, and Mental Illness,* ed. Albert C. Gaw. Washington, D.C.: American Psychiatric Press, 75–99.

Simoons, Frederick J. 1978. The Geographical Hypothesis and Lactose Malabsorption: A Weighing of the Evidence. *Digestive Diseases* 23:963–80.

Singer, Merrill. 1986a. Developing a Critical Perspective in Medical Anthropology. *Medical Anthropology Quarterly* 17(9)5:128–29.

———. 1986b. Toward a Political Economy of Alcoholism: The Missing Link in the Anthropology of Drinking. *Social Science and Medicine* 23(2):113–30.

———. 1987. Cure, Care, and Control: An Ectopic Encounter with Biomedical Obstetrics. In *Case Studies in Medical Anthropology,* ed. H. Baer. New York: Bordon and Breach.

———. 1989a. The Coming of Age of Critical Medical Anthropology. *Social Science and Medicine* 28(11):1193–203.

———. 1989b. The Limitations of Medical Ecology: The Concept of Adaptation in the Context of Social Statification and Social Transformation. *Medical Anthropology* 10(4):218–29.

———. 1990a. Critical Medical Anthropology in Question. *Social Science and Medicine* 30 (2):v–viii.

———. 1990b. Postmodernism and Medical Anthropology: Words of Warning. *Social Science and Medicine* 12 (3):289–304.

———. 1992a. Biomedicine and the Political Economy of Science. *Medical Anthropology Quarterly* 6(4):400–3.

———. 1992b. The Four Fields: A Medical Anthropology Perspective. *Anthropology Newsletter* (October):15.

———. 1993. Knowledge for Use: Anthropology and Community-Centered Substance Abuse Research. *Social Science and Medicine* 37:15–25.

———. 1995. Beyond the Ivory Tower: Critical Praxis in Medical Anthropology. *Medical Anthropology Quarterly* 9(1):80–106.

Singer, Merrill, C. Arnold, M. Fitzgerald, L. Madden, and C. von Legat. 1984. Hypoglycemia: A Controversial Illness in U.S. Society. *Medical Anthropology* 8:1–35.

Singer, Merrill, and Hans Baer. n.d. Why Not Have a Critical Medical Anthropology? Unpublished manuscript.

Singer, Merrill, Lani Davison, and Gina Gerdes. 1988. Culture, Critical Theory, and Reproductive Illness Behavior in Haiti. *Medical Anthropology Quarterly* 4:370–85.

Singer, Merrill, Lani Davison, and Fuat Yalin, eds. 1988. *Alcohol Use and Abuse among Hispanic Adolescents.* Hartford: Hispanic Health Council.

Singer, Merrill, Ray Irizarry, and Jean J. Schensul. 1991. Needle Access as an AIDS Prevention Strategy for IV Drug Users: A Research Perspective. *Human Organization* 50:142–52.

Singer, Merrill, Freddie Valentin, Hans Baer, and Zhongke Jia. 1992. Why Does Juan Garcia Have a Drinking Problem? The Perspective of Critical Medical Anthropology. *Medical Anthropology* 14:77–108.

Singer, Merrill, Zhongke Jia, Jean J. Schensul, Margaret Weeks, and J. Bryan Page. 1992. AIDS and the IV Drug User: The Local Context in Prevention Efforts. *Medical Anthropology* 14: 285–306.

Singer, Phillip, ed. 1977. Introduction to *Traditional Healing: New Science or New Colonialism? Essays in Critique of Medical Anthropology.* Buffalo, N.Y.: Conch Magazine.

Singh, Har Gopal. 1977. *Psychotherapy in India: From Vedic to Modern Times.* Agra: National Psychological Corporation.

Siskind, Janet. 1988. An Axe to Grind: Class Relations and Silicosis in a 19th Century Factory. *Medical Anthropology Quarterly* n.s. 2(3):199–214.

Skinner, Elliott P. 1960. Labour Migration and Its Relationship to Socio-Cultural Change in Mossi Society. *Africa* 30:375–401.

Skocpol, Theda. 1979. *States and Social Revolutions.* Cambridge: Cambridge University Press.

Slome, C., D. R. Brogan, S. J. Eyres, and W. Lednar. 1986. *Basic Epidemiological Methods and Biostatistics: A Workbook.* Boston: Jones and Bartlett Publishers.

Slomka, Jacquelyn. 1992. The Negotiation of Death: Clinical Decision Making at the End of Life. *Social Science and Medicine* 35(3):251–59.

Smith, Carol. 1983. Regional Analysis in World System Perspective: A Critique of Three Structural Theories of Uneven Development. In *Economic Anthropology: Topics and Theories,* ed. S. Ortiz. New York: University Press of America, 307–60.

Smith, Robert V. 1983. *Japanese Society: Tradition, Self and the Social Order.* Cambridge: Cambridge University Press.

Snow, Loudell F. 1974. Folk Medical Beliefs and Their Implications for Care of Patients. *Annals of Internal Medicine* 81:82–96.

———. 1993. *Walkin' over Medicine.* Boulder, Colo.: Westview.

Sobo, Elisa J. 1991. Reports That U.S. Tried to Control Third World Population Spark Probe. *National Catholic Reporter* 20 (September): 5.

———. 1993. Bodies, Kind, and Flow: Family Planning in Rural Jamaica. *Medical Anthropology Quarterly* 7(1):50–73.

Sobolik, Kristin D., and Deborah J. Gerick. 1992. Prehistoric Medicinal Plant Usage: A Case Study from Coprolites. *Journal of Ethnobiology* 12:203–11.

Sofowora, Abayomi. 1982. *Medicinal Plants and Traditional Medicine in Africa.* Chichester: J. Wiley.

Sofowora, Abayomi, ed. 1979. *African Medical Plants: Proceedings of a Conference.* Ile-Ife: University of Ife Press.

Sohoni, Neera Kuckreja. 1988. *Parava Seva Sanstha.* New Delhi: Ford Foundation.

Solomon, Robert C. 1984. Getting Angry: The Jamesian Theory of Emotion in Anthropology. In *Culture Theory: Essays on Mind, Self, and Emotion,* ed. R. Shweder, and R. Le Vine. Cambridge: Cambridge University Press.

Sommerfeld, Johannes. 1994. New Diseases: A Challenge for Medical Anthropological Research. *International Health and Infectious Disease Study Groups* (Society for Medical Anthropology) *Newsletter* n.s. 1(1):1–3.

Sontag, Susan. 1978. *Illness as Metaphor.* New York: Farrar, Strauss and Giroux.

Sotiroff-Junker, J. 1978. *A Bibliography on the Behavioural, Social and Economic Aspects of Malaria and Its Control.* Geneva: World Health Organization.

Southall, Aidan. 1961. Population Movements in East Africa. In *Essays on African Populations,* ed. K. Barbour and R. L. Prothero. London: Routledge & Kegan Paul.

Souza Brito, R. M. Alba, and Antonio A. Souza Brito. 1993. Forty Years of Brazilian Medicinal Plant Research. *Journal of Ethnopharmacology* 39:53–67.

Sow, Alfa Ibrahim. 1980. *Anthropological Structures of Madness in Black Africa.* New York: International Universities Press.

Spallone, Patricia, and Deborah Lynn, eds. 1987. *Made to Order: The Myth of Reproductive and Genetic Progress.* Oxford: Pergamon Press.

Spector, Rachel E. 1979. *Cultural Diversity in Health and Illness.* New York: Appleton-Century-Crofts.

———. 1985. *Cultural Diversity in Health and Illness.* Norwalk, Conn.: Appleton-Century-Crofts.

―――. 1991. *Cultural Diversity in Health and Illness.* 3d ed. Norwalk, Conn.: Appleton-Century-Crofts.

Spencer, Robert. 1949–1950. Introduction to Primitive Obstetrics. *CIBA Symposium* 11(3):1158–88.

Spindler, George, ed. 1978. *The Making of Psychological Anthropology.* Berkeley and Los Angeles: University of California Press.

Spiro, Melford E. 1965. *Context and Meaning in Cultural Anthropology.* New York: Free Press.

―――. 1978. Culture and Human Nature. In *The Making of Psychological Anthropology,* ed. George D. Spindler. Berkeley and Los Angeles: University of California Press, 331–60.

―――. 1982a. *Buddhism and Society.* 2d exp. ed. Berkeley and Los Angeles: University of California Press.

―――. 1982b. *Oedipus in the Trobriands.* Chicago: University of Chicago Press.

―――. 1986. Cultural Relativism and the Future of Anthropology. *Cultural Anthropology* 1(3): 259–86.

Spitzer, Robert L., and Janet B. Williams. 1983. International Perspectives: Summary and Commentary. In *International Perspectives on DSM-III,* ed. Robert L. Spitzer, Janet B. Williams, and Andrew E. Sokol. Washington, D.C.: American Psychiatric Press, 339–53.

Spivak, Gayatri. 1995. North and South: The Cairo Conference. Lecture presented at Columbia University Institute for Research for Women and Gender, October 13.

Spree, Reinhard. 1988. *Health and Social Class in Imperial Germany.* Oxford: Berg. (German ed. 1971)

Spring, Anita. 1986. Women Farmers and Food in Africa: Some Considerations and Suggested Solutions. In *Food in Subsaharan Africa,* ed. Art Hansen and Della E. McMillan. Boulder, Colo.: Lynne Rienner Publishers, 332–48.

Stacey, M. 1992. *Regulating British Medicine: The General Medical Council.* Chichester: J. Wiley.

Staiano, Kathryn V. 1981. Alternative Therapeutic Systems in Belize: A Semiotic Framework. *Social Science and Medicine* 15B:317–32.

Stall, Ron. 1988. The prevention of HIV Infection Associated with Drug and Alcohol Use during Sexual Activity. *Advances in Alcohol and Substance Abuse* 7(2):773–88.

―――. 1989. Alcohol, Drug Use and AIDS: An Anthropological Research Agenda. *Newsletter of the Alcohol and Drug Study Group, American Anthropological Association,* no. 23.

Stall, Ron, ed. 1985. Anthropology, Epidemiology, and Substance Use. Abstracts published in *Drinking and Drug Practices Surveyor* 20:54–59.

Stall, Ron, Suzanne Heurtin-Roberts, Leon McKusick, Colleen Hoff, and Sylvia Wanner Lang. 1990. Sexual Risk for HIV Transmission among Singles-Bar Patrons in San Francisco. *Medical Anthropology Quarterly* 4(1):115–28.

Stamm, L., and A. Ong Tsui. 1986. Cultural Constraints on Fertility Transmission in Tunisia: A Case Analysis from the City of Ksar-Hellal. In *Culture and Reproduction: An Anthropological Critique of Demographic Transition Theory,* ed. W. P. Handwerker. Boulder, Colo.: West-view.

Stanworth, Michelle. 1987. *Reproductive Technologies: Gender, Motherhood and Medicine.* Minneapolis: University of Minnesota Press.

Stark, Evan. 1982. What Is Medicine? *Radical Science Journal* 12:46–87.

Starr, P. 1982. *The Social Transformation of American Medicine.* New York: Basic Books.

Stavenhagen, R. 1971. Decolonizing Applied Anthropology. *Human Organization* 30(4).

Stebbins, Kenyon R. 1986. Curative Medicine, Preventative Medicine, and Health Status: The Influence of Politics on Health Status in a Rural Mexican Village *Social Science and Medicine* 23(2):139–48.

―――. 1987. Tobacco or Health in the Third World: A Political Economy Perspective with Emphasis on Mexico. *International Journal of Health Services* 17(3):521–36.

―――. 1991. Tobacco, Politics and Economics: Implications for Global Health. *Social Science and Medicine* 33(12):1317–26.

―――. 1993. Garbage Imperialism: Health Implications of Dumping Hazardous Wastes in Third World Countries. *Medical Anthropology* 15:81–102.

———. 1994. Making a Killing South of the Border: Transnational Cigarette Companies in Mexico and Guatemala. *Social Science and Medicine* 38(1):105–15.

Steedly, Mary Margaret. 1988. Severing the Bonds of Love: A Case Study in Soul Loss. *Social Science and Medicine* 27:841–56.

Stein, Howard F. 1973. Cultural Specificity in Patterns of Mental Illness and Health: A Slovak-American Case Study. *Family Process* 12(1):69–82.

———. 1974. Envy and the Evil Eye among Slovak-Americans: An Exploration into the Psychological Ontogeny of Belief and Ritual. *Ethos* 2(1):15–46.

———. 1978. The Slovak-American "Swaddling Ethos": Homeostat for Family Dynamics and Cultural Continuity. *Family Process* 17:31–45.

———. 1980a. Medical Anthropology and Western Medicine. *Journal of Psychological Anthropology* 3(2):185–95.

———. 1980b. Clinical Anthropology and Medical Anthropology. *Medical Anthropology Newsletter* 12(1):18–19.

———. 1982a. Adversary Symbiosis and Complementary Group Dissociation: An Analysis of the U.S./U.S.S.R. Conflict. *International Journal of Intercultural Relations* 6:55–83.

———. 1982b. Ethanol and Its Discontents: Paradoxes of Inebriation *and* Sobriety in American Culture. *Journal of Psychoanalytic Anthropology* 5(4):355–77.

———. 1982c. The Ethnographic Mode of Teaching Clinical Behavioral Science. In *Clinically Applied Anthropology: Anthropologists in Health Science Settings,* ed. Noel J. Chrisman and Thomas W Maretzki. Dordrecht: D. Reidel, 61–83.

———. 1984. The Scope of Psycho-Geography: The Psychoanalytic Study of Spatial Representation. *Journal of Psychoanalytic Anthropology* 7(1):23–73.

———. 1985a. Principles of Style: A Medical Anthropologist as Clinical Teacher. *Medical Anthropology Quarterly* 16(3):64–67.

———. 1985b. The *Psychodynamics of Medical Practice: Unconscious Factors in Patient Care.* Berkeley and Los Angeles: University of California Press.

———. 1985c. The Culture of the Patient as a Red Herring in Clinical Decision Making: A Case Study. *Medical Anthropology Quarterly* 17(1):2–5.

———. 1985d. Therapist and Family Values in Cultural Context. *Counseling and Values* 30(1): 35–46.

———. 1985e. What the Patient Wants; What the Patient Needs: A Dilemma in Clinical Communication. *Continuing Education for the Family Physician* 20(2):126–35.

———. 1985f. Whatever Happened to CounterTransference? The Subjective in Medicine. In *Context and Dynamics in Clinical Knowledge,* ed. H. F. Stein and M. Apprey. Charlottesville: University Press of Virginia, 1–55.

———. 1986a. Cultural Relativism as the Central Organizing Resistance in Cultural Anthropology. *Journal of Psychoanalytic Anthropology* 9(2):157–75.

———. 1986b. Social Role and Unconscious Complementarity. *Journal of Psychoanalytic Anthropology* 9(3):235–68.

———. 1987a. Culture and Ethnicity as Group-Fantasies: A Psychohistoric Paradigm of Group Identity. In *From Metaphor to Meaning: Papers in Psychoanalytic Anthropology,* ed. H. F. Stein and Maurice Apprey. Charlottesville: University Press of Virginia, 122–55.

———. 1987b. *Developmental Time, Cultural Space: Studies in Psychogeography.* Norman: University of Oklahoma Press.

———. 1988a. AIDS as Lethal Metaphor. *Transcultural Research Review* 25(3):231–36.

———. 1988b. The Influence of the American Group-Fantasy upon Contemporary American Biomedical Education and Practice. *Journal of Psychohistory* 15(3):281–93.

———. 1995. Cultural Demystification and Medical Anthropology: Some Answers in Search of Questions—A Commentary on Singer. *Medical Anthropology Quarterly* 9(1):113–17.

Stein, Howard F., and Robert F. Hill. 1988. The Dogma of Technology. In *Psychoanalytic Study of Society,* ed. L. B. Boyer and S. Grolnick. Hillsdale, N.J.: Analytic Press, 149–79.

Stein, Howard F., and S. Kayzakian-Rowe. 1978. Hypertension, Biofeedback, and the Myth of the

Machine: A Psychoanalytic-Cultural Study. *Psychoanalysis and Contemporary Thought* 1(1): 119–56.

Stein, Howard F., and William G. Niederland. 1989. *Maps from the Mind: Readings in Psychogeography.* Norman: University of Oklahoma Press.

Stein L. 1967. The Doctor-Nurse Game. *Archives of General Psychiatry* 16:699–703.

Steiner, Richard P., ed. 1986. *Folk Medicine: The Art and the Science.* Washington, D.C.: American Chemical Society.

Stenning, Derrick J. 1957. Transhumance, Migratory Drift, Migration: Patterns of Pastoral Fulani Nomadism. *Journal of the Royal Anthropological Institute* 87:57–73.

Stepan, J. 1985. Traditional and Alternative Systems of Medicine: A Comparative View of Legislation. *International Digest of Health Legislation* 36(2):283–341.

Stephen, Lynn. 1988. Zapotec Gender Politics: The Creation of Political Arenas by and for Peasant Women. Paper presented at Annual Meeting of the American Anthropological Association, Phoenix, Arizona.

———. 1991. *Zapotec Women.* Austin: University of Texas Press.

Stephen, Michelle. 1989. Self, the Sacred Other, and Autonomous Imagination. In Gilbert Herdt and Michelle Stephen, eds., *The Religious Imagination in New Guinea.* New Brunswick: Rutgers University Press, 41–66.

Sterk-Elifson, Claire, and Kirk W. Elifson. 1993. The Social Organization of Crack Cocaine Use: The Cycle in One Type of Base House. *Journal of Drug Issues* 23(3):429–41.

Stern, J. 1981. *Unemployment and Its Impact on Morbidity and Mortality.* Discussion Paper 93. London: Centre for Labour Economics, London School of Economics.

Sternberg, Robert J. 1985. Human Intelligence: The Model Is the Message. *Science* 230:1111–25.

Stevens, J., S. K. Kumanyika, and J. E. Keil. 1994. Attitudes toward Body Size and Dieting: Differences between Elderly Black and White Women. *American Journal of Public Health* 84:1322–25.

Stevens, R., L. W. Goodman, and S. S. Mick. 1978. *The Alien Doctors: Foreign Medical Graduates in American Hospitals.* New York: Wiley.

Steward, Julian, Robert Manners, Eric Wolf, Elena Padilla, Sidney Mintz, and Raymond Scheele. 1956. *The People of Puerto Rico.* Urbana: University of Illinois Press.

Stierlin, Helm. 1973. Group Fantasies and Family Myths: Some Theoretical and Practical Aspects. *Family Process* 12:111–25.

Stigler, James W., Richard A. Schweder, and Gilbert Herdt. 1990. *Cultural Psychology. Essays on Comparative Human Development.* Cambridge: Cambridge University Press.

Stini, William A. 1969. Reduced Sexual Dimorphism in Upper Arm Muscle Circumference Associated with Protein-Deficient Diet in a South-American Population. *American Journal of Physical Anthropology* 36:341–352.

———. 1975. Adaptive Strategies of Human Populations under Nutrition Stress. In *Biosocial Interrelations in Population Adaptation,* ed. E. S. Watts, F. E. Johnston, and G. W. Lasker. The Hague: Mouton, 94–41.

Stock, Robert. 1980. Health Care Behavior in a Rural Nigerian Setting. Ph.D. dissertation, University of Liverpool.

———. 1987. Drugs and Underdevelopment: A Case Study of Kano State, Nigeria. *Studies in Third World Societies* 34:115–40.

Stocking, George W. 1982. Afterword: A View from the Center. Special issue of *Ethos* 172–86.

Stoller, Paul. 1989. *The Taste of Ethnographic Things: The Senses in Anthropology.* Philadelphia: University of Pennsylvania Press.

———. 1994. Embodying Colonial Memories. *American Anthropologist* 96:634–48.

Stover, Eric. 1987. *The Open Secret: Torture and the Medical Profession in Chile.* Washington, D.C.: American Association for the Advancement of Science.

Strathern, Andrew, and Marilyn Strathern. 1971. *Self-Decoration in Mount Hagen.* London: Gerald Duckworth.

Stratmeyer, Dennis, and Jean Stratmeyer. 1977. The Jacaltec Nawal and the SoulBearer in Concepcion Huista. In *Cognitive Studies of Southern Mesoamerica,* ed. H. L. Neuenswander and D. E. Arnold. Dallas: S. I. L. Museum of Anthropology, 126–59.

Straus, Robert. 1982. "From the Ground Up": Medical Behavioral Sciences at the University of Kentucky. *Medical Anthropology Quarterly* 14(1):23–25.

Stein, Howard. 1995. Cultural Demystification and Medical Anthropology: Some Answers in Search of Questions. *Medical Anthropology Quarterly* 9(1):113–17.

Strickland, Bonnie. 1992. Women and Depression. *Current Directions in Psychological Science* 1(4):132–35.

Strug, David L., Dana E. Hunt, Douglas S. Goldsmith, Douglas S. Lipton, and Barry Spunt. 1985. Patterns of Cocaine Use among Methadone Clients. *International Journal of the Addictions* 20(8):1163–75.

Suarez-Orozco, Marcelo. 1989. *Central American Refugees and U.S. High Schools: A Psychosocial Study of Motivation and Achievement.* Stanford: Stanford University Press.

Sullivan, Earl L., ed. 1984. *Impact of Development Assistance on Egypt.* Cairo Papers in Social Science, vol. 7, monograph 3. Cairo: American University in Cairo.

Sullivan, Harry Stack. 1953. *Conceptions of Modern Psychiatry.* New York: W. W. Norton.

———. 1962. *Schizophrenia as a Human Process.* New York: W. W. Norton.

Susser, Ida. 1985. Union Carbide and the Community Surrounding It: The Case of a Community in Puerto Rico. *International Journal of Health Services* 15(4):561–83.

———. 1988. Directions in Research on Health and Industry. *Medical Anthropology Quarterly* n.s. 2(3):195–98.

Susser, M. 1988. Falsification, Verification and Causal Inference in Epidemiology: Reconsideration in the Light of Sir Karl Popper's Philosophy. In *Causal Inference,* ed. Kenneth J. Rothman. Chestnut Hill, Mass.: Epidemiology Resources, 33–57.

Suzuki, D. T. 1960. Lectures on Zen Buddhism. In *Zen Buddhism,* ed. D. T. Suzuki, E. From, and R. Demartino. New York: Grove Press.

Swagman, Charles F. 1989. Fija: Fright and Illness in Highland Yemen. *Social Science and Medicine* 28:381–88.

Swartz, Harold M. 1983. The Future Development and Role of Clinical Anthropology—The Perspectives of a Medical Educator. In *Clinical Anthropology,* ed. Demitri Shimkin and Peggy Golde. Lanham, Md.: University Press of America, 15–25.

Swartz, Leslie. 1991. The Politics of Black Patients Identity: Ward-Rounds on the "Black Side" of a South African Psychiatric Hospital. *Culture, Medicine and Psychiatry* 15(2):217–44.

Swedlund, Alan C., and George J. Armelagos, eds. 1990. *Disease in Populations in Transition: Anthropological and Epidemiological Perspectives.* New York: Bergin and Garvey.

Symposium. 1955. Projective Testing in Ethnography (Jules Henry, S. F. Nadel, William Caudill, John J. Honigmann, Melford E. Spiro, Donald W. Fiske, and A. I. Hallowell). *American Anthropologist* 57:245–70.

SYSTAT. 1988. SYSTAT Manual. Evanston, Ill.: Systat.

Talbot, Lee M. 1986. Demographic Factors in Resource Depletion and Environmental Degradation in East African Rangeland. *Population and Development Review* 12:441–51.

Tambiah, Stanley. 1977. The Cosmological and Performative Significance of a Thai Cult of Healing. *Culture, Medicine, and Psychiatry* 1:97–132.

———. 1985. (1981). A Performative Approach to Ritual. In *Culture, Thought, and Social Action.* Cambridge: Harvard University Press.

Tausig, Mark. 1982. Measuring Life Events. *Journal of Health and Social Behavior* 23:52–64.

Taussig, Michael T. 1978. Nutrition, Development, and Foreign Aid: A Case Study of U.S. Directed Health Care in a Colombian Plantation Zone. *International Journal of Health Services* 8(1):101–21.

———. 1979. Food and Development Policy: Some Tough Questions for Anthropologists. *Anthropology Resource Center Newsletter* 2(2).

———. 1980a. Reification and the Consciousness of the Patient. *Social Science and Medicine* 14B: 3–13.

———. 1980b. *The Devil and Commodity Fetishism.* Chapel Hill: University of North Carolina Press.

———. 1981. Nutrition, Development, and Foreign Aid: A Case Study of U.S. Directed Health Care in a Colombian Plantation Zone. In *Imperialism, Health and Medicine,* ed. Vicnete Navarro. Farmingdale, N.Y.: Baywood Publishing.

———. 1984. Culture of Terror—Space of Death: Roger Casement's Putumayo Report and the Explanation of Torture. *Comparative Studies in Society and History* 26(3):467–97.

———. 1987. *Shamanism, Colonialism, and the Wild Man: A Study in Terror and Healing.* Chicago: University of Chicago Press.

Taylor, C. 1970. *In Horizontal Orbit.* New York: Holt, Rinehart & Winston.

Taylor, Charles. 1990. *Sources of the Self: The Making of the Modern Identity.* Cambridge: Harvard University Press.

———. 1992. The Politics of Recognition. In *Multiculturalism and "The Politics" of Recognition,* ed. Charles Taylor and Amy Guttman. Princeton: Princeton University Press, 25–73.

———. 1995. Two Theories of Modernity. *Hastings Center Report* 25(2):24–33.

Taylor, Katheryn M. 1988. Physicians and the Discourse of Undesirable Information. In *Biomedicine,* ed. Margaret Lock and Deborah Gordon. Boston: Kluwer Academic Publishers, 441–63.

Taylor, Rex, and Annelie Rieger. 1985. Medicine as Social Science: Rudolph Virchow on the Typhus Epidemic in Upper Silesia. *International Journal of Health Service* 15(4):547–59.

Tedlock, B. 1987. An Interpretive Solution to the Problem of Humoral Medicine in Latin America. *Social Science and Medicine* 24:1069–83.

Teicher, M. I. 1960. *Windigo Psychosis.* Seattle: University of Washington Press.

Temkin, Oswei. 1963. The Scientific Approach to Disease: Specific Entity and Individual Sickness. In *Scientific Change: Historical Studies in the Intellectual, Social, and Technical Conditions for Scientific Discovery and Technical Invention, from Antiquity to the Present,* ed. A. C. Crombie. New York: Basic Books, 629–58.

Ten Have, Henk. 1994. The Hyperreality of Clinical Ethics: A Unitary Theory and Hermeneutics. *Theoretical Medicine* 15(2):113–132.

Teno, Joan, T. Patrick Hill, and Mary Ann O'Conner. 1994. Advance Care Planning: Priorities for Ethical and Empirical Research. *Hastings Center* 24(6): Special Supplement.

Tesh, Sylvia Noble. 1988. *Hidden Arguments: Political Ideology and Disease Prevention Policy.* New Brunswick: Rutgers University Press.

Therborn, Göran. 1987. Migration and Western Europe: The Old World Turning New. *Science* 237: 1183–88.

Thoits, Peggy A. 1981. Undesirable Life Events and Psychophysiological Distress: A Problem of Operational Confounding. *American Sociological Review* 46:97–109.

Thomasma, David C. 1984. The Context as a Moral Rule in Medical Ethics. *Journal of Bioethics* 5:63–79.

———. 1994. Clinical Ethics as Medical Hermeneutics. *Theoretical Medicine* 15(2):93–112.

Thomasma, David, and Glenn Graber. 1990. *Euthanasia: Toward an Ethical Social Policy.* New York: Continuum.

Thompson, D. 1939. *Report on an Expedition to Arnhem Land 1936–39.* Canberra, Australia: Government Printer.

Thompson, E. P. 1967. Time, Work, Discipline, and Industrial Capitalism. *Past and Present* 38:56–97.

Thompson, F. E., and T. Byers, eds. 1994. Dietary Assessment Resource Manual. *Journal of Nutrition* 124 (11 suppl.).

Thompson, J. A. 1981. Translation: The Impact of Reactionary Perspectives in Transcultural Nursing. In *Developing, Teaching and Practicing Transcultural Nursing: The Proceedings of the*

6th Transcultural Nursing Conference, ed. P. Morely Salt Lake City: University of Utah, College of Nursing and Transcultural Nursing Society, 34–36.

Tierson, F. D., C. L. Olsen, and E. B. Hook 1985. Influence of Cravings and Aversions on Diet in Pregnancy. *Ecology of Food and Nutrition* 17:117–29.

Tiglao, T. V. 1982. Health Knowledge, Attitudes and Practices Related to Schistosomiasis. *Hygie* 1:31–38.

Todd, Harry F., and M. Margaret Clark. 1985. Medical Anthropology and the Challenge of Medical Education. In *Training Manual in Medical Anthropology,* ed. C. E. Hill. Washington, D.C.: American Anthropological Association, 40–58.

Tomlinson, Tom. 1994. Casuistry in Medical Ethics: Rehabilitated, or Repeat Offender? *Theoretical Medicine* 15(1):5–20.

Toombs, S. Kay. 1992. *The Meaning of Illness.* Dordrecht: Kluwer Academic Press.

Topley, Marjorie. 1976. Chinese Traditional Etiology and Methods of Cure in Hong Kong. In *Asian Medical Systems: A Comparative Study,* ed. Charles Leslie. Berkeley and Los Angeles: University of California Press, 243–72.

Torrey, E. Fuller. 1973. *The Mind Game: Witchdoctors and Psychiatrists.* New York: Bantam Books.

Torstendahl, Rolf, and Michael Burrage, eds. 1990. *The Formation of Professions: Knowledge, State and Strategy.* London: Sage.

Toulmin, Stephen. 1982. *The Return to Cosmology: Postmodern Science and the Theology of Nature.* Berkeley: University of California Press.

Toussignant, Michel. 1984. Pena in the Ecuadorian Sierra: A Psychoanthropological Analysis of Sadness. *Culture, Medicine, and Psychiatry* 8:381–93.

Tran, Thanh Van. 1987. Ethnic Community Supports and Psychological Well-Being of Vietnamese Refugees. *International Migration Review* 21:833–44.

Traweek, Sharon. 1993. An Introduction to Cultural and Social Studies of Sciences and Technologies. *Culture, Medicine, and Psychiatry* 17:3–25.

Trevathan, W. 1988. Childbirth in a Bicultural Community: Attitudinal and Behavioral Variation. In *Childbirth in America: Anthropological Perspectives,* ed. K. Michaelson et al. South Hadley, Mass.: Bergin and Garvey, 216–27.

Trigg, Heather B., Richard I. Ford, John G. Moore, and Louise D. Jessop. 1994. Coprolite Evidence for Prehistoric Foodstuffs, Condiments and Medicines. In *Eating on the Wild Side: The Pharmacologic, Ecologic, and Social Implications of Using Noncultigens,* ed. N. L. Etkin. Tucson: University of Arizona Press, 210–23.

Tripp-Reimer, Toni. 1980. Clinical Anthropology: Perspectives from a Nurse-Anthropologist. *Medical Anthropology Newsletter* 12(1):21–22.

———. 1983a. Retention of a Folk Healing Practice (Matiasma) among Four Generations of Urban Greek Immigrants. *Nursing Research* 32:97–101.

———. 1983b. Human Variability and Nursing: A Neglected Aspect of Clinical Anthropology. In *Clinical Anthropology,* ed. Demitri Shimkin and Peggy Golde. Lanham, Md.: University Press of America, 245–59.

———. 1984a. Cultural Assessment. In *Nursing Assessment: A Multi-dimensional Approach,* ed. J. Bellack and P. Bamford. Monterey, Calif.: Wadsworth Health Sciences, 226–46.

———. 1984b. Reconceptualizing the Construct of Health: Integrating Emic and Etic Perspectives. *Research in Nursing and Health* 7(2):101–9.

———. 1984c. Research in Cultural Diversity. *Western Journal of Nursing Research* 6(3):353–55.

Tripp-Reimer, T., and P. J. Brink. 1985. Culture Brokerage. In *Nursing Interventions: Treatments for Nursing Diagnoses,* ed. G. M. Bulechek and J. C. McCloskey. Philadelphia: Saunders, 352–64.

Tripp-Reimer, T., P. J. Brink, and J. Sauders. 1984. Cultural Assessment: Content and Process. *Nursing Outlook* 32:78–82.

Tripp-Reimer, T., and M. M. Schrock. 1982. Residential Patterns and Preferences of Ethnic Aged:

Implications for Transcultural Nursing. In *Focus on Transcultural Nursing: Arching the Domains of Practice: The Proceedings of the 7th Transcultural Nursing Conference,* ed. J. Uh Salt Lake City: Transcultural Nursing Society, 144–57.

Trostle, J. 1986. Anthropology and Epidemiology in the Twentieth Century: A Selective History of Collaborative Projects and Theoretical Affinities, 1920 to 1970. In *Anthropology and Epidemiology,* ed. C. Janes et al. Dordrecht: D. Reidel, 59–94.

Trostle, J., et al. 1989. Fostering Research Capacity in The Developing World: Problems and Prospects for Medical Anthropology. Symposium at American Anthropological Association Annual Meetings, Washington, D.C.

Trotter II, R. T. 1985. Greta and Azarcon: A Survey of Episodic Lead Poisoning from a Folk Remedy. *Human Organization* 44:64–72.

———. 1987. The Case of Lead Poisoning from Folk Remedies in Mexican American Communities. In *Anthropological Praxis: Translating Knowledge into Action,* ed. R. M. Wulff and S. J. Fiske. Boulder, Colo.: Westview Press, 46–159.

Trotter II, Robert T., Anne M. Bowen, and James Potter, Jr. 1995. Network Models for HIV Outreach and Prevention Programs for Drug Users. In *Social Networks, Drug Abuse and HIV Transmission,* ed. R. Needle, S. Coyle, S. Genser, and R. T. Trotter II. NIDA Monograph Series, 151. Washington, D.C.: National Institute on Drug Abuse, 144–80.

Trotter II, Robert T., and Juan Antonio Chavira. 1978. Discovering New Models for Alcohol Counseling in Minority Groups. In *Modern Medicine and Medical Anthropology in the United States–Mexican Border Population,* ed. Boris Velimirovic. Washington, D.C.: Pan American Health Organization.

———. n.d. Personal communication.

Trowell, H. D. 1975. Obesity in the Western World. *Plant Foods for Man* 1:157–65.

Trowell, H. C., and D. P. Burkitt 1981. *Western Diseases: Their Emergence and Prevention.* Cambridge: Harvard University Press.

Trowell, H. D., J. N. Davies, and R. F. A. Dean. 1954. *Kwashirorkor.* London: Edward Arnold.

True, William R. 1984. Perspectives on Postdoctoral Public Health Training for Medical Anthropology. *Medical Anthropology Quarterly* 15(4):95–96.

True, William R., Mary Anna Hovey, John Bryan Page, and Paul L. Doughty. 1980. Marijuana and user Lifestyles. In *Cannabis in Costa Rica,* ed. William E. Carter. Philadelphia: Institute for the Study of Human Issues.

Trussell, T. James. 1979. Natural Fertility: Measurement and Use in Fertility Models. In *Natural Fertility,* ed. Henri Leridon and Jane Menken. Liege: Ordina, 29–64.

———. 1980. Statistical Flaws in Evidence for the Frisch Hypothesis That Fatness Triggers Menarche. *Human Biology* 52:711.

Tseng, W. S., and J. Hsu. n.d. *Psychotherapy: Origins and Methods.* N.p. Waterbuffalo Publishing Co. (In Chinese).

Tsing, Anna Lowenhaupt. n.d. Premature Mothers: Cultural Meanings of Infanticide. Unpublished manuscript.

———. 1990. Monster Stories: Women Charged with Perinatal Endangerment. In *Uncertain Times: Negotiating Gender in American Culture,* ed. Faye Ginsberg and Anna Lowenhaupt Tsing. Boston: Beacon Press, 282–99.

Tuchman, Barbara W. 1984. *The March of Folly.* New York: Knopf.

Tucker, Gisele Maynard. 1986. Barriers to Modern Contraceptive Use in Rural Peru. *Studies in Family Planning* 17 (6, pt 1):308–16.

Tully, James, ed. 1994. *Philosophy in an Age of Pluralism.* Cambridge: Cambridge University Press.

Turnbull, Colin. 1962. *The Forest People.* New York: Simon & Schuster.

Turner, Bryan. 1984. *The Body and Society: Explorations in Social Theory.* Oxford: Basil Blackwell.

———. 1986 Personhood and Citizenship. *Theory, Culture and Society* 3:1–16.

Turner, Edith. 1992. *Experiencing Ritual: A New Intepretation of African Healing.* Philadelphia: University of Pennsylvania Press.

Turner, Terrence. 1980. The Social Skin. In *Not Work Alone,* ed. J. Cherfas and R. Lewin. London: Temple Smith, 112–40.

Turner, Victor. 1964. An Ndembu Doctor in Practice. In *Magic, Faith, and Healing,* ed. A. Kiev. New York: Free Press.

———. 1967. *The Forest of Symbols.* Ithaca: Cornell University Press.

———. 1968. *The Drums of Affliction: A Study of Religious Processes among the Ndembu of Zambia.* Oxford: Clarendon.

———. 1969. *The Ritual Process: Structure and Anti-Structure.* Chicago: Aldine.

Turshen, Meredith. 1977. The Impact of Colonialism on Health and Health Services in Tanzania. *International Journal of Health Services* 7(1):7–35.

———. 1984. *The Political Ecology of Disease in Tanzania.* New Brunswick: Rutgers University Press.

———. 1986. Health and Human Rights in a South African Bantustan. *Social Science and Medicine* 22(9):887–92.

———. 1989. *The Politics of Public Health.* New Brunswick: Rutgers University Press.

Twumasi, P. A. 1975. *Medical Systems in Ghana.* Tema: Ghana Publishing Corporation.

Twumasi, P. A., and D. M. Warren. 1986. The Professionalisation of Indigenous Medicine: A Comparative Study of Ghana and Zambia. In *The Professionalisation of African Medicine,* ed. M. Last and G. L. Chavunduka. Manchester: Manchester University Press for the International African Institute, 117–36.

Tylor, Edward B. 1871. *Primitive Culture.* Boston: Estes & Lauriat.

Ulijaszek, S. J. 1990. Nutritional Status and Susceptibility to Infectious Disease. In *Diet and Disease in Traditional and Developing Societies,* ed. G. A. Harrison and J. C. Waterlow. Cambridge, Cambridge University Press.

Ulin, P. 1992. African Women and AIDS: Negotiating Behavior Change. *Social Science and Medicine* 34(1):63–73.

UN Advisory Committee for Co-ordination of Information Systems. 1992 *ACCIS Guide to United Nations Information Sources on Health.* New York: United Nations.

Underhill, Ruth M. 1965. *Red Man's Religion.* Chicago: University of Chicago Press.

Unschuld, P. U. 1975. Medico-Cultural Conflicts in Asian Settings. *Social Science and Medicine* 9: 303–12.

———. 1979. *Medical Ethics in Imperial China: A Study in Historical Anthropology.* Berkeley: University of California Press.

———. 1980. The Issue of Structured Co-Existence of Scientific and Alternative Medical Systems. *Social Science and Medicine* 14B:15–24.

———. 1985. *Medicine in China: A History of Ideas.* Berkeley: University of California Press.

Urdaneta, M. L. 1975. Fertility and the "Pill" in a Texas Barrio. In *Topia and Utopias in Health: Policy Studies,* ed. S. Ingman and A. Thomas. The Hague: Mouton, 69–83.

USAID. 1989. *Status Report: United States Economic Assistance to Egypt.* Washington, D.C.: United States Agency for International Development.

U.S. Institute of Medicine. 1979. *Health in Egypt: Recommendations for U.S. Assistance.* Washington, D.C.: National Academy of Sciences.

Van der Geest, Sjaak. 1987a. Unequal Access to Pharmaceuticals in Southern Cameroon: The Context of a Problem. *Studies in Third World Societies* 34:141–68.

———. 1987b. Pharmaceuticals in the Third World: The Local Perspective. *Social Science and Medicine* 25(3):273–76.

Van der Geest, Sjaak, and Susan R. Whyte, eds. 1988. *The Context of Medicines in Developing Countries: Studies in Pharmaceutical Anthropology.* Dordrecht: Kluwer.

Van der Kuyp, E. 1961. Schistosomiasis in the Surinam District of Surinam. *Tropical and Geographical Medicine* 13:357–73.

Van Schaik, Eileen. 1989. Paradigms Underlying the Study of Nerves as a Popular Illness Term in Eastern Kentucky. *Medical Anthropology* 11(1):15–28.

Vaskilampi, Tuula, and C. P. MacCormack, eds. 1982. *Folk Medicine and Health Culture: Role of Folk Medicine in Modern Health Care.* Kuopio: University of Kuopio.

Vaughn, Christine. 1989. Annotation: Expressed Emotion in Family Relationships. *Journal of Child Psychology and Psychiatry* 30:13–22.

Vaughn, Christine, and Julian Leff. 1976a. The Influence of Family and Social Factors on the Course of Psychiatric Illness. *British Journal of Psychiatry* 129:125–37.

———. 1976b. The Measurement of Expressed Emotion in the Families of Psychiatric Patients. *British Journal of Social and Clinical Psychology* 15:157–65.

Vaughn, C., K. Snyder, S. Jones, W. Freeman, and I. H. R. Fallon. 1984. Family Factors in Schizophrenic Relapse: A California Replication of the British Research on Expressed Emotion. *Archives of General Psychiatry* 41:1169–77.

Veatch, Robert M. 1981. *A Theory of Medical Ethics.* New York: Basic Books.

———. 1984. Autonomy's Temporary Triumph. *Hastings Center Report* 12(5):38–40.

———. 1985. The Ethics of Critical Care in Cross-Cultural Perspective. In *Ethics and Critical Care Medicine,* ed. John C. Moskop and Loretta Kopelman. Boston: D. Reidel, 191–206.

———. 1989. *Cross-Cultural Perspectives in Medical Ethics: Readings.* Boston: Jones and Bartlett Publishers.

———. 1995. Abandoning Informed Consent. *Hastings Center Report* 25(2):5–12.

Veatch, Robert M., and William E. Stempsey. 1995. Incommensurability: Its Implications for the Patient/Physician Relation. *Journal of Medicine and Philosophy* 20(3):253–69.

Vega, William A., Bohdan Kolody, and Juan Ramon Valle. 1987. Migration and Mental Health: An Empirical Test of Depression Risk Factors among Immigrant Mexican Women. *International Migration Review* 21:512–30.

Velimirovic, R. 1984. Traditional Medicine Is Not Primary Health Care. *Curare* 7:61–79, 85–93.

Vermeer, D. 1971. Geophagy among the Ewe of Ghana. *Ethnology* 10:56–72.

Verpoorte, R. 1989. Some Phytochemical Aspects of Medicinal Plant Research. *Journal of Ethnopharmacology* 25:43–59.

Veterans Administration Study Group on Anti-Hypertension Agents. 1970. Effect of Treatment on Morbidity in Hypertension: II. Results in Patients with Diastolic Blood Pressure Averaging 90 Through 114 mm Hg. *Journal of the American Medical Association* 213(7):1143–52.

Vieille, Paul. 1978. Iranian Women in Family Alliance and Sexual Politics. In *Women in the Muslim World,* ed. Lois Beck and Nikki Keddie. Cambridge: Harvard University Press, 451–72.

Villa Rojas, Alfonso. 1947. Kinship and Nagualism in a Tzeltal Community, Southeastern Mexico. *American Anthropologist* 49:578–87.

Villerme, L. R. 1840. A Description of the Physical and Moral State of Workers Employed in Cotton, Wool, and Silk Mills. In *The Challenge of Epidemiology: Issues and Selected Readings,* ed. C. A Buck, A. Llopis, E. Najera, and M. Terris. Scientific Publication, no. 505. Pan American Health Organization.

Vingerhoets, A. J. J. M., and F. H. G. Marcelissen. 1988. Stress Research: Its Present Status and Issues for Future Developments. *Social Science and Medicine* 26:279–91.

Vogel, Virgil J. 1973. *American Indian Medicine.* New York: Ballantine Books

Vogt, Evon Z. 1969. *Zinancantan: A Mayan Community in the Highlands of Chiapas.* Cambridge: Belknap Press of Harvard University Press.

———. 1970. *The Zinacantecos of Mexico: A Modern Mayan Way of Life.* New York: Holt, Rinehart & Winston.

Volkan, Vamik D. 1976. *Primitive Internalized Object Relations.* New York: International Universities Press.

———. 1988. *The Need to Have Enemies and Allies.* New York: Jason Aronson.

Von Mering, Otto. 1985. On Doing Anthropology in Clinical Settings: A Commentary. *Medical Anthropology Quarterly* 16(3):71–73.

Vries, M. W. de, et al., eds. 1982. *Use and Abuse of Medicine.* New York: Praeger.

Waddell, Jack O. 1988. Playing the Paradox: Papago Indian Management of Reservation/Off Reservation Prohibition Policies. Paper presented at the International Union of Anthropological and Ethnological Sciences Congress, Zagreb, Yugoslavia.

Waddell, Jack O., and Michael W. Everett, eds. 1980. *Drinking Behaviors among Southwestern Indians: An Anthropological Perspective.* Tucson: University of Arizona Press.

———. 1984. Alcoholism-Treatment-Center-Based Projects. In *Recent Developments in Alcoholism,* vol. 2, ed. Marc Galanter. New York: Plenum.

Waitzkin, Howard. 1979. The Marxist Paradigm in Medicine. *International Journal of Health Services* 9(4):683–99.

———. 1983. *The Second Sickness: Contradictions of Capitalist Health Care.* New York: Free Press.

———. 1986. Micropolitics of Medicine: Theoretical Issues. *Medical Anthropology Quarterly* 17(5):134–36.

———. 1989. Introduction. Marxist Perspectives in Social Medicine. *Social Science and Medicine* 11:1099–1101.

Wallace, A. F. C. 1956. *Tornado in Worcester: An Exploratory Study of Individual and Community Behavior in Extreme Situations.* Washington, D.C.: National Academy of Sciences/National Research Council.

———. 1959. Cultural Determinants of Response to Hallucinatory Experience. *Archives of General Psychiatry* 1:58–69.

———. 1961. *Culture and Personality.* New York: Random House.

Wallace, Anthony F. C., and Robert E. Ackerman. 1960. An Interdisciplinary Approach to Mental Disorder among the Polar Eskimos of Northwest Greenland. *Anthropologica* 2(2):249–60.

Wallerstein, Immanuel. 1979. *The Capitalist World Economy: Essays.* New York: Cambridge University Press.

Walsh, Anthony, and Patricia Ann Walsh. 1987. Social Support, Assimilation, and Biological Effective Blood Pressure Levels. *International Migration Review* 21:577–91.

Walsh, Julia, and Kenneth Warren. 1979. Selective Primary Health Care: An Interim Strategy for Disease Control in Developing Countries. *New England Journal of Medicine* 301(18):967–74.

Ward, Martha. 1990. The Politics of Adolescent Pregnancy. In *Births and Power: Social Change and the Politics of Reproduction,* ed. W. Penn Handwerker. Boulder, Colo.: Westview Press, 147–65.

Ware, Norma. 1992. Suffering and the Social Construction of Illness: The Delegitimation of Illness Experience in Chronic Fatigue Syndrome. *Medical Anthropology Quarterly* 6:347–65.

Ware, Norma, and Arthur Kleinman. 1992. Culture and Somatic Experience: The Social Course of Illness in Neurasthenia and Chronic Fatigue Syndrome. *Psychosomatic Medicine* 54:546–55.

Warner, Richard. 1985. *Recovery from Schizophrenia: Psychiatry and Political Economy.* London: Routledge and Kegan Paul.

———. 1992. Commentary on Cohen: Prognosis for Schizophrenia in the Third World. *Culture, Medicine and Psychiatry* 16(1):85–88.

Warner, W. L. 1958. *A Black Civilization: A Social Study of an Australian Tribe.* New York: Harper & Row.

Warwick, R., ed. 1977. *Nomina Anatomica.* 4th ed. Amsterdam: Elsevier, Excerpta Medica for the International Anatomical Nomenclature Committee.

Waterman, P. G. 1984. Food Acquisition and Processing as a Function of Plant Chemistry. In *Food Acquisition and Processing in Primates,* ed. D. J. Chivers, B. A. Wood, and A. Bilsborough. New York: Plenum Press, 177–211.

Watson, J. D. 1968. *The Double Helix.* New York: Signet Books.

Waxler, Nancy. 1974. Culture and Mental Illness: A Social Labeling Perspective. *Journal of Nervous and Mental Disorders* 159:370–95.

———. 1977. Is Mental Illness Cured in Traditional Societies? A Theoretical Analysis. *Culture, Medicine and Psychiatry* 1:233–53.

Webel, Charles P. 1983. Self: An Overview. In *International Encyclopedia of Psychiatry, Psycho-analysis, Psychobiology, and Neurology,* ed. Benjamin Wolman. New York: Aesculepius Press, 398–403.

Weber, M. 1946. Class, Status, Party. In *From Max Weber: Essays in Sociology,* ed. H. H. Gerth and C. Wright Mills. New York: Oxford University Press.

———. 1947. *Theory of Social and Economic Organization.* New York: Free Press.

Wegrocki, Henry J. 1953. A Critique of Cultural and Statistical Concepts of Abnormality. In *Personality in Nature, Society, and Culture,* ed. Clyde Kluckhohn and Henry A. Murray. New York: Alfred A. Knopf, 691–701.

Weibel-Orlando, Joan. 1984. Substance Abuse among American Indian Youth: A Continuing Crisis. *Journal of Drug Issues* (Spring):313–35.

———. 1987. *Culture-specific Treatment Modalities: Assessing Client-to-Treatment Fit in Indian Alcoholism Programs. In Treatment and Prevention of Alcohol Problems: A Resource Manual.* New York: Academic Press.

———. 1988. Hooked on Healing: The Anthropologist's Role in Substance Abuse Intervention. *Newsletter of the Alcohol and Drug Study Group, American Anthropological Association,* no. 21.

Weidman, Hazel H. 1980. Comments on "Clinical Anthropology." *Medical Anthropology Newsletter* 12(1):16–17.

———. 1982a. Introducing Transcultural Perspectives in Medical Training. *Medical Anthropology Quarterly* 14(1):25–26.

———. 1982b. Research Strategies, Structural Alterations, and Clinically Relevant Anthropology. In *Clinically Applied Anthropology: Anthropologists in Health Science Settings,* ed. Noel J. Chrisman and Thomas W. Maretzki. Dordrecht: D. Reidel, 201–43.

———. 1983. Research, Service and Training Aspects of Clinical Anthropology: An Institutional Overview. In *Clinical Anthropology,* ed. Demitri Shimkin and Peggy Golde. Lanham, Md.: University Press of America, 119–55.

———. 1985. Stylistic Aspects of Clinical Anthropology: A Mirrored Description. *Medical Anthropology Quarterly* 16(3):63–64.

Weil, Peter M. 1986. Agricultural Intensification and Fertility in the Gambia (West Africa). In *Culture and Reproduction,* ed. W. Penn Handwerker. Boulder, Colo.: Westview, 294–320.

Weisner, Thomas S. 1983. Putting Family Ideals into Practice: Pronatalism in Conventional and Nonconventional California Families. *Ethos* 11(4):278–304.

Weiss, K. M., R. E. Ferrell, and C. L. Hanis. 1984. A New World Syndrome of Metabolic Disease with a Genetic and Evolutionary Basis. *Yearbook of Physical Anthropology* 27:153–57.

Weiss, M. G. 1988. Cultural Models of Diarrheal Illness: Conceptual Framework and Review. Special issue of *Social Science and Medicine* 27(1):5–16.

Weiss, M. G., D. R. Doongaji, S. Siddharta, David Wypij, S. Pathare, M. Bhatawdekar, A. Bhave, A. Sheth, and R. Fernandes. 1992. The Explanatory Model Interview Catalogue (EMIC): Contribution to Cross-Cultural Research Methods from a Study of Leprosy and Mental Health. *British Journal of Psychiatry* 160:819–30.

Weisz, George, ed. 1990. *Social Science Perspectives on Medical Ethics.* Boston: Kluwer Academic Publishers.

Welch, M. L. 1989. Trauma Recovery: An Ethnography. Ph.D. dissertation, University of Connecticut.

Wellenkamp, Joseph. 1988. Notions of Grief and Catharsis among the Toraja. *American Ethnologist* 15(3):486–500.

Weller, Susan C. 1980. A Cross-Cultural Comparison of Illness Concepts: Guatemala and the United States. Ph.D. dissertation, University of California, Irvine.

———. 1983. New Data on Intracultural Variability: The Hot-Cold Concept of Medicine and Illness. *Human Organization* 42:249–57.

Weller, S., and A. K. Romney. 1988. *Systematic Data Collection.* Qualitative Research Methods, vol. 10. Newbury Park, Calif.: Sage.

Wellin, Edward. 1977. Theoretical Orientations in Medical Anthropology. In *Culture, Disease, and Healing,* ed. David Landy. New York: Macmillan, 47–54.

Werner, David. 1977. The Village Health Worker—Lackey or Liberator? Paper presented at the International Hospital Federation Congress, Tokyo, Japan, May 22–27.

———. 1983. Health Care in Cuba: A Model Service or a Means of Social Control—or Both? In *Practicing Health for All,* ed. David Morley, Jon Rohde, and Glen Williams. Oxford: Oxford University Press, 17–38.

———. 1988. Empowerment and Health. Presentation to the Christian Medical Commission/CCPD Joint Commission Meeting, Manila, Philippines, January 12–19.

Westermeyer, Joseph. 1982. *Poppies, Pipes and People: Opium and Its Use in Laos.* Berkeley: University of California Press.

———. 1985. Hmong Drinking Practices in the United States: The Influence of Migration. In *The American Experience with Alcohol,* ed. L. Bennett and G. Ames. New York: Plenum.

———. 1988. DSM-III Psychiatric Disorders among Hmong Refugees in the United States: A Point Prevalence Study. *American Journal of Psychiatry* 145:197–202.

———. 1989. *Psychiatric Care of Migrants: A Clinical Guide.* Washington, D.C.: American Psychiatric Association Press.

Westermeyer, Joseph, J. Neider, and T. F. Vang. 1984. Acculturation and Mental Health: A Study of Hwang Refugees at 1.5 and 3.5 Years Postmigration. *Social Science and Medicine* 18: 87–94.

Wethington, Ethel, and Ronald C. Kessler. 1986. Perceived Support, Received Support, and Adjustment to Stressful Life Events. *Journal of Health and Social Behavior* 27:78–89.

Wheaton, Blair. 1983. Stress, Personal Resources, and Psychiatric Symptoms: An Investigation of Interactive Models. *Journal of Health and Social Behavior* 24:208–29.

White, Geoffrey. 1992. Ethnopsychology. In *New Directions for Psychological Anthropology,* ed. T. Schwartz, G. White, and C. Lutz. Cambridge: Cambridge University Press.

White, Geoffrey, and John Kirkpatrick, eds. 1985. *Person, Self and Experience: Exploring Pacific Ethnopsychologies.* Berkeley: University of California Press.

White, Geoffrey, and Catherine Lutz. 1992. Introduction to *New Directions for Psychological Anthropology,* ed. T. Schwartz, G. White, and C. Lutz. Cambridge: Cambridge University Press.

White, Kerr L. 1988. *The Task of Medicine: Dialogue at Wickenburg.* Menlo Park, Calif.: Henry J. Kaiser Family Foundation.

White, L. 1986. Prostitution, Identity and Class Consciousness in Nairobi during World War II. *Signs* 11(21):255–73.

———. 1990. *The Comforts of Home: Prostitution in Colonial Nairobi.* Chicago: University of Chicago Press.

Whiteford, Linda. 1986. Economic Diversity, Family Strategy, and Fertility in a Mexican-American Community. In *Culture and Reproduction,* ed. W. Penn Handwerker. Boulder, Colo.: Westview, 237–48.

———. 1993. Child and Maternal Health and International Economic Policies. *Social Science and Medicine* 17(11):1391–1400.

Whiteford, Linda M., and Marilyn Poland, eds. 1989. *New Approaches to Human Reproduction: Social Science and Ethical Dimensions.* Boulder, Colo.: Westview Press.

Whiteford, Linda M., and Michael Sharinus. 1988. Delayed Accomplishments: Family Formation among Older First-Time Parents. In *Childbirth in America: Anthropological Perspectives,* ed. Karen Michaelson. South Hadley, Mass.: Bergin and Garvey, 239–53.

Whiteford, Scott, and Laura Montgomery. 1985. The Political Economy of Rural Transformation: A Mexican Case. In *Micro and Macro Levels of Analysis in Anthropology,* ed. Billie R. DeWalt and Pertti J. Pelto. Boulder, Colo.: Westview Press, 147–64.

Whiting, Beatrice B. 1950. *Paiute Sorcery.* Viking Publications in Anthropology, no. 15. New York: Viking.

Whiting, John W. M. 1961. Socialization Process and Personality. In *Psychological Anthropology: Approaches to Culture and Personality,* ed. F. L. K. Hsu. Homewood, Ill.: Dorsey Press, 355–80.

Wiedman, Dennis. 1990. Big and Little Moon Peyotism as Health Care Delivery System. *Medical Anthropology* 12:371–87.

Wiesenfeld, S. L. 1967. Sickle-Cell Trait in Human Biological and Cultural Evolution. *Science* 157: 1134–40.

Wikan, Uni. 1990. *Managing Turbulent Hearts: A Balinese Formula for Living.* Chicago: University of Chicago Press.

Wilbert, Johannes. 1987. *Tobacco and Shamanism in South America.* New Haven: Yale University Press.

Wilcox, L. 1981. Social Support, Life Stress, and Psychological Adjustment: A Test of the Buffering Hypothesis. *American Journal of Community Psychology* 9:371–86.

Wiley, Andrea S. 1992. Adaptation and the Biocultural Paradigm in Medical Anthropology: A Critical Review. *Medical Anthropology Quarterly* n.s. 6(3):216–36.

———. 1993. Evolution, Adaptation, and the Role of Biocultural Medical Anthropology. *Medical Anthropology Quarterly* 7(2):192–99.

Willett, Walter. 1990. *Nutritional Epidemiology.* New York: Oxford University Press.

Williams, Celcily D. 1933. Nutritional Disease of Children Associated with a Maize Diet. *Archives of Disease in Childhood* 8:423.

———. 1935. Kwashiorkor: Nutritional Diseases of Children Associated with a Maize Diet. *Lancet* 2:1151–52.

Williams, M. A. 1972. A Comparative Study of Post-surgical Convalescence among Women of Two Ethnic Groups: Anglo and Mexican American. In *Communicating Nursing Research: The Many Sources of Nursing Knowledge,* ed. M. Batey. Boulder, Colo.: Western Interstate Commission on Higher Education, 5:59–73.

Williams, Roger J. 1956. *Biochemical Individuality: The Basis for the Genetotrophic Concept.* Austin: University of Texas Press.

Williams, T. R., and M. Williams. 1959. The Socialization of the Student Nurse. *Nursing Research* 8:18–25.

Wilmsen, Edwin. 1986. Biological Determinants of Fecundity and Fecundability: An Application of Bongaarts' Model to Forager Fertility. In *Culture and Reproduction,* ed. W. Penn Handwerker. Boulder, Colo.: Westview, 59–89.

———. 1989. *Land Filled with Flies: A Political Economy of the Kalahari.* Chicago: University of Chicago Press.

Wilson, Monica. 1977. *For Men and Elders: Change in the Relations of Generations and of Men and Women among the Nyakyusa-Ngonde People, 1875–1971.* New York: Africana.

Windom, R. E. 1987. Seeking Answers to the Slowing Progress in Lowering Infant Mortality. *Public Health Reports* 102(2):121–22.

Winikoff, Beverly. 1988. Women's Health: An Alternative Perspective for Choosing Interventions. *Studies in Family Planning* 19:197–214.

Winnicot, David. 1971. Le Corps et le self. *Nouvelle revue de psychanalyse* 3:37–51.

Winslow, C. E. A. 1951. *The Cost of Sickness and the Price of Health.* Monograph Series, no. 7. Geneva: United Nations.

Wisner, Ben. 1988. GOBI versus PHC? Some Dangers of Selective Primary Health Care. *Social Science and Medicine* 26(9):963–969.

Wolf, Eric. 1956. Aspects of Group Relations in a Complex Society: Mexico. *American Anthropologist* 58:1065–78.

———. 1982. *Europe and the People without History.* Berkeley: University of California Press.

Wolf, Susan M. 1994. Health Care Reform and the Future of Physician Ethics. *Hastings Center Report* 24(3):28–41.

Wood, James W., and Maxine Weinstein. 1988. A Model of Age-Specific Fecundability. *Population Studies* 42:85–114.

Woolgar, Steve. 1992. What Is ''Anthropological'' about the Anthropology of Science? *Current Anthropology* 32:79–81.

World Agricultural Research Project. 1980. The Political Economy of Food and Agricultural. *International Journal of Health Services* 10:161–70.

World Health Organization. 1973. *The International Pilot Study of Schizophrenia.* Geneva: WHO.

———. 1974. *Glossary of Mental Disorders and Guide to Their Classification.* Geneva: WHO.

———. 1976. *African Traditional Medicine: A Report of an Expert Group.* AFRO Technical Report Series, no. 11. Brazzaville: WHO Regional Office for Africa.

———. 1978a. The Alma-Ata Conference on Primary Health Care. *WHO Chronicle* 32(11):431–38.

———. 1978b. *The Promotion and Development of Traditional Medicine: Report of a WHO Meeting.* WHO Technical Report Series, no. 622. Geneva: WHO.

———. 1979a. *Schizophrenia: An International Follow-up Study.* Chichester: John Wiley and Sons.

———. 1979b. *Workshop on the Role of Human/Water Contact in Schistosomiasis Transmission.* WHO Technical Report Series, no. 79.3. Geneva: WHO.

———. 1992. *The Global AIDS Strategy.* Geneva: WHO.

———. 1993. *Global Programme on AIDS. The HIV/AID Pandemic: 1993 Overview.* Geneva: WHO.

Worsley, Peter. 1966. The End of Anthropology? Paper prepared for the Sociology and Social Anthropology Working Group, Sixth World Congress of Sociology.

———. 1981. Social Class and Development. In *Social Inequality: Comparative and Developmental Approaches,* ed. Gerald D. Berreman. New York: Academic Press.

———. 1982. Non-Western Medical Systems. *Annual Review of Anthropology* 11:315–48.

———. 1984. *The Three Worlds: Culture and World Development.* London: George Weidenfeld and Nicolson.

Wrangham, R. W., and T. Nishida. 1983. *Aspilia* spp. Leaves: A Puzzle in the Feeding Behavior of Wild Chimpanzees. *Primates* 24:276–82.

Wright, Anne. 1982. Attitudes toward Childbearing and Menstruation among the Navaho. In *Anthropology of Human Birth,* ed. Margarita Artschwager Kay. Philadelphia: F. A. Davis Co., 377–94.

Wright, A. L., and T. M. Johnson. 1990. Preface to Symposium on Critical Perspectives in Clinically Applied Medical Anthropology. *Social Science and Medicine* 30 (9):v.

Wrigley, E. A., and R. S. Schofield. 1981. *The Population History of England, 1541–1871.* Cambridge: Harvard University Press.

Wulf, Robert M., and Shirley J. Fisk, eds. 1987. *Anthropological Praxis: Translating Knowledge into Action.* Boulder, Colo.: Westview Press.

Wunsch, G. J., and M. G. Termote. 1978. *Introduction to Demographic Analysis.* New York: Plenum.

Yamahara, J., S. Miki, H. Murakami, T. Sawada, and H. Fujimura. 1985. Screening Test for Calcium Antagonists in Natural Products and the Active Principles of *Cnidii monnieri. Yakugaku Zasshi* 105:449–58.

Yáñez, Leticia, Lilia Batres, Leticia Carrizales, Martha Santoyo, Virgilio Escalante, and Fernando Diaz-Barriga. 1994. Toxicological Assessment of Azarcon, a Lead Salt Used as a Folk Remedy in Mexico. I. Oral Toxicity in Rats. *Journal of Ethnopharmacology* 41:91–97.

Yap, P. M. 1962. Words and Things in Comparative Psychiatry, with Special Reference to the Exotic Psychoses. *Acta Scandinavica* 38:163–69.

———. 1974. *Comparative Psychiatry: A Theoretical Framework.* Toronto: University of Toronto Press.

————. 1977. The Culture-Bound Reactive Syndromes. In *Culture, Medicine and Healing: Studies in Medical Anthropology,* ed. David Landy. New York: Macmillan, 340–49.

Yesilada, Erdem, Gisho Honda, Ekrem Sezk, Mamoru Tabata, Katsumi Goto, and Yasumasa Ikeshiro. 1993. Traditional Medicine in Turkey IV. Folk Medicine in the Mediterranean Subdivision. *Journal of Ethnopharmacology* 39:31–38.

Young, Allan. 1978. Rethinking the Western Health Enterprise. *Medical Anthropology* (Spring):1–10, 34.

————. 1980. The Discourse on Stress and the Reproduction of Conventional Knowledge. *Social Science and Medicine* 14B:133–46.

————. 1982. The Anthropologies of Illness and Sickness. In *Annual Review of Anthropology* 11: 257–85.

————. 1983. Relevance of Traditional Medical Cultures to Modern Primary Health Care. *Social Science and Medicine* 17(16):1205–11.

————. 1987. How Medicine Tamed Life. *Culture, Medicine, and Psychiatry* 11:107–21.

————. 1988. A Description of How Ideology Shapes Knowledge of a Mental Disorder. In *Analysis in Medical Anthropology,* ed. S. Lindenbaum and M. Lock. Dordrecht: Kluwer Academic Publishers.

————. 1990. Moral Conflicts in a Psychiatric Hospital Treating Combat-Related Posttraumatic Stress Disorder (PTSD). In *Social Science Perspectives on Medical Ethics,* ed. George Weisz. Boston: Kluwer Academic Publishers, 65–82.

Young, J. C. 1980. A Model of Illness Treatment Decisions in a Tarascan Town. *American Ethnologist* 7:81–97.

————. 1981. *Medical Choice in a Mexican Village.* New Brunswick, N.J.: Rutgers University Press.

Young, J. C., and Linda Garro. 1982. Variation in the Choice of Treatment in Two Mexican Communities. *Social Science and Medicine* 16:1453–65.

Yu, M. C., J. H. C. Ho, S. H. Lai, and B. E. Henderson. 1986. Cantonese-style Salted Fish as a Cause of Nasopharyngeal Carcinoma: Report of a Case-Control Study in Hong Kong. *Cancer Research* 46:956–61.

Zahan, Dominique. 1979. *The Religion, Spirituality, and Thought of Traditional Africa.* Chicago: University of Chicago Press.

Zatuchni, G. I., J. J. Sciarra, and J. J. Speidel, eds. 1979. *Pregnancy Termination.* New York: Harper & Row.

Zhong, Y. B. 1988. *Chinese Psychological Analysis.* Shenyang: Liaooning Peoples Publishing Company.

Zinsser, Hans. 1943. *Rats, Lice and History.* Boston: Little, Brown and Co.

Zola, I. K. 1972. Medicine as an Institution of Social Control. *Sociological Review* 20(4):487–504.

Zumstein, A. 1983. A Study of Some Factors Influencing the Epidemiology of Urinary Schistosomiasis at Ifakara (Kilombero District, Morogoro Region, Tanzania). *Acta Tropica* 40:187–204.

Zussman, M. 1992. *Intensive Care: Medical Ethics and the Medical Profession.* Chicago: University of Chicago Press.

Index

About the Editors and Contributors

LINDA A. BENNETT is professor and chair of anthropology at the University of Memphis; she received her Ph.D. in anthropology from American University. As a research faculty member in the Department of Psychiatry and Behavioral Sciences, George Washington University Medical Center, she conducted more than a decade of research on family culture and the intergenerational transmission of alcoholism and other pathology. She has carried out a series of alcohol studies in Yugoslavia in the areas of treatment, alcoholism, and depression and has worked with the temperance movement.

PETER J. BROWN is professor of anthropology at Emory University, Atlanta. He holds additional appointments in the divisions of Behavioral Science and Health Education and in International Health at the Rollins School of Public Health at Emory University. He has conducted research on the effects of endemic malaria and its eradication on the biology, demography, economy, and culture of Sardinia, Italy. Another research interest is the evolution of biological and cultural predispositions to obesity. Currently, he is working on an ethological study of an Alzheimer's special care unit, a qualitative case control study of infant diarrhea-dehydration deaths, and a project to improve communication between medical caregivers and people infected with tuberculosis. He is editor-in-chief of *Medical Anthropology* and coeditor of the textbook *Applying Anthropology*.

CAROLE H. BROWNER is professor in the Department of Psychiatry and Biobehavioral Sciences and the Department of Anthropology at the University of California, Los Angeles. She received a Ph.D. in anthropology from the University of California, Berkeley, and an M.P.H. in health administration and planning from the same institution. She has conducted research in Colombia, Mexico, and the United States on how power, as it is structured and enacted in everyday activities, influences reproductive behavior.

NOEL J. CHRISMAN is professor in the Department of Psychosocial and Community Health, School of Nursing, University of Washington, with adjunct appointments in anthropology and family medicine. He received his Ph.D. in anthropology and an M.P.H. from the University of California, Berkeley. His research interests include ethnicity, social networks, and voluntary associations as elements in urban adaptation; the relationships of health beliefs and social networks with health care seeking; American health beliefs; the role of community organization interventions in cancer prevention; and application of anthropological knowledge in clinical settings.

PAUL W. COOK, JR., received his M.A. in anthropology in 1989 from Memphis State University. He studied medical anthropology, with an emphasis on drug research and mental health. During his graduate work, he conducted research at Northeast Community Mental Health Center, the Memphis city school system, and the Veterans Administration in Memphis. He is a research associate with the University of Tennessee Medical Group, Department of Psychiatry.

THOMAS J. CSORDAS received his B.A. in anthropology from the Ohio State University and his Ph.D. from Duke University. He is associate professor of anthropology at Case Western Reserve University. Dr. Csordas has conducted research among Catholic charismatics and Navajo Indians, and his interests include psychological and psychiatric anthropology, comparative religion, phenomenology of bodily experience, and rhetorical dimensions of language use.

WILLIAM W. DRESSLER is professor of behavioral and community medicine, University of Alabama School of Medicine—Tuscaloosa Program, and adjunct professor of anthropology, the University of Alabama. He received his Ph.D. in the medical anthropology program at the University of Connecticut. He has conducted research on social factors and cardiovascular disease in the Caribbean, Mexico, Brazil, the United Kingdom, and the southern United States, as well as on psychiatric disorder in the rural South. He is currently carrying out research on cardiovascular disease risk factors in southern Brazil and the southern United States.

NINA L. ETKIN is professor of anthropology at the University of Hawaii, Manoa. She received the B.A. in zoology from Indiana University and the M.A. and Ph.D. in biological anthropology from Washington University, St. Louis. Her research interests include indigenous medicine, ethnopharmacology, nutrition, and human variation and adaptations to infectious diseases.

MICHAEL R. HASS has an M.A. in psychology from California State University, Northridge, and is a candidate for the doctorate in social science at the University of California, Irvine. In addition to coordinating a program for disturbed adolescents, he is conducting research on the social and cultural dimensions of tuberculosis among Mexican immigrants in southern California.

CHARLES C. HUGHES is professor, Department of Family and Preventive Medicine and professor, Department of Anthropology at the University of Utah. He is also director of Graduate Programs in Public Health. He received his Ph.D. from Cornell University. His research interests include psychiatric issues in medical anthropology, and he was a member of the Diagnosis and Culture Group that developed proposals for the inclusion of the concept of culture in the fourth edition of the American Psychiatric Association's *Diagnostic and Statistical Manual.* Currently he is involved in an extensive analysis of the life history of an Eskimo shaman.

MARCIA C. INHORN is assistant professor in the Department of Anthropology at Emory University. She received her B.A. from the University of Wisconsin–Madison and her M.P.H. and Ph.D. degrees from the University of California at Berkeley. She has conducted research in Egypt and is the author of two books on the experiences, causes, and consequences of infertility among poor urban Egyptian women. Her research interests include women's health, ethnomedicine, the interface of anthropology and epidemiology, the anthropology of infectious disease, and gender and health issues in the Middle East.

JANIS H. JENKINS is associate professor of anthropology and psychiatry and director of the Women's Studies Program at Case Western Reserve University. She is an anthropologist who has conducted National Institute of Mental Health–sponsored studies of culture, gender, and mental health among Latino and Latin American populations, and published articles and book chapters on related issues.

THOMAS M. JOHNSON is professor of family medicine in the School of Primary Medical Care of the University of Alabama School of Medicine–Huntsville. He received his Ph.D. in anthropology from the University of Florida and an M.A. in clinical psychology from Southern Methodist University. As an applied medical anthropologist who has worked for the past twenty years in community mental health and medical education settings, he has emphasized clinical teaching, including supervision of medical students and residents in obstetrics and gynecology, internal medicine, psychiatry, and family medicine. He has served the Society for Medical Anthropology as editor of the *Medical Anthropology Quarterly* and was elected president of the society for 1993–1995.

ARTHUR KLEINMAN is professor of anthropology and psychiatry at Harvard

Medical School and the Faculty of Arts and Sciences, Harvard University. Educated at Stanford and Harvard universities, he has conducted medical anthropological research in Taiwan, China, and the United States. He received the Wellcome Medal for Medical Anthropology from the Royal Anthropological Institute of Great Britain and Ireland and is a member of the Institute of Medicine, National Academy of Sciences. He is the author of numerous books and articles.

BARBARA A. KOENIG is senior research scholar and executive director of the Center for Biomedical Ethics, School of Medicine, Stanford University. An anthropologist engaged in the study of Western biomedicine, her past research has focused on the use of advanced medical technology, physician education in care of the dying, and the impact of the AIDS epidemic on the training of physicians in internal medicine. Koenig is currently engaged in two research projects relevant to "anthropology and bioethic": a study of end-of-life decision making by culturally diverse patients (and families) with cancer and AIDS, and a study of the social and ethical impact of presymptomatic DNA testing for breast and ovarian cancer.

SANDRA D. LANE is assistant professor of anthropology, bioethics, and international health at Case Western Reserve University. From 1989 to 1995 she was a member of the Steering Committee on Operations Research for Tuberculosis Control at the World Health Organization. She is co-chair of the international health and infectious disease study group of the Society for Medical Anthropology. Her research interests include international health policy, infectious diseases, and women's reproductive health. She has conducted research in rural and urban Egypt, Liberia, the United States, and Canada.

MURRAY LAST is professor of medical anthropology and the ethnography of West Africa at University College, London. He received his M.A. degree from Yale University and his Ph.D. from the University of Ibadan, in history. He is the editor of the International African Institute's journal *Africa*. He has conducted fieldwork in Nigeria and is completing research on non-Muslim Hausa medicine and culture.

MARGARET LOCK is professor in the Department of Social Studies of Medicine and the Department of Anthropology at McGill University. She is the author of *East Asian Medicine in Urban Japan: Varieties of Medical Experience* (1980) and *Encounters with Aging: Mythologies of Menopause in Japan and North America* (1993), which won the Eileen Basker memorial Prize and the Canada-Japan Book Award, and was a finalist for the Hiromi Arisawa Award. Lock has edited three other books and written over one hundred scholarly articles. She was the recipient of a Canada Council Izaak Killam Fellowship for 1993–1995 and is a fellow of the Royal Society of Canada, a member of the Canadian Institute of Advanced Research, Population Program, and currently participates in two strategic network research teams funded by the Social Science and Humanities Research Council of Canada.

PATRICIA A. MARSHALL is associate professor of medicine and associate director of the medical humanities program at Loyola University of Chicago, Stritch School of Medicine, in Maywood, Illinois. She received her Ph.D. in anthropology from the University of Kentucky. She is a recipient of the Kellogg Foundation National Fellowship for leadership. Her research interests have focused on medical ethics, clinical ethics consultation, fear of AIDS in medical settings, and organ transplantation. She is currently involved in a study of cultural diversity and bioethics in the United States.

SOHEIR A. MORSY serves as a consultant to specialized agencies of the United Nations. She received her B.S. in bacteriology from Florida State University and her Ph.D. in anthropology from Michigan State University. She has taught anthropology at Michigan State University, the American University in Cairo, and the University of California, Berkeley. In recent years her work with the UN has addressed issues of agrarian development, health and nutrition, and gender equity in Africa and Asia. Her current concerns include child labor, gender and technology, and the politics of science.

GRETEL H. PELTO received her Ph.D. in anthropology from the University of Minnesota. She is professor of nutritional sciences and anthropology at the University of Connecticut. Dr. Pelto has conducted research in Mexico, the United States, and Finland, and her research interests include infant and maternal nutrition, dietary change, and research methods in primary care.

PERTTI J. PELTO received his Ph.D. in anthropology from the University of California, Berkeley. He is currently Professor Emeritus of Anthropology and Community Medicine at the University of Connecticut. He has conducted research in Finnish Lapland, rural Mexico, India, Bangladesh, and rural and urban United States. His interests include research methodology, primary health care in underserved areas, and the impact of technological change and modernization.

SARA A. QUANDT is associate professor in the Department of Public Health Sciences, Bowman Gray School of Medicine of Wake Forest University, as well as adjunct associate professor of anthropology. She received her Ph.D. in anthropology from Michigan State University. Her research interests include nutrition and aging, infant feeding practices, and hunger in the United States. She is currently engaged in research on the nutritional strategies of older adults in rural communities and participates in clinical trials of dietary interventions for a number of chronic diseases.

LORNA AMARASINGHAM RHODES obtained her Ph.D. in anthropology from Cornell University. She has done research in South Asia and in the United States, where she is interested in psychiatric institutions and practice. She teaches at the University of Washington, Seattle.

ARTHUR J. RUBEL is research professor. Department of Family Medicine, and research professor, Department of Anthropology, at the University of California, Irvine. He received his Ph.D. from the University of North Carolina, Chapel Hill. His research interests include ethnomedicine, tuberculosis, and the epidemiology of folk illness. He has done research in Mexico, along the U.S.-Mexico border, and in the Republic of the Philippines. He is currently involved in studies of tuberculosis in Mexico and southern California.

ROBERT A. RUBINSTEIN is associate professor of anthropology and director of the Program on the Analysis and Resolution of Conflicts in the Maxwell School of Citizenship and Public Affairs, Syracuse University. He is co-chair of the international health and infectious disease study group of the Society for Medical Anthropology. His interests are in international health, epidemiologic and anthropological methods, peace and international security, and the health of populations in civil conflict. He has conducted research in urban and rural Egypt, Belize, Mexico, and the United States.

CAROLYN F. SARGENT is professor of anthropology and director of women's studies at Southern Methodist University. She received an M.A. from the University of Manchester, England, where she studied as a Marshall Scholar, and a Ph.D. in anthropology from Michigan State University. She has conducted fieldwork in West Africa, Jamaica, and Dallas, Texas, and her research interests include the management of women's health, gender and child health, and the Khmer refugee experience in Dallas.

NANCY SCHEPER-HUGHES is professor and chair of the Department of Anthropology at the University of California, Berkeley. She has taught at the University of Cape Town (1993–4), the University of North Carolina, Chapel Hill (1979–1982), and Southern Methodist University (1977–1979). Scheper-Hughes is the author of numerous publications including: *Death without Weeping: The Violence of Everyday Life in Brazil; Saints, Scholars and Schizophrenics: Mental Illness in Rural Ireland; Psychiatry Inside Out: Selected Writings of Franco Basaglia* (edited with Anne Lovell). She is the editor of *Child Survival: Anthropological Perspectives on the Treatment and Maltreatment of Children*. She is the recipient of several book awards, including the Margaret Mead Award for *Saints, Scholars and Schizophrenics* and the Eileen Basker Prize (Society for Medical Anthropology), the Bryce Wood Award (Latin American Studies Association), the Harry Chapin Media Award (World Hunger Year), and the Pietre Prize (Centro Internazionale di Etnostoria, Italy), all for *Death Without Weeping*.

She is writing a book, *To Cape Town and Back,* on the year of the democratic transition in South Africa.

DANIEL J. SMITH is a Ph.D. candidate in the Department of Anthropology at Emory University in Atlanta, Georgia. He is a graduate of Harvard University and holds an M.P.H. from Johns Hopkins University. He served for three years as a health project adviser in Nigeria. His dissertation field research examines the cultural context of fertility decision making in Igbo-speaking southeastern Nigeria.

WILLIAM R. TRUE is associate professor of community health at the School of Public Health of St. Louis University and of anthropology in psychiatry at the School of Medicine. He is also a research anthropologist in the research service of the St. Louis Department of Veterans Affairs Medical Center. He has a Ph.D. in anthropology from the University of Florida and an M.P.H. in epidemiology from the University of North Carolina in Chapel Hill. His research is focused on studies of adult male twins who were veterans of the Vietnam era. He is working on genetic aspects of drug and alcohol use, health services utilization, posttraumatic stress disorder, and other psychiatric disorders. He is currently funded by the National Institute on Alcoholism and Alcohol Abuse (NIAAA) with colleagues from Washington University in St. Louis, Harvard University, the Department of Veterans Affairs, and the University of Illinois.

ISBN 0-313-29658-8

90000>